The WAR DIARIES of WEARY DUNLOP

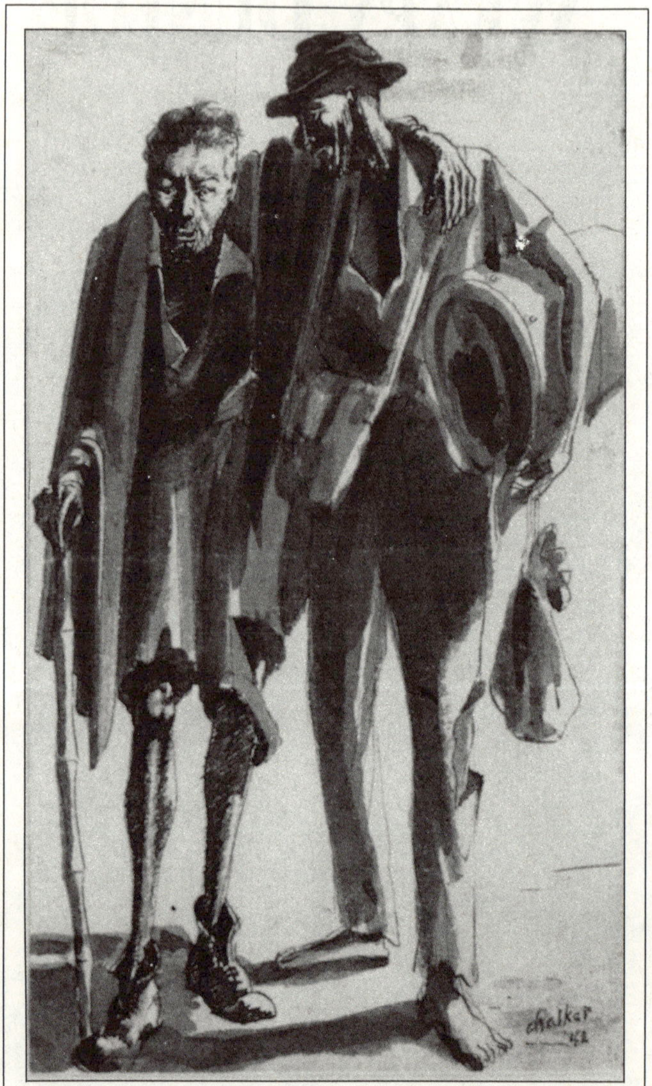

The WAR DIARIES of WEARY DUNLOP

JAVA AND THE BURMA-THAILAND RAILWAY 1942-1945

E.E. DUNLOP
CMG, OBE, KSJ, MS, FRCS, FRACS, FACS,
D. SC. PUNJABI (HON.)

NELSON

Nelson Publishers
Thomas Nelson Australia
480 La Trobe Street Melbourne Victoria 3000

First published 1986
Reprinted 1986

National Library of Australia
Cataloguing in publication data:

Dunlop, E.E. (Ernest Edward), 1907-
The war diaries of Weary Dunlop.

Includes index.
ISBN 0 17 006667 3.

1. Dunlop, E.E. (Ernest Edward), 1907- . 2. Burma-Siam Railway. 3. World War, 1939-1945 – Prisoners and prisons, Japanese. 4. World War, 1939-1945 – Personal narratives, Australian. I. Title.

940.54'72'520924

Jacket design: Tom Kurema
Text design: Sharon Carr
Illustration design: Carley Lau
Typeset in Hong Kong by Best-set Typesetter Ltd

Printed in Australia by Impact Printing

Frontispiece: 'Working men'. This first version by Jack Chalker has never been published until now. The second version is already well known 'Only two drawings survived from the first batch I did at Konyu river camp. These were discovered by a Korean guard while I was preparing a new "hide" in a section of bamboo, and the drawing above [was] not seen and survived the ensuing unhappy few days,' says Jack Chalker. 'I would be privileged if it could be used for "Weary's" book only.'

Dedication

To those prisoners-of-war of several nations whose courage and fortitude uplifted me during dark days.

The many dead are hallowed in my memory and the friendship of those living is one of life's precious gifts.

I pray that 'they shall hunger no more, neither thirst any more; neither shall the sun light on them nor any heat'. *(The Revelation of St John the Divine vii.16)*

Acknowledgements

I am deeply indebted to the many old friends and fellow prisoners who have contributed to this book.

To Col. Sir Laurens van der Post, CBE, I owe not only the foreword, but much inspiration and a treasured friendship.

I have drawn most heavily for the illustrations upon three men of multiple, remarkable gifts who shared my captivity: Ray Parkin, RAN, Gnr J.B. (Jack) Chalker, RA, and Sheriff Principal G.S. (Stanley) Gimson, QC (Edinburgh). Two line drawings from *Mark Time*, the camp magazine, Bandoeng, are by Sid Scales. R. van Willigen NEIA drew the author and Maj. A.A. Moon, RAAMC in Bandoeng. There are Thailand camp drawings and greeting cards by P. Meninsky, Old, T. Elsey, and R.G. Brazil, all British prisoners of war.

Murray Giffen gave me the photograph of his portrait of me many years ago; the original hangs in the Australian War Memorial; plates 135 and 137 are reproduced from photographs in the Australian War Memorial. Some photographs have their origin in those given to me by Bill Lovelock and Helen Ives (Lifetime Associates Pty Ltd) from my *This is your Life*, 1979.

The work of my editor, Lady Ebury (Sue), in assembling and organising material, has been invaluable. Much of the typing of the manuscript has been an arduous task carried out by my secretary, Mrs Valda Street, and Miss Caroline Bagworth.

Some more recent photographs I owe to a tour of Java, Singapore, and Thailand organised by Keith Flanagan of Western Australia in which I, along with Blue Butterworth, was a guest of previous members of 'Dunlop Force', following our *Via Dolorosa* of the past. The map of the Burma-Thailand Railway is from *Burma-Thailand Railway of Death* by E.R. (Bon) Hall, published by Graphic Books.

Foreword

by Colonel Sir Laurens van der Post

These diaries of Sir Edward Dunlop are of great human and historical importance. They are concerned with an aspect of the War in the East, a sort of war within the externally more dramatic and momentous War of which the world knows far too little and of which those who were most intimately and authoritatively concerned have not yet adequately rendered account. This war within a War was that which the hundreds of thousands of European, American and Australian prisoners of war and internees of the Japanese army, had to fight not only for physical survival but for sanity of mind and wholeness of spirit. To be compelled to surrender and be imprisoned in the best of wartime circumstances is difficult enough for the male spirit to accept. However good and compelling the reasons for doing so, there is something instinctively humiliating about giving up the battle and letting oneself be incarcerated in apparent safety while one's countrymen and allies lay down their lives in hundreds of thousands. In Europe, as far as military prisoners of war were concerned, this instinctive reaction was mitigated by the fact that prisoners of war were not dishonoured in the code of their captors, and allowed certain minimums of decency and self-respect. In the Far East, or more particularly the South-East Asia of which I can personally speak, it was a totally different story. This feeling of humiliation and, in my own case, guilt even that I had not done enough to stay in the battle however unfair to myself, was heightened to an almost unbearable degree by the contempt in which Japanese held all prisoners of war. It was a contempt that one could not ignore and dismiss merely as an archaic prejudice of a mediaeval military élite, because the Japanese themselves practised what they preached and died in their hundreds of thousands rather than submit to what they regarded as the ultimate degradation of surrender. For them, surrender was the final depravity which deprived the human being of the right to live with honour, and a life without honour with onself and one's society, I knew from my own pre-war experience in Japan, was utterly impossible. So one started one's life as a Japanese prisoner-of-war with this complex poison of guilt, shame and dishonour already subtly at work in one's system and one's state of mind unusually vulnerable to the helplessness and apparent hopelessness of one's physical situation.

Apart from the one gallant action by 'Blackforce', an ad hoc Australian brigade under Brigadier Blackburn, at a place called Leuwiliang, there was no serious resistance to the Japanese invasion by land. Barely within a week of the two-pronged attack of the Japanese on the island the Allies surrendered. Thousands of British and Australian soldiers, airmen and sailors, who had been rushed from other theatres of war to the defence of the Dutch East Indies, were imprisoned without having fired or even heard a shot being fired. It all happened so suddenly that there was no one to explain the why of it to all those confused and frustrated thousands. It seemed to them almost as if they had been needlessly betrayed by their own kind and they went into imprisonment sullen with resentment, disillusioned and suspicious of the high military authorities and the visible officer hierarchy who represented them in prison, for abandoning them so casually and needlessly – as they saw it – to so desperate and dishonoured a fate.

Once in Japanese prisons, this toxic compound of feelings among men of a British complex of nations of a long, proud and heroic military tradition and as collects of men go, unusually sensitive and imaginative, there seemed no obvious defence against the undisguised contempt of the Japanese and the indignities and brutalities inflicted on them in a rapidly accelerating measure. It was as if, utterly disarmed, a greater kind of courage was now expected of them than had been when, fully armed, they flocked to various military centres to withstand the Japanese invasion. Yet what sort of courage was this to be and who was to set the example of something not taught in military textbooks nor recorded in the long traditions they had inherited? Authority already discredited for them, they were not inclined to seek it among officers whom they did not even know and who were in their heart of hearts as confused as they themselves. For what made matters infinitely worse, was the fact that all these thousands had been surrendered in no coherent military pattern or form. With the exception of a few Australian units, they were of all sorts of military conditions and departments with no common experience or external frame of command to unite them. Externally they seemed as leaderless and disintegrated as they were powerless and dismayed within.

Within two months of the surrender, this disintegration had gone so far that, on the first morning on which I went to join a parade of officers the Japanese had suddenly called at Bandoeng, I was profoundly shocked to hear them booed by some privates, LA/Cs, sailors and non-commissioned officers watching the scene from the windows of the cantonments and open areas on the fringes of the camp. Wing Commander W.T.H. Nichols, one of the great prison commanders of the War, and I had arrived in Bandoeng only the night before on a roundabout way from a place in Java called Soekaboemi, which is the Malay for 'the desired earth'. Soekaboemi, a Dutch hillside station and refuge for the Dutch from the fever and heat of the coastal regions, was a Japanese military centre for what they called the 'bad men' of our forces. They called them so because the men interned there consisted of men of various branches of the armed forces, both Australian and English and even one lone American, who had tried to join me in the jungles of Bantam to carry on a guerilla war against the Japanese despite the overall command to surrender. Almost without exception they had been intercepted on their various ways before they could do so, and had been exceedingly fortunate indeed in not being executed instantly for their pains.

When I joined them at Soekaboemi after I had walked into a Japanese trap one morning on a mountain in the far west of Java called Djajasempoer – the 'mountain of the arrow' – they had already, despite the fact that they were curious assortments of military pattern and strata, of life and race – army, air force, navy – managed to become singularly at one. A common experience and endeavour, the fact that surrender had been imposed on them and not entered into voluntarily, enabled them to transcend humiliation and maltreatment. Paradoxically too we were enormously helped by the fact that all the while I was with them, their lives and mine were in the balance, and we were fortunate to leave Soekaboemi alive, and nothing helps the human imagination more to separate the false from the true, the illusion from reality, and heighten a sense of universal kinship than living under a common threat of instant death. That and the feeling they had all done their utmost to carry on the battle, made them one of the most united and unique groups of men I have ever known, and gave one an inkling that no matter what the odds against them, these men and their kind were of a quality to surmount them.

Accordingly, we exchanged Soekaboemi suddenly one day for the larger sprawling military prison at Bandoeng, a truly coherent and disciplined unit. I remember, therefore, as though it were yesterday, how startled we all were by the sour and fragmented atmosphere of the prison, and to me personally this display that morning not merely of hostility, but contempt for the abnormally large numbers of unemployed officers marching on to the parade ground, was profoundly shocking.

The parade dismissed, I spent the rest of the day going round the camp and talking to the men and immediately was moved and uplifted to find how quickly this lone act of recognition abolished barriers and how shallow, for all its effusiveness, was the manifestation of hostility we had witnessed on parade. As a result, Wing Commander Nichols and I called a meeting of all the senior British officers in our prison quarters that evening. The Japanese had already ordered us in the afternoon to present them the following morning with the names of the officers who would be in charge of each group of men in the prison. Nichols and I had already talked over the idea that whatever the other nationalities did in prison we all from the Commonwealth should be represented in prison as we had fought without, as one, and that we should have only one senior officer to represent us all in the eyes of the Japanese. We both felt that such a demonstration of unity as far as the British were concerned would not merely impress the Japanese as a dignified and desirable disciplinary measure, but far more would begin in the imaginations of all the incoherent fragments of men a unifying process of its own. But the question was who could best fill so militarily unorthodox a role?

According to our own King's Regulations, our prison commancer was supposed to be the senior combatant officer in the camp which happened to be Nichols. And when we first discussed the idea, Nichols, who had served in the Royal Air Force with distinction without break from the time he joined it as a boy, was inclined to interpret Regulations strictly and literally. However, the sensitive and imaginative person he was, acknowledged that we all found ourselves in a situation which King's Regulations, despite the long, pooled experience of many generations in problems of command and war that had gone into their framing, had never confronted a situation like the one in which we now found ourselves. I remember quoting to him one of my favourite texts from this Bible of the armed forces which I had used many times before during the War when, as the commander of small independent units behind enemy lines, I had to vary orders with which I had been issued at the outset from High Command at base. It was the clause – and I quote from memory – which implies something to the effect that when an officer carries out an order knowing that by carrying out the order he will defeat the purpose for which the order was issued he shall be considered as not having carried out the order. We both managed to raise a good laugh over this and by the time we had our meeting of senior officers were extremely flexible in our own minds as to how our own 'senior' officer for dealing with the Japanese should be appointed.

It was at this meeting that I first met Sir Edward Dunlop, then a lieutenant-colonel in the Royal Australian Medical Corps, and affectionately known as 'Weary' to his unusual and highly skilled medical team and orderlies. I was as impressed with him as Nichols was and in one inspired flash we both knew that, even if all the precedents and all the military regulations and conventions in the world argued against it, he should be commander of all the Commonwealth and English-speaking units in prison. Our only problem was Colonel Dunlop himself, who was as modest as he was gifted in all else. We insisted, however, and argued that, as our short prison experience already showed, we were going to be engaged in a new war, a war for physical and moral survival, a war against disease, malnutrition and most probably a protracted process of starvation as well as against disintegration from within by the apparent helplessness and futility of life in the prisons of an impervious, archaic and ruthless enemy. It would be a war for sanity of mind and body, and who, we asked Weary, could be more fitted to conduct such a war than a doctor and healer? Reluctantly he accepted the difficult role and neither Nichols nor I ever regretted the step. Our one regret was to be that our prison régime with Weary in overall command lasted for so short a time.

It lasted barely three months, but in those three months an astonishing transformation took place in our camp. All traces of confusion, bitterness and incohesion vanished. We rounded up all the public money we could find in the possession of senior officers in the camp, established contact with Chinese merchants outside prison and bought food on the advice of the Australian medical team to supplement inadequate and unbalanced prison rations. I remember one of our greatest investments was in ducks' eggs. We saw to it in the course of those three months, which were to become a kind of golden prison age in the totality of our prison memories, that every man had half a duck's egg every day to give his diet its minimum protein ingredient. We knew that we had to invest in the promotion of the physical well-being of our men as a matter of life-and-death urgency.

At the same time, we evolved a vast educational system where at one end of the scale an English officer of a fashionable Hussar regiment was in charge of a kindergarten, in which the illiterate among us came to learn the alphabet, to write and to read, rising up to a high school, agricultural and technical colleges, and even an open university where a classics don from Cambridge, 'Don

Gregory', serving as a batman in the Royal Air Force, became a kind of Warden of All Souls beginning a steady process of preparing middle-aged military and naval students for graduation in the arts and sciences. This don was a particular favourite with the Australians in our midst, who flocked to his public lectures given under some flambouyant tree in a corner of the camp with the high equatorial sun sizzling like the surf of a boiling sea around them and tree lizards from time to time gliding over their attentive heads from out of the summit of green above them. And their intellectual curiosity, love of learning and discussion, which sometimes would continue long into the day and night as a private argument in the barracks, was endless and, for me, one of the most marked and endearing characteristics of the Australian soldier. Not a day passed without a dozen or more Australians stopping me on my rounds in the camp and saying, 'Colonel, would you mind coming and settling an argument for us?' And this classics don seemed designed by life itself, with his own endless diversity of knowledge of the Greek and Roman past, to be the ideal centre for this unsatisfied hunger of our Australian fellow prisoners to know and learn more. They were, I remember, particularly interested in the *Iliad* and the *Odyssey*. It is one of my most moving recollections of the insatiable need man has for myth, legend, story and art to administer to his sanity and to secure his spiritual survival, as well as of a not sufficiently recognised mainstream of the Australian national character of the time. Our Australians, I felt, saw themselves quite rightly as having something akin to the Greek expeditionary force fighting on the great plain of Troy for a Greek Commonwealth cause. They were, it seemed, a contemporary version of the same immemorial and constantly recurring pattern and in the authentic line of succession of all men who had ever left their homes to fight for a cause greater than themselves.

The *Odyssey* in particular, as expounded by their Cambridge professor, seemed to draw them even more than the *Iliad*, I suspect because they knew that, like Odysseus and his men, they had a long and perilous journey through time and circumstance before the lucky few among them would come home again to their own version of Penelope. In addition to schools, classes and lectures, we had a college of art and published a daily newspaper; and none of us, officers or men, had ever worked harder or more to a true purpose, because when we were not all at work in this battle for physical survival and what had become not merely spiritual sanity but more meaningfully an increase of mind and imagination, we had to field large working parties for the Japanese every day.

We had also established, in a wooden chair, a radio, where at night a few of us could listen in secretly to BBC, Australian and American broadcasts on the progress of the War. In those early months of incarceration, this could not have made more cheerless listening. And in the establishment of this radio, Weary Dunlop played a role which provides one illustration of the many-sided qualities of the man. We had put word out to our Chinese suppliers that we needed a radio. And after some days a radio, concealed under a pile of fruit and vegetables, passed safely through the Guard at the entrance of the camp. The Guard, of course, drew a commission from our Chinese suppliers in those 'golden days' and encouraged this form of exchange. Yet one radio, particularly so dangerously large and gleaming a cabinet radio as came out from underneath the bananas, the beans and sweet potato leaves we ate as spinach, was quite enough for our purposes. To our horror, however, radios continued to come in every day for three more days. The four days that had gone by without methodical search of the supplies were a record in our experience. In fact, we thought the situation appeared so critical on the fifth day that Weary Dunlop and I went to watch the arrival of the handcarts bringing in our purchases from the Chinese. The handwagons were barely through the gates when a private rushed out of the Guardroom, halted them and declared that he would summon the Corporal of the Guard to conduct a search of our supplies. Our Chinese providers had grown so careless that we could see, through the ragged screen of fruit and vegetables, shining streaks of the deep red-brown sides of another mahogany radio cabinet. If the Japanese found, as they could not fail to, the radio among our supplies, it would mean not only the end of a vital source of food, but judging by what had happened in other camps, the execution of the people concerned in the smuggling of the radios. Weary, seeing that the Guard had his back turned to him in hurrying up to the office where the Corporal and rest of the Guard were sitting in comfort, instantly walked up to the relevant handcart and whisked out the cabinet radio. He did it as lightly and easily as if he were merely extracting a rugby football from another ruck on an international rugger ground where he had played for Australia and acquired considerable fame before the War. He tucked it under his arm and proceeded to walk smartly past the Guard towards the prison hospital. I followed as fast as I could. I saw a sleepy corporal coming out of the room, stopping him, and in the rudest of Japanese demanding to know what it was that he carried under his arm.

'Medical supplies,' Weary answered, with a ring of authority in his voice that was so irresistable that the moment I translated for the corporal, adding that he was the doctor in charge of the sick people in the hospital, the corporal waved us on and the incident was closed. But it could easily have been the end of Weary as well as some half dozen of the rest of us.

I remember, too, how enthusiastically Weary had joined us in setting up a microcosm of a Commonwealth Parliament in prison. It seemed criminal to us that the peoples of the Commonwealth should need catastrophes like world wars to unite them as we were united at that moment. We felt that there should be some kind of overriding political institution to express this profound sense of identity and purpose which we seemed to recognise as the greatest gift from Britain's imperial past. We thought it essential to set up a prison model of the macrocosm of the institutions we thought necessary to express what we had come to recognise as the supreme political value. We appointed an RAF officer who had resigned his seat in the Westminster Parliament to fight in the War, Squadron Leader – later Sir – Ian Horobin, to be our prison prime minister. He was charged with the duty of selecting a prison government, complete with cabinet and the relevant equivalents of Royal Commissions to investigate the various special problems the creation of such a body would call into being. This prison parliament was as great and therapeutic an attraction as the rest of the prison educational and cultural activities, and it did a great deal to maintain a feeling of continuity with some worthwhile purpose pitched far beyond prison walls which the act of imprisonment daily tried to refute. The minutes and reports of proceeding of this parliament, faithfully kept on the precious lavatory paper with which the Japanese provided the camp in strange and uncharacteristic abundance, unfortunately were lost. I say unfortunately, because they were of such a quality, keenness of thought and width of vision that I believe they would be a source of healthy shame to the British and Commonwealth governments who today are betraying the values fought for in the War as well as the precious breathing space of peace gained by the sacrifice of so many millions of young lives.

In addition to such a multiplicity of duties and interests, of which these are only a few illustrations, it is hardly necessary to add that Weary Dunlop and his team of doctors built up a model prison hospital in which the most advanced operations were successfully performed on men who would have died otherwise.

When, ultimately, Weary and the majority of our Australian fellow prisoners were suddenly ordered to prepare to leave the camp for an undisclosed destination, the physical state of health of every British prisoner in the camp was better than it was at the beginning – in fact, far better than it was ever to be again. But far more, we had discovered a way of living in prison as if it were not a prison and instead an immense opportunity for re-educating ourselves and freeing our minds and imaginations for life in a way they have never been free before. We had discovered, as I put it to the Japanese General who announced his surrender to me in September 1945 in urging him to emulate the example, how to lose in a way that losing became another kind of winning.

Although this is little more than a bare summary of our time together, it is enough, I hope, to explain why all of us who remained behind felt so singularly bleak when our Australian fellow prisoners under the command of Weary Dunlop left Bandoeng early one wet and black Javanese morning. Nichols and I had got up to say goodbye to Weary. I remember, walking between the low barracks and cantonments, under the dripping wet trees towards the prison gates, how the stars had just re-emerged from the clouds and in the puddles we trod underfoot were reflected the great constellations like Orion, stars like Sirius and Aldebaran and the planet Jupiter which had newly taken over the role of morning star from Venus. And whenever I think back to that walk and that moment when Weary, undismayed and even at so gloomy an hour, extracting a laugh from his overburdened men, met us at the great gate, all the adjectives personified in the *Pilgrim's Progress* and so unfashionable today occur to me as the only ones precise enough for the occasion; adjectives like 'valiant', 'standfast', 'tell-true', 'great-heart' and so on, but also joined to those some not to be found in Bunyan's vocabulary, like Weary's unfailing sense of humour and his light and classical use of irony as a means of defeating self-pity and reducing the intrusions of fate in the life of himself and of those under his command to bearable human proportions. It was, we all three knew there in the dark at the gate, the end of an era in our prison lives, and the beginning of a new one in which we were all to be tried and tested in a way we had never been before in our own lives and for that matter in the lives and memories of any men we knew. As far as Weary and his men were concerned, the test was to be almost more than flesh and blood should have been asked to endure because, although none of us knew it at the time, they were on their way to start work on the Burma-Siam

Railway, where most of them were to die and many to be maimed for life.

I cannot testify out of personal experience to the role Weary played on that scene of almost unmitigated cruelty and horror, and the height of challenge to which he raised his own spirit and those of his men. His fellow countryman and our mutual friend, Ray Parkin, gives some idea of the stature of the man in those days in his book, *Into the Smother*. I know only that I have the testimony of hundreds of Australians who had served with me and who accompanied Weary to Burma and Siam that he was both the inspiration and the main instrument of their physical and spiritual survival. I know, moreover, from the letters I get every year from the rapidly diminishing number of those who shared our prison experience, that the memory of the unique service Weary performed for them all remains with them, as it does for me, as though it were not something in the past but a forever 'now' in our beings.

Who can doubt, therefore, that the detailed, day to day evidence of such a man, recorded in these diaries, is an event of immense significance?

Laurens van der Post

Preface

I have shrunk from publishing these diaries for over forty years. It seemed that they might add further suffering to those bereaved, and add to controversy and hatred. What at the time was maintained simply as a military duty was in no sense designed for publication or to have any literary merit.

Further, I have distrusted the judgements I made at the time under harsh circumstances which were viewed only as black and white with no shades of grey. On the one hand, I felt that in the annals of human suffering, Australians had written something very special of their own, and handed on a precious legacy to the future. I formed the opinion that even the humblest of men have quite a lot of God in them. On the other hand, I reacted harshly to those few who shed all decency in their preoccupation with self preservation. Also, there were those who bore the badges of leadership, even men of proven valour in action, who reacted to imprisonment with an irritating inertia reflecting suspension of purpose.

It was, of course, a startling situation for British officer prisoners to find that rejection of all conventions of war did not isolate them from the suffering of their men, yet gave them little or no authority or resources to intervene effectively on their behalf.

Those in the medical services had the stimulus of the stark needs of a deluge of piteously ill men, and most doctors were fearless in approaches to our captors. However, much of the salvage of sick and broken men was achieved by securing the involvement of the whole stricken force in the sharing of slender resources, money and food, and contributing ingenious improvisations and gifts of labours of love out of their ebbing energy.

Who could forget one of my devoted medical staff (S/Sgt Alan Gibson), who was himself reduced to a near-naked skeleton, shivering with chronic malaria and racked with dysentery, yet when confronted with a man naked and tormeted with cholera, dropped his last shred of comfort in the world – his blanket – over the dying man.

Only those ill, emaciated and thin, who slept on exposed and rough services in all weathers, could comprehend his depth of sacrifice.

Brooding over all other diffidence and sensitivity has been the unfinished business of judgement upon the Japanese. I sustained for most of my time in captivity a burning hatred of them with only a few exceptions.

In time, I learned that unflinching controntation was not in the interests of those for whom I cared, and a few Japanese won my respect and even liking. In the closing phase of the war, I was confronted with a train-load of Japanese casualties of the Burma campaign, in wretched condition, on a chaotic, over-crowded and often interrupted journey via the Burma-Thailand Railway.

I paused before a man whose wretchedness equalled the plight of many of my own men – one leg had been hacked off at the mid-thigh and the bony stump projected through gangrenous flesh; his eyes were sunken pools of pain in a haggard, toxic face. With indomitable spirit he had hopped through hundreds of suffering miles without care. Some bombs fell and soldiers desperately fought for a place on the moving train. I moved to help him when he was trampled under in the rush, but his hand was limp and dead and the tortured face at peace.

The memory dwelt with me as a lingering nightmare and I was deeply conscious of the Buddhist belief that all men are equal in the face of suffering and death. This conviction has grown during long years of preoccupation with Australian-Asian relationships generally and with several visits to Japan itself. On one of these, I was honoured to be able to escort a dying Japanese diplomat, who was my patient, on an eventful journey back to Japan and the comfort of his loved ones.

Surely some increased understanding should emerge from a tragic conflict in which when all is said and done, Japanese losses vastly exceeded our own. If not, I reflect with Macbeth as to what is life:

> It is a tale
> Told by an idiot, full of sound and fury
> Signifying nothing.

There was much to admire in Japanese courage and deadly earnestness of purpose. Their contempt for those who surrendered to an enemy steeled me to a resolve to at least never show them fear in facing death and, still more testing, not to flinch as it came.

We can find much to admire in modern Japan in the way of industry, integrity, ability and patriotic fervour, which has rebuilt a shattered country and transformed a wrecked economy. This has lessons for the 'Lucky Country', where old and proven virtues appear to be declining whilst we trend the perilous path down which other civilisations have gone whose fault was 'giving too little and asking too much'.

In Japan there is much of sensitivity and creativity, but I have sensed that the single-minded loyalty gives the system some of the defects of an insect society, with a pattern of blind, unswerving acceptance of leadership whether towards good or evil.

This, too, marches with the Germanic brooding madness of the *Götterdämmerung*, 'The Twilight of the Gods', with desperate overtones of self-immolation. It is difficult for those with such intensity of purpose to temper their actions or to direct humour to them.

Some years of involvement with Asia, including the Colombo Plan work in Thailand, Sri Lanka and India, surgical work for the tragic civilian population of South Vietnam, and post-graduate medical exchanges with most of the Asian-

Pacific countries, has left me with the conviction that all the races of mankind bear some special mark of God's tenderness, some unique contribution to human kind. I deeply admired the leadership and prized friendship with Lord and Lady Casey, who steered Australia towards new and exciting relationships with 'friends and neighbours'.

It is also with deep emotion that I pay tribute to the bonds that I formed with men of numerous nations in captivity, many of whom died in alien lands, and to men of the 'underground', like Boon Pong, who risked their lives to help our lot. Most uplifting of all is the timeless, enduring, special brotherhood shared with all survivors of prison camps whose devotion and pride smacks of the St Crispin's Day of Henry V. There can be no gift so rich as the gratitude and love of such men and women. To them I attribute any good there may be in this book and commend their unquenchable spirit to their children, to their children's children and to those yet unborn.

'In thy face I see the map of honour, truth and loyalty.'

E.E.D.

Contents

List of Plates

Introduction

My years between the ages of seven and twelve that I spent on my father's farm, Summerlea, about the Sheepwash Creek at Stewarton, coincided with the momentous events of World War I. Scores of sturdy, heroic men, including four Dunlops, donned the ANZAC garb to seek high adventure or death. It was a bitter frustration to my burning ardour that my participation was largely limited to The Young Gardeners' League, for my heart yearned for the high romantic ground of adventure in strange lands, and the challenge of death.

Later, I was to reflect upon the advice of a Spanish proverb: 'Never wish for anything too much. It might come true.'

I served enthusiastically in cadets and Citizen Forces with yearly camps and some training in the Lee-Enfield mark 3 rifle, and Lewis gun. After qualifying as a doctor in 1934, I speedily obtained a commission as Captain RAAMC attached to the Coburg-Brunswick Battalion whose annual camps were at Numurkah. This rank I took to England in 1938 during further post-graduate training. I obtained my FRCS England after a ten-week course at St Bartholomew's Hospital in London.

The outbreak of World War II found me on the staff of the British Post-Graduate Medical School at Hammersmith and the qualification MS (Melb.) FRCS (Eng.) brought me posting to St Mary's Hospital, Paddington, as a specialist surgeon to the Emergency Medical Service. Arriving at St Mary's we heard Mr Chamberlain make his formal declaration of war, eerily punctuated by the first mournful air raid warning.

Chamberlain and the appeasers of those monstrous dictators, Hitler and Mussolini, had long filled me with shame and disgust. The British spirit was stirring to Churchill's growling bugle call to war. Life at St Mary's was a charmed circle, with we surgeons led by Mr Arthur Porritt, athlete and surgeon, (later Lord Porritt and Governor-General of New Zealand). The legendary miler, Jack Lovelock, was a friend, and I played poker at times with Alexander Fleming. The usual stream of London surgery persisted and blackout accidents were common.

The St Mary's rugby union team in which I played, along with another international, Tom Kemp, was superb and unbeaten. I received invitations to play with the British Barbarians, and for the British Commonwealth versus Combined Services. My one frustration was that a commission in the British services depended upon release from the Emergency Medical Service by the leader of the West London Sector, Sir Charles Wilson, Dean of St Marys and later better known as Churchill's physician, Lord Moran. A great rugby fan, he seemed reluctant to let me go.

Enlistment in the 2nd AIF required that I first return to Australia, which seemed to me a tortuous way to get to a war in Europe. However, an exchange of cables with my old Children's Hospital Chief, Major-General Rupert Downes, DGMS Australia, resulted in an unorthodox and probably unique posting direct to Australian Overseas Base which was later revealed as Jerusalem, Palestine. My commission to 2 AIF as Captain VX 259 was dated 13 November 1939.

Shedding my *tenue de ville*, I donned a picturesque Australian militia uniform with corduroy riding breeches, boots, leggings, spurs, tunic and a crowning slouch hat with emu feathers. The enthusiasm of the crowd that gathered to welcome the coming of a 'digger' to Fleet Street so embarrassed me, that I fled down Shaftsbury Avenue into Morris Angel's Shop to be equipped as an officer and gentleman! I emerged indistinguishable from British officers, save for a keen inspection of the bright buttons worn by Australians in World War I.

I departed my beloved London sadly as the midnight clamour of the Savoy Hotel greeted New Year's Day, 1940, and in deep secrecy as to destination, joined S. S. *Mantola*, in the frozen Tilbury Docks, as the only soldier. An eventual voyage through the Channel, the wide Atlantic, Gibralter, Malta and Port Said ended in the Sinai Desert train to Palestine. I was met by the only other Australian Medical Officer as yet in the Middle East, Col. H. C. Disher, ADMS, Australian Overseas Base. This old and admired teacher claimed me as his DADMS and driven by Pte Harry Crowe we swept through the Bab-el-Wad up the Judean Highlands to Jerusalem.

I seemed chained to arduous staff work successively at Australian Overseas Base (Jerusalem), HQ Aust. Corps (Gaza) and HQ 2 AIF (Alexandria and Heliopolis). This involved endless travel, not only in what I termed the 'wholly unholy Holy Land' but in Lebanon, Syria, the then Transjordania, Egypt, and later Libya. Close liaison was necessary with the British Forces; I came to know the leaders of the AIF from General Blamey down and, in consequence, those who led the army for many years to come. I was, however, concerned to return to surgery and, with the secret planning of the Greek campaign 'Lustre Force', was granted at last a field appointment.

To my chagrin, my boss, Major General Burston, DMS then cajoled me that I become Medical Liaison Officer to British Army HQ under General 'Jumbo' Maitland Wilson. The job at least proved most exciting, and under chaotic conditions of communication I lived dangerously by staff car and later motor cycle between Athens and the hard pressed Australians and New Zealanders under General Blamey.

Eventually, after running a personal ambulance service, Athens to the beach, I was evacuated from Nauplion, Peloponesus, by caïque, and the gallant HMS *Calcutta* to Crete.

Ignominiously, I departed from Crete with an aftermath of hepatitis, sticking to my clothes with boils and carbuncles, and a throbbing middle ear infection, to eventually reach hospital at El Kantara on the Suez Canal. When offered a position on the staff as lieutenant-colonel, I begged a return to surgery, and nominated a vacant post as major with the 2/2 Aust. CCS located in besieged Tobruk. No competition! After the fall of Crete things looked bad.

Alas, within months the unit was withdrawn to Cairo and I was given a whirlwind appointment to raise and command a mobile Field Hospital along the lines of my report. This I arranged at the highest level to be tested in battle with General Auchinleck's Offensive into Libya. This hastily improvised unit of 50 beds moved about the desert in standard transport and could establish anywhere in tents with casualties reaching theatre twenty minutes after arrival at a site. Sadly, we were forgotten on the order of battle, and avid for action, stayed stranded in Sinai while our forces suffered another reverse.

After a brief and unofficial tour to Syria with the unit, I relinquished command in disgust, and returned to 2/2 Aust. CCS. I declined command of that unit, prefering to remain in a surgical post as major. Highly equipped, trained and experienced, we departed Beit Jirga on 30 January 1942 to join the momentous departure of 1 Aust. Corps from Suez. The main body of 2/2 Aust. CCS totalled 87. All ranks were clad in winter battle dress with a pack for personal possessions, and we had a sole first aid pannier for medical equipment. The rest of the unit were scattered over the convoy accompanying light and heavy equipment and motor transport in separate ships. As Unit Embarcation Officer, my stubborn refusal to embark on a lighter to HMT *Orcades* without packs, officers' valises, nurses' trunks, and even the first aid pannier saved these last crumbs. No further baggage reached us before sailing, accompanied by the baggage of those who sailed a day before.

Months of patient work in organising stores to a high pitch of efficiency and sectionalised packing, to assist efficient and rapid unit function, foundered on the intricate bungling of 'movement control'.

God help the highly trained 1 Aust. Corps if Churchill had succeeded in throwing them into collapsing Burma in this scrambled state with essential weapons on other ships! However, with Curtin's insistence, all reached Australia except our fast, ill-fated *Orcades* on which I was travelling.

Malaya was rapidly gobbled up by the Japanese and Singapore fell whilst we were off Sumatra. HMT *Orcades* carried as principle units the main bodies of 2/3 Machine Gun Bn, 2/2 Pioneer Bn, 2/1 Anti Aircraft Bn, 2/6 Field Company Engineers and 2/2 Aust. CCS, all without weapons and equipment.

On 15 February 1942 we were called upon to land at Oesthaven, Sumatra, for a desperate stand against the Japanese. The extreme shortage of arms and ammunition led to our even borrowing some ships mausers and ship's medical stores to add to our pannier.

Mercifully, this spirited, ill-armed, scratch force, largely sweating in winter dress, was withdrawn and we reached Tanjongpriok unsunk by 17 February 1942. At the same time some heroic nursing sisters arrived from Singapore in the battered and holed *Empire Star*.

After two days of indecision with repeated landings and return to ship, the die was cast. Units other than the specialised 2/1 Anti Aircraft Bn finally disembarked. Included amongst them was Private Beverly, whose appendix I had removed five days before. Some two weeks later he was again on my hands, near dead, with a great deal of his jaw and carotid artery blown away.

1 Bandoeng February 1942

Our main CCS body entrained and, bemused by the greetings of civilians in Dutch, were transported through green fertile paddy-fields, large rivers, mountain and jungle to the bracing upland city of Bandoeng. Here we were allotted the herculean task of converting a large empty school, the Christelijk-lyceum into a big general hospital. This task devolved upon me, as Lt-Col. N. Eadie became SMO of the rapidly improvised 'Blackforce' commanded by the legendary Brig. A.S. Blackburn VC, who was promoted from Command of 2/3 MG Bn.

DMS 2 AIF Major General S.R. Burston CBE, DSO, ED, my old boss, welcomed us and authorised the equipping of the hospital with any stores available and the help of a generous imprest account.

We were to come under the administration of HQ British Forces Java (Maj.-Gen. Sitwell). We related also to RAF details under the command of Air Vice-Marshal Maltby, a hero of the defence of Malta, and liaised with HQ Netherlands East India Army (Medical).

On 22 Feb 1942 1 Aust. Corps staff departed along with the disappearing residue of General Wavell's South-East Asia Command. General Burston carried from me two brief letters: one to my hapless and long-separated fiancée, acquainting her of our impending fate, and one to the ship's sister of HMT *Orcades*, committing him to her tender care.

Sadly protesting, our unit nursing sisters were also evacuated.

Now with the distraction of almost daily air action, we bent ourselves feverishly to equipping and staffing what became 1 Allied General Hospital. Equipment was gathered from most diverse sources, such as the debris lying about the docks after timely diversion from Singapore, scattered minor Medical Centres, salvage from Sumatra, purchases from shops and very generous donations from our Dutch allies. Our slender staff required to expand to at least 200 and this was met by urgent appeal to the RAF Medical Service and RAMC, who responded grandly.

Casualties began arriving with staff and stores and frequently in greater numbers than the unpacked beds. I was provided with some Dutch Liaison Staff, and recruited 80 Dutch 'Helpsters' or VADs, admirably commanded by Matron Borgmann-Brouwer de Jonge, a valiant daughter of the second last Governor-General of the Indies.

The ultimate staff less VADs was 206 including 23 officers. In keeping with a General Hospital Command, my rank became Temporary Colonel. Casualties handled totalled 1351 sick and wounded, largely British and Australian army, navy and airforce with only 9 deaths.

Among those who passed briefly through my hands was Lt-Gen. Gordon Bennett in the course of his arduous and controversial escape, and his acompanying staff included my old rugby playing friend Maj. Charles (later Sir Charles) Moses. Moses at the time was injured with broken ribs and pneumonia and I detached a nursing party to care for him.

I found my lengthy staff experience invaluable in dealing with the Netherlands East Indies Army, and rather divided responsibilities to several British headquarters.

At this time of sick apprehension, the unfortunate Dutch, overrun and occupied in their homeland, and with their cosy world falling apart, seemed paralysed with fear. Nevertheless, the generosity of Dutch citizens was evidenced by the flow of comforts to the hospital: fruits, flowers, delicacies, tobacco, assorted drinks and English books.

The Helpsters, though from luxurious homes with ample servants, buckled down cheerfully to menial tasks and basic nursing, the challenge of mangled and blood-stained bodies, the stench, dirt, and helplessness of sick men.

The tide of disaster flowing from Singapore brought sensational news of rape and mass killing including the Alexandra Hospital massacre of staff and patients. We were too busy to feel much fear. The daily flow of casualties due to air action swelled heavily on 4 and 5 March 1942 with a spate of casualties from a spirited Australian action on the Leuwiliang River. Casualties included two rugby union Wallaby friends, Cliff Lang (who died on the way back), and Denny 'Scrub' Love, who reached hospital.

On 6 March 1942 I was informed by ADMS Lt-Col. 'Pete' Maisey that the Dutch were about to capitulate and that the British Forces would retire past Bandoeng towards the south coast. The hospital must continue functioning and would be captured. I at once said that I would remain with the hospital. I hoped that some staff and fitter patients should have the opportunity to move.

A confusing order was later received to retain all staff and patients 'until the order to cease fire for British Troops was given'. I was able to make contact with Maj. Gen. Sitwell and Brig. Blackburn on the outskirts of Bandoeng and had this order promptly rescinded and permission given for me to retain a skeleton staff and discharge others and selected patients to retire with the main force.

I went back to the hospital with the offer that I would guide those eligible and willing to escape to a night rendezvous with the column twenty miles south of Bandoeng, and then return. To my surprise, all said that they would prefer to remain with me. Consequently, I made the lone journey to the rendezvous through jumpy road patrols, and left the following letter to GOC with Maj. H.G. Greiner 2/3 MG Bn.

> Following conversation this day with GOC AIF, all ranks were informed that only 4 medical officers and 60 ORs were required to remain with patients at 1 Allied General, but that the decision to depart or remain was voluntary. All ranks notified their intention of remaining with the patients in their care, but expressed their complete willingness to undertake any

> further medical services which 'Blackforce' might require. Thus all personnel are being held at the hospital awaiting further instructions.

After my return, final preparations were made for capture. All documents likely to give useful information to the enemy were burned and unit designations erased or obliterated. All weapons in the hospital store including rifles, Bren guns, tommy guns, pistols and grenades were put out of action and deeply buried or thrown into ponds. All ranks were addressed, congratulated on their performance, and urged to face captivity in the same brave spirit. They were cautioned to give only name, number and rank on questioning.

For three peaceful but tense days our flags flew bravely before the formal occupation of Bandoeng by the Japanese. These, the last British flags to fly in Java, survived the march of occupation to finally descend at sunset.

During the Japanese Triumphal March of the occupation a remarkable Dutch lady drove through the ranks and up the drive to the hospital steps, and importuned me to come to her house to rescue two Dutch VADs from rape. With a fully loaded 38 pistol in each side pocket of a bush jacket, I accompanied her like a glum Garry Cooper at High Noon, in defiance of Japanese clearance of all streets. I retrieved the unraped ladies from the lawn of the house filled with tired Japanese. I was pawed and inspected whilst the nurses packed a few things, but with a loud-voiced pantomime avoided the critical discovery of the pistols. All Dutch VADs then moved into the overcrowded hospital and, at their insistance, slept on the floor.

1 Allied General Hospital continued to function under great difficulties after the Capitulation of Java 8 March 1942 to 18 April 1942. In the early days of occupation the busy Japanese ignored us officially, though a few individuals sought medical or dental attention. Supplies to the hospital, at first clandestine for two weeks, resumed under Dutch arrangement, controlled by the IJA. The stringent ration scale of the latter was ignored by the Dutch, and gifts flowed in.

I was successful in gaining an interview with the Japanese Commander at the Bandoeng HQ Preangor Hotel, accompanied by Dutch Liaison Officer John Disse. We managed to obtain two passes for movement about the town, one for me as CO and one for the interpreter. These,with authority for 7 days, were extended by forgery. This enabled me to conduct some very useful negotiation for supplies and money, and I was also able, by a confidence trick, to secure the transfer of wounded British servicemen in *kempi* gaol to the hospital. These included a man bayonetted through his chest and arm whilst tied up.

After an initial fortnight of fairly autonomous activity our troubles began. Staff officers, extremely truculent and offensive, began visiting and screaming demands to me using the surname only, rendered DUNROP! They issued a string of unreasonable demands, including the removal or obliteration of Red Cross identification and causing red crosses to be scraped off the walls. Perimeter guards were placed on the hospital and at Capt. Nakazawa's orders Dutch VADs were ejected, and all outside contact forbidden.

The local International Red Cross representative, a Swiss, proffered help, but then had smuggled in to us a letter to the effect that the Japanese rejected all conventions, were ill-treating Swiss, and had taken his car. I discussed this disregard of conventions with my patient Air Vice-Marshall Maltby RAF, and GOC AIF. Air Vice-Marshal Maltby showed me a letter signed by Nipponese Commander General Muriamo at the Capitulation promising that the Japanese would not only behave as a signatory to the Geneva Convention; but also observe the Hague Convention for POWs to which they were not a signatory.

Discipline of staff and patients, previously excellent, was breached by certain isolated VD patients with a clouded military record in Singapore. Certain offenders disposed of hospital blankets and stores through the fence, and when caught by a warrant officer, D. Topping, threatened him with throat cutting. I paraded them all and dealt out prompt field punishment with solitary confinement on rice and water to principle offenders, and appealed for co-operation and good behaviour in the interest of safety of all patients. Behaviour thereafter was very good.

On 17 April 1942 the increasing harshness of the Japanese flared to extreme brutality. Capt. Nakazawa demanded the immediate break-up of the hospital with most of the patients to go to prison along with those medical staff not needed for the few remaining. All were required to move at once. In order to dissuade him, I conducted him with his guard to demonstrate the serious illness of many patients. First amongst these LA/C 'Bill' Griffiths, blind with a shattered face, amputated hands, and a broken leg. Together with him there was another blinded lad and two patients paralysed from the waist down.

Capt. Nakazawa motioned to the bayonets of his guard. There was a tense moment as I interposed my body before Griffiths and glared at Nakazawa.

The threat was then transferred to the paraplegics whose eyes were dark with fright in their sweating faces.

Sick patients with chest and abdominal wounds had their legs struck contempuously: 'Man walk'.

I drew Capt. Nakazawa's attention to General Muriamo's promise on Capitulation with an offer to produce a copy of the letter. Repeatedly he said, 'General Muriamo sign no such letter'.

Finally I said, 'Well, Capt. Nakazawa, if you will name those responsible for these illegal actions I shall ensure that the British, Australian, and American Governments will hold them responsible; if you do not do so, I shall hold you responsible, and I have little doubt that I shall have you hanged.'

"Good,' he said. 'Now you will lead the march to gaol.'

My only concession gained was one night to break up the hospital instead of ten minutes. First we reclassified the absurd Japanese classification of Stretcher Case, Sitting, and Walking, redistributing the cards.

It was a night of desperate and feverish activity. Plaster casts were hurriedly made for several patients on fracture extension, and special measures to make movement of patients as comfortable as possible were taken.

Nominal rolls of all in hospital were made out together with essential documents such as those recording promotions, postings, burial returns, recommendations for awards, and the admission and discharges book was brought up to date. Bulky records and some valuable instruments we were not allowed to carry were smuggled out by Disse together with field medical cards of discharged patients. We were not allowed to remove medical stores, but I arranged distribution of essential drugs and instruments over patients and staff in small inconspicuous packages. I carried a haversack of instruments, a pannier, and some heavy medical books, and numerous books were carried for a future library.

The hospital accounts were audited as correct and a residue of funds amounting to £3947 in gulden equivalent was distributed over the force.

Rations were distributed, together with one blanket and at least one serviceable set of clothing. Water bottles were filled.

A movement order was prepared with allocation of staff to parties of patients and instructions as to their care. In the early dawn all ranks were complimented on their devoted work within the hospital and wished good fortune.

The stage was set for a new incalculable experience. Life had been too busy for us to feel the sadness of captivity, and something tinged with guilt and shame that our lives were in the hands of men who despised prisoners. I pledged myself to at least face them unflinchingly at all costs.

⋆ ⋆ ⋆ ⋆ ⋆

On 17 April 1942 I recorded: 'Jan. 30th '42.2/2 CCS departed Beit Jirja. Embarked Suez 1 Feb. 1942. Arrived Batavia 18 Feb. 1942. On Feb. 26th 1942, I was promoted to command 1 Allied General Hospital. On 28th Feb. '42 received first patients.

'*1 Allied General Hospital*

Admissions 27 Feb. 1942 to 17th April, 1943 inclusive.

British Army	639
RAF & RAAF	347
AIF	342
Royal Navy	9
US Navy	2
US Army	2
Dutch	4
Civilians	6
Grand Total	1351
Total Deaths	9

'Help was acknowledged from Maj. King, RAMC. Motor Ambulance Convoy. and Capt. Ellsback, NEI Army.

'The Nipponese Officers in control of the hospital after our capture:

Col. Minamoto
Adjutant 1st Lt Sumiya
Lt-Col. Odakura, Head of Medical Service
Capt. Nakazawa, Medical Staff officer
Mr Abe, Nip Gen. HQ.'

18 April 1942 was an extremely busy night devoted to the break up of the hospital and diary entries became rather fragmentary. I was up all night. I recorded: 'None of the staff have had much sleep. Three hip plaster spicas were applied to cases of fracture of the femur. Arrangements for medical records were that all patients take their own, including X-rays. The unit retained the Admission and Discharges book and this, together with Field Medical Cards of discharged patients, were given to John.*

I decided that I would try to contact Matron Borgmann-Brouer to seek her help in hiding and preserving my war diary, part 2 orders recording promotions, my citations recommending awards and a couple of special instruments. I carried these to the sentry gate on the Dagoweg (main street) and when confronted by an armed sentry, I employed a ruse which I had learned from F/0 Cicurel, a resourceful American citizen who had joined the RAF.

'His advice for all crises was: "Have something to recite with great emotion (I always use Lincoln's speech at Gettysburg!) Then brush aside any resistance and walk through." I selected the Shakespearean sonnet beginning "When I have seen by times fell hand defaced, the rich proud cost of outworn hurried age". This I recited with great emotion and gesticulation, then, pushing the sentries bayonet gently aside, I walked on firmly. My back felt exposed and uneasy, until I glimpsed him turning and calling out to his Commander for guidance as I crossed the street and gained a doorway which led to my objective.†'

We selected the worst patients for transfer to some sort of hospital at Tjimahi. This party was composed of:

Lying patients	63
Sitting	123
Walking	143
	329 (Includes officers 28)

of which Australians 120; British 209.

Those who were to march to gaol were as follows:

Staff of Hospital	*Patients*	
17 officers including	Officers	27
Sqn Ldr MacGrath, RAAF	Sgts & WOs	74
	Other Ranks	376
	Total	477

As many instruments as possible, sulphanilamide, quinine, emetine and important drugs, were spread over the patients. Also, every person was en-

* Lt J.G. Disse, our Dutch Liaison Officer, made several gallant sorties to hide these and other sensitive material outside the hospital.

† I was alas many years later to find that poor 'Mickey' Borgmann-Brouwer became active in the Dutch Resistance and was later taken with all documents to suffer torture from which she only just recovered.

trusted with one book which later contributed to the godsend of a circulating library. We finally assembled outside the hospital for movement. Some separate patients from Sol Sana, a convalescent section, arrived at 0830. Lt Kikooka arrived at 0930 and called for a count.

He was requested to let us hire a cart to take some cooking gear and a little medical equipment, but this he refused, even refusing to allow one of our three remaining ambulance cars to accompany the party to pick up those falling by the way. I instructed the officers to carry their own baggage.

'The party moved off at approximately 1015 with a Japanese escort in command, for a march of about 7 km in intense heat. 300 of those discharged were quite sick and only about 50 were fit for a march with all gear. If, however, they fell by the wayside, boots and bayonets were applied and this was a strong deterrent to weakness.'

Lillie and Nini, two of our attractive Dutch VADs, waved and greeted us on the way and the latter was kicked for taking a snap and her camera confiscated. Boys and others offered help with packs but were kicked off. It was a bit of a *Via Dolorosa* for pale, wilting wrecks. Fortunately there were rests.

I carried a medical pannier, a side haversack of essential instruments and a valise stuffed with medical gear, medical books, and some clothing which weighed about 250 lb in all. 'Blue' Butterworth, my batman of better days, gallantly bore some of the weight with a bamboo pole between us. Our necks and shoulders ached painfully and knees wobbled.

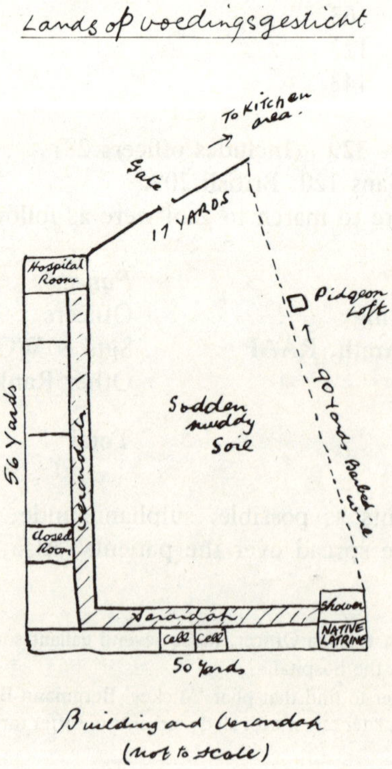

We arrived about midday at *Landsopvoedingsgesticht*, a penal institution designed for Javanese 'bad boys'. This was a formidable, walled, stone building with confining iron bars. At this stage, sentries insisted we leave our baggage, and seized mine. I adopted an 'over my dead body' stance and was belaboured with a rifle by a frantic sentry, until realisation dawned on me that were to be inspected by a visiting general and must all stand to attention without gear. Our possessions were then searched with special attention being given to weapons, steel objects, helmets, compasses, maps, etc. Some cameras and gramophones were taken.

We finally made an exhausted entrance into the rear of the gaol which is outlined on the sketch plan.

Inside, we met Lt Rintoul with 107 others. When every square foot of floor and the verandah were covered with bodies, there were still 150 approximately obliged to take turns out on the sodden earth in the rain.

The gaol was originally designed for 500 Javanese criminals and some 250 still remained, together with over 1200 Dutch, and now our British party became infinitely the worse off for space. I sought out Overste van Lingham, the POW Commandant, and eventually it was conceded that a party of approximately a hundred, with sleeping gear, might pass through the gate at 2130 hours to occupy a line of verandah until 0730. The 27 officers were concentrated, 17 in a small cell (or room) and the adjacent verandah for the rest. There were 12 each of showers and latrines, both very primitive. The latrines were of the open squatting type which blocked repeatedly and were unsuitable to use with paper. These were common to all. I wrote:

'The last meal was at 0800 hours today. A little rice is available for a few invalids – the rest a slice of bread and some tea by courtesy of the Dutch who were individually very kind. More old friends are in sight, including Major Sarabaer. The Dutch all seem most optimistic as to the length of their troubles and pin much faith to an old Javanese legend that "Java would be conquered for 100 days!" There are countless rumours of bombings and invasions by allies. Today, it is Batavia that is said to be bombed, and there are rumours of invasion of the islands by Americans. Also, bombs on Tokyo and Yokohama!

'My troops are in amazing fettle, singing to the theme of an accordion. Favourite: "You'll get no promotion this side of the ocean so f. . . 'em all!" The small NEI RAP room offers assistance. A sample of people who marched out today is my goitre patient, eight days after thyroidectomy. His neck is bleeding from the chafing and pull of his pack though it looked healed before. There are 20VD patients with active syphilis and about 60 in all.'

* * * * *

19 April 1942

Slice of bread for breakfast. I paraded troops and addressed them re:

1 To show no spirit of sullen resistance. To stand to attention on all inspections and show seeming deference.

2 Latrines to be kept spotless. No paper to be used.
3 All kit to be laid out by 0900. Parade at 0930.
4 To remain within the area. Nipponese soldier this morning waved his automatic at my chest with finger on trigger and said he would shoot all outside the wire. This to be taken up with Dutch Commander.
5 Spotless cleanliness of body. Wash once a day.
6 Sick parade at 1000. One room cleared for sick bay and RAP. Maj. Moon in charge.
7 Orderly officer appointed and order NCOs.
8 No firewood to be used by individuals. If this rule observed, Dutch officer in charge of kitchen may be able to lay on two hot meals daily.
9 Fatigues peeling vegetables etc. to be supplied from NCOs with officers' picquets.

I arranged a parade each day with daily routine orders appointing fatigues and orderly duties. I saw the Camp Commander (Overste van Lingham) about our cramped quarters, who said that he would take up the matter with N authorities today. 'Meantime stay inside the wire.' (This prevented some 180 men getting cover at night.) I mentioned the plight of one Indian and caste difficulties. The Dutch sick room gave us drugs and dressings and our sick room is established (no drugs to be given without order of an MO). Major Sarabaer offered me 100 gulden weekly which I refused.

Church parade 1130. Chaplain Camroux and Chaplain Elliott – early morning mass.

A hot meal arrived at 1530. As it was then 36 hours since the last real meal, all were famished. Short supply and poor distribution resulted in only about two-thirds being fed. The officers, who were last, and some NCOs and troops went hungry.

Later, a Nipponese officer arrived on an inspection. Inattentive troops were kicking a soccer ball which was booted in his direction. The chaplain was having 2015 service with hymns (services and any singing were forbidden). A general parade was called by the mortally offended Lt Sumiya, who had taken his guard out, given a 'pep talk' and and ensured that magazines were full and bayonets fixed.

He then gave an inflamed address to the troops through the Dutch interpreter, beginning by saying that morale was very bad and suffered much in comparison with the Dutch. We must all try to capture something of the magnificent discipline of the Nipponese army! We were such whose lives had been spared and we were being well cared for, yet like rats we bit the hand that fed us! He seemed to come to a close and the interpreter instructed me to dismiss the troops, which I did in British fashion, the troops turning to the right, as I moved to the Nipponese officer saluting. To my astonishment, he swung a 'haymaker' which hit me heavily on the jaw. I narrowly avoided being felled by moving my head back a little. I raised my open hands and gave him an angry look.

Lt Sumiya ripped out his sword and lunged at my throat with a deadly tigerish thrust. I avoided the point with a boxer's reflexes, but the haft of the sword hit my larynx with a sickening thud and I could not temporarily breathe or speak. The troops muttered angrily and began moving forward. The guards levelled their rifles and thrust their bayonets menacingly towards them. The scene was tense with the impending massacre. I put up my left hand towards my troops, motioning 'don't move!', and then turned to the officer, gave a coldly formal bow, pointing to the sword with the right hand, implying, 'You are the brave man with the sword!'

I stood to attention too coldly furious to flinch, whilst he swung the sword about my head, fanning my scalp and ears and bellowing loudly. Finally, he sheathed the sword but poked down Lt Durieu and one or two others with thrusts in the throat with the sword in the scabbard, seemingly for deficiency in their position of attention. The lecture then resumed as before:

'The brave and generous Nipponese army do not ill-treat the sick and the weak!' (We were being admirably treated!) 'The British, on the other hand, had committed foul atrocities and had whipped and beaten starving prisoners. Let us take heed!' Instance a soldier this morning crawling through the fence did not heed the warning. In future we were to suffer for such actions by death. Singing and games were forbidden. We were at length allowed to dismiss and I gave the order warily.

A sympathetic cluster surrounded me and a gallant officer of Hussars (Pat Lancaster) produced a whisky flask saying, 'Take a swig of this sir!' I croaked, 'It is hardly that bad, Pat', but took his advice.

The Dutch Commandant, van Lingham called at this stage and said that at his conference with the Nipponese Colonel, the adjutant (Lt Sumiya) had reported to the latter that we had been inspected and were in a satisfactory state!

We were thus left to our existing squalor. The menace of epidemics was acute. Depression reigned. My breathing was still very laboured. Some soup was served at 2230 hours and so to 'bed'.

20 April 1942

Breakfast two slices bread, a little margarine and coffee. John Disse reported that he would endeavour to get out by using his pass and offered to buy a few things for our troops. Dutch officers who go out pulling carts for rations stated that they were able to purchase a little food and comforts outside and would share these equally with our troops. We would, of course, share the expenses.

General parade. Troops all warned to pay more seeming respect to inspecting N officers and to stand to attention. Games and singing are off.

Overste van Lingham called to see me with good news: we are to spread into the reformatory next door, thus taking over a further area equal in size to the present one. A barbed wire fence is first to be erected by our troops and the area cleaned up – all seats, beds and creature comforts being removed! A party of 22 ORs was detailed for the work and a fence was built of spare timber and barbed wire under the direction of a Dutch engineer officer and N soldier busybody, who directed the laying of every strand of barbed wire and the driving of every nail and was most annoyed at the finish when a soldier was about to crawl through it back into the enclosure. This new portion of the building has three very large rooms and each would take 50 troops with one metre per head plus an additional small room for half the officers. 196 men, including 16 officers moved in. Two filthy latrines in this area will be used for infectious cases when made to function.

21 April 1942

General parade called by me anounced impending inspection and ordered thorough layout of kit in neat lines, scrupulous cleanliness and punctilious attention to compliments. Maj. Morris organising the details smoothly. 1300 hours I was called to the commander's office where cordial N officer asked for the numbers of officers, NCOs, ORs, and Red Cross personnel. This is a tall order, so he finally gave us until 2000 hours for completion. Nominal rolls are being made and checked today. 'Did we have any wireless sets?', he asked.

I conferred with D officers on matters of importance – information as to buried weapons, automatics, grenades etc.; plans for emergency rising and commando platoon. Food situation much better today.

Inspection carried out in late afternoon – troops put up a very good show. Morning PT at 1100 hours continues. Food at present 2 slices bread and margarine in the morning, a rice dish at around 1500, soup at 2000.

Maj. Morris is arranging a comprehensive series of lectures by officers and other ranks on matters of interest from 'Commercial airlines in America', 'Malaria', 'The London Stock Exchange', to morse code. Organisation of troops on a service basis [Army, Navy, Airforce] is considered for administration etc. An officers' picquet is maintained on the gate. Apart from those on fatigues to kitchen, all ranks remain inside area.

22 April 1942

Ground is very wet. Food is not to be consumed before 0900 hours in accordance with the N custom, so distribute usual time, eat later. Yesterday D were inspected thoroughly re wireless sets. These and torches, cameras etc. confiscated. *NB*: news from our point of view much better, even allowing for D rumours.

	Red Cross	Non-medical	Total
Officers	16	16	32
NCOs	30	63	93
ORs	64	347	411
Total:	110	426	536

Today whole D camp stunned and depressed by action of N – 3 men caught escaping. Tied to poles and bayoneted to death like pigs before their comrades. On being asked re last request, first man asked for eye bandage to be removed and said firmly 'Long live the Queen' which all then said in turn. A Dutch officer who fainted on witnessing the scene was severely rebuffed by N officer for his unmanliness.

The formal salute to the dead was given by the Nipponese. N Captain inspected camp with troops standing by. Finally ordered that in future parades to be at 0830 am and 1900 hours – orderly officers to report at Japanese Police HQ 0900 and 2130 hours. Capt. Rintoul first to make trip on bicycle accompanied by N escort. I had to make report in Nipponese, '*Ijo arimasen*' (nothing to report). More prisoners at HQ roped together on floor.

N officer also expressed pained(?) surprise at our unclipped heads. A barber will come tomorrow to show us how it should be cut in N style (ORs only). I was questioned re resistance of British troops to this; said none would be opposed.

I am to attend all conferences at Police HQ at 1800 hours along with other officers to hear the Emperor's orders. Warned re any man escaping – captain going through the motions with bayonet at my 'tummy'.

23 April 1942

One slice of bread and coffee.

Warning given last night by Overste van Lingham re any weapons and other contraband.* 1500 hours all knives etc. handed in and troops laid out gear in readiness, but no inspection after all. Weather wet and whole area is a quagmire. Troops doing well in making most of things.

Lectures begin today. To Police HQ where I was rather on the outer among twelve Dutch officers, as Dutch captain interpreter, who spoke fluent Japanese, intepreted to Dutch officers but not to me. I obtained a bicycle for trips. Two white soldiers seen roped on floor awaiting doom; they were kicked by Lt Sumiya (I believe our friend of other night who attacked me).

No inspection today.

24 April 1942

Breakfast: coffee and slice of bread. At general parade I warned troops of risks taken in escape, also danger of holding any weapons. Best for our cause to wait. Emperor's decree re discipline and saluting of all ranks conveyed. Saluting to be done according to N army style: all ranks salute those above.

Lt-Col. van Lingham called today, and congratulated me on good behaviour and discipline of British troops 'which was so much better than the Dutch'. Lecture by Lt Lancaster on 'The tank in modern warfare' much appreciated. Also Maj. Morris on Morse code. Heavy thunderstorm in pm with lashing rain which drenched and flooded camp area. It is difficult to keep mud out with men so herded together.

At Police Bureau I heard words of the Emperor. Ye Gods, the difficulties of finding out what everybody is saying. Geneva crosses are not to be worn any more. I am to submit numbers of officers, NCOs, ORs, English, Australian, American, active or reserve.

Court Martial of the two Dutch soldiers. Defence put up was that N had shown such leniency and generosity that the two unfortunately had been lulled into false security, and would not have offended if they had known the serious view N would take. To secure their release, all commanders raised the right

* Contraband included wireless sets, written records, compasses, maps, also anything which could be used as a weapon. Needless to say, I did not part with my pistols.

hand and promised to do all possible to prevent escapes. I unfortunately also raised my hand as I thought it was a vote for release of the prisoners. The D commanders are a supine lot.

Incidently, Emp. explained death by the bayonet most merciful and honourable of all. It was a personal thrust, not a cowardly striking from afar as in shooting. Officers however, were to be beheaded! So we need have no worries. Home in drenching rain. Numbers given in for all as 'reserve'.

25 April 1942

ANZAC day in squalor, but the 3 minutes silence observed at 1100 hours Java time. It is too utterly mucky for PT or any outdoor activity at present. 'The modern news press', an interesting lecture by Corporal Clarke. All Geneva crosses taken off today. Breakfast, 1 slice bread and coffee 0900; Lunch, rice and soup 1530 – one feels hungry all the time. N medical officers recommended supply of fresh fruit, but this is not forthcoming. No canteen arrangements or private purchases permitted.

Lighting has been requested for rooms of new quarters. Heavy rain again today. Today's rumours: Finland has 'toweled it', Sweden has come in with allied powers, Colombo has fallen. Timor fallen to Americans and Australians. Some action! Russians have surrounded Smolensk. At conference Overste Willikens appealed re loss of Red Crosses, but told nothing doing. Americans, it seems, had sunk a hospital ship. He also requested help re dysentery in camp and this was promised. We are told we may have church services tomorrow. D have no army chaplains and priests are not allowed to come in, hence Tom Elliott, our Catholic chaplain, is in demand.

F/O Cicurel returned tonight with N news given out at Police Bureau. Advised not to listen to Bandoeng rumours and learn the truth. N statements always 'truth' and show that aircraft carrier *Hermes* sunk, also 46 American transports recently. Bataan Peninsula surrendered. Troops in a bad way.

26 April 1942

Inspection by N officers and soldiers at 0230. All Red Crosses to be collected and handed in by 1000 hours. No Red Crosses to show on panniers etc. (It will make interesting reading one day if someone is shot for being in possession of the Red Cross!)

Mass at 0800 and communion 0830, C. of E. Service 1200. Breakfast: rice porridge and coffee. The Dutch living conditions contrast most favourably with ours. Infinitely more space – seats everywhere to sit on, tables, chairs etc. Every officer has a bed or mattress. Commandant has excellent office and typewriter etc. Thus it is possible for D officers to retain some privilege of officer class. Maj. S informs me food supplied has calorie value 1800 daily per man, basic requirements for Europeans being over 2000. Our troops in tents are having a miserable time. Lunch: beans and meat; tea: rice and soup. All civilian clothes are to be handed in tomorrow. British troops in rear of building have no lights. Lights out time laid down: 2200 ORs, 2359 officers.

27 April 1942

No more bread henceforth: rice, plain and unadulterated for breakfast, and coffee, which is said to be finished soon. At approximately 1030 N bomber and fighter planes collided in mid-air with explosion and dissolution. Maj. Corlette lectured on malaria. D officers are forbidden to communicate with wives and relatives outside on pain of death to both. All respirators, steel helmets, knives, cameras, binoculars, civilian clothes collected today. John Morris requested return of gramophones, with no luck.

Those troops who were well on admission look fairly healthy; those who were ill on admission look sick and emaciated. Sqn Ldr Cumming very thoughtfully brought sufficient N.A.B. with him to carry on the treatment of syphilis for a little while longer.

Today Emperor says all officers to lose their hair tomorrow – will allow us 1mm length! Moderate amount of music goes on now in the evening with a piano accordion (squeeze box). Rumours really 'fruity' tonight. Timor and Bali fallen. Colossal bombardments in European Lubeck and Rostic-Heinkel works flattened. Great bombardments of coastal France, Holland and Germany; Russians moving into Sweden and up to 1939 borders!

28 April 1942

Moderate amount of rice three times a day. Nobody feels much like exercise. There is tendency to slight giddiness and stars flash at times when one rises to the vertical. Two inspections by N officers early this morning and notice served of big inspection at 1600 hours by Lt Owihara. Everyone to be in rooms standing by kit. All steel helmets, respirators, binoculars, compasses, cameras, knives and daggers and ribbons of decoration to be handed in by 1400 hours. Inspection finally occurred at approximately 1800 with full layout of kit. Some minor confiscations, compasses, pliers etc.

All officers' hair clipped. Maj. Moon went full measure with shave. Flagrant insubordination by Sgt Leach, who claims to be a flight sergeant but is probably bogus; he has repeatedly broken out of compound and provoked N sentry (addle-pated lad). I admonished him strongly and 'reduced him to ranks', then promised him a cell if he gave any more trouble. Can only hope that if there is an 'after the war' the GOC would back me up.

Maj. Moon complimented by N officers on a good show and promised (if possible) some help re a few beds and blankets for hospital; also enquiries to be made about medical stores. At Police HQ I was informed that a special parade would take place tomorrow in honour of the Emperor's birthday. All troops to assemble at 1015, face the NE and salute. Felt a bit poor about this. I stated my complete disinclination to ask our troops to salute the Emperor of an enemy people and refused to give such an order. The Nipponese captain borrowed a rifle and bayonet from his sentry and prodded my abdomen menacingly. I looked down and said 'I see your point. I shall discuss the matter with the British troops'. These I told I was prepared to defy the order. Capt. Pat Lancaster summed up: 'Please don't get killed for such a thing. If you live with madmen you must humour them'.

29 April 1942

Everyone on parade 1015. In the event it was set up with some childish compass bearings on the north-west (London); I took the parade with many highly-armed sentries watching. I said – 'Gentlemen you are about to receive a very extraordinary order, to salute an Emperor. On the command: "To your front, Salute". You will be saluting an Emperor – I refer, of course, to the King Emperor – if you don't know who that is you bloody well should! "To your front salute"!' This gesture was well received by beaming guards, and the quiet grins of our soldiers! Perhaps a little dignity was saved. D salved consciences by discovering that Canada and Princess J. were in that direction. All damn nonsense anyway.

Quiet day. Lecture on 'The trend of the modern stage' by Bell. Opportunity to buy a few more citrus fruits and a little native sugar on the way to Police HQ and these were distributed to the 'needy'. Talked to interpreter about N mentality, their seeming childishness and inconsistencies. He is half Jap and said that trouble is we try to translate N thought into our own terms, but are usually completely wide of the mark. Nipponese in general are starkly mediaeval, the greater part of the country believing implicitly in the divinity of the Emperor. What we call mysticism they call history. One N historian who introduced ideas of western scepticism was dismissed and lucky to emerge with his life.

Bushido, for example, we elect to translate as chivalry, but bushido and chivalry have nothing in common. Bushido is compatible with the ill treatment and killing of prisoners or with a cowardly attack from the back (any means to an end). There is considerable unhappiness in life and suicide is common. Underneath the hotch potch of mediaevalism, mysticism and racketeering, there is a firm core of tough stuff; Japan is probably ruled more by fanatical idealists who are not rich men and most Nipponese consider it worthwhile to die for Emperor. Most of common soldiery about Bandoeng are farmers.

30 April 1942

Today is Princess Juliana's birthday and D are observing the day as a Sunday, each dressed as neatly as possible and wearing the Orange emblem.

Today D officers came to see me re electric lighting – our needs to be used as a lever to enable them to send a purchasing commission down town. Yet the Dutch commander tells me that we are a separate camp and must deal separately with N and particularly will not supply me with brooms, cleaning materials etc. I saw van Lingham in presence of this officer and was not offered a chair. D commander was put very smartly in his place by me and gave with the blow, saying that he would do his best for us with the Ns and we could try ourselves as well. I do not entirely trust this man.

I then wrote a formal letter thanking him for previous efforts on our behalf (negligible), stating our desire for full co-operation, and to that end requesting representation on all executive bodies common in interest to the two camps and including rations – supply and cooking etc.; electric light; water supply; camp sanitation. Also medical (particularly supplies), clothes and personal requirements. A reply was requested in writing. This is a step to stop this business of the D having all control of stores and rations and according us 'charity'.

Today the sons of Amata Asu o mi Kami (the mythical sun goddess) require all staff maps to be handed in. On our way to the Police Bureau, D Commander in a rather supine way asked if I was angry with him this morning. I shared my long-stored little silver flask of Johnny Walker with three Dutch officers including Maj. Sarabaer and Tom as loving cup to drink to Peace Time.

1 May 1942

Rain every late afternoon or at night. Otherwise, excellent sunny weather and nights just a little cold for one blanket. Some mosquitoes and ye gods! how hard the floor, which necessitates many changes of position during the night, slithering around on smooth tiles. A few troops are recalcitrant, particularly re breaking bounds, and there are the inevitable groans about food, about which I can do damn all. The diabolical nature of things is that just across the road there is an enormous store of tinned food (military), but nothing is released. I think there is bad management in this camp, as other camps report they are at least getting as much rice as they want to eat and they cook it more attractively (baked, etc.) Our cooking apparatus, however, is inadequate. Have been endeavouring to obtain the keys of two cells to be used for delinquents. These cells were opened today.

Emperor today says that we must give numbers possessing money and amounts: i.e. up to 1 gulden, 1–5, 5–10, rising in 5s to 50, 10s to 100, 50s to 500, 100s to 1000. I did not comply. We are advised to have no anxiety about this (like 'ell no!). I was told of one camp which, in making a similar request, said each soldier should have at least 10 gulden and each officer 20 gulden. If they did not, it would be made up. Most of the camp agreed to declare their money, which was checked and handed back to the commander. Then the blow fell. The N Commander said, 'Very sorry – higher orders come that all money now be handed to me. You have, of course, X gulden'.

POWs are to be organised in groups of 50 ORs under one NCO with relieving NCO, ten such groups (500) to be under an officer of rank not higher than captain – relieving Lieut. Camp Commander however to remain (small source of consolation to this unfortunate).

There has been a demand for gunners to show Ns how to work our guns. These I have stalled off (temporarily), by saying that the soldiers have all come from hospital and I do not know of any. Our interpreter, who seems to be a young man of easy conscience, warns me that there will be trouble and that I will be responsible. He says that International Convention lays down that prisoners may be called upon to give information, but not to instruct. I sneeringly told him that I failed to see where he drew the line, and that we, at any rate, did not feel disposed to help shoot down the planes which no doubt would be welcomed in these parts. Further, that British troops contented themselves with giving number, rank, name.

Food is now largely rice, rice, rice and not enough of that. Meat and vegetables negligible.

2 May 1942

I gave one soldier 24 hour solitary confinement in cell. I dislike this very much but there is no alternative. There is considerable petty pilfering in the camp but no one has been caught as yet. Lecture, 'Forgotten Theories of Science', by Sgt Baker, one of the 'unwashed intelligentsia'.

Emperor decrees today no gambling for money permitted, also all bugles to be handed in. In benign mood and allowed me to take a battered Royal typewriter. N sentries not bad chaps if no officers about – occasionally allow me a snap purchase, e.g. got some jam for the hospital today and one or two personal oddments. [These purchases were made in Indonesian shops whilst on escorted cycle visit to Nippon HQ.]

3 May 1942

Food remains the great worry. Personally have lost 25 pounds since leaving Middle East and was under weight then. Now 13 stone 8 lb. One great worry is that the D, who have plenty of rice, put up a damn bad show as to cooking it, and, in any case, as they are nearly all officers with local contacts, they do better than us.

Revolting spectacle has been seen of our lads salvaging D scraps from refuse bins. Interviewed deputation today as to the dishing out of food – all troops are watching this most minutely.

The officers are conducting daily debates. Today, a spirited one on 'Is religion necessary?'. This on a Sunday, too! Emperor has sweet FA to say today.

4 May 1942

Chess tournament began. No meat or vegetables delivered today. Plain rice for breakfast and lunch. Typical D management. They are providing a small bread roll tonight, so propose no rice, since too much trouble to cook it. We at once announced that we would lay on a team for cooking for the whole camp. D now have illicit sources of milk, butter and cheese. Have contributed 1 gulden a head – ask will we do the same and share 43 per cent. This is an excellent offer, but the troops choose apparently to withold money under the impression that the officers are rolling in oof. The first issue was made by D tonight without any money as yet – a little butter and cheese. This with bread and rice was best meal for some time.

5 May 1942

Conversation with Lt-Comm. Smits and Lt Naarhuis re food situation; now there is a food committee of practically all naval men to deal with the problem. Naval pay officer Lt-Comm. Siegers; Lt-Comm. Smits; Dr Postmuis. Our representative is Lt Ian Cameron. Calories at present supplied: 2073, but given the difficulties in cooking rice and lack of cooking gear, less than this is available. In daily life here Europeans require 3400; N soldier at rest gets 3000; at work soldier gets 3000 ++. N checked our figures and agreed with 2073; we then asked for eight additional items, headed by *fresh* fruit. This refused absolutely, also potatoes: reason being danger of infectious disease!

It is possible that we will get a little bread and native sugar added to the diet. Meat and vegetables come from Tjimahi. Meat varies from 30–70 grammes including bone and is distributed according to bill of lading. No meat or vegetables were sent yesterday.

Rail and all other transport is in a hell of a mess. Ns are using what there is, presumably to get foodstuffs back to ports to Japan. Attempts made to get adequate cooking gear unsuccessful. People who go out for food are 'spoiling the show' with small personal parcels and letters. Trying to arrange a permanent quota of about ten people who have no homes or people in Bandoeng and can thus concentrate on real business and contact with outside world. A large-scale smuggle is going on at present e.g. 200 lb coffee, 200 lb onions, possibly 600 lb sugar. We received the first benefits last night.

Problems in Java – enemy making a horrible mess of the economy of the country, presumably on purpose. Banks closed on 8 March and remain so. All civil and government officials, European and natives, are now dismissed. No one has any money. Houses deserted, people beginning to live in communities of, say, about twenty to a house where there was one family before. Rice crops etc. are rotting; it begins to look like starvation soon for the 80,000,000 inhabitants. Natives are already becoming rebellious and some killings have occurred. It is noted that Ns are obviously short of supplies; they like to eat their own white rice, but here they are obliged to eat Java rice which they dislike. They are trying to secure information re use of D bombs, explosives, arms etc., and it is alleged this is due to their own shortage. Cheese and butter again in evidence at today's lunch.

6 May 1942

Weather now fine and the area is drying up a little. The food purchases continue – obviously known to N commander but nothing is done at present. D officers are now allowed to play tennis and football. The days pass very slowly but one gradually becomes accustomed to perpetual squatting on the floor and sleeping en masse on the floor.

M [morse] code and lectures continue; all very interesting. Officers play cards a good deal at night.

7 May 1942

Continued purchases of butter, cheese, milk etc. produce a reasonable diet, only thing missing being fresh fruit. Expense however is going to be beyond us (approx. 110 gulden daily).

Orderly room for insubordinate soldier who, when given an order by F/O Cicurel, said: 'I will consider it' (3 days solitary confinement).

8 May 1942

Same old routine continues. It seems like months since we were imprisoned. A soldier was beaten about today by a N soldier. Nobody quite knows why, but it seems likely that N soldier asked about butter and cheese – our laddy, not understanding, did not stand to attention.

A number of the officers in the British camp have been beaten and knocked about at one time or another.

Emperor today decrees that all badges and marks of distinction or rank are to be handed in – Australian rising sun badges, badges of rank etc. This applies to D as well as ourselves, and the D colonel squad are as stricken as though a fox had got into the fowls' roost. When asked how we were to maintain discipline, Capt. Kawakatta said that the Emperor had thought of that and we were later to get some distinguishing marks acceptable to His Highness. What is the reason? Ideas: 1 humiliation; 2 cupidity – possible sale of badges; 3 having made us all privates now easy to plunder us further.

9 May 1942

The extra supplies of fatty food continue. Ft-Lt Peach lectured today on 'Bird Photography'. All distinguishing badges and tokens of rank handed in 'like hell'.* The D colonels etc. look rather like plucked fowls and are depressed. I tell them it is better to be a private in the service of the Emperor!

Col. van Lingham protested about badges to the higher command and was told that, meantime, commanders may wear badges of rank inside the camp. That is the one place I don't care particularly about. The men are reacting by showing more courtesy than usual.

Emperor approached to give us some Vitamin C which has been estimated to be very deficient. Nothing doing, but we are requested to supply numbers of men needing it specially. Also it seems we could get newspapers each day (not stated who will pay – the available newspapers are printed in Jap and Malayan so perhaps one will be sufficient).

10 May 1942

Sunday, Chaplain Tom Elliott takes mass at 0800 looking a very dignified figure in white and purple. Candles burning. D take part in service on other side of the fence. Fred Camroux takes three services during the day. He has no surplice but has somehow preserved his books for troops' service. Both are excellent fellows who can 'take it' and are a credit to the church.

Lt Chadwick, who has had a recurrence of malaria recently, had a fit this morning and fell heavily. The absence of serious illness is surprising and there are only about twelve patients in the hospital. A weekly medical inspection is held; the last one revealed about eighty cases of tinae of the feet or cruris, and one case *pediculosis pubis*. Instructions issued re prophylaxis. The extras – butter, milk, cheese, sugar etc – have greatly increased the vigour of the troops.

News today is big stuff: battle said to have occurred in Coral Sea near the Solomons with heavy losses by N fleet – damage being done first by planes. Seventeen enemy ships said to be sunk including at least 1 aircraft carrier, 2 battle cruisers, 6 cruisers, rest destroyers and transports; action said to be continuing. Chinese said to be counter-attacking near Mandalay. Prize rumour is that local Italian residents are being interned!

* Many, like myself, hid most of them.

11 May 1942

Fine clear weather and ground drying up. General parade at which I outlined food position to troops: cheese and butter too much for general fund and must stop. They are available for purchase by 'rooms' who can raise the money and order through Sgt Ian Cameron. Milk, it is hoped, will continue, also extra sugar, jam, condiments, fish, and occasionally chocolate. A debt of 250 gulden plus for cheese and butter was met from hospital reserve fund. Tobacco to be sold to troops; this was supplied in quantity today, with papers for cigarettes. Troops congratulated on good morale and those concerned with games and recreations were thanked. More exercise urged. Endeavoured to encourage a spirit of optimism.

Further lecture by Major Moon, 'Pioneers of Medicine'. News today is an extraordinary mixture and mostly tripe, e.g. 9 American naval ships said to be sunk in above action (sounds possible but less likely) and: Hungary, Rumania, Bulgaria capitulate to Russians!; Germans have marched out of Holland – (this one for D Consumption!); Anthony Eden has made a speach giving an ultimatum to Germany to surrender completely. (To this, Hitler is said to have replied evasively!) Chinese have captured Mandalay.

Just as a counter, it has been rumoured that Australia has repeatedly been invaded north, south and west!*

12 May 1942

Heavy rain again in evening. Staff Sgt Baker's lecture, 'The Trend of Modern Literature'. We are seldom bothered by N inspections these days. The local N commander spends much of his time in camp talking to Overste van Lingham and leaves us severely alone. D in this camp said to have 3 cases of scurvy. This may be so, due to dislike of soup which is the only possible source of vitamin C. Representations to local command and *Kebetai* who allow purchase of citrus for *those suffering only*. Prevention is apparently not important.

Only news from Emperor today is that the number of the British camp is 13. (Perhaps there is something in this superstition business.)

13 May 1942

Cpl Clarke gave excellent lecture on 'English Lakes District'. Strong rumour today of N Cabinet changes, Prince Konoye replacing Tojo. Nobody knows quite what this would mean. I am trying to arrange the transfer of two sick men to Tjimahi to hospital and saw Overste Willikens to that end.

Bill for milk and other odds and ends mounting rapidly, so I gave Mr Cameron 100 gulden from my own little reserve; am afraid that troops will have to buy milk in future, as camp funds will not stand the racket.

* There was said to be one reliable source of information in the place: a hidden wireless in Dutch hands used twice a week, and the naval 'news' was said to come from this. It proved quite *unreliable*.

14 May 1942

N officer arrived this morning with motor lorry to take sick men to Tjimahi. Quinn (paratyphoid fever); W/O Ellis (malaria and renal colic); Sgt Bennett (dysentery). Beds were carried out and placed in lorries and later returned. Maj. Moon sent as 'nursing orderly' to get information at Tjimahi. He met McSweeney, who reported things going fairly well, no cases lost. Plaster spica cases travelled well. Kinmonth doing a good job; operating 3–4 times a week. They too, have been deprived of hair, Red Cross brassards, badges of rank and so forth, and get the same orders that we do. Living conditions and food are much better and, of course, they have work to do. Sgt Gibson also seen – his normal self – they have lost a little weight.

Spelling and general information competition in vogue, also language courses.

15 May 1942

N officer (medical) along to make enquiries about patients who have gone to hospital, in particular paratyphoid fever; required facts of contacts, clinical history, etc., also whether I had carried out disinfection. Reported this impossible since no disinfectant; he thought possibly this might be got and left with Ov. Willikens to that end.

Emperor today benign: reports that we may obtain fresh fruit and some milk twice a week upon production of a medical certificate, provided we pay. Decent fresh fruit and vegetables are not considered necessary for the rest. The great food smuggle has now come to an end. D not allowed out for the purpose and searches much stricter. Personally obtained some foodstuffs today, including some bread and jam for the hospital. N today opened some closed cupboards in rear of our quarters, revealing many tools, one of these more innocent, which the soldier allowed us to retain. Amusing thing was that we had used the cupboard to conceal a few odds and ends, contraband etc.

The days are pleasant now, with plenty of sunshine, and the troops are very tanned but thin.

16 May 1942

Required by two N medical officers and questioned re 'medical matters'. First question: number of field hospitals to a division. Refused to answer. Questioned why: 'My general forbids me'. Who is your general? 'General Blackburn'. Where is he? 'A prisoner in Java'. Laughter. Then why put us in a position of having to punish you? (Gestures re removal of head.) Here I pointed out that N officers no doubt appreciated a point of honour. I could do nothing till released from my word. Would not the honourable gentlemen of the N army not do the same in my circumstances? Much going into a huddle after this. Finally asked me if I would answer questions re hygiene.

Of course! No doctor would withhold such information from another, but as I was purely a specialist surgeon appointed for that purpose, I regretted that I knew 'sweet FA' about hygiene.

Much discussion about my rank and appointment and disappointment that I was not an 'army surgeon'. I said that I had come straight from Australia to Java in January, had seen nothing, knew nothing, heard nothing (and was just about sunk into pit of lies). Finally, was given headings for a report on Australia which was to be as comprehensive as possible, embracing geographic details on the country, mountains, plateaux, plains, rainfall, deserts, seaside resorts, cities, hospitals, roads, effect on roads and railway trains, waterworks etc., drug manufacture, and everything to notable sights! This I was given two days to complete and I promised to do so, since I did not want to bring displeasure on my troops by direct refusal. Said all the information would be in Baedaker anyway.

Some more technical information is required re army organisations which will cause more worry. Information also asked re diseases and distribution and Civil Health organisation.

All officers (Australian) are sharing in the report and imaginations are working well. It should be a masterpiece of school essays. I directed them to draw heavily on *Talking Points for Australian Soldiers*. I was told that they proposed to put me in jail until the report was completed. I said, 'Alas, I am temperamental and could only do the report in my quarters!'

Concert today organised by AC2 Solity (a cockney humourist); quite a good show, but was interrogated in middle of show by further N officers who wished to known particularly where Australians and British 'had their homes in Java'. That one was easy to answer. Also stressed that all the officers were doctors and knew nothing, except a few young fellows (mostly air force), who also knew nothing. Sqn Ldr Cummings was then produced – the next senior officer for interrogation – very unfruitful.

17 May 1942

Report now drafted by several officers is amusing reading. I prepared the answers to more difficult questions, such as organisation of the Army Medical Services. I believed that we had a Director-General in command somewhere in Australia and that he had help from one or two staff officers. However, as a surgeon called in late, I was not really informed!

Rumours of N attempting a further attack on A[ustralia]; can the report required be significant? Emperor not receiving yesterday or today (bad for the larder). N soldiers have suddenly begun to show a barrage of friendship and are thronging the camp with only side arms, carrying on brisk barter with the troops on a very fair basis. Of course, a few asses are trading in watches and other personal gadgets of value. Is this change of attitude inspired? The large-scale smuggle has stopped but in the last two or three days we have had some chocolate and some tobacco. D still play tennis and football and talk vaguely of extending the privilege to us. John Disse is now teaching the troops Malay. What with Dutch, French and Malay classes I find the going a bit tough.

18 May 1942

The fourth day Emperor is not receiving. Reformatory is being cleared of 'bad boys' (the Indonesians)! Some fresh move of prisoners here; something is afoot.

N soldiers still romping round like little baa lambs. Curious tragic declamations resound in corners of the camp where *Julius Caesar* rehearsals go on.

General parade: troops warned that there are some anophyline mosquitoes and to use nets where possible. Butterworth – who has borrowed mine – did not take the hint. They are a real pest.

More outrageous rumours: Germans now making big drive in south, particularly Crimea; Russians counter-attacking and would seem to be having things their own way in the north; rumours of heavy boming – particularly Berlin; British credited with having retaken a town or two in Burma. Churchill credited with having made a speech in which he says 'the end is in sight – Germany now to have the blood and toil, tears and sweat'.

19 May 1942

Change in command today: Lt Owihara was replaced by another officer (1 pip) – Captain at Police Bureau. Kiwakata replaced by '2 pipper' Our camp inspected by the new commander accompanied by Kiwakata and Ov. van Lingham – approximately 1000 troops standing to. To Police Bureau at 1200 hours for the 'hand over', where a colourful monkey show. First, both officers took several pictures of the captive commanding officers on the steps, British CO (me) showing his natural modesty by standing in the gutter behind a fat Dutch colonel until dragged out with laughter, and then buried his nose under the peak of his cap and chin in his shirt. Next, assembled and did our attention and saluting display and were addressed by the old commander, who expressed his gratification at our previous relations and the way we had carried out the orders. (My comment: bayonets are useful!) He then expressed the trite hope that we would continue to accord his successor the same enviable behaviour. The latter introduced, a picturesque character with a villanous shaven brachycephalic pol, a long drooping moustache, spectacles, a white tennis shirt, white cotton gloves – dandy what! He addressed us less eloquently, felicitating us upon the good reports given to him of our behaviour towards the departing and abjuring us to continue the good behaviour with him. Curtain, with more bowing and a very successful sortie [obtained food] on the way home. Rest of day somewhat uneventful.

20 May 1942

All troops have been worried that there is fifth-column activity in camp. I witnessed the departure of a certain hidden radio certainly not known to Ns. Little incident today of D officer (junior?) calling to 'warn me' that he had heard that I had a radio and that he felt it was 'his duty to warn me'. The reply, 'why your duty?' did not produce any satisfactory reply. Of course I emphasised, no radio, but no one ever believes the truth. The only answer to my queries was that he was a friend of van Telenburg, an officer for whom I sometimes bring in parcels.

N guards were changed today and the new lot are not full of joy and lightness. Guard with Ov. van Lingham and me seemed a nasty type and cut up rough at me whilst waiting for van Lingham who takes tea and gossips endlessly with other colonels about sweet FA. Not being satisfied with my response the soldier began grunting and making gestures of physical violence, whereupon I rose to my feet and rather foolishly struck a fighting attitude and told him to go to hell and generally bawled him down.

Similar scene on the way home, where searched by N soldiers and had my coat thrown at me. Good types! Fortunately nothing in my coat, for once.*

M. Schaub teaching officers contract bridge; pass my time in chess, languages and bridge and some sun baking.

21 May 1942

Rations, despite promises, instead of rising from 2200 calories to 2500, having actually fallen to 1800. Less large-scale swindling, but there has been much more activity of late in individual purchase, in which Ns are co-operating. Yesterday, however, saw the amusing racket of the seven baskets for vegetables whereby 160 kg vegetables were obtained instead of eighty. Seven baskets full on roadside, each journey replacing one empty with a full. N very active in trying to catch officers passing letters – even some shooting in the air and waving of automatics but no luck – letters passed satisfactorily.

Recently a D juggler was giving a display when the senior N soldier in charge of guards announced that he was an escapologist and could not be restrained by ropes or handcuffs etc. Upon invitation, D trussed him up like a fowl preparatory to his escaping display. At this moment the N commander arrived, found senior soldier all trussed up, gates open and guards mingling with prisoners without weapons. Finally he could do nothing but join in the laughter.

'News': Americans definitely in Timor. Battle of Coral Sea – both sides suffered heavy losses but Ns between 60 and 70 ships; lost the battle and admiral recalled to Nippon. Admiral Hellige took part in this affair and, of course, knows these seas like his hand, so was said to be responsible for a decoy withdrawal leading N ships on to the rocks by turning in the dark.

Local: All the big importing firms have been commanded to send foodstuffs etc. to Tanjongpriok and ports. This definitely looks like a major shift of stuff to Nippon and the fact that food figures so prominently would seem significant. Ns are definitely very short of everything – automatic weapons – one sees damn-all transport. Cannot even organise a transport service from Bandoeng to Batavia.

Uniforms are patched and tattered. Australian officers are obtaining raincoats to have made into uniforms (this actually done by me).

Fed up with van L. re the vacated camp accommodation at the back. Van L. informed me that of this the N had given us a negligible amount, although already Dutch have more than two-thirds of camp. However he was prepared to be generous! He would give us more if the Ns agreed. I inspected what the proposed arrangement would include, which was for the most part cells fit for dogs, and told van L so in forthright terms. Then he, as usual, shuffled a bit and said that all he wanted was a recreation hall, a kitchen, a store-room and a new office, as he has to sleep in the present one. I told him that we were all

* It was then obvious that my guard had advance knowledge that I would be searched and did me a great favour in not letting me purchase anything.

sleeping with heads three feet apart, 50 men in damp tents and that we were interested in living space not recreation halls, offices or store-rooms, since being British we had been given nothing to store. Perhaps this was because we are still at war with the Ns!

Later in day van L. saw the guard to protest against his officers being used for manual labour and was told that they must obey. He protested and said he would go to *Kebetei*. Whereupon five soldiers took him into the guard room and beat him up. Good heavy stick for beating – twisted his arms and tore his clothes about. Damage to his head and hands. Later called him back and beat him again, then a third time, when he was informed that it was enough – but that he must at once carry out all orders and that if he reported the incident to the *kebetei* worse would follow. Accordingly he instructed his officers to get on with the work and made no report. No notice was taken of his obvious bashings.

22 May 1942

Warned of inspection but none came. Van L. is obtaining the necessary wire for fence and shift held up until available. Weather is brilliant sunshine in am, still frequently rain in pm. Nights rather hot in crowded quarters, where air is very fuggy and mosquitoes thick. Lectures, language class, debates, spelling and intelligence competitions, bridge, chess and other games continue. Somehow the days seem full. Asked N to shift four men to hospital yesterday. They sent a medical officer to enquire today. Present commander fears to come into our camp! Organised PT began today. Van L. called with a little *horse flesh* for the officers for tomorrow (Pentecost).

23 May 1942

Pentecost – special mass and services. Maj. Arthur Moon to Tjimahi with four patients. Patients 317. No deaths. Receiving a few from Tesigmalaya, mostly RAF and RAAF. No news of Blackburn force, Batavia, but 2/3 M.G. Bn said to be still at Heles. Patients being discharged to 6 Bn Camp (D). Troops at 'Tesig' being moved to Surabaya. Conditions pretty good, with canteen and can get milk, fruits etc. No over-crowding. Big troop movements going on on that side.

'News'. Confirmation of Churchill's optimistic speech re blood and toil and tears and sweat on the other side and prophecy of big naval battle in Pacific. Local: Ns get still tougher – we are now told that if we do not carry out the orders of any N soldier we can be shot or bayonetted on the spot – a start made with four Dutch who, on encouragement of sentry, bought food but were then betrayed by sentry, food confiscated, and bayonets then used. (Nice little chaps!) Fortunately, those concerned were not killed but are in hospital. 1600 Javanese soldiers said to have signed declaration of allegiance and are to return home tomorrow. Officers, I believe, are not signing.

Amongst other soldiers who have been manhandled is W/O Ellis, who had his moustache pulled, was cracked about, and threats made to cut off his tatooed Union Jack with bayonets.

24 May 1942

My general parade: troops warned about new powers of N sentries. All soldiers now to be saluted and orders to be carried out as if given by officers.

Began the move into new quarters from which D have already annoyingly seized many of the comforts and furniture. Crowning annoyance reached when Maj. Morris in my company took back a box from their area which was previously ours. Dutch officer rudely seized this from him. I protested and Overste Drough (2IC) came up and apparently supported him in the action. I gave him the full blast of my wrath, comparing his officers to carrion birds and refused to speak to him any more in the presence of other ranks.

25 May 1942

Troops working hard moving into new quarters and making themselves more comfortable. Things are certainly much better. Some of the cells even have been made almost comfortable with 'curtains' and shelving. N officers looked in. An orderly room is now a *fait accompli* with a sleeping portion screened off for Maj. Morris and me. Officers now occupy three rooms instead of the two in which they were very crowded indeed.

Messing is as before and seems to be fairly satisfactory now. Most of things acquired by the move rather bug-ridden, particularly an old cupboard, bed boards etc. A very ornate altar for Tom is included.

Troops being weighed today and height taken. Idea is that if below standard weight for height (e.g. 6 foot man 80 kg), or if lost over 25 lb since admission, we can recommend to Nips that milk be supplied – for which, of course, we pay. Disturbed to find my own weight now 85 kg = 12 st 10½ lbs = 38 lbs lost.

26 May 1942

Splendid hot sunny days with rain in late afternoon and evening. Further call of N officers this morning who threatened the camp with 400 more troops. It was originally for maximum 500 boys, but now 1300 troops here. 1700 was explained as just about an impossibility. They talked usual patter about seeing what they could do – ominous expression always. Meantime, things are looking up with almost feasible *sleeping* space.

'News' of the day. N said to have admitted fall of Timor (a temporary withdrawal), Queen Wilhelmina said to have made a speech promising relief within six months and meantime telling Dutch East Indies not to be rash. Gawd! *Later*: the great naval battle is said to have started near New Guinea. I wonder?

Nasty guards back and poking their noses around. Van L. very strict about his officers coming in. (N guards a cross between children and devils. Entertained by those outside 15 Bn Barracks who indulged in all sorts of buffoonery and amongst other things had me showing them how a kangaroo jumps. They admired my legs but struck a note of resistance and alarm on my part on their wanting to see an adjacent organ.

They meantime urinated publically outside their own quarters.

Dutch astrologer is in danger of losing this reputation. He promised something dramatic by 25 May. The following is typical of amusement efforts:

GALA NIGHT
IN ROOM 2
26/5/42
DANCE DANCE DANCE
TICKETS FREE
GOOD PRIZES (PRESENTED BY THE RICE KING)
ALL INVITED. BRING YOUR GIRL FRIENDS
NOVELTY DANCES
FIRST CLASS BAND
BROOK AND HIS HARMONICA PLAYERS
LIGHT REPRESHMENTS AT INTERVAL
RICE RICE RICE (BRING YOUR OWN)
DANCING FROM 6.30 TILL RICE TIME. ROLL UP BOYS
AND ENJOY YOURSELVES
SARONGS AND DRESS SUITS

M.C. Prisoner W. Millward

Amusing exhibitions were given, Apache dancing etc.

27 May 1942

Discussions with Lt-Comm. Smits (Royal Netherlands Navy) re food question and reported our difficulties in raising 75 cents per head. D quite willing to 'carry' us until their own money ran out.

This I refused because there is definitely enough money in the camp for the levy, and the Dutch have families reaching the starvation point, too. With no money coming in, many will not get as good a diet as even the prisoners. They have a devil of a job getting supplies in, with frequent threats, slappings and standing at attention with glasses of water on head and threats of death. In any case, if it is on a charity basis, we lose all control in this and other matters.

Assembled all officers and section NCOs and put the question to them: what was it going to be like with a diet of rice three times a day relieved only by one lot of soup? No coffee, no bread rolls (since no oil to use with the flour supplied by Ns), no flavouring or any of the extras. Following proposals discussed:

1 Reasons given for refusing charity.
2 Policy re possible cessation of all supplies.
3 If so, propose to stop purchases of supplies extra to levy brought in by D (cheese, milk, butter etc.).
4 Question as to whether those willing to subscribe should receive routine supplies; or only be allowed to purchase such extras from camp sources.

Considered it would be unfair and cause trouble to give extras only to those willing to subscribe. (Some of the others have already given their all.)* The

* This incident is illustrative of the intimidating difficulty of regulating the supply of foodstuffs available for purchase so that the sick got some, and as many as possible derived some benefits. We were largely dependent on the Dutch parties who went out and pulled ration carts, making purchases both official and 'under the lap'. They ran most of the risk. We then purchased a set share from the Dutch out of camp funds, which had to be subscribed by the prisoners, who were

position seems to boil down to either raise the money, or confiscate all money, giving a receipt, and then only authorise approved purchases.

The following policy was determined:

1 Special parade of all troops to launch a new blitz and explain the position to them.
2 All troops to declare the amount of money they hold.
3 Section commanders to report suspected false declarations.
4 Supplies to be stopped as from tomorrow unless money raised.
5 A committee to be appointed to enquire into the financial state of the camp.

27 May 1942

Ns in bad mood today. Twenty-nine officers on the way to the dentist talked and smoked, so were slapped and hit on heads with stick. They are now padding their caps. Van L. and I accordingly rode like good boys on our bicycles to the *kebetai* in silence and, as for the last few days, cast no side glances at shops, even though the sentry tried to lure van L. into one. He said, '*Arigato*' and rode on again.

28 May 1942

Committee of Sqn. Ldr R.A. Cummings, Maj. Moon and Lt Rintoul to investigate the financial state of the camp. Terms of inquiry: to interview soldiers suspected of having made false declarations of money held and to ask whether they were prepared to make statements on oath. All evidence to be voluntary. Committee began working this morning. Of course, no soldier at present will be actually required to make sworn statements (but unsatisfactory birds will be noted). As the officers have made big contributions and the goal is in sight, supplies will not be stopped. Thank the Lord!

Still bright sunny days with rain in the evenings. All tents now struck. To *kebetei*, where lieutenant with long moustache drilled us commanders in 4s interminably with much *kiotské*, *keré*, *yasumé*, calling upon us each to give the commands. I yelled something loud and hoarse which got by; several poor wretches were kept at it for many repetitions.

Nip requirement last night was:

1 Obey all orders at *kebetei*.
2 Obey the guard – same as *kebetei*.
3 Must not order goods through guard soldier (actually the little sods occasionally do this purely on their own volition and we must obey them!).
4 More returns of Australian information etc., 'active', 'reserve', 'conscripts'.

Nip commander of camp called me to office today re return of this sort and I

receiving pay at the time. Officers were expected miraculously to find the money, but few had such resources, and we found, as is recorded above, that we were out of funds to pay our way. I refused to contemplate accepting charity from our allies.

The task before me was to create a moral climate in which men would recognise that foodstuffs could only decently be got to them through our camp organisation and, that having shared benefits derived from the money subscribed by others, it was up to them to put in money too. Naturally, it was proposed to keep a record, in the hope that Governments would make post-war repayment.

told him no permanent soldiers ('active'). On the way out he picked a soldier with a much-tatooed chest and asked him when it was done, to which he repled, 'Before the war'. 'What did you do before the war?'. 'I was a soldier!' (What?!!!) Frantic signals from me nigh unto collapse and he then denied all knowledge of soldiering in any form. [I suspected that declared professional soldiers would be under pressure to instruct in use of weapons and to disclose military matters. Thus I portrayed my charges as war-time volunteers – 'babes in the wood' in military matters.]

29 May 1942

0830 Ov. van L. called to suggest that 1000 hours. Ov. Drough and I look into question of allottment of mutual property, seats, tables, etc. I obtained 50 school desks which, when cut in two, make a seat and table. Also one table and a promise of further consideration re tables. Everybody quite friendly.

N Commander called to request me to supply personnel who understood bombs. My regrets – how particularly regrettable for this inferior person that he cannot oblige noble commandant – alas we fear bombs and do not understand them. No sirree!

30 May 1942

Called to *kebetei* at 12 noon with van L. We were informed that all troops from Landsopvoedingsgesicht were to move tomorrow to Tjimahi on foot. 17 kilometres.

I protested that many men were not fit enough for such a march, and was told details to be discussed with local commandant. Local commandant arrived at 1400 and I discussed the move with him and van L. Total British and Australian troops: 529. Thirty-two officers including 13 Australian, 1 Canadian, 1 NZ, 17 British (including one RAF officer, Cicurel, who is really an American). Total: Australian 228, English 297; British Indian: 1.

Reported 11 'lying sick'. Excess given so that extra beds and mattresses might be shifted. Total unable to march to Tjimahi: 96. Unfortunately, D had already 'batted' strongly on this first morning, saying about 300 unable to march, and final figure settled on was 100 for lorries. Remainder to march without equipment; consequently, we did not do so well. Agreement was reached as to the 11 lying cases but it was ruled that only 46 would be taken by motor transport, the remaining 40 to march without equipment, and all of remainder to march with full equipment. I stressed that the troops had been in hospital prior to prison and many were unfit.

Assembly was to take place the following morning at 0800 on the area east of *Landsop* – in front of the tennis court.

Transport: five lorries to be available for sick troops and excess baggage. Rest to be taken by hand carts (approx 5 men per cart), 10 carts to be available for British. N said they would move excess baggage for us if clearly labelled and put in a separate room from the D.

A movement order was then drafted by John Morris and I – Maj. Moon to be in charge of the sick and stay with them for the move, all remaining troops to be on parade at 0715 ready for the move to assembly area. Hand carts to be loaded and drawn out onto the road opposite the assembly area. Attention to be given to Japanese etiquette and warning given re N command. Lt Cameron to arrange for cooking today of a ration sufficient for tonight's meal and for two meals tomorrow (append this order). A concert was given by the 'Rice Revellers', organised by A/C Solity. Two Dutch officers took part in this excellent show. It included the two RSMs in a sketch, another one 'The price we pay', a 'Hill-billy band', and some excellent musical and vocal items.

The evening meal finally arrived at midnight N time; meantime there was an orgy of packing and cleaning up. Large fires for the burning of rubbish lit this pitiful scene. The hand carts were loaded by the baggage party under the command of Maj. Clarke and finally we turned in for an hour or two of sleep before the 0545 reveille.

Solemn warning that any contraband found would lead to execution on the spot: I decided to take a chance on my maps and compass in present spot [behind scrotum]. Badges of rank scattered about in out-of-the-way corners of my clothes and a further compass sewn into the bottom of my shirt. Thought of putting it at bottom of tin of sugar but was unhappy about this lest sugar confiscated – or tipped out. Devil of it all was that I had arranged today to obtain a 'sparks' and had arranged a hiding place for it.*

* The wireless set. I was actually reticent about this in my diary. There was a search for such contraband sprung by the *Kempis* (Nippon Military Police) a day or so before the move. In the middle of this tense situation, W/O 'Rod' Allanson trotted into my almost bare cell bearing a large parcel wrapped in camouflage sheeting about 2 feet by 1 foot by 9 inches. Urgent message: 'Compliments of Lieutenant Naarhuis of NIA and would you please hide this!' (Imagine my embarrassment at being handed the baby in our bare rooms when the Dutch had so much more space and resources to hide things. I said ironically: 'Rod, I don't suppose you could find the perisher to give it back?' He smiled and said, 'You're dead right!'

I was obliged to stroll innocently out amongst the searching Japanese. scratch earth out of a revettment behind my back and to push the six-valve wireless set in – all in a leisurely, careless style but with my heart decidedly racing. It rained during the day and that night, and I had to smear mud over the exposed parcel which stuck out like a whale's rib.

When the move was made the following day, I simply carried it under my left arm with a ground sheet draped over it, and gave a crashing salute to the guard. My all too early confident reaction was: 'all one needs is a bit of cheek'.

2 Tjimahi

May 1942

31 May 1942

Early breakfast; filled our dixies with rice and had also 4 flour pancakes for the trip (cooks having worked all night). Said farewells to van L., John [Disse], Schank (who gave the excellent bridge lessons) and Kingman, our French teacher, also many other who have been very kind.

On parade at 0715 carrying packs, haversack, water bottle and respirator haversack filled with odds and ends). Addressed the troops re trip, warning them to go easy on water at first and to help each other out as much as possible and mentioned Japanese commands re saluting. Our assembly area was reached before 0800. Finally the right number of heads was counted and at 0935 we left behind Landsopvoedingsgesticht with no regrets but with little optimism as to the other end. Order of the march: D handcarts: 51, 5 D to a cart (British definitely done in the eye there by D who even tried to get away with giving us eight only, one without a wheel; eventually produced 10); then D troops – army first, air force, then navy. Next British handcarts: 10 – British troops, Australian troops, other Dominion troops with JaggerNa British India, dead last. Maj. J.E. Clarke in charge of our handcart – six men per cart.

It was a most extradordinary cavalcade, with the streets of Bandoeng lined by families of those marching, almost as though a triumphal march. Sentries accompanying us rode on bicycles, many of them with waddies and canes of various sorts to deal with offenders. As the various citizens crowded around a bit, blows and kicks were freely handed out, one burly sergeant seemingly deriving much enjoyment from knocking people off their bicycles and inflicting blows and kicks, occasionally making a sortie chasing people. Lillie and Nini, Dutch VADs, were amongst the crowd. British and Australians sang lustily 'Tipperary', 'Roll Out the Barrel' etc. and such expressions as 'Good Luck', 'Not for long' and the victory sign were much in evidence. Many women were crying. Eventually Ns served notice that if crowd followed any further there would be shooting and safety catches were adjusted. Visse (interpreter) was made to ride up and down to explain this to the crowd.

It was very hot, and after leaving the city the singing died away and sweat rolled forth.

A few kilometres along the road the column was halted, ostensibly for a rest, when to my alarm, alert sentries had all baggage deposited on the ground and ordered us all to strip naked whilst our effects were searched. Each man stood by his baggage and was thus identified. My own baggage was fortunately down the line of search.

I constituted myself unofficial 'ombudsman' to plead the innocence of various articles being confiscated, picking things up, waving them and putting them down, then at times in disgust going back to my original position. In this way, I managed to transfer the six-valve wireless set and other contraband piece by piece to the searched area. During this confidence trick my original jaunty optimism fell to a low ebb.

Ns gave comic relief by falling off bikes frequently. We reached Tjimahi assembly ground at 1330 – a large open space near the railway line, which caused some alarm. British and Australian troops again raised a song on reaching Tjimahi, though many were swaying in their tracks and just about all in.

A few swastika emblems were seen on the arms of one or two gentry about the assembly area, causing no particularly pleasant expectation, since fear of N ferocity and German efficiency.

Troubles then began on the assembly ground, where it was hot as hell. D interpreters and a horde of N soldiers and NCOs began forming us in 4s and 8s with and without equipment, here and there reducing tired troops to a confused state. I was alternately called upon to give commands and then hauled back into ranks by N soldiers who struck and kicked soldiers fairly freely.

During one of these episodes, when I had been kicked into the centre of the back row, and again restored to Command position by calls of 'No. 1!' there appeared an amazing speciman of the Master Race who rose in this confused scene like Aphrodite from the waves. I was confronted by a smooth, bland face, a splendidly proportioned lithe frame poured into a superbly tailored uniform tapering to shining jack boots. I noted the swastika armband, the gentian blue eyes at my 6 ft 4 in. level and the cultured English 'Perhaps I can be of use to you sir,' accompanying the Hitler salute.

The humiliation of the day simmered in my blood and I thought, 'Here at last is someone I can sting.' I returned the salute carelessly and without enthusiasm, coldly sweeping my eyes from his head to his feet. 'Yes,' I said, 'Perhaps you can. Suppose you explain to these Japanese (whom I understand your Fuhrer refers to as "lacquered yellow monkeys", but with whom you seem to have something in common, which is denied to me and my men) that if they give some sensible order we will endeavour to carry it out.'

This insult produced a dull flush to his face and I saw him fight for control. He said, 'You must see that I am trying to help you.' I replied, 'Under these painful circumstances, that is all the help I can accept from you.'

He accomplished miracles of liaison with the Japanese in a fluent language exchange and brought about order to the parade at last. He returned to give me the Hitler salute and was returned a perfunctory touch to the cap. My experience in the western desert had made me feel that a splendid arrogance in adversity was the best approach to the German race.

At 1520 hours at last satisfied as to our numbers. We marched through lines of N barracks to our camp, a much more spacious affair with a soccer ground. We were not searched (D were before starting).

We were then paraded before N commander in 4s and the same business of N command drill and counting of heads began. N soldiers chased up and down the lines inflicting a smack, a slap or a kick, but after a long session of this men began to collapse here and there – about eight in all passing out and eventually reaching the camp hospital.

We were unfavourably received as to length of hair and all hair is to come off by tomorrow. After breaking off, D then conducted us to our barracks, explaining that they were to administer the camp. Twenty officers allotted a smaller barrack, but rest (12) placed in barrack with men.

I protested strongly; eventually, I saw Major de Vries and expressed my disgust in forthright terms, not disguising my opinion that we were being played off as usual with the N bogey. He gave me a solemn assurance that it was an N instruction and begged me to try only twenty officers together for a couple of days to see how they took it. Eventually we were given another room, at present used by D as a classroom, 'on my own responsibility' – whatever the hell that is. This implied that I must be responsible to the Japanese. Major Moon found Dutch hospital staff a good bunch, treating our sick mostly excellently from the start.

Amazing news: there is actually a canteen in the camp and a meal is laid on for us from camp sources this evening. Coffee (4c) can be purchased in the evenings.)

Troops have put up an excellent show. Many have blistered feet and are stiff and sore. Lights out 2200 hours – one light per barrack must stay on all night and one inhabitant must be always on piquet (not dressed) to account for everyone in the barracks at any time during the night.

One of our number was taken to a wrong camp and has not marched in – thus strength coming in 528 – though check was finished on 529 (trouble tomorrow). Total British troops in camp: 585.

1 June 1942

Reveille at 0645 N time. Breakfast 0730, tea and rice porridge. Called on the camp hospital – good crowd and I arranged to share in arrangements, seeing our patients after theirs, using our own doctors and orderlies and sharing hospital accommodation when required. It is easy to transfer cases, particularly if you say 'dysentery' or 'enteric', but Ns are in a bad temper today and we can not transfer our seven cases. At 0930 hours paraded by N commander Lt Susuki, who called me forth and told me that I must detail Japanese drill and commands to the troops. He and D officers explained commands to me and I detailed them to the troops with frequent interruptions. Then he took over. His strident voice echoed all over the parade ground but the commands as given did not sound anything like the previously spoken or written words and we kept making mistakes, although assisted by signs from N soldiers and D officers.

A touch of humour was then added by his asking those who did not understand the commands to raise the hand. N soldiers looked round and indicated to us right thing to raise the hand (of course, I couldn't as an 'instructor' even though I was equally at sea). A few officers waited with me while the rest were fallen out for further drill. We, of course, waited in great trepidation, expecting to be asked first to exhibit our skill before the rest, but the mass of troops moving covered up the score remaining and we quickly sat down out of the way. Meantime, the rest were given a stiff lesson with much marching about, running and doubling, but only a few fell out *hors-de-combat*.

I was called to see D camp commander in his office (Maj. Doornbos), who was fairly pleasant but impressed me as a rather cold, pompous individual holding his chin more or less in the 'Musso' style. He regretted that we were to be under D admin. and hoped that I would bear with that. I said yes with no great enthusiasm, and intimated that all communications from our troops would come through me, as a hint that the reverse procedure would be appreciated. I assured him that the troops would co-operate and try to appease the Tiger and maintain the *status quo*.

Meals for troops are well organised at fixed hours. Today 0800, 1300, 1800. D camp commander said that there was a 'do' on because now that the soldier who had gone astray had returned we were one soldier over and the commandant was angry. He had directed that British and Australian *Buitenlanders* [foreigners] were to drill two hours a day in N style.

Much ceremonial attends the visits of N officers and inspections, senior officer calling *Kiotské*! [attention!], *Kashira naka* (eyes to officer) – salutes himself and only when salute returned giving *Naoré* (as you were). Outside, one must never be without head gear, since it is an insult to salute without it out of doors; conversely, insult to have one on inside, where you do the *keré* by the N bow and must hold the bow until senior officer following N officers' return of salute gives *Naoré*. Inspecting soldiers and officers pay great attention to cleanliness, particularly cigarette ash trays or tins which must be empty and with some water in the bottom when inspected. Cigarette butts or ash on floor earn a kick or a smack. Floors must be swept clean both in the morning and also for the 2200 round.

Afternoon sees a count-the-heads parade by D at 1530, when we consistently have one missing. This proved to be a rather insolent 'swab', Sgt (Driver) Thomson, who turned out only on my special message and gave cheek, but it seems he has a private arrangement with the Dutch! It took about two weary hours to sort out this tangle and relations are generally strained – I am beginning to hate D guts, also one or two of our own fellows.

As we are not in administrative command, we put out a Routine Instruction No. 1 Concentration Camp No. 4 Tjimahi, to British and Dominion Troops to try to secure co-operation and give advice.

Canteen arrangements are excellent with coffee, bread, fruits, butter, tobacco (native), toothpaste, soap, possibly chocolate and cocoa. All very reasonable. I appointed the following committee to administer the troops common fund: Lt Rintoul (British Army); W/O 2 Allanson AIF; Sgt Haddon AIF; Cpl Clarke RAF.

We formed a mess of our part of 20 officers: 1st contribution 2 gulden all round. I provided Binstead, Ryan and Glowry with funds – 45 gulden.

Thus, for the first time in ages, we had a supper of fresh fruit bananas and oranges, bread and coffee. N inspection at 2200 hours. No trouble.

Troops who have not one blanket or a mosquito net are to be supplied with these. I tried last night to sleep on a straw palliasse given to me by the Dutch, but did not make a go of it, so back to old sleeping bag with excellent results. Bed boards great improvement on a stone floor.

2 June 1942

By arrangement of the D officers, huts each have four orderlies who are excused other duties. They bring food and do some of the cleaning up. These include Butterworth [Pte 'Blue' Butterworth, acquired by me as batman during the evacuation of Greece] who is always good value. Parade at 0900 hours for N commandant, with more N drill and counting of heads. Unfortunately two short, Sgts Harrison-Lucas and Williams, who were typing nominal rolls out of earshot and were not called. They arrived after a long delay and when their excuse was made to commander he let then down lightly with six solid slaps in the face apiece. This was rather a relief, as there is in the compound a barbed wire enclosure where Ns put people, clothed only in trousers, for periods of, say, two days, on half rations. Last two were so burnt up that on removal they were taken straight to hospital.

Two men were executed in this camp for breaking bounds to visit their family (said to be about thirty executed in Tjimahi in all). Method: *single shot*. These two were cleanly executed, but in one case recently four soldiers to execute six – one required 17 shots, first one hitting him in the knee. After several shots he asked for water. He is an Ambonese and the natives now regard his grave with reverence, making pilgrimages to it.

Drill is a frightful affair, troops being pushed about all over the place, here there and everywhere. D still administering us by barracks and I quite believe that is more their own idea than that of the Ns. They continue to make direct approach to the troops in everything and their orders refer to the *Buitenlanders*. Afternoon free for sport which is at present ill organised.

N sentries inspected at 2200 and said we must be in bed. We had hoped officers might be allowed 2400, but did not feel like arguing the toss. Ns at present do not permit our medical officers or Dutch officers to work officially. Dental work is especially urgent, since troops have had not dental attention for ages. 'Unofficial' work is going on. It is still not permitted to transfer the sick to hospital.

3 June 1942

Conditions now fairly tolerable – continual rumours of further troops coming to camp. British and Australian sick transferred to hospital.

Two-hour session of N drill this morning with troops divided into batches of 50. This they carried out very well. D officers etc. acting as advisers. I believe Ns were favourably impressed by inspection of our quarters. There is a 1630 session of P.T. given by a D instructor – very tough, advanced stuff, but good if you can take it. Also some shot putting and field games if interested. Football is played each day with little skill. A request has been made for a rugger ball. Mike Visse calls in frequently and is a very pleasant fellow. He seems to be able to 'manage' the Nips. A friendly D officer took me round today to show me the 'theatre' etc. This is the gymnasium, and an excellent stage with spotlights, microphone etc. has been produced by the D.K.K.K. (*kale koppen kampement*), an enthusiastic company. D have a room where they do fine arts – some elegant calendars, playing cards etc. being beautifully painted. Junior officers fairly friendly.

4 June 1942

Fine and warm. Surrounding hills rise up steeply, with their tops nosing into the clouds, and some beautiful trees can be seen. Ns are pleased with us and accordingly state that if we go on improving we are to be given the 'privilege' of going out on *corvée* (fatigue parties), also to wear the N white cloth insignia of rank. Doctors and dentists now allowed to work. Sentries do not worry us very much. Night inspection, no cards after 2200 (we are warned not to play for money). That's not hard, with so scarce a commodity.

D soldier who has been 'out' since the capitulation gave himself up today. Wife went to *Kebetei* and begged for his life. Surprising result: given only two days in our cage, and when Mike Visse rang up and told them it was too cold at night he was taken out, pretending to be on the point of collapse, teeth chattering etc.

Maj. Morris attended a conference of sport, dramatic bodies etc. and arranged committees for recreation purposes. We are to continue with D in such activities.

5 June 1942

'Big do' of drill today, Lt Susuki in attendance. He is a rather taller than average N, very regimental, and looks as though poured into his clothes of very smart tropical drill. Much instruction in the 'parade step' – the goose step used in saluting – commands when on the march '*hotiotaré*', '*kashira migi*' etc., *naoré*, then '*hotiojamée*' (back to original). Demonstration finish by Nippon NCO then by a squad of D soldiers. Then our troops drilled by D officers and I must say they performed very well indeed, pleasing the lieutenant a lot. The things we do for Nippon!

The news is all odds and ends at present and nothing seems reliable. Samples of rumours today: three submarines got into Sydney harbour and were sunk; five landings in Australia met with disaster (100,000 N prisoners)! Rumours of bombings here and there. We still hear of the old legend of Java conquered for the duration of the rice crop or 100 days, but in general there is far less blatant optimism here, and the feeling is that it will at least be many months. Optimistic think perhaps of being out for Christmas.

Language classes will soon begin again. An impossible mountebank who claims to be a famous sergeant pilot, is again in trouble – today definitely identified as having sold a stolen watch. Propose now to court martial him.

6 June 1942

Fine clear day. Saturday – all hands out to wash and sun their floor boards which are fairly freely bug-ridden. No drill.

N commander Lt Susuki round inspecting in afternoon. Arrival of a party of

British and Australian troops from Sukabumi by train. Officers include Lt-Col. van der Post (British Army), Wing Commander Nichols RAF, Majors Woods and Wearne AIF and a remnant of about 70 of the missing Pioneer Battalion. They consist largely of parties who went bush and were ultimately rounded up by Ns. Laurens van der Post is the most impressive character. South African in origin, he speaks English, French, Dutch, German, Russian and Malayan, some Japanese and numerous African languages. He is an 'intelligence wallah' and is not in his usual costume piece.*

His guerilla party was well equipped and organised in an inaccessible spot and are still 'out', but he himself was caught in an unguarded moment without weapons. He has acted as doctor and father confessor to his lads and knows them all intimately. Wearne is, of course, sterling value, but Nichols is 'nervy' and a bit jumpy.† This party have been fairly well fed but rather badly handled and slapped about. They are all well grounded in N drill and can even number in Nip. Many have begun lessons in the language and understand N characters with some ability at writing. Their outside information dovetails fairly well with ours, but is not as recent.

Discipline: our RAF *bête noire*, was charged under section 40 'Conduct Prejudicial' and given one week solitary, but when referred to D commander, no room was available. He thinks Ns would find out and cut off his head or hand, so we have to be content with enforcing daily fatigues *ad infinitum*.

I have, of course, at once notified van der Post and Nichols that one of them must become camp commander as senior combatant officers.

7 June 1942

One hour's drill in the morning, which was not a good show. Church parades were attended. Sport in afternoon included baseball. Dutch P.T. instructor who is 440, 800 and mile champion of Java, gave some instruction in running followed by strenuous session of P.T. Wet weather now in afternoon and we are mystified to hear that the wet season has now begun in Tjimahi (it is just finishing in Bandoeng!). New British and Australian inhabitants of camp are fairly uniformly equipped with two pairs of shorts and shirts each, D native hats and boots. All possessions were collected except the clothes they had on and they were then re-issued in a haphazard way to the above standard. *All money* was confiscated by Ns so they are in a poor way for canteen purchases.

D inform us of *corvée* duties for us tomorrow.

* The following information was given to me by Ingaret Gifford, Laurens van der Post's wife, in September 1979. Many years before in South Africa, Laurens had befriended two Japanese visitors who had been ejected from a 'white' hotel or eating house. He made them his personal guests and cared for them. Later they invited him to Japan. He learnt Japanese and delved deeply into the literature and legends of Japan.

As the guerilla leader, he went personally to negotiate with the Kampong leaders about food supplies. Highly armed Japanese soldiers in ambush dropped out of trees and surrounded him with bayonets poised for the kill. He said calmly in elequent Japanese, 'Pause an honorable moment gentlemen'! Surprised, they hesitated, and after talks his life was spared for further investigation.

† I subsequently found that Nichols' diffident style cloaked a dedicated, brave and virtuous officer.

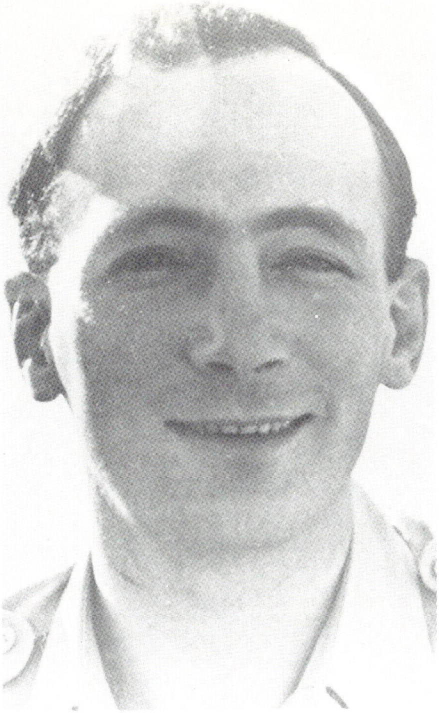

1 The author in the western desert, Middle East, 1940

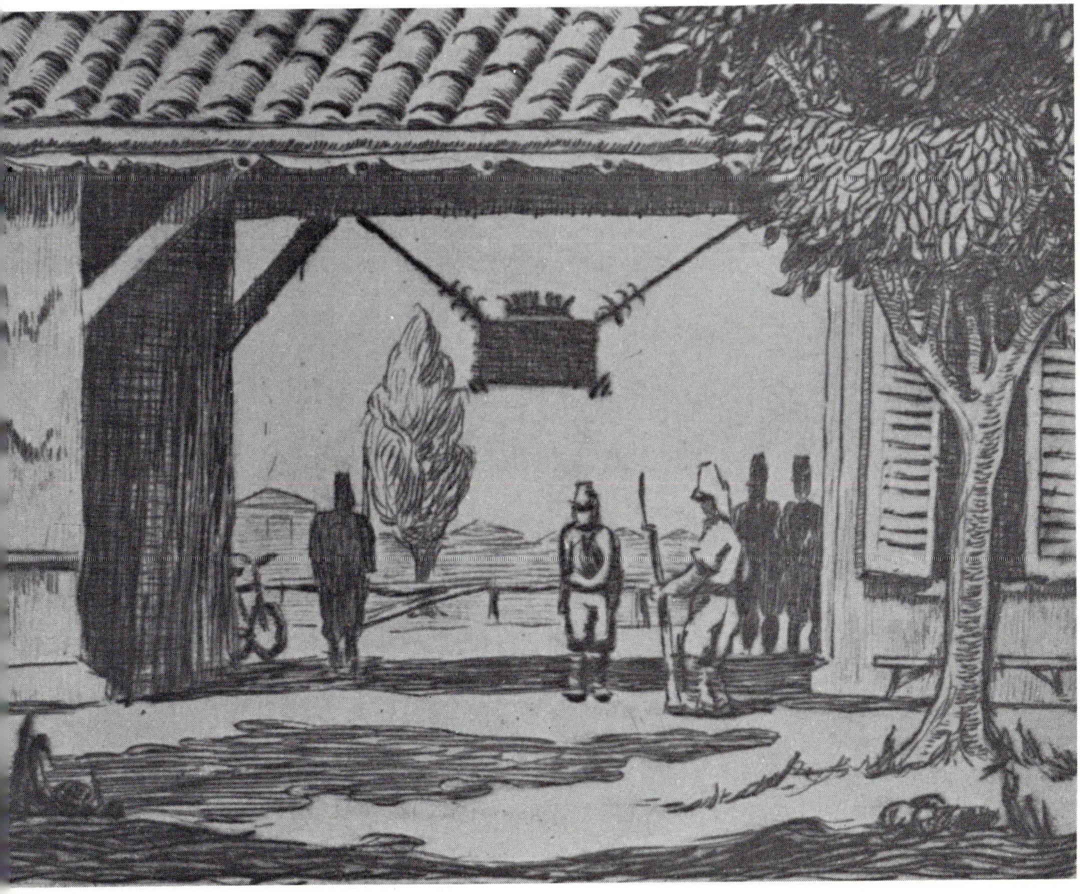

: gates, Bandoeng POW Camp (*Ray Parkin*)

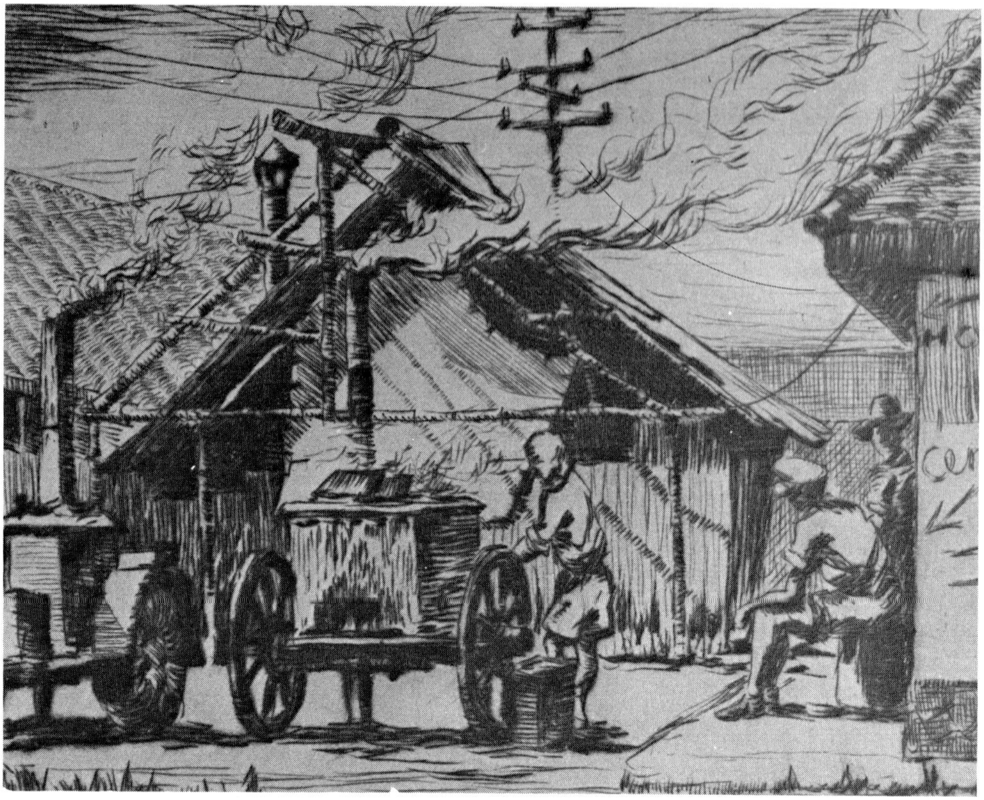

3 Hot water service, Bandoeng (*Ray Parkin*)

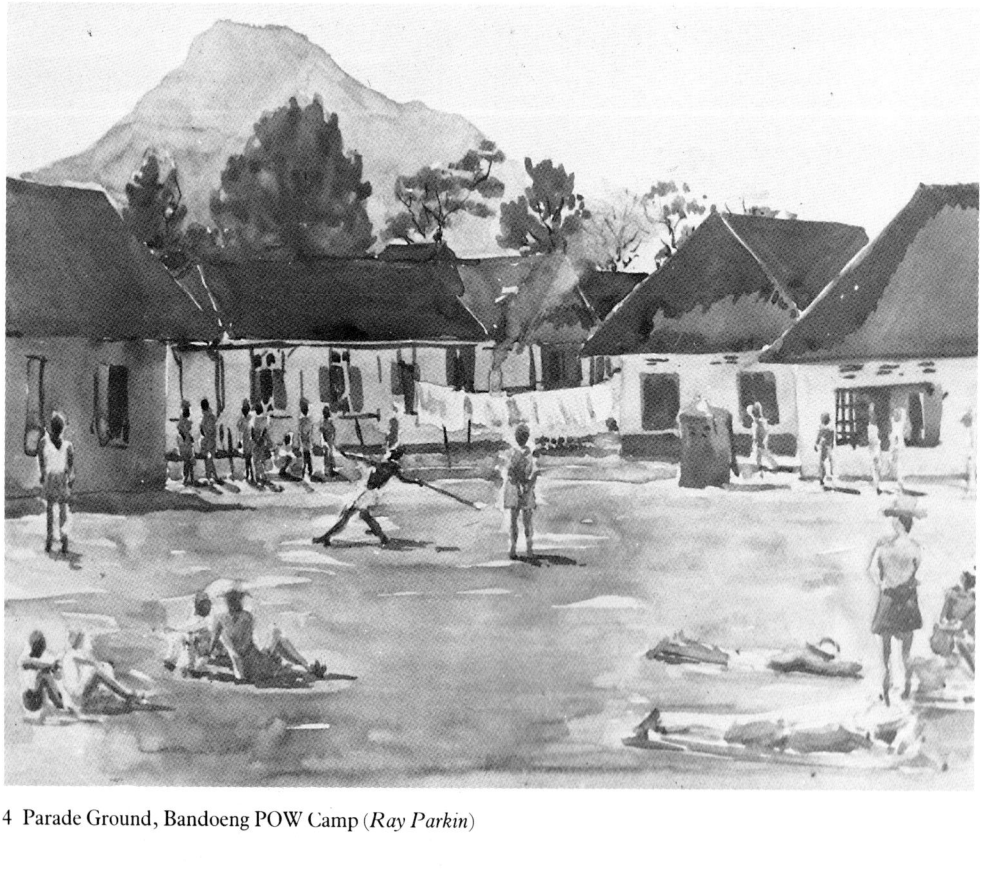

4 Parade Ground, Bandoeng POW Camp (*Ray Parkin*)

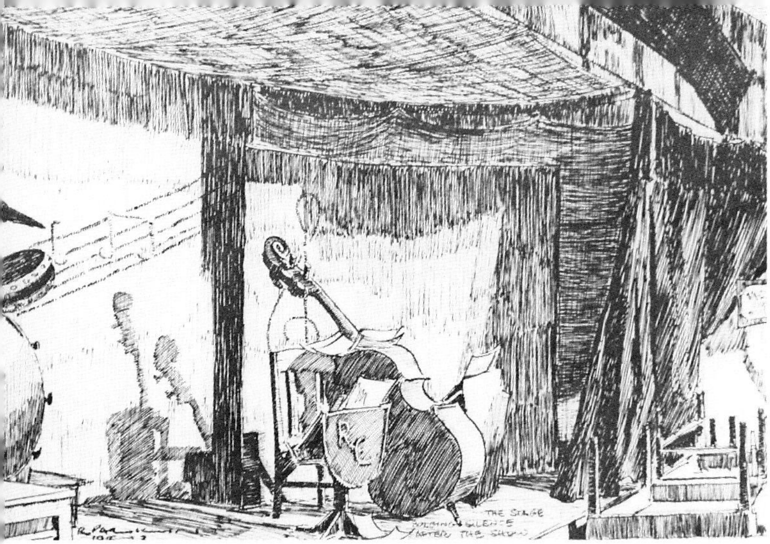

5 The stage in Radio City – a converted gymnasium for entertainment (Ray Parkin)

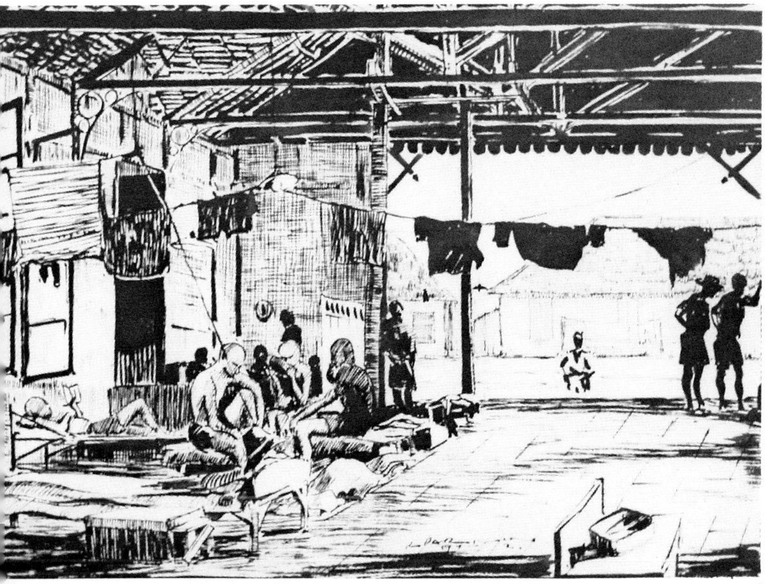

6 Australian barracks, near cookhouse, Bandoeng (*Ray Parkin*)

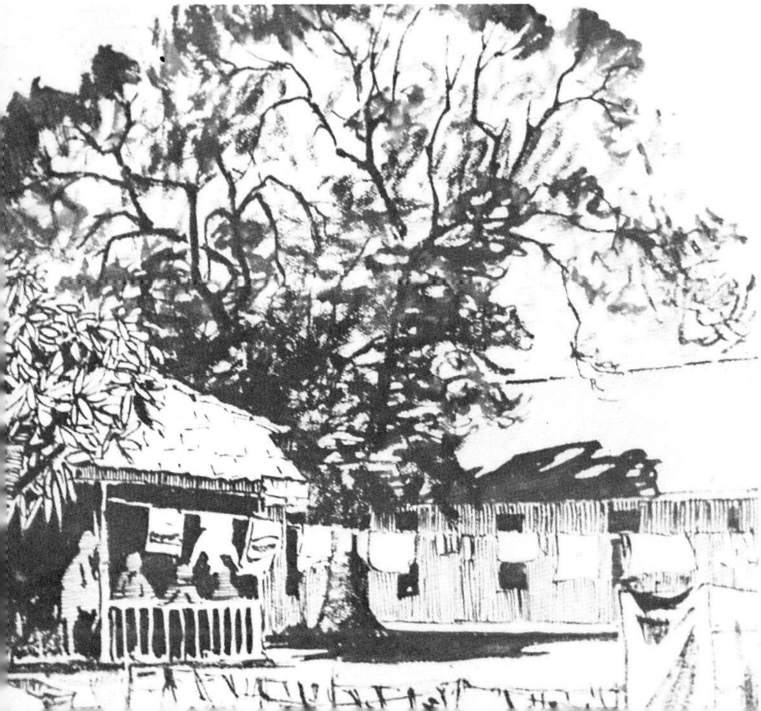

7 Barrack, officers' area, Bandoeng (*Ray Parkin*)

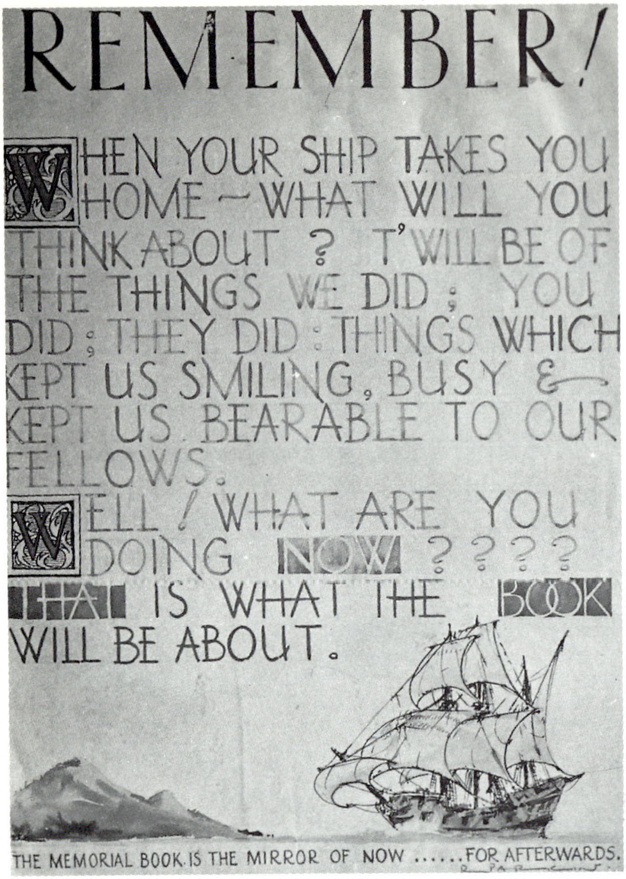

8 Poster exhorting contributions, Memorial Book, Bandoeng (*Ray Parkin*)

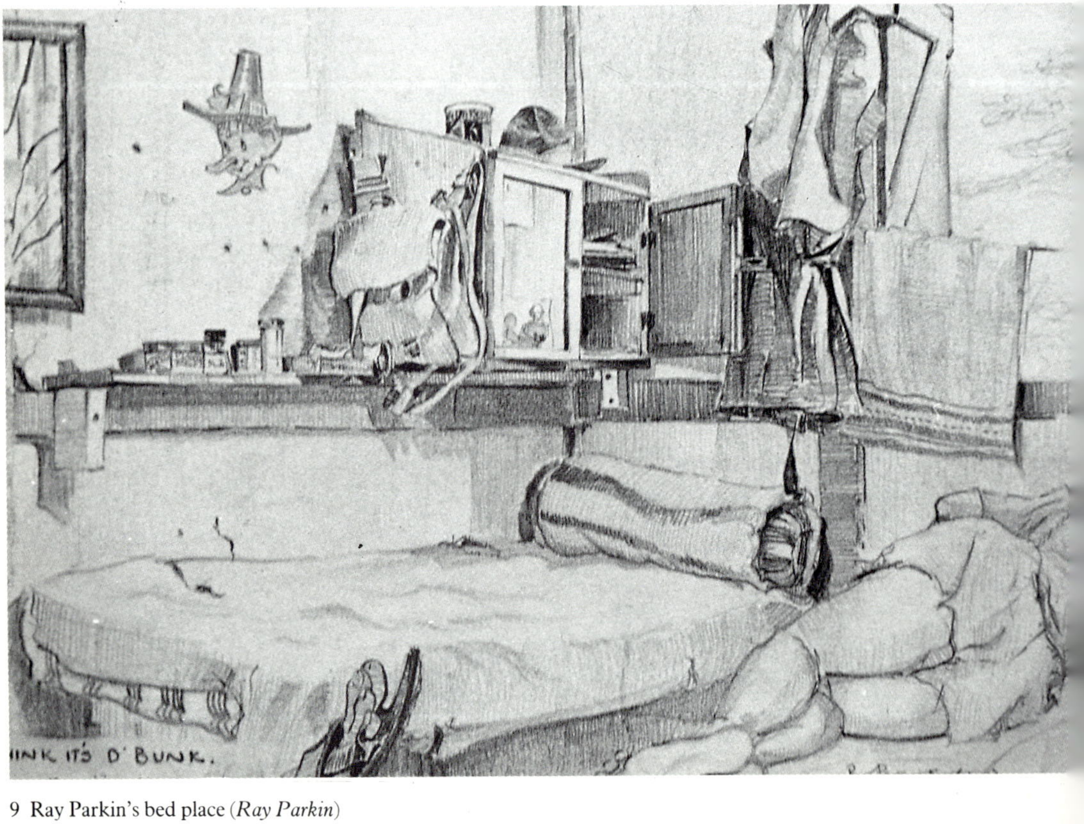

9 Ray Parkin's bed place (*Ray Parkin*)

8 June 1942

Conference with Lt-Col. van der Post and Wing Commander Nichols who, for confidential reasons advanced, requested me to carry on with the command of British troops. This anomalous position I accepted under protest. Don't care a hang about the Ns or 'the responsibility', but think that is is not correct army procedure.

Large sick parades. Men out on *corvée* duty all day reported that this was very pleasant and they were able to engage in pleasant conversation with Dutch (ladies for most part), also to make purchases.

D up to their usual finicky nonsense. The big bad wolf (IJA) has said that we are to have nothing to do with the treatment of the sick and are getting two doctors in from outside, yet we 'assist' with sick parades, do the VD clinic and carry out dental work. Told Maj. Moon to declare a 'sit down strike' of all hands. Lt-Col. van der Post reports conversation with the jolly old D majors who report their discomfort that with many more D troops arriving, Ns will of course want the British to give up their bed boards!

9 June 1942

Absence of our doctors from the sick parade and the sight of about 150 men caused a prompt change in the interpretation of the N commands and once more we treat our sick. There is sufficient space for plenty of outside exercise and the troops are relishing the change. Soccer is the most popular and cricket has a keen following. The P.T. class grows. Lt S. has decreed that all spare ground round the camp is to be converted to vegetable gardens, also the slit trenches are to be filled in, although we have a big ammunition dump 150 yards away. Tokyo is said to have broadcast warnings to Java of possible air raids, but all air raid shelters were long ago removed by order.

Lectures have not begun as yet and contract bridge is popular. Troops do not carry out N drill with any particular enthusiasm unless Lt S. is about. Majors Wood and Wearne introduce a note of enthusiasm with doubling and 'O'Grady says' (keen fellows). Morris remains my adjutant.

10 June 1942

Corvée duty again, carried out locally. Some of the troops obliged to move ammunition about and are not particularly pleased. D are having an exhibition of work of the 'playing cards factory'. Some of the calendars are quite delicate little works of art, and many of these works exhibit considerable artistic skill and feeling. Amongst the games is one new invention whereby 'counters' are moved about a barbed wire maze. Money raised goes to camp benefits (all proceeds of the exhibition etc.). Another money raiser is by lottery – articles submitted by soldiers first valued by a 'commission', then allowed to sell tickets up to the value. Five per cent of proceeds go to camp funds. Cooking and food remain fairly good. At present it is possible to obtain occasional fresh bread, fruit, peanut butter and jam through ordinary camp sources.

11 June 1942

Morning drill one hour – rather slovenly. Inspection by Lt S. in afternoon – he appears to be very interested in the garden. Saluting outside I find is made by all coming to the *keré* – not *kashira naka*, which is a parade ground affair.

Afternoon quite astonished to find 71 personnel arriving from 1 Allied General Hospital who were tipped out with three hours' notice, which of course gave no reasonable time to 'hand over' patients or to collect useful medical kit. Number arriving included all seven officers, Alan Gibson, Ambrose Etherington and many CCS personnel, most of whom are fairly well. Only one patient had been lost and not from the originals, most of whom are doing very well.

The move from Allied General Hospital might have been worse and, for a time, purchasing and canteen arrangements were possible. These came to an end with a concert permitted by local commander but unfortunately the 'hall' jutted out near a public thoroughfare and a passing N officer, allegedly rather bibulous, conceived the whole thing one great insult to Ns – maintained he heard insults to the Axis in three languages! He stormed through or over two barbed wire barricades and burst upon the scene, dissolving all in confusion. A reign of slapping and kicking followed, several being imprisoned. In an effort to get all on parade, patients were slapped and pummelled from their beds and some collapsed on the way.

Reg Withers was imprisoned for a time and N soldier cheered him up by sharpening a sword suggestively. The hospital had wireless access but news not as good as we had been led to believe: Timor has not fallen, according to this source, nor has there been any land fighting about these parts. Talk in the Melbourne press of Macarthur being ready for his push in two months' time. From all sides news of a sea battle, near Wake and Midway! With heavy N losses: 16 ships including 2 small aircraft carriers, 2 battleships. Russia: all goes well. More fighting in the desert west of Tobruk. Amusing theory in the camp that Lt S.'s ill humour is due to the loss of two brothers in the Midway battle.

Dutch cabaret an excellent show. Maj. Moon and I were unfortunately late through receiving incoming troops. Several excellent sketches in Dutch and music provided by mouth organs and violins. Vocal items included '*J'attendrai*' with mouth organ and violin accompaniment. (This made me think painfully of Beirut, and of dancing in that magic moonlight on the roof of the Gaza Club. Sentimental...)

12 June 1942

Early morning arrival of Capt. Alting van Geausau, adjutant to the modern Caesar. The latter mounted the dais last night and made the newly-arrived British troops treat him to N drill and *kashira naka* etc. Capt. Alting van Geausau now requested new arrivals to move in with the other officers into the same three rooms to make space for expected arrivals. Show down! I went up in smoke with the following contentions: that there was plenty of time to move when the necessity should arise; that D officers had made no such move and were very comfortable, thank you; that where N administered directly, British officers had never been particularly crowded or forced to live with ORs.

Could I please receive any definite assurance that the Ns had ordered such a move? *Specifically*. And by the term *Buitenlander*, did he refer to British, Australian and American army soldiers? I then followed hotfoot to Maj. de Vries with Lt Col. Van der Post and Wing Commander Nichols. Former poured marvellous gutteral oil on the troubled waters. Maj. de Vries said no such order was given concerning the officers.

Later, commander came to my quarters with Maj. de Vries and discussed the whole question, denying that he had given the order and seemingly quite friendly: Van der Post is an ideal go-between, very fluent in the Dutch language.

N search of the incomers yesterday was much more looting than a search and was carried out by private soldiers with no officer. A kit bag was confiscated and filled with desirable articles of food, writing cases, trinkets etc., even private photos. Overcoats, torches, cameras, and the usual items all taken. Today I asked commander to request return of greatcoats and personal items.

At the N inspection this morning they noticed some soldiers had more than one blanket; these extra blankets ordered to be handled in.

13 June 1942

In the course of conversation between the WO and D commandant and the interpreter, Mike Visse, it now appears that all troops are being concentrated by nationality into different areas.

The problem of two old Portuguese African sailors who came with the troops from Sukabumi is most interesting. These were employed on an Axis ship (Hungarian *Nyuugat*) which was seized in Batavia earlier in the war, and these two old 'coloured gentlemen' found themselves in a Dutch concentration camp. When, however, the Ns took the island, the Ns – seemingly a bit careless of the interests of 'neutrals' – imprisoned them along with British and Australian troops. On one occasion they were released but rounded up by *Kempis* and subjected to the water torture. They made their protests, saying always that they were 'non combatant gentlemen' but these do not seem to have reached their consular representative (if such still exists). The Ns still seem to regard them as in the British ambit. Can this be because Portugal is our oldest ally? Curiously enough, too, the part of Africa they name is a Spanish possession (San Vincente Cape Verde). They are nicely spoken, white-haired, old Uncle Tom's Cabin negroes. Our faithful Stephen Xavier spends much time in conversation with them (he is half Portuguese, half Chinese). Anyway, in the course of further conversation, it transpired that all British and Australian troops were to move tomorrow to Bandoeng! This just incidental. I made hurried mention of the sick and lame and requested at least twenty carts for the movement. These surprisingly look like being forthcoming. Later in the day, by consultation with Major Moon and phoning to the Ns, it was agreed that 67 of our sick troops (including 32 in hospital) would be taken by lorry. This is a fair provision.

D are alarmed by the proposition of many more troops coming to Tjimahi Camp, but are playing up splendidly with us and laying on food in a big way. In the morning arrangements are: reveille 0530, carts to be loaded by 0600, breakfast 0630 and extra food (rice) for the troops. On parade 0730. Camp to be cleaned up. A mixed concert was hurried on '*kale Koppen Kampament*' – Major Doornbos and Major de Vries and other Dutch officers attending with me. The singing was good and several amusing sketches were put on, including A/C Bell as a super bad villain in *The Maid of Freetown*. At the interval a D barrack commander made a speech in which he said that all canteen food available was to be turned over to us and a collection was being made for those with 'no dough'. I thanked the Dutch for this fine gesture and for the excellent way they had received us and looked after us in the camp. The subscriptions actually reached 67 gulden and a good deal of food and cigarettes was also donated. I also thanked the administrative officers of the camp. Maj. Doornbos replied with a charming and friendly letter (all rather emotional).

Maj. de Vries and Maj. Doornbos with some other D officers gave a little farewell supper to me, Lt-col van der Post, Wing Commander Nichols and Maj. Moon. Most excellent mock turtle soup, bread and onions, real butter and some tinned fruit. Lt Col van der Post proposed a toast to our comrades (once) in arms.

3 Bandoeng

June 1942

14 June 1942

The move – 0530 reveille – stone dark until 0730. Everything worked to the schedule and troops paraded satisfactorily at 0800 when Lt Susuki arrived to receive a crashing '*kashiri migi*' Then the counting of heads went merrily on.

The two old Portuguese were commanded to fall in with Dominion and US 'odds and sods' and to march. Their luggage (rather expensive suitcases etc.) placed on our handcarts. Poor old boys – over 60, one with varicose ulcers on shin and not their bloody war, anyway.

Marched off at 0845, moving off on a 'back road' near Tjimahi.

A misty morning ideal for marching, country looking lovely with mists bathing the mountains, clumps of jungle, palms and paddy fields, some gorgeous big green trees with great red blossoms recalling England's unforgettable horse chestnuts. A much larger number of escorts than usual frisked about on bicycles with fixed bayonets and rifles loaded in a business-like way. Guards, however, not behaving badly.

Carts were right in the rear. Twenty in number: ten for English, ten Australian with 50 men to each party. Maj. Clarke in charge, pulling one cart with 'Fred' and Tom and Ian Cameron amongst the five officers concerned. We moved in a sort of semi-circle about Tjimahi, moving eventually along a road to Tjimahi a little way and, after marching until 1030 hours, were still very near to the barracks we had left.

A halt was then called and some 5000 Indo-European troops passed us (Eurasians with a sprinkling of whites, since apparently the Ns regard D born in the country in this group). These were carrying the most strangely assorted goods and chattels and tugging grossly overloaded carts. They were straggling and staggering and sweating and looked the picture of broken men. Hardly a chin lifted off the chest and a sort of dull hopelessness pervading all. Physique dreadful too – one got the impression they were half starved and yet they said food was fair enough. One of the bright boys in the English column grunted at them in the N way and promptly received a crashing smack on the head from a sentry's rifle, and I was very surprised that he did not go 'out' to it. I suppose that was asking for it.

During this rest we had our lunch and no further activity until 1255 when Lt 'Bushy Whiskers', the rather cheery little adjutant from the Kebetai, arrived and began the counting, running along the 4s and putting out each tenth man as marker. He recognised me cheerfully and seemed pleased with my grasp of N drill (remember he gave me my first lesson at the *kebetei*). A little while later the guards arrived on bicycles from Bandoeng to take over from the Tjimahi guards. Many of these I recognised.

The march moved off at 1320, still in sight of the barracks we had left, with Ambonese and Menadonese troops in front who set quite a cracking pace since, of course, we had much heavier kit for the most part. We marched steadily for over two and a half hours without a stop until we arrived at the XV Bn barracks, right against the *kebetei*.

All the way the streets were completely cleared of people back for at least fifty yards from the road and almost lined by N soldiers with fixed bayonets. Bandoeng has become dreary, dirty and ill kept, with scarcely any Europeans in sight. Even the fine houses lining the streets of the European quarters looked deserted and locked up. One could see no one looking out of the windows or doors. What a difference from the riotous scenes of previous marches! The troops moved in a good order and I personally felt strong as a horse (PT and better food), shoulders much harder so that the pack caused little worry. Some of the Ns tried marching with us, but made frequent changes to bicycles and wry gestures as to their short legs. New innovation: one guard had an automatic weapon which looked like N equivalent of Bren gun.

Arrived in barracks. 'Bushy Whiskers' already there and *kebetei* chief seated idly in a chair puffing a cigarette. Counting began again but no search. Maj. Moon and lorried sick had already arrived and he had been over the allotment of accommodation with D commandant Major Link of Camp No. 11, our new neighbours. He was very friendly, going to some pain to help our move in.

No N drill in this camp and things said to be rather slack. The whole place is filthy dirty. Only annoying incident was Dutch ORs causing a stampede by handing out buns to some troops in rear. When parade was dismissed, the move into quarters was quite rapid and fairly smooth. I, along with Wing Commander Nichols, am to have a little 'flat': two rooms plus a 'bath room'! (Bathroom, however, a dirty little annex with a lavatory pan with flushing system – not working – and a tap in the wall leading to a petrol drum. Water said only to run early in the morning, in any case.) No bed boards – back to the tiled floor, but one is used to that. Rumours of a further move in two to three days.

Rice laid on for troops so everyone happy enough. Ambonese and Menadonese are in the same barrack area and were dismissed first. But there are also a number of D troops. These go out on working parties and are allowed to buy freely, but are searched carefully for notes (this is now said to be a shooting matter). Message received in evening from *kebetei* demanding Commander British troops and adjutant for orders. Wing Commander Nichols rather dubious whether I should go – after all, should he, as senior officer, leave this to a medical officer? My reply, of course, is, 'That is for you to decide. I am very willing to withdraw in your favour'. Van der Post, however, with tactful remarks, called a truce until the conference tomorrow morning and off I went. Damn all required of us; just told that adjutant must attend at 0900 hours and 2130 hours and CO at 1800 hours as in the previous régime.

15 June 1942

Morning conference with Wing Commander Nichols and van der Post who contrived last night to talk 'Nick' into a submissive frame of mind – latter stressed he did not want to assume job of camp commander, but felt he would be shirking his duties as senior officer and not fair to me. Van der Post is a natural leader and diplomat, very persuasive with both D and Ns. I wish he could take over the job.

Administrative parade at 1100; addressed the troops about the camp routine with special mention of hygiene and cleanliness, sick parades, roll call parades and mess parades, daily administrative parades (at which everyone is required *to dress and behave like soldiers*); recreation organisation, saluting Nippon soldiers (order of *kebetei*) and avoidance of noise after lights out, which must be observed (2200 ORs, 2400 for officers). Importance of discipline and duty was stressed, also of remembering that they were still British soldiers. The posting of officers for this parade was accompanied by a rather nasty little demonstration at the back of the parade, clapping of hands and a few remarks to which Major Morris naturally replied with a few stern words. As usual a few specimens attribute all troubles to the officers, who are no doubt responsible for it all!

New camp administration is now worked out. Wing Commander Nichols to take over British troops with Sqn Ldr Cummings as 2I/C plus several barrack commanders who will do roll call parades etc., W/O Axell as company sergeant major. AIF Details under Maj. W.W. Wearne, 2I/C Maj. Woods, W/O Allanson and barrack officers. Camp commandant and adjutant, Dunlop and Morris. W/O Ellis to replace Dave Topping as RSM as a further concession to British troops on camp administration. All purchasing of food, whether from common fund or by individuals, now to be handled by Lt Rintoul and his committee. They will make a profit on individual purchases to go to the common fund, and also decide what to purchase. Ian Cameron is thus relieved of a good deal of worry; he has had a thin time attending all meal parades for weeks and just being a target for abuse. Orders of the *kebetei* are a repetition of previous ones, really, with some additions:

1 If any one escapes, whole camp to be wiped out from above down. Special mention of COs and adjutants!
2 Passing of notes – much the same as above. There must be no communication with the outside world.
3 Troops must not gather in groups anywhere (on special request can do so for games or concerts).
4 Special areas must be set aside for smoking and ash trays provided.
5 No naked bodies, though troops may take off shirts if working or for sunbathing. Must not walk about naked.

Two cycles, two typewriters, and armbands for CO and adjutant automatically issued. (Purchasing of food seems to be now freely permitted to D, at any rate, and working parties are allowed to purchase.) Much stress of death to CO (me), but all very friendly with much laughing. I, of course, laughing more like a man with a brick dropped on the toe.

Stir at No. 2 camp where a man said to be missing, so if not found tomorrow

CO and adjutant to be shot! (At present moment we, too, are *two* men light and are trying very hard to account for them by the morning roll call. What cheer!) Lt 'Bushy Whiskers' remembers me a little too well I fear, knows my name, and talks of giving me a photo of myself at the *kebetei*.

16 June 1942

(Said to be approximate ration of camp at present N sources: Lt Stoeffel)

Potatoes or Rice	500 g
Sugar	20 g
Meat	50 g
Flour	± 22 kg a day for 500 men
No butter	
No coffee	
No tea	– but D have some in store
Vegetables	± 25 kg for 200 men
Salt	5 g
Coconut oil	5 g

Capt. Moraki: *kebetei*; Lt Matsuda: adjutant. Conversation this morning between Maj. Morris and Matsuda, who said some interesting things about execution of whole camp as punishment for escaping. 'It is all very well for some ass on a desk at Div. HQ to order these things but if we try to kill the whole camp we get killed too! We believe that COs will realise it is not possible to escape and therefore will not help escapees; but they will be expected to find out who assisted and all concerned will be shot. Of course, the escapee too.' Stationery request of Ns promptly supplied.

Numbers:

Dutch:	1360
English and Australian:	846
Ambonese:	365
Menadonese:	761
Chinese:	46
Malay:	2
Total:	3380 and 150 officers across the board

Ambonese and Menadonese have two kitchens, Dutch have three. As usual, we are the unfortunates with one only. Lt Kroesan is in charge of D kitchens. D soldiers man the *corvées* which go out for food – rice, meat, flour, vegetables. In addition, coffee – one or two items are to be sold by *kebetei* and there is a racket whereby a party goes out each day to buy milk, cheese, ham, butter, bread etc. which is then sold back to troops. N soldiers accompany the party and it is an unofficial but sanctioned affair. Mr Hannenie, Mr Johansen and a small party of old *Landstormers* who have plenty of money in this way live merrily, getting meat, wine etc., and include in their armaments an excellent frigidaire, hot plates, electric kettles etc. We call them 'the smugglers' and they have actually managed to introduce bribery.

Purchase System: Goods said to be distributed on a *per capita* basis and all troops share in the profits, e.g. milk distributed to a camp commander at cost price 22c a litre, commander takes 1c for a camp maintenance scheme, brooms etc. and milk is then sold at 26c; rest of profits go to troops' common fund. This sounds all right, but actually the camp is one great racket, supplies (which obviously come from N sources), such as flour, being retailed back to our troops. No bread supplied to our troops but many D 'firms' offer pancakes at 15c each. Also, no wood for our kitchen purposes, yet all over the place private coffee stalls retailing a cup with sugar and so forth at, say, 5c; also numerous sources of hot water. Anyway, commander says that Ian Cameron will attend arrival of all supplies and see that distribution is fair. Lt Stoffel and Lt Driessen are in charge of Quartermaster's store. Lt Fey, who has lived 23 years in Japan, is camp interpreter. He must have some ability to handle Ns because he still wears long hair. Mr Kamerling (a broker) acts as English interpreter, but he is hardly necessary with a fellow like van der Post about. He manages the D with the greatest of ease and gets all sorts of things out of them.

The camp is very dirty and the latrines and showers are a nightmare, shared with the Dutch, Ambonese and Menadonese who slop their clothes around in the showers (taps three feet from the ground). Two British soldiers (Cpl Smith RAF and L/Bdr Pullin) who have been with D for a long time, today requested transfer to our force.

Ns mentioned that our efforts to clean up the camp had been noticed.

Administration: Now a clear-out English group under Wing Commander Nichols and an Australian group under Maj. Wearne. Camp HQ staff: myself, Maj. Morris adjutant and W/O Ellis (3rd Hussars). Administrative parade is very formal at 0930 hours, followed by sick parade. Each group parades separately and has their own orderly room. Roll call parades are at 0730 and at 0530 before breakfast and tea respectively. Troops are to be warned not to go about bare-footed – hookworm etc. rampant!

This incoming party now have long hair and seem to effect beards. They have not been badly treated at Tjilatchap, except for usual slapping down. They have felt the heat and malaria and dysentry. (Incidentally, van der Post and W. Wearne are both suffering malarial recurrence.) The party were tucked away quickly and we managed a good big hot meal for all concerned, with coffee for the officers. All were glad to see English faces.

17 June 1942

Many rumours of D movement. Called to *kebetei* at 1000 and notified that approximately 120 British troops arriving at around 1800 hours. Must prepare quarters and food. This makes us terribly crowded and the kitchen arrangements almost impossible, but Dutch said to be leaving any day now. Our old *Landstormer* friends, 'the smugglers', have thrown several rather good parties, including one with red madeira. Soccer is all the go. We have damn all in the way of furniture but commander No. 10 camp has given us a chair and a table or two. Ns appear friendly.

Party from Tjilatchap arrived in dark approximately 2000. Total: 139, made up of 23 English officers and 99 ORs plus 19 Australians (2 officers, RAAN; 15 ORs RAAN, and 7 ORs, RAAF, Sqn Ldr Harrison (RAF) in charge, all their property on their backs as they came by train. RAN survivors are from HMAS *Perth*. Many of this party were the survivors of two train loads who got into trouble about Tjilatchap. Sqn Ldr Harrison's train was heavily ambushed and shot up, a lot of petrol wagons on the back catching fire. Of the two train loads (at least 600), less than 100 are accounted for. One unpleasant story of a party of Ns headed by an NCO falling upon 23 wounded and exhausted men in a carriage with bayonets. Only two known to escape – one who crawled out and hid in the garden during the melée and another, already severely wounded in the leg, who received two bayonet wounds in the chest causing haemothorax. He was covered by two other bayonetted men and left for dead but later crawled into fields where he was found by a native who put a halter over his head and began tugging him along. He called weakly to a passing car and a N officer took pity on him and drew his sword on his escort. He made a recovery.

18 June 1942

D know they are going tomorrow by train, probably to Tjilatchap, and can only take what they can carry on the back, so there is a great desire to trade with the whole camp. Our fellows hanging off since they know the stuff will be left anyway. I saw Commander Linck this morning and requested that his kitchen supply 300 of our men at present. Request for separate latrine and showers thought not possible (lack of control, I guess). He had nice proposition to put forward. His own accumulated stores from ordnance issue (rice, potatoes, sugar, oil, margarine, flour, salt, tinned foods etc.) offered to us for *sale* with the preliminary warning that if we did not buy, he would feel it his duty to *give* the stores first to his own troops, next the Ambonese and Menadonese, *lastly* to us. Regrets of course but must do the best for his troops! (Kamerling, his interpreter, said *sotto voce* he had never had any benefit from the stores and thought it rather a poor show.) He would not even state a price but asked us to say what we would pay; the same proposition put up to Ambonese and Menadonese. Eventually, we raked up about 150 gulden and gave a promise on the British and Australian governments for the additional 150 gulden required. Smiling 'Van' was able to get sum of 150 gulden for the troops' fund by giving a promise on behalf of British and Australian governments which he and I signed cheerily. (This sum, by the way, from the rich but good old 'smugglers' who, incidentally, think the N soldiers are not bad little chaps at all. Ft/Lt McSweeney has 350 gulden of the Imprest fund of the hospital with him and has handed over 150 gulden for the Tjimahi Hospital troops and Sqn Ldr Harrison 100 gulden for the group fromTjilatchap. So the fund is not doing badly.

Ns have warned us our troops must keep in the area, but Ambonese and Menadonese come freely into our lines to latrines, showers etc. Back road, however; is being closed by barbed wire. Maj. Moon, 'the Doctor', is allowed to go to the hospital in this back area and even has a special armband. Ns say people crossing the area will be shot but the doctor will not be shot!

Farewell to our new friends, particularly the old 'smugglers', who told Van the whole plan and lay-out of their illegal activities (ice cream and milk best bribe for guard apparently and note passing the thing which brings trouble e.g. case of of one of their number who consented to bring in a cake of soap for a soldier. This Ns looked at carefully and it contained three letters. Hence he was beaten up and put in the 'chicken coop' without clothes.

Smith and Pullin, the two British soldiers, were formally transferred to me by *kebetei* and they expressed disappointment at having to return to fellow British soldiers as they preferred the Australians. Details given to Van and I concerning certain dumps [ammunition, weapons etc.]. 5 + 124; 1 gross; O.P. ++* Preparations were made to piquet all Q stores, offices, barracks etc. in the morning at 0530 hours in view of departure of Dutch, to try and insure furniture etc. used to best purpose. Our own troops and Ambonese and Menadonese will all be on the job like tigers.

19 June 1942

Rose at 0600 N Time. Pitch dark. Find party of Dutch about to move out and farewell Maj. Linck. All key points guarded by our best NCOs but 'pillage' is rampant. D leaving quarters like pigsties, too. Next party leaving at 1000. Lt Matsuda supervising. I told him of our overcrowding and asked if we might use some of the barracks after cleaning them up. He inspected one or two of our barracks in a rather friendly way but said wait until tomorrow. In the evening I was informed that by tomorrow I must devise a scheme for the complete division of the camp into English and Australian elements, with talk of barbed wire between. I at once drew attention to sporting and parade ground activities and lack of ground available, and was told that both would be given an entrance to the oval. There was much discussion of the subdivision with Wing Commander Nichols who will, of course, become camp commander of the British camp. Further large movements of D troops are going on – it is rumoured to Tjilatchap. Menadonese are being shifted from near to us and all Ambonese being concentrated adjacent to us. I have met the Menadonese doctor who is a pleasant little chap.

20 June 1942

Arrival of the warrant officer from the *kebetei*, who at once set about the division of the camp. First we were taken across to a street behind the *kebetei* to a line of houses (fine double houses excellently furnished and in good order, though very dirty following Dutch moving out). These he said were for the officers. Australian strength: 20 officers, total 449; English: 51 officers, 51 warrant officers, total 549; 1 Canadian, 1 NZ, 1 American officer to be included with the British; Australians to have three double houses, rest to British.

I then pointed out that it would be necessary to retain doctors with the troops.

* Refers to Weapons. Bren guns, rifles, grenades etc.

He grinned and said, 'But you are are a doctor' (perhaps information of my medical treatment of a N NCO listening to the chest with *ichi ni san* had got around). Nevertheless, said no difficulties would be made about the doctors going in and out. Then when asked about the discipline of the troops by officers 'to please the Emperor' said that all officers were free to pass to the men's camp. A breach would be made in the wire at 1400 today and officers to move into houses with baggage. Wire then to remain cut.

Troops' quarters then clearly defined by a drain running north and south, cutting the camp in two just east of the present administrative block. Canadians and NZs to be with British troops, the others and the Portuguese with us. Wing Commander Nichols and adjutant Lt Christmas to be responsible to the Ns for 'English', though they said that socially etc. they did not mind us mixing and were not particularly interested in our administration. They then looked at the cottages on the south of the camp and picked out two, one for each commander and adjutant. These each have a second room with a small kitchen and shower and quite a bit of furniture, but they were even quite apologetic and asked us if they would do! Ye Gods, what next! We were then instructed to get on with the business of moving, this occurring without a hitch.

Ambonese etc. are ranging through our camp seeking what they may devour and carry away. Also, when the officers did move to new quarters, the 'rats' had already been in with a vengeance, tearing lights out of the ceilings, stoves off the pipes etc. Rapid conference of COs, adjutants, and Lt-Col. van der Post to decide whether the central 'mixed' administration was to continue for all our own activities as apart from the Ns, or whether we separate. I supported 'mixed' strongly, with Maj. Morris and van der Post, stating that I did not care who ran the show. It was decided that the present administration carry on our own affairs.* *Corvées* of our troops out again. Today very well treated and given as much food as could eat and had a quite excellent time.

Meeting with Major Morris in the chair to discuss arrangements for camp sport and recreation, latter including lectures, debating, dramatics, chess, cards, library etc. This is to be run under camp HQ common to British and Australian groups.

An Australian soldier who gave trouble defying officers was given three days solitary, according to rules drawn up for solitary confinement, including 1 hour's pack drill daily.

21 June 1942

Everybody settling comfortably in new quarters. Ambonese still raiding like demons – they are everywhere. *Kebetei* now playing up well and canteen arrangements permitted. D are very loath to let our parties take over the work of going out for these stores, as it gives them contact with their wives! (Also some control over profits!) *Kebetei* notifies us that some 600 plus Australian and some English troops are to arrive tomorrow at 1730 hours and they also request returns of all personnel who can ride and handle horses. We have sent in only

* This is explained in the Foreword by Laurens van der Post.

seventeen Australians who have been either breakers or trainers etc. – real horsemen. P/O Glowry, for example, was for seven years a race horse trainer. In the evening I called to *kebetei* at 1230 hours with Wing Commander Nichols, where we were given new armbands.

New camp numbers: 3 English, 4 Australia. Wing Commander Nichols, Lt Christmas (Engineer *chusai* and adjutant) report separately. We were told British and Australian troops good boys, cut hair always short; Ambonese and Menadonese please take notice. This from cadet officer of *kebetei* who suffers from incipient baldness. Several of *kebetei* clerks anxiously feeling the hair and grimacing. Much laughter.

22 June 1942

Warned of inspection between 1400 and 1700 by officer of *kebetei*. Camp Commanders' Parade (Wing Commander Nichols did not attend). Troops notified of good impression caused by cleanliness of camp, good behaviour of *corvées* and the cropping of the hair. Requested to help newcomers as much as possible by clearing ground on arrival and sharing out camp furniture to a common level. Parade was well organised and no slackness. Troops now nearly all have either bed boards or mattresses, some both.

Capt. Marika accompanied by friendly cadet officer arrived at 1700 and did a complete camp inspection. He noticed the canteen and asked if it was the canteen. This gives it the official recognition, so to speak. Troops' quarters were excellent but there was some slight lack of system in the indoor '*kere*' in that the whole room usually gave the initial bow – did not hold it until *Naoré* – and then began individual bowing as the inspecting officer went about.

Garoet party arrived approximately 1730; first to arrive Capt. Godlee and 28 sick (dysentery and malaria for the most part). Troops in general had had rather bad food but otherwise good treatment, very little slapping down and good relations with Ns. They all have their hair on and looked surprisingly untidy with long, dirty locks, beards etc. (am I becoming Nipponised?). They knew little or nothing about N drill and rather expect to be saluted by the Ns! Officer party very large, 50 plus, includes 2 wing commanders, a *Group Captain* Nicholetts, Lt-Col. Lyneham, CO 2/3 M.G. Bn. Lyneham cheery and co-operative in every way; spent the night with me and chatted away, *actually* producing a bottle of whisky, 'Doyles whisky' from Perth, Australia, which tasted just fine to my now neglected palate.

He slept cheerily on his valise on the floor without worries. Meantime the Group Captain and friends were making all sorts of querulous fuss about their *house* – their beds, their position and two Bofers cases full of 'grub' they were paying Australian soldiers to carry for them – but they failed to make the distance. Lyneham says these birds have lived on chickens and delicacies in splendid isolation by means of ample public funds. He has run the camp and rates them same as Ds. The machine gunners are a well-organised show with comprehensive lecture and entertainment programme and classes in bookkeeping, languages etc. Says he has only a few 'bad devils' who are not from his own unit.

Malayan local paper (N inspired) says today Tobruk has fallen and Germans 16 kilometres from Mersa Matruh. Also Sebastopol has fallen. Pacific situation seems to have the confidence of Americans who say Dutch East Indies now effectively blockaded from N. who has lost 2,000,000 tons of shipping.

23 June 1942

Australian group now to be commanded by Lt-Col. Lyneham who is working them into a company organisation with a purely combatant basis. Maj. Wearne and Maj. Woods are assisting in this work. Garoet group turned out on parade at 1000 today for the necessary sorting out. Personnel interview with Group Captain Nicholetts in presence of Wing Commander Nichols. He said that the situation was difficult: he felt that it was really his wish *not* to take any prominent job which brought him in contact with the Ns, as fellows of his rank were all taken away. Nevertheless, felt that is was his responsibility: sort of bad show not taking things over, perhaps on the whole better than I carried on for the present while the situation was under consideration. I replied meekly that I was willing to hand the job to any officer or combatant of equal rank, but rather thought that it was a matter which might be of some interest to Lt-Col. Van der Post representing British Army and to the rather large Australian group with some senior officers. Not to mention the Ns. Meantime the Group Captain very interested in getting a suitable house, suitably furnished, well out of the way. Lt-Col. Lyneham has given me a word or two of warning re certain personalities in the party.

Our own *corvée* now going out for milk etc. which is a momentous forward step as far as canteen arrangements concerned. Our idea is now if possible to order stores directly from Captain Segars of the Intendance branch* (working for *kebetei*) or send party out direct to retailers, as in case of milk party. Suggested today to the Dutch hospital group that we obtain our stores (bread etc.) on a strict cost basis and pay them a *per capita* rate for our soldiers in their hospital. They realise now that otherwise it will be easy to obtain the stores direct.

Major Morris today spoke to Ns re soldiers' shortage of blankets. They promised prompt supply of one per man. He also obtained a promise of furniture, piano etc. to make the gym into a theatre. (N officers asked to be permitted to come to concerts.)

Kebetei informed camp commanders today that the time for future afternoon reports is to be 1700 hours, and 'lights out' from now on are to be 2100 for NCOs and men, 2200 for officers. This seems to be a blackout precaution. Important that no lights to show outside. There are signs of anti-air raid activity in Bandoeng – sand bagging etc. British and Australian troops were also admonished re compliments to be paid to N officers. We promised further instruction.

Rather large numbers of troops for one parade now, so Lt-Col. Lyneham's group have a separate parade at 1000 after British group. They are doing half an hour's compulsory P.T. each day but will exempt those doing special classes.

* Dutch Ordnance.

24 June 1942

Canteen to take over some 1600 gulden worth of stock today, including cigarettes and tobacco. A loan of 1300 gulden floated, 1100 gulden EED (me), 1100 gulden Lt-Col. Lyneham, 1100 gulden Sqn Ldr Harrison. This stock obtained directly from Capt. Segars (*kebetei* representative). Parades today – British first, with Group Capt. Nicholetts standing upstage from Wing Commander Nicholls in a rather embarassing way, Australians later at 1000 hours, followed by company P.T. Officer in charge of group including 2/2 CCS made an unfortunate speech in which he referred to the fact that such people had not been as fortunate as to be with the 2/3 M. G. Bn and accordingly their discipline could not be expected to be as good. Calls of 'Cock!' from the ranks and W/O D.J. Topping stepped from the ranks with 'I resent those remarks', followed by a little homily on the question of service and discipline in general. This sort of comparison is definitely odious. Sgt Bill Aldag's class is being rushed, since there is to be exemption from doing P.T. parade. Arrangements made to give them a special session of Aldag medicine tomorrow with a roll call. This should reduce the class to enthusiasts. Boxing and wrestling classes are in session daily.

Meeting of group commanders, Dunlop, Morris and Lts Rintoul and Cameron to discuss rations, canteen arrangements, type of issue of food etc. which could be given troops. An attempt is to be made to lay on a special hot drink in the evening as a camp enterprise and to scrap private coffee stalls. These actually are making little or no profits.

25 June 1942

Kebetei have warned that in the next two days approximately 200 troops are to be expected, 100 English and 100 Australian from Tjimahi hospital. Australian group is now well organised and is working in a very regimental way, which is causing little comment amongst troops in general. The only real difficulty caused up to date is by a party of RAAF sergeants who do not like to get up for the 0730 hours morning roll call. Lt-Col. Lyneham is attending to these and they are in good hands.

Ns are now using large working parties about the town to cut grass, clean streets, buildings etc. and small groups are being used for technical jobs: car repairing, bicycle repairing and so on. One soldier who has been repairing Lt Marika's car has actually been asked if he would take on the job of chauffeur. He said he was not a good driver (pity – this is a good job for our purposes). Another peculiar happening today is that A/C Gray (RAF) who was Air Vice-Marshall Maltby's driver, Air Com. station, and who hid the car away before entering the Christylijk Lyceum was required by the *kebetei*. He was taken out to locate the car and retrieve the property of two high air force officials from the car. This is to be sent to Batavia to the officers concerned. This is a remarkable change in attitude, which seems to be general. There is a quite evident desire to please at present. For example, when Maj. Morris went to D theatre for the concert, the 'props' piano was missing and an N officer said he knew another camp that had a piano and that he would go himself and get it and give it to us. There is a most happy liaison between the N cadet officer and Maj. Morris.

26 June 1942

Air raid precautions are now evident in Bandoeng. Bags of sand here and there, machine guns on buildings and spotters, air raid gongs and sirens. The siren was sounded today, presumably as a test. This cheered the troops considerably. 600 troops out on *corvée*, mostly moving food from store near 'Landsop' to *kebetei* store. *Kebetei* requested also 15 horsemen to be ready at *kebetei* at 0800 hours with kit, mosquito nets etc. ready for job lasting approximately eight days. ORs to go, not NCOs or officers. It was, however, arranged that Sgt Montefiore be included in the party for intelligence purposes, and I had a talk to him re this matter. Also today three cooks were requested as cooks to Kawakatso, who is in Bandoeng. His company are said to have many sick following exercises. Official inspection of camp at 1600 hours by a high N officer (captain). Apparently equivalent to Lt Marika in Batavia. He considered that we (the officers) here had more luxury than at that place. As usual, the inspection had a *Mikado* touch: more and more the *kebetei* becomes a joy with 'Moon Face', Clown Face' and 'Stupid'. Malayan press states Tobruk fallen, 35,000 prisoners.

27 June 1942

Kebetei warned us that we do not pay adequate compliments to Ns; we have ourselves introduced N drill one hour daily for those not specially engaged in other work. Ns wish to know if we have any prominent Australian personages in camp, particularly admin., political or entertainers, musicians etc. This sounds like a propaganda snare, so we say there are no prominent Australians – they are all in Australia. *Kebetei* pays us the compliment of doubting this.

Today the Nip W/O in charge of our carpentry party at *kebetei* rushed up behind me and sprang on my back suddenly with a horrifying yell, then rode piggyback in triumph whilst I pretended to buck him off'.

The British and Australian officers seem to be very confident and are settling down to an easy-going life of gardening, reading, bridge playing and making marmalade jam. Col. van der Post in particular turns out to be a good marmalade cook.

There has been much electrical activity, Lt Smedley (in particular) doing a house-to-house search 'to inspect the roses'. Major Corlette and Capt McNamara think they know where there is a leak in the ceiling.* (D say so.) Leak detected. No aural arrangements yet. Housing arrangements discussed with Van and are difficult. At this stage Sqn Ldr Cummings produced another, more serious leak, and Van found out that there was still another one known to RAF officers.

Canteen business still brisk, but prices are almost completely prohibitive: e.g. milk 30 cents a litre, bread 35 cents a loaf. I saw Capt. Segars and told him our feelings about this, frankly hinting at a 'ramp' which I politely assumed to be entirely Nipponese. He say that he is only permitted to deal with one Chinese firm under *kebetei* arrangements and he knows prices to be very dear. We still deal through the doctors in all things other than milk and they make a small

* Each 'leak' is a wireless set.

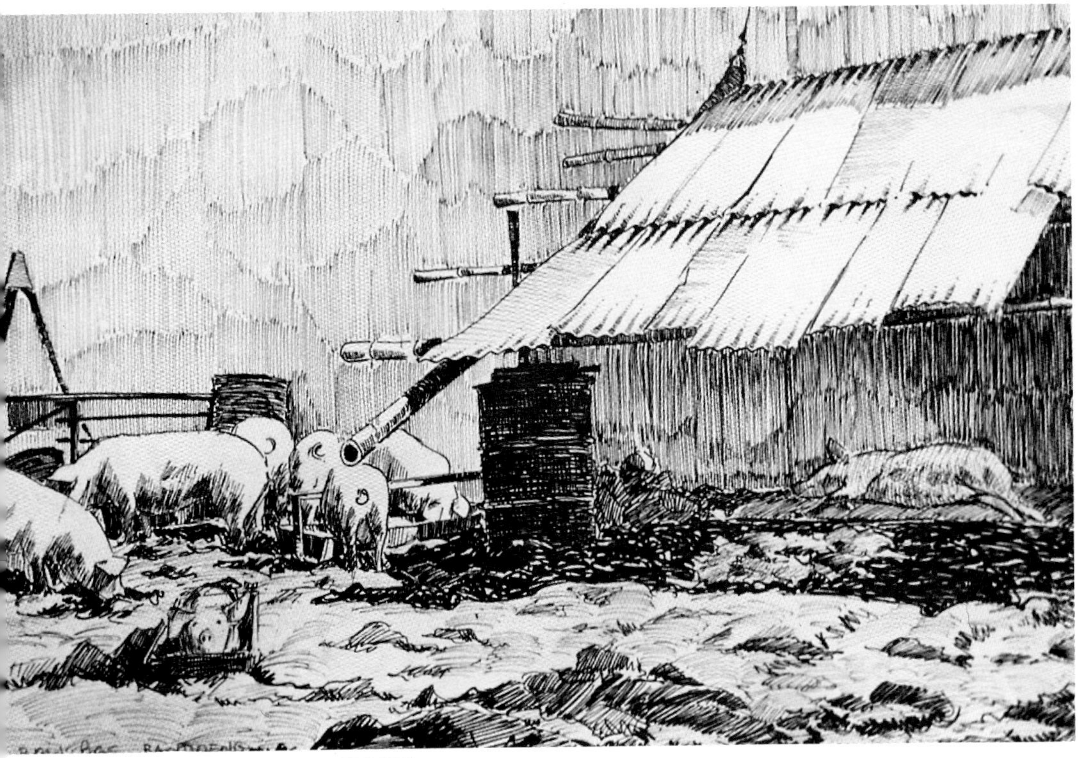

gery, Bandoeng (*Ray Parkin*)

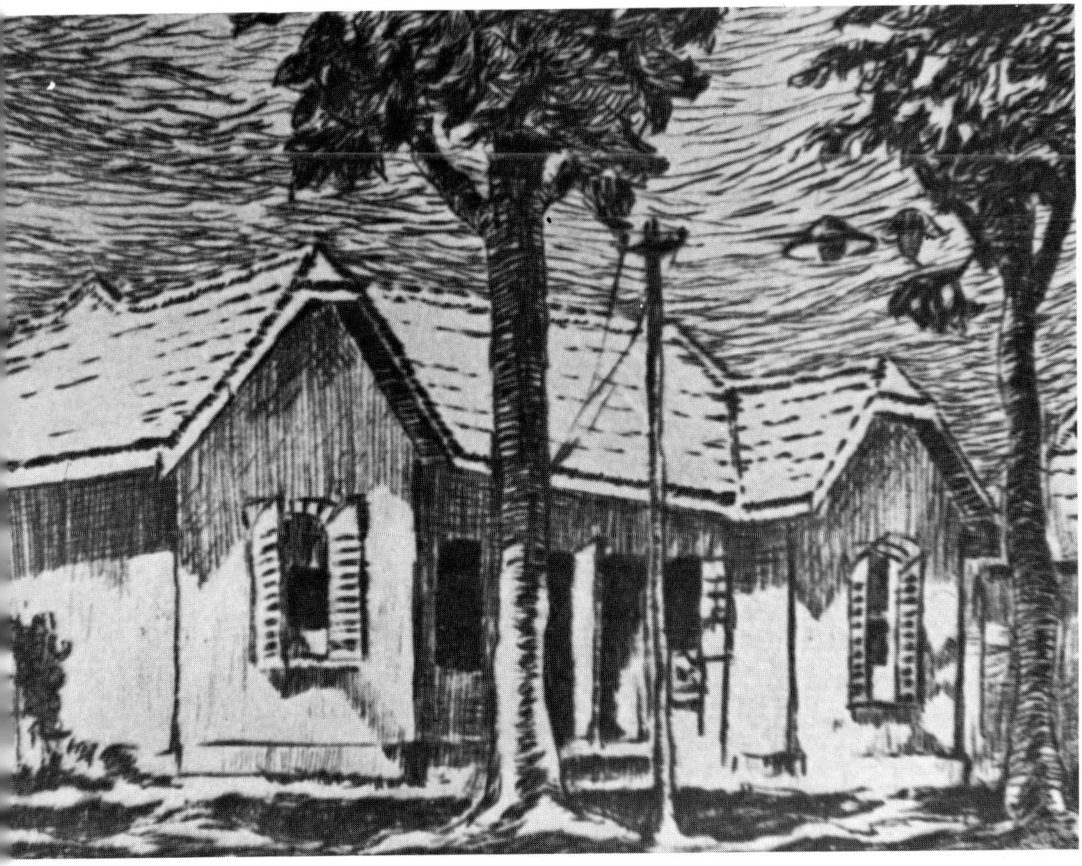

uren's cottage – a place of wise counsel (*Ray Parkin*)

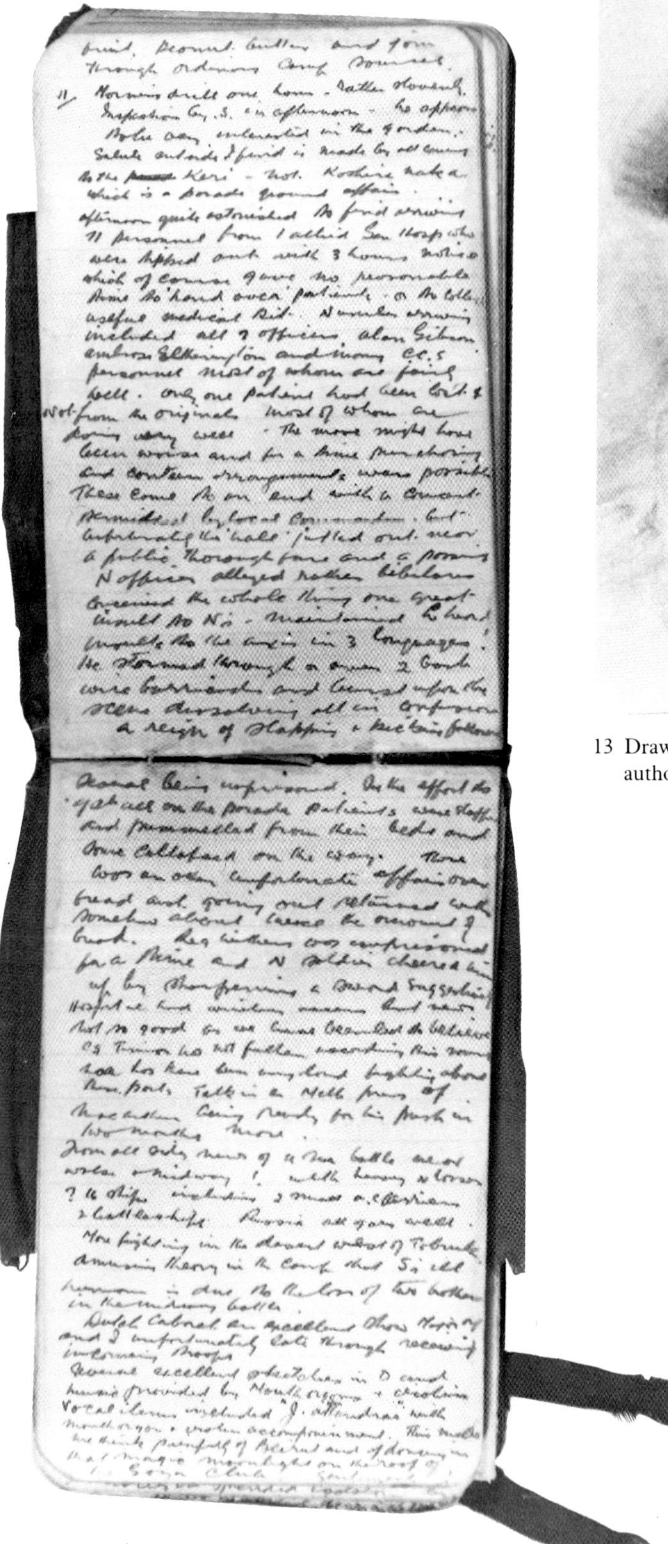

12 Two pages of an early diary, Java, 1942

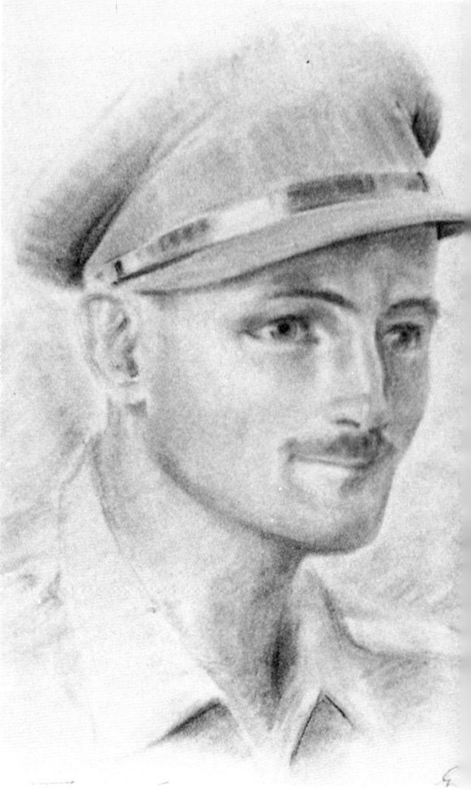

13 Drawing by R. van Willigen, 3 August 1942, of the author as Commander, Bandoeng POW Camp

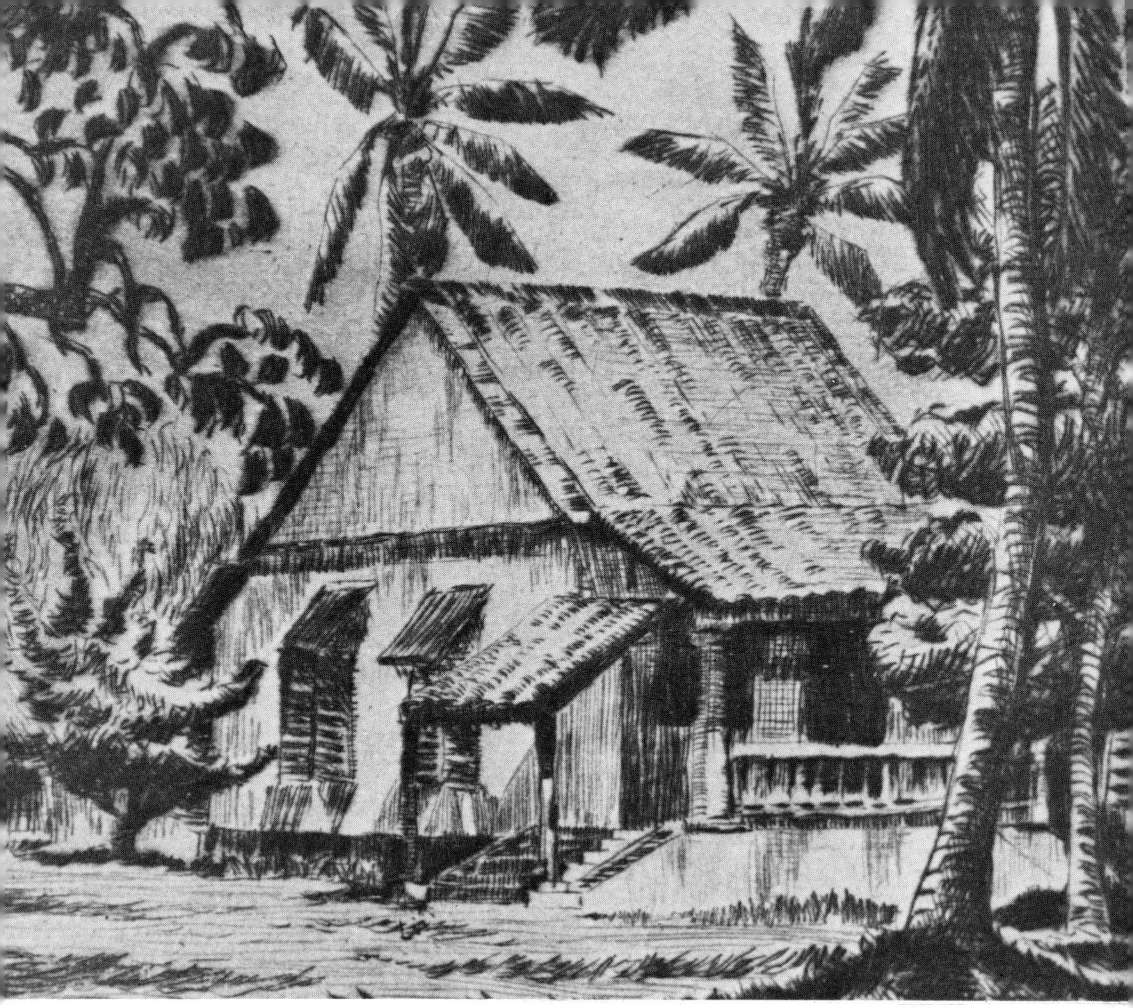

14 Japanese commander's house, Makasura, Java (*Ray Parkin*)

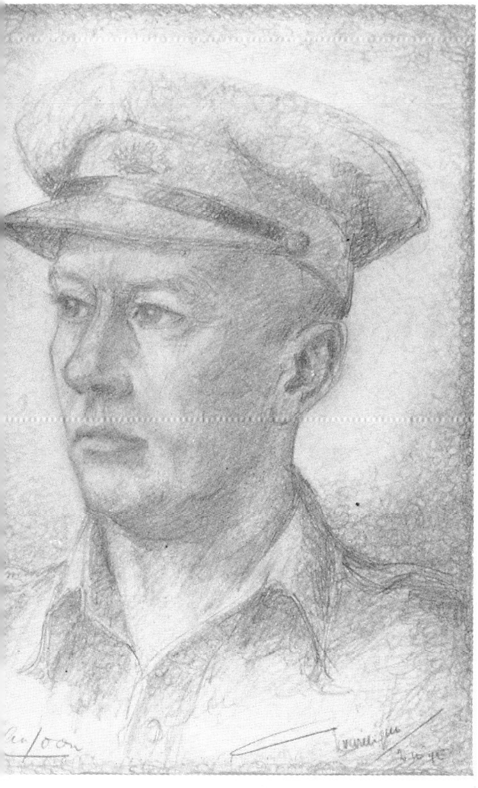

15 Major Arthur Moon OBE, RAAMC and beloved surgeon. Drawn by R. van Willigen, Java, 2 October 1942

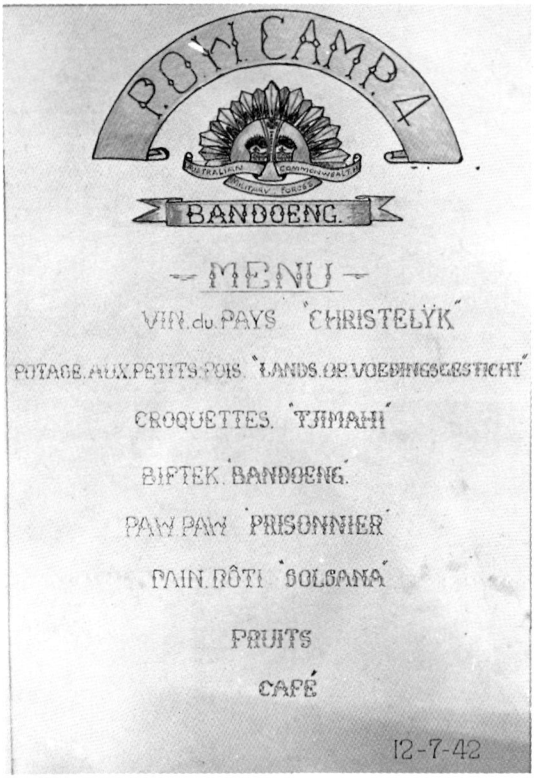

16 The author's birthday dinner, Bandoeng, 1942

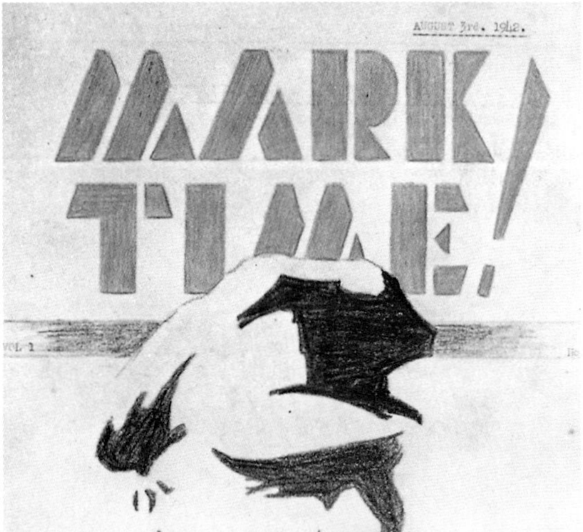

17 *Mark Time*, first issue 3 August 1942. Cover sketch of Maj. J.C. De Crespigny by Sid Scales.

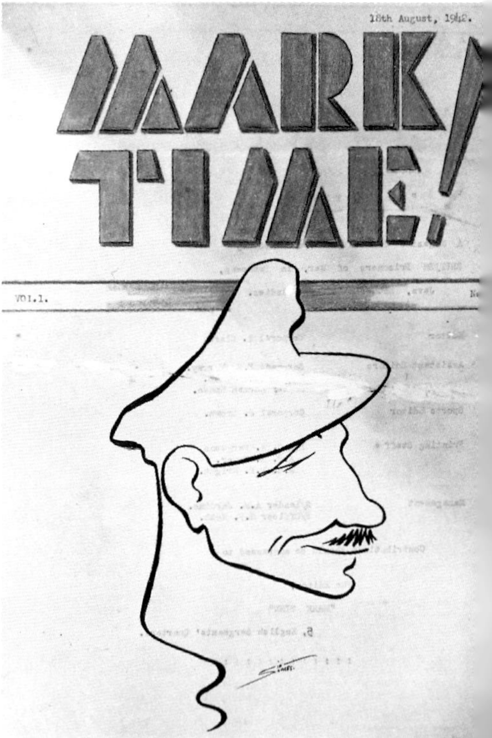

18 'The Colonel' – cover sketch for issue 2 of *Mark Tim*
by Sid Scales

profit. Though we say we prefer a flat rate per head per day for hospital patients (25c a day).

*XXXX** Germans holding a line west of Matruh six miles from escarpment to sea. It is expected to strike now at either Alexandria, Cairo or both. Kerkov has fallen and Gs driving to east; Sebastopol appears next. Mr Churchill is in America with Roosevelt. House of Commons tabling a motion of lack of confidence in the central prosecution of the war to meet him on return. Far east, damn all happening. Ns raiding Port Moresby etc. This is rather different from the glorious news produced today by a 'paranoic' from Tjimahi hospital who 'listened to the news himself'.

28 June 1942

Church parade in gym today where the National anthem was sung, probably rather unwisely. In the evening the 'Brains Trust' entertained.

29 June 1942

COs parade, British and Australians separately. Really felt my position frightfully – inspecting rows of senior British officers in particular. And, incidentally, the parade was a ghastly show, both as regards procedure and turnout of ORs. Surprisingly enough the Australian parade was almost like a regimental parade – I inspected them by companies with Lt-Col. Lyneham. Really excellent work. I suppose this inspection business will 'get the troops' goats' but what the hell. Lt-Col. Lyneham sentenced two really bad devils today to three days in the cells. They are prison birds. One is a heavyweight boxing aspirant and gym work offered him for one hour each day in lieu of pack drill. Nothing doing!

Kebetei today rather amusing. Was having tea with interpreter when Lt Matsuda came along and said that a captain from division had taken exception to Dutch *corvées* going out (with opportunity to contact their relatives), also commenting on them sitting about eating ice cream. Ruling no more *corvées* for D and if they are not very careful, rest must go also to Tjilatchap.

X [Wireless] Mersa seems to have fallen. N soldiers patrol the front of our cottage very vigorously at night with moonlight glinting on bayonets. And tuning down is difficult!

30 June 1942

Routine.

1 July 1942

Called to *kebetei* at 1030 by Capt. Marika who gave me tea and interrogated me at great length.

Q: I was an Australian – what had I done before the war?

A: Not a professional soldier but a surgeon.

* My wireless now functioning and referred to with this mark.

Q: Did I not as an Australian regret British conduct of the war and the behaviour of British statesmen?
A: Was afraid as one who had lived in England for a few years before the war, I was a bit out of touch with Australian opinion and politics. I was not aware of any significant body in Australia entertaining that opinion.
Q: Did I hope and believe that Britain would win the war?
A: Ah, when I came to Java I had high hopes. Now I know nothing and cannot give a sound opinion. (Laughter!)
Q: What do I think of the N army?
A: Admired discipline, considered western powers surprised by efficiency.
Q: How do you think N soldiers compare with British or Australian?
A: Afraid I have no real data to base a comparison. Considered that N soldiers perhaps helped by conditions under which fought in Hongkong and Malaya etc. Perhaps Britain failed to secure the harmonious combination of forces needed.
Q: Have you not as an Australian soldier noted a difference in the way British treat you to their own soldiers?
A: Have been under Australian admin.* In medical service all are brothers etc. Noted no difference.
Q: Do you not think Britain responsible for war in Australia?
A: No – Australian government declared war and must share responsibility.
Q: Do not Australians now resent the fact America encouraged them and led them on with promises of help.
A: No – think Australia and America have grown closer together in recent years.
Q: Given the following information: Mr Churchill has been to America to meet the warmonger Rooseveldt (sic) and beg for more help from him amongst the shoal of disasters. This gambler's throw is futile. Both these statesmen have deceived the people and conceal great losses and people now finding out. Egypt had now fallen and Germans about to drive down to the south. Mr Churchill returning to England with 'lost face'. Rooseveldt also lost face. What do our soldiers think now they find themselves misled.
A: Soldiers do not worry about politics – obey officers and are loyal to the army and the Crown.
Q: What do you think of my treatment of prisoners-of-war?
A: Begged to thank Capt. M. for the very great improvement in our treatment, which in most respects I found satisfactory. One source of worry to all was absence of any knowledge that information had been given to Australian government and relatives as to our fate and no letters could be written.

Maj. Morris and Lt-Col. Lyneham were then called and questioned in a similar way. Gave occupations as refrigerator salesman and fruit grower (I think a shade of distate crossed the delicate, truly military countenance; Morris a professional soldier AIC). They gave similar replies.
Q: If we wrote letters, would we say 1 We were well treated; and 2 Express political opinions against British government and war.
A: Yes – 2 Difficult for us, since political opinions of soldiers difficult to estimate or control. Most of them just soldiers with no political feelings. It was

* A lie on my part.

felt that the receipt of letters in Australia would be a shining example of N good care of prisoners, helped by our statement that we were well treated. Political utterance might not be understood and spoil gesture. At this stage Matsuda came in, listened, and finally made a long speech in which he said we might write one letter each, in which we could say personal things (nothing military) and we promised to censor such letters ourselves.

A clerk went out and with remarkable celerity produced paper. (This was 'Clown Face' who had taken notes throughout the interview in a sort of shorthand.) I was stricken with the thought that in a recent return required I have given wife 1, children 7, therefore address difficult re my fiancée Helen. Therefore asked could I write to more than one person on the slip of paper given. Answer: Yes, but only one address top left corner, OK!* Troops given one and a half days to complete letters.

A recent return, obviously propaganda, was also requested re prominent sportsmen. Had a consultation with Group Capt. Nicholetts, van der Post, Wing Commander Nichols, who said best decision to send in one or two carefully selected names, then if broadcast might be able to get some information out to distressed relatives. This we know to be against orders of governments but feel that in the unusual circumstances justified. Names given: Lt Rymill (Australian cricket); E.E. Dunlop (Rugby football).

Cadet Lt Yamita to afternoon tea, very friendly, imbibing huge quantities foul tea with sucking noises and belching. He said we must have some china, must have more electric lights, must have more chairs and did all the officers have beds? (No – well, party must go out right away for 20 stretchers etc. etc.) Questions re wife and family, age etc. (He is also 34–2 children so not up to my 7.)

2 July 1942

Inspected camp; not frightfully good show. Troops slipping a bit in barracks from 'Landsop' days and certainly do not stand to in fashion regarded as appropriate for N officers or indeed NCOs.

'Radio City Revels' opened by me who declared 'Radio City' open. Interesting soccer British v. Ambonese: good class football. British: 3, Ambonese: 2.

Troops ration

Rice or potatoes in lieu	500 g	(1797)
Sugar	20 g	(82)
Flour	50 g	(185)
Meat (fresh)	50 g	(57)
Salt	5 g	(nil)
Coconut oil or margarine in lieu	3 g	(28)
Tea	4 g	(nil)
Vegetables	100 g	(24)

Total calories per day: 2173, enough only for rest or very light work.

* Prestige required me to have a larger family.

Minimum 2400–3000 required for soldiers performing duties. (Authority: Atwater and Bryant, quoted in W.H. Howell's *Textbook of Physiology* 14th ed. 1940, page 988 etc.) The calorific value of this ration, assuming half rice and half potatoes, is approximately 1600. If the full amount of rice was given instead of potatoes, this would increase the value to the above. Atwater stated that a man doing no work required 2040; moderate muscular work needed 2900. Basal metabolic rate in round numbers, 1600 calories, so theoretically we are just about alive. Can this be a tougher generation than that when his work was done in 1889? Dutch rather interesting on this point and say that Russians who were prisoners in Germany in last war actually lived and worked on 1400 calories a day! Allowing 2/3 rice, 1/3 potatoes, the total calories per day is actually 1715. Rice 333g: 1197 cals; potatoes 167g: 142 cals. Possibly some 60 per cent of the staff supplement the ration diet in one way or another.

3 July 1942

It was decided that educational facilities should be expanded and given full camp control. (There has been a little tendency for 2/3 M.G. Bn to continue in a sectional way.) Lt-Col. L.J. van der Post and Maj. W.W. Wearne will control the *educational branch*, all classes, lectures, library etc. There is a galaxy of teachers available – languages, history etc., e.g. Gunner Rees MA Cambridge (a teacher). An immense number of languages can be tackled, history (ancient and modern), English, Classics, engineering and technical subjects, navigation, agricultural science, medical and scientific subjects. The syllabus is being prepared and requirements are being worked out.

X [Wireless] Western desert still terribly critical. 'The Auk' somehow holding on about eighty miles from Alexandria. Russian news bad – Sebastopol gone and now fighting back behind Kharkov, which has been a bastion.

Maj. Morris at *kebetei* tonight; he is worried that several N officers are coming to the boxing and wrestling display tomorrow at my invitation, also to cabaret show 'Radio City Revels'. To his astonishment, Capt. Marika sent out a challenge to any British or Australian to appear in the ring against him so that he could demonstrate the superiority of Ju Jitsu as a 'gentle art'. I invited Capt. Marika and officers through John Morris. The latter came back with a message for me which ran: 'Captain Marika accepts challenge of Camp Commander or other champion to appear in boxing ring against him. Condition two rounds boxing and two rounds Ju Ju.'

As a past Australian universities champion heavyweight, I was embarrassed not by any threat from the lightweight Marika, but by the inhibitions imposed by the situation. Soon 'Jimmy Starr' and Bill Belford were around seeking the job. I said, 'Go away, I don't want him killed.' John Morris was sent back to say 'I think you have misunderstood the Colonel's invitation. He desires you to attend as an honoured guest, but if you really desire to compete yourself, only he could contend against you!' He came back beaming and said 'Yes, he will.' I never saw a more relieved man. Capt. Marika was tactfully dissuaded by the interpreter that it would upset the programme! In case this challenge is repeated tomorrow, I intend to say that we are all keen for the honour and that I myself am available, though if he would prefer the best exponent one Mounsey, a pro who boxes under the name of Starr, will perform.

4 July 1942

Saturday. Wing Commander Nicholls and I to *kebetei* where we are asked to inform by 2130 hours how many pigs we can take and raise and materials required! Pigs will be tenderly nurtured and raised under *kebetei* patronages – who will eventually say when pigs are to be killed, but if pig disappears or is killed *you will be killed* (roars of laughter from the guards at this edict from Lt Macheda who laughed merrily).

Wrestling began at 1745 hours with a most excellently roped ring and improvised matting; huge audience of troops. Capt. Marika and officers arrived at 1800 hours and after compliments were paid went to their ringside seats. Capt. Marika as usual sartorial perfection and spotless white cotton gloves, Macheda rather untidy and merry and running round, taking ciné films. Marika sat stiffly, almost immobile and rarely changing facial expression, occasionally removing his white gloves to applaud. The last wrestling bout was six-round, beautifully staged affair between two experts, 'Bull Mountana' and one other who applied 'excrutiating' hold after hold in continuous brilliance. Real stadium-type showmanship. Ns enjoyed this, as did all. Marika then thanked those concerned and left.

Macheda and others went to the show. This was real low variety for the most part with cockney humour, naturally beyond the Nips – and I suppose most people. They enjoyed, however, the female impersonation, the music and the sort of obvious drama of 'The New Deal' and 'Freetown Bumboat', with its exaggeration – gross villains, pure young hero and young virgin and fairies etc. After the concert finished OCs of groups, their adjutants, Maj. M, orderly officer Major Beaney, P/O Cicurel, Lt-Col. van de Post and the two D interpreters came to my house for supper with Sub-Lt Yamida, Capt. Hoto and another cadet officer. Steve and Blue put on a wonderful show of food: fried rice and nasi goreng with eggs and spices and all sorts of little toast and potato dishes. Balls of rice cake etc. N officers played up and rushed out producing 4 bottles of port (2 Portuguese, 2 Aust.) 2 bottles of beer, one for Aust. Commandant, one for English. Also some excellent mandarin oranges. The food was consumed with singing and appropriate expressions of N etiquette. Terrific intaking of breath, succulent noises and belches! Van and the little cadet officer has much interesting conversation in N and English and songs sung included opera, 'Oh Solé Mio' (Capt. Hoto), Nipponese songs and English and Australian songs. And the 'Internationale'! The little cadet officer, who is a school teacher, showed comic dismay when we pointed out that it was funny to hear him on the 'Internationale' and shook his head from side to side saying, 'No! No! – No good'!

It really was a vastly entertaining affair and P/O Cicurel summed up my feelings by saying that 'you cannot hate for 24 hours a day.' Sub-Lt Yamida is always helpful and told me that if we sent a party the following day he would 'lay on' many boots and other articles of clothing (100 boots). Relations at present are really quite cordial. We almost fear that we may lose our cooks, Blue and Steve, after their performance.

5 July 1942

Sunday – usual services in gym – Yamida laid on the boots and other articles as promised. Very good spirit prevails.

6 July 1942

The officers who are interested, especially Van and Billy Wearne, have a Japanese class in the afternoons given by Lt Jongehan's, the interpreter. This I am attending sporadically. A grand beat up of educational talent for our 'school' is being done. There's plenty available and much enthusiasm.

7 July 1942

Camp library functioning well under Van; much bookbinding etc. in progress. Special references in Routine Orders re fire precautions: no smoking after lights out in barracks and no improvised lights or candles.

8 July 1942

Arrival of some new troops from Djogjakarta, consisting of about 800 Dutch but also some UK troops, RAF and Navy, 21 in all (senior officer, F/O Duffy (medical); 5 Australians, senior Lt (Fred) Airey, 2/4 M.G. Bn. These troops report conditions have been pretty tough, with no possibility of obtaining outside food, cigarettes or tobacco. They are in poor condition.

Airey escaped from Singapore in a small boat five days after the capitulation and got across to Sumatra. He eventually crossed somehow to Padang where, after Sumatra was taken, he put to sea with some other persons in a lifeboat. They wrecked the boat on an island off Sumatra but eventually had it repaired and set off for Australia with about three weeks' rations.* Unfortunately, they could not get out through the first main ocean current and were eventually nine weeks at sea, getting no further than the south coast of middle Java. Having had nothing to eat for ages but small handfuls of uncooked rice, they were just about all in. Friendly natives carried them up into the hills in chairs and litters. Airey had beriberi badly and still has gross oedema of feet. Duffy and Airey came to my house for some food including a couple of fried eggs, some toast and coffee. They were obviously famished and it was a pleasure to see them tuck in. Airey must go to hospital. He was in World War I.

9 July 1942

There is now some possibility of obtaining outside financial relief; apparently there is some back-door business being done by the banks (though not officially open).

Lt Smedley's [wireless set] passed to Lt-Col. Lyneham, who has an expert to

* He was the sole survivor of a massacre and left the island in a child's canoe.

help and 'ears' [headphones]. Our own mincer [my set] functions intermittently. Some difficulties of central command of the camp arise in that the UK discipline differs a little from that of the rest of the camp. 'Confined to camp 4 days' is a typical sentence. Also some differing ideas about having a uniform reveille and muster roll call in morning. Troops not getting out of bed too well. Also some trouble re wearing of shirts. With a little tactful help from Van, all these matters were settled once more.

An excellent new variety show opened today: 'On the Air', with John Morris as compère at the mike. Some Shakespeare from *Othello* and a most excellent monologue written and delivered by A/C Bell entitled *The Story of Paul Clandelle*; some 'Crazy Song' items; one joke by the 'Two Loose Screws' – 'What is this C.B. 4 days?' 'It means you must not escape from the camp for 4 days!' We have now quite a good selection of instruments and are developing a jazz band.

10 July 1942

Discipline question may be a little clarified by the publication of the following from the manual of military law 1941 – quoting AMR and R 76 'an officer or soldier, although he has become a prisoner-of-war, remains subject to the provisions governing the military relations of superior and subordinate and the military duty of obedience'. This in ROs may clarify the position.

11 July 1942

Weather is now excellent with rarely any rain. 'On the Air' is a great success and many Dutch have attended.

12 July 1942

My birthday: presents received; and one large beautiful loaf of bread specially cooked by the camp bakery. I entertained the officers of the CCS (less Tom Elliott who had dysentery) at morning tea, also the sergeants at afternoon tea. Was myself given a dinner by Moon, Macnamara, Cameron, Glowry etc. in their house. Most excellent show actually, with an astonishing menu which I am retaining as a souvenir – even included some wine (sauterne) and *steak* and eggs. Many courses, finishing with paw paw dessert, bananas. I quite forgot about being a prisoner-of-war.

In the morning was called to the *kebetei* at approx. 1000 where Lt Marika was handling over to his successor Lt Sato of Kawakatsos company. Sato san is said to be an Olympic athlete and the Dutch speak highly of his humane attributes. He spoke to me, saying that he had spent four months in England at Brighton. Did I know Brighton? etc.

The usual *kebetei* hand-over occurred: speech from that little dandy M in white gloves – pleased with our behaviour and the way we had carried out the orders – now introduced Lt Sato and hoped we would do the same under him. Sato then expressed himself pleased with our reported conduct under M. He must now see that we obeyed the orders of the N army as before but he would endeavour to interpret the orders as humanely as possible (good start). Then an orgy of photography by Marika, Macheda and Sato. 'Moonface' and 'Clownface' ran about in a friendly way with beaming faces. It will be awfully distressing to me if 'Moonface' should one day get shot whilst he's fumbling around in a pleasant way trying to find his gun. He is a sort of N equivalent of our Altman, and a nice fellow. Macheda is a most humorous little man: when at tea with the interpreters the other day he came in and began a most entertaining impersonation of hypnotism and tricks with swords under hypnotism in N. Fix the eye – flick the hands and BIM! He is hypnotised. Then he can be made walk on sharp swords. Hands bandaged tightly to shart sword blade and sword drawn. Person made to draw a sword 2 metres long – yet disastrous to do so unhypnotised. All this looked extremely funny illustrated by a yard ruler.

Macheda's last act was to go to much pains to obtain for John Morris some make-up required for his 'shows'. (Cost £15.)

Yamida, who was not at the handover, made a special trip down to say good-bye and said he was going back to Japan where he had not been for seven years. He seemed to be almost sorry to be leaving us and exchanged addresses with John Morris. He is the most friendly of the bunch and has been kind in every way.

K.P. Durieu, an Australian in RAF, was with troops near Maos on the Friday before capitulation attempting to reach Tjilatchap for evacuation and he received information that the railway bridge near Maos was to be blown up. With a number of others, he seized a little gear and was running across the bridge but the explosion occurred when he was almost directly over the charge, so that his ear drums ruptured, he was knocked unconscious and suffered a great number of small flesh wounds. An incredibly lucky escape. He came to to find himself on the wrong side of the partly submerged bridge and was helped back. Two trainloads of people then on the wrong side of the bridge were told that the Japs were coming and they must get across. This was done somehow by getting a wire across the gap and getting a slippery foothold on the tottering bridge remains. Some 22 unable to be got across had to be left behind and are said to have been 'polished off' by Japs – one soldier escaped by feigning death. (Sqn Ldr MacGrath knows the story).

Durieu and several companions, at this stage all in and collapsing, reached a Dutch field hospital. Tjilatchap at this time was being bombed to hell. The party had their wounds dressed and lay all day in a village, with sounds of battle raging about, under the care of an amazing Dutch doctor who cheered them up with tales that it was only a few local looters. Eventually they secured a lorry and had a terrible trip to a station across paddy-fields. At one stage the doctor walked ahead of the lorry and took pot shots with his revolver at snipers.

The sick British and Australians, nine in all, were eventually got on to a train and taken with the doctor to be admitted to a native hospital at Tjimahi. There they lay until Ns came on Wednesday, the day after capitulation. Shortly after this they arrived one morning and forced all British troops to walk out to a lorry, despite one with fractured bones of the feet; one fractured patella (bad); one with eye wound etc. Here they saw the ominous sight of a N officer cleaning and polishing his sword, others practising bayonet thrusts, and four shovels placed abroad. Now a controversy arose. The nine soldiers were obviously not fit to dig their own graves. Another small car was brought along and the shovels placed in it, the party then going into jungle area behind the hospital. Meantime, the wounded lay in the lorry in the sun, while the doctor of the hospital frantically tried to get in touch with the local Japanese army HQ. After what seemed hours, a car arrived with a higher N officer, Col. Matsu. Eventually, the culprits were 'pardoned' and re-admitted to hospital, where they lay listening to an impatient tooting in the wood from the gravediggers. Later the party was shifted to Tjibatoe and finally to Bandoeng with Maj. Calder's party where, having no passes regarded as satisfactory, they were thrown into Bandoeng goal and remained there for 36 hours.

In the first hospital affair, whilst 'outside', their kit and money was 'confiscated'; there were further losses in Bandoeng goal and unpleasant threats from a gentleman who made sword play. Finally they arrived in Bandoeng Allied General Hospital after I intervened to have them released. Of this party, Durieu still has much ear trouble, but wounds are almost healed.

HMAS *Perth* in vicinity Surabaya 27 Feb. Five cruisers (*Perth*, *Houston*, *Exeter*, *Java*, *De Ruiter*), 10 destroyers. Brisk action in the morning very satisfactory. Night action not so good: *Exeter* badly damaged, attempted to get back to Surabaja; *Java* and *De Ruiter* sunk by torpedoes. Submarines caused a good deal of the bother. *Perth* and *Houston* put back to Batavia with some damage to gun turrets, where unable to get a full load of shells etc. and oil. *Houston* the worse off. Pushed on through the Sunda Strait where became involved in a grim affair with large N convoy – outnumbered completely but fought it out though hit by several large shells and own ammunition nearly running out. Finally three torpedoes – after that everything raining on them and a case of 'take to the drink'.

The party coming here from Tjilatchap consists of 5 officers, 7 ORs. They were in the sea for approximately ten hours, with a fairly strong current pulling people out to sea, but finally landed on an island; only about sixty of ship's company accounted for. Mort Tymns and Stenning* known to have got off into water but no more heard of them. This small party had a metal lifeboat which they tried to sail to Australia but after eight days had only got round to Tjilatchap where they were imprisoned.

F/Lt Miller, 84th squadron, in vicinity of Tjilatchap, tried to escape on a D corvette. This was forbidden. Corvette was used in a further attempt to block the harbour. The party put to sea in two lifeboats and a launch, but these were too heavily laden in the rough sea so decided to put back and landed on Tjilatchap Island, the 'Island of Long Grass', at a remote point near lighthouse. CO then put out to sea on the 6th in a lifeboat with a party of eight in an attempt to reach Australia. It is not known if he got through. Rest of party continued on the island until 21 April when they gave themselves up after being discovered by a Malayan sergeant. Two reconnaisance parties were sent to Tjilatchap at one stage to find out what was doing. The first, of 4 persons, landed at Tjil. and ran up against a N soldier and shot him. Other N soldiers ran out. Two of ours got clear; other two, when last seen, were trying to help up N soldier. Never seen

* Medical officers, HMAS *Perth*.

again. The two who ran got a boat and eventually reached main body after two terrible days hiding up.

Of the other party of 8, two ran into a N lorry, were taken prisoner and beheaded after a beating-up a couple of days later (apparently connected with death of some N soldiers). Two others decided to give themselves up (one had VD); remainder ran away and hid, eventually getting back to the island by boat. Miller was one of those. When eventually they gave themselves up there was a terrific slapping down of them all and threats of beheading or shooting. They chose shooting. Nevertheless, from then on, treated fairly well.

13 July 1942

A full educational syllabus began today with all classrooms in full swing and the greatest prevailing enthusiasm. At approximately 1030 hours, numerous officers arrived, obviously staff, several speaking most excellent English and showing signs of very quick wits. One major and three of 1st Lt rank, two obvious but one with stars on the shoulders and five green stars on the chest – ? air force. In addition, a local captain, probably Divisional Staff, and Lt Sato.

First they demanded all Australians on parade, then separately those from West Australia and Queensland. They they dismissed those from Fremantle, Perth and Brisbane, beginning a quick-fire interrogation at two tables. The places of main interest seemed to be north Queensland and northern West Australia, Cairns, Townsville and many small towns. Large-scale maps were produced and many very detailed questions were asked, beginning often with openers about where born, what occupation, then attention to roads and beaches, aerodromes, power houses, hydro-electric works, fortifications, etc. The only answers I heard were very vague and misleading. After a quick once through, individuals were picked for more detailed examination.

Meantime, some fireworks were provided by the N captain who declaimed that the compliments paid on arrival were most unsatisfactory and made a scene, talking explosively and gesturing with his sword. To avoid further trouble, I began seeing him and Sato off the premises when the usual B.F. did not stand in spite of a stentorian *kiotské* which had to be repeated with gestures. The Nip officer advanced on him very menacingly and the Dutch interpreter and I had to talk him out of striking him by the lie that he had not heard. He then passed the British orderly room where Nick called everyone up, but there was a lack of uniformity because some had no hats, so there was further trouble. Damn all fools who will insist on getting slapped.

The following were ordered to attend at 1430 hours: myself, Maj. Wearne, Ambrose and Mould, two CCS boys with no special intelligence but who had enlisted in Cairns. I noted one particularly smooth-voiced Nipponese who spoke most excellent English with a slightly American accent, 'You may dismiss them now, I guess.' He had a long, thin face with rather European features, excellent teeth and thin hair (with a close clip of course), a very smooth noice and gesture and a habit of fluttering the eyelids in a sort of ecstatic spasm. I christened him 'Bird on the Bough'.

In the afternoon, Sato was very pleasant. Another interpreter was present, who I think of as one of the *kebetei* crowd, civilian khaki dress and 'golf socks'. He speaks a little English. Spent about two hours with Sato sipping weak, dilute tea and smoking endless cigarettes, talking of sportsman, race horses and racing events, the virtues of Australian race horses and considerable talk of rugger (I am firmly established as our rugger representative at the *kebetei*, damn it). Both Ambrose and Mould were taken away to a small house and interrogated, Ambrose not looking so well, and then Wearne disappeared and had not come back after two hours. 'Bird on the Bough' then wanted to see me. Much preliminary politeness. Talk of family, sport, rugger and then to business. He was a psychologist and interested in the psychology of prisoners, also a specialist in psychiatry. It would help him enormously if I were to write a screed on the personnel feelings of a prisoner of war – a purely personal favour, of course!

One other little matter – he was a very junior officer and most not think it definite but he would like to do his best to communicate with higher authority. Would I like to send a message to Australia? Definitely. Write it on a separate piece of paper. I might be required to broadcast it. Now suggested that no privacy in the camp. Better that I remain at the *kebetei* to do the work. I said, 'Many thanks, but I was sensitive to atmosphere and my own room back at the camp suited me better.' This was finally conceded. The others, Wearne, Ambrose and Mould were kept at the *kebetei*. It was said that they had received some food and that bedding had been arranged. I do not like this.

Further interrogation going on today of those retained at the *kebetei* who have not returned and I am naturally very worried about them. It is rumoured that threats have been made against them and that Maj. Wearne had not co-operated and quarrelled. All COs, adjutants and two senior officers from each camp were called to the *kebetei* and marched to our parade ground and drilled in the *keré* and matters of etiquette for some two hours. This by a Nipponese NCO who was quite polite. I was selected to give the commands. Directly afterwards, the Nipponese called and asked for my memorandum and was told it would be finished at 1400 hours.

A. Personal feelings of a prisoner of war
B. Message to friends in Australia.

The latter might conceivably have some propoganda value but it is agreed by all our officers that it was desirable to get a message through. Interrogation also continued of troops today and Lt Hamilton of north-western Australia had also disappeared. I was again called to the *kebetei* where greeted cordially by 'Bird on the Bough' who has read my memorandum with great interest. I told him that he was indeed fortunate in his occupation as psychologist and must have some interesting material! I conclude he is on higher intelligence staff. He also talks of such things as the clipping and growth of the hair – a remedy for baldness requested! The only real intelligent question was where had I come from. Answer: 'Egypt via the Suez Canal.' Had not most Australians come from there? Answer: No. Some from the Middle East. Some from Malaya. Some from Australia. Much further flap with weak tea and Sato arrived. Then the rest of staff. Asked a few questions about rugger and summarily dismissed.

I saw the interpreter and asked for help re Wearne and the two Queensland boys. They are known to be locked up but are being fed. The guards are kindly and some chocolate and cigarettes to be taken in by the Dutch doctor. Sato assured the interpreter that they were at present OK and he would do anything in his power to help to get them back to us without very serious trouble. Van, in particular, is worried re Billy and has got me a bit too. I will see the *kebetei* officials and state the deplorable effect likely to be caused as regards co-operation if any threat or actual violence occurs. Actually, I used the words, 'There will be hell to pay.'

15 July 1942

The lads are still away. Sato hoped that the two ORS would be back today and has been very helpful. In the RAP O.R. De Longe, who has been in poor health with an infected thumb, today has had a cerebral catastrophe with a left hemiplegia and Cheyne Stokes' breathing etc. A cerebral disaster in one aged 24. He is about to die. I arranged that certain fellow Jews attend for the last rites and funeral arrangements which are being considered in advance since difficult to arrange. P/O Cicurel, Sgt Baker, L.A/C Altman are keeping vigil by his bed.

16 July 1942

De Longe died in the early hours of the morning. It is arranged that the Rabbi come in today for the inside service over the body in the hospital, which a few fellow Jews will attend, and the coffin, which has to be made from old boards in the camp, will be carried to the *kebetei* for embussing to the cemetery.

It was an impressive little ceremony at 1400 hours. A small party of mourners bore the coffin followed by some other special friends and senior officers, including Nick and I. Sqn Ldr Jardine, AFC, was in charge of the squadrons of RAF who slow marched in the rear as far as the *kebetei*.

On reaching the *kebetei*, Sato came out and saluted the dead and the wreaths were placed on the coffin. He accompanied Nick and the small party of personal friends of the deceased to the cemetery. An argument had ensued as to Jewish burial rites, P/O Cicurel saying that it was usual at the graveside to remove the body from the coffin and place it in the earth. Altman, however, maintained that many Jews in England were buried in the coffin. This problem was settled by the nailing up party who clouted the lid down too securely for further argument! Sato took part in the service by sprinkling a few clods on the body of the deceased.

At 1500 hours, I obtained an interview with Sato, Jongehans as interpreter, and expressed my view that immense concern had been caused the British camps by the failure of the Australian officers to come back from interrogation. One further small request, that since the officers were my personal friends, could I send them some cigarettes and tobacco.

Answer: Yes, if I brought them to the *kebetei*, Sato would arrange delivery. I immediately sent six packets of cigarettes and ten bars of chocolate.

Ambrose and Mould were returned this morning. They were interrogated on the first day and asked questions as to Cairns, about which neither knew anything of military value, Ambrose having spent only a fortnight's holiday there and Mould, an English boy, also a short time in search of work. They were questioned as to such things as the beach, the coastline road, and rivers between Townsville and Cairns. After a time, both were locked up, first separately and then together, one blanket only, no changes of clothes, their beards growing. Food, however, was given to them. Finally today, the fourth day, they were taken back for interrogation and no longer the higher staff but simply 'Golf socks' (who I gather was previously at Garoet) assisted by Russell, one of our officers, a Malay interpreter. There was talk of failure of co-operation and what the Nip army did to those who failed to co-operate – definite talk of shooting – however, on long discourse by Russell and much talk, shooting was wiped out. Eventually, they were allowed to return to the camp without further ill treatment but an appeal was first made to their sportsmanship – not to talk to anyone in the camp about what happened to them! They were busy telling me the full story when someone came in to say the Nipponese interpreter is outside. I shot both of them and Russell quickly out the window but when I opened the door found only Jongehans!

17 July 1942

My inspection day. Conditions of the camp are fair now. The Nipponese then announced they were inspecting the camp today and would expect evidence of the benefits of Nipponese drill instruction. They were to come at 1500 hours and at 1330 hours, it was announced that two guards were to be supplied to give a demonstration of Nipponese drill, i.e. one from each camp. Hurriedly, we named them, selecting as many Soekaboemi persons as possible. The Australians can number in Nipponese and understand the drill very well. They put on fine show but unfortunately only the Warrant Officers turned up to see it. Lt Sato was too busy.

18 July 1942

Slapping is rather in vogue again. About eight of the Australian *corvées* coming in today were slapped down for bringing in cigarettes, though this is often permitted. They were allowed to retain the cigarettes. The Nipponese who slapped them was very short and had to swing wildly, far uphill. The results were rather devastating actually – a ruptured eardrum, a broken tooth plate and a tooth knocked out. We have not had this sort of thing for some time.

19 July 1942

Attend today some of the lectures for the first time. Gunner Rees is excellent in French and A/C 2 Gregory MA a fellow of New College, Cambridge – Ancient History (Salamis & Thermopylae, etc.) – a most entertaining lecture.

One or two others nearly slapped down this morning neglecting to salute a private soldier when they passed behind. Still no return of Wearne and Hamilton but reports that they are still in the vicinity in the *kebetei* and locked up. This is solitary confinement with a vengeance. Until they were told they did not even know the other one was next door.

There is a bridge competion amongst the officers. I am paired with Christmas and we are playing fairly often now.

20 July 1942

We hear that Major Wearne and Lt Hamilton are still in this area and that their health is satisfactory. An annoying theft of flour occurred from the canteen bakery last night – one whole bag. Half of this was later recovered from a cooker in the rear of the bakery which is not in use. The bakeries are operating very well, producing excellent bread. Messrs Leach and Carter are now found to be rich in flour.

R74782 Sgt James, W.H., Royal Canadian Air Force died today at 1400 hrs. He has been in low health with malaria and amoebic dysentery and to cap this an acute gangrenous instruction of a loop of the small bowel due to old peritonitis from appendicitis. The Dutch actually operated on him in the small hours of the morning without telling anyone in the camp and made a most shocking mess of the case, deciding that it was a diverticulum of the bladder which they actually considered they drained when they were really in the peritoneal cavity. Something simply must be done to get more control of hospital arrangements.

21 July 1942

Funeral arrangements: specially constructed coffin brought down on a carriage by the chief mourners, accompanied by slow marching escort parties supplied by RAF, British Army and AIF. This procession passed from the hospital to the parade ground, where the troops were drawn up ready to pay the necessary compliments and a service was conducted by Padre Camroux finishing with 'The Last Post'. Wing Commander Nichols, Sqn Ldr Jardine and a few personal friends then accompanied the body to Bandoeng cementery. Lt Sato sent apologies and was represented by his W/O Hoshina. Wreaths were laid before the service by Nick and I, one of which is really from Japanese. A wreath costs 5 gulden. Poor James was just a youngster – a sergeant pilot. His effects were sent to *kebetei* and a letter written as usual by Nick.

22 July 1942

Ns requesting names of personnel who can act for radio direction location. Radio transmitter location. The N NCO found difficulty in explaining what he wanted to interpret. Surabaya was mentioned as the area for operation. We of course replied that we do not have such personnel, similarly Ambonese and D.

Menadonese are far more compliant and gave many names of men said to be radio experts, though I think they would be useless for this job. They have also handed over a number of 'ack ack' personnel to work guns of various calibre and showed no objection to this work. The D regard their present spirit and loyalty as poor. Almost all D males between the ages of 18 and 60 appear to be now in gaol. Landsopvoedingsgesticht is again occupied.

A meeting today was attended by representatives of all companies and squadrons, and all sorts of ideas were presented as to how the camp fund should be handled. There is the grossest misapprehension as to how far a few hundred gulden will go amongst 1500 men. The camp fund is hardly in the same category as regimental funds in general, since portions of it have been raised by such devices as signing on behalf of British and Australian governments and the CO must have the final responsibility. It was, however, explained that the meeting might make recommendations and criticise.

23 July 1942

The third death in a few days: 1017040 Gunner Abraham. This was one of my patients at the Lyceum on the Dagoweg.

With Maj. Moon I interviewed Overste Willikens and the SMO of the hospital, stating our case for our doctors to work on the staff and look after our own sick. (Nothing to do with the deaths, of course! In fact apologies for raising it at such a time!) Also vague reference to Nips, as we know that the Dutch grasp on Bandoeng depends on the Ns letting them run the hospital and they are very frightened they may lose the privilege. We assured them we wanted no official status and would work under their administration and use the same drug economy they practised. They capitulated readily.

Some good ideas came forth today, both of them from Maj. J. Champion de Crespigny (Geoff's cousin), a commercial artist – thick-set, fair, Norman blue of eye, full of life and the lusts thereof. An arts and crafts society for all who can make things to be followed by an exhibition and sale of products; and a memorial sourvenir book to parallel the old *ANZAC* volume – dedicated to comrades in arms in Java. We are producing a newspaper now and probably there will be good stuff forthcoming from it. Artists such as P/O Ray Parkin are hard at work on the camp, and now a series of portraits is to be done with the help of a Dutch artist. I hope that it will be a true record of the manner in which the human spirit can rise above futility, nothingness and despair, since truly we were left here with nothing.

A strong drive was made in Routine Orders today re dysentery, which has reached mild epidemic proportions. Ewan Corlette is most enthusiastic about sulphaguanidine and states that you can get in at the *pain* stage and have practically no blood, mucus loss and dehydration.

Julius Caesar opened tonight, with modern dress; audience very sympathetic with absolutely no frivolity.

Ns had all Australian companies on parade today to check their organisation, absentees etc. One soldier in D company smacked for laughing and talking. W/O Hoshina, melancholy, thicknecked N whom I call 'Pig's eyes', in charge. He also inspected the kitchens (last night he did the British and went round the whole camp looking at the naughty nudes on the walls with assumed disfavour). In this process went into canteen and asked prices charged and costs. This is the result of a bit of propaganda going on between Van, Russell, and 'golf socks'. It becomes increasingly apparent that the D supply officers are slugging us for a handsome profit. They have openly admitted to making profits on certain lines. Hoshina expressed his comparative disgust with the way our soldiers saluted (justifiable). They avoided saluting by appearing not to see him, but crowning disgust was that when they did salute, they did so in a slovenly, half-hearted way without looking at him. (True – same when they salute anybody!)

There is an Australian outside named Douglas, who calls himself Smidt. He is always contacting our *corvées* on the street and trying to get them to take information in and out as to our 'organisation' etc. I am told Brig. Blackburn put this chap on charge (or posted him) as a deserter. We hold no truck with him and do not reply. I seem to remember him as the lad who always had a vehicle and a free pass after the capitulation. He may well be an enemy agent.

25 July 1942

Held a meeting of trustees of the Christelijk Lyceum fund and said the time had come to hand the money over to central control. Probable amount approx. 450 gulden; each officer to still hold 10 gulden. This money given over to John Rintoul.

26 July 1942

Mumps reported. Newspaper *Chronicle* being prepared. Sittings of prominent camp officials begun. Church services very popular.

27 July 1942

Shoe leather removed from QM store by some Ns on 24 July. Letter written to *kebetei* protesting. Nothing ever comes of these protests, but it seems apt that we ask for a return of our propety. Meantime S/Sgt Armstrong and the Q staff are rather anxious lest I let them in for a beating.

29 July 1942

A meeting of group OCs and adjutants, Q staff, John Rintoul etc. to discuss the monotonous nature of the diet and growlings of the troops. Variety is to be introduced with two soups a day for a certain number of days a week, ground rice porridge at times, cooking the free milk into the rice, coconut and cinnamon as flavouring for rice – possibly a fried bread roll of '*Landsop*' type once a week as a change from baked bread roll. Maggoty rice causes much comment. Ground rice is used to thicken soup etc.

Anyone with sulphaguanidine is asked to hand in this life-saving drug for hospital use. Three N officers, 2 captains and 1 lieutenant made an exhaustive inspection in the late evening. N officers were particularly amused by an Ambon band which, when first heard, was playing 'God Save The King' on an amazing assortment of flutes and pipes cut from crude bamboo sticks – one of these most diverting, consisting of one large hollow pipe fitting into another and giving trombone-like or sonorous organ notes. Wily Ambon is rather an amusing soul.

30 July 1942

Kebetei still making a great deal of trouble about our failure to pay adequate compliments and our lamentable *keré*ing, also warning that there is too much contact with outside people by our *corvées* who make illegal purchases. Severe punishments are promised if these practices continue.

Volunteers called for Camp police and Camp barbers, the former a vexed question which cannot be postponed longer since the average soldier will not look after prisoners satisfactorily and there is slackness in enforcing orders. D called a meeting in the doctors' quarters to raise the big storm of the Ambon independent canteen. I attended to grind my own sullen axe with Van, John Rintoul for company. D supply officers, Major of intendance,* present and Jongehans as peacemaker. Simons and Prouse and the other doctors opened the big row by stating already three *corvées* going out, 2 Dutch, 1 Australian. Now this additional Ambon one not really authorised by Ns probably meant trouble. Eventually fixed that the Ambon continue his rather irregular buying under the supervision of D 'morality' (which will, however, no doubt destroy some of his bargaining efficiency!) For once it was not suggested that we give up our *corvée*.

The question of iniquitous prices charged through regular supply channels came up but general opinion seemed to be divided, making this a side issue.

I chose be rather cold and generally insulting and said that it was no wonder that the Ambons had started something embarrassing, as the prices were the limit and at once raised bluntly the question of profits by the supply officers, stating in forthright terms what we thought of that sort of thing in an army at any time, still more when unfortunate prisoners-of-war were involved. A statement from the supply officer was definitely required.

In the hullabaloo of D and Ambon squabble, this point of view was determinedly put aside. Eventually if was decided that *corvées* were to purchase for the camp as a whole, not to profit from other camp sections, but to distribute at cost on a *per capita* basis; all retail sales to be at standardised prices; and there was to be a combined D and Ambon *corvée*.

I then ground my axe with scraping discord, at long last getting to the bottom of things. Big profits have been made. Supply officers originally given 2000 gulden for trade increased to 2500 gulden, but when D camps moved and took with them all but 700 gulden, supply officers without consulting us have gone on to make heavy profits out of us in order to build up a trading balance. Profits at first 28 per cent falling lately to a mere 12 per cent. I said some rather bitter things about not knowing whether I was dealing with an officer of intendance or a shopkeeper, but that in any case I thought that a self-confessed trustee of our money should at once produce the books and let us know how much of our money he held – also expressed extreme dissatisfaction with the whole principle involved. I have no doubt that if we had marched out of the camp without inquiry we would never have seen this sum. We are, however, to some extent held responsible by D since we had never bothered to find out the method of trading from the major. (Recall my unproductive talk with Capt. Segars). Perhaps the D now will regard me as a 'whip of scorpions'. I think Van was a little shaken by my absolute departure from tact and diplomacy. The only reason I have held off this long is fear of bitching his loan. As we have traded some 3,400 gulden through D, there must now be a bonus of at least 400 gulden. John Rintoul is therefore pleased and amused.

31 July 1942

Camp coffee stall opened today with Sgt Stewart (AIF) in charge. Private enterprises closed down. Today, canteen conditions still much the same,

* Dutch ordnance.

Ambon holding the field and D raising the price of 'eggs' to John. (This to cover breakages they say.)

1 August 1942

International sports! in the morning with Dutch teams, Ambon and Australian. Australia rather foolishly entered two teams (UK prudently none at all). Australia lost both relay races, the first by bad stick work,but won both tugs-of-war, contrasting massively with the light, squat Ambons.

It was a curious occasion, with a great crowd of enthusiasts, Ambon and Dutch and Menados (in green for most part) and our strangely assorted and bearded troops all cheering wildly. Also, of course, the inevitable N soldiers straying from the guard room and Sato and the new officer from the *kebetei*, who watched. Sato took special interest in the high jump and insisting on the uprights being further apart – but soon left.

A solitary N did a camp inspection today (strange officer); slapping down and bashing prevalent. Four UK soldiers caught it hot and strong for bringing in tobacco. Tonight, at *kebetei*, Dutch and Menado returns wrong; Hoshina in a towering rage, and struck them both a punch, coming up nearly from the floor. This received by the Menado with tears of pain, D in stolid, silent contempt.

News [my wireless]: Russian front.Germans 150 miles south of Rostov, pushing on to the Black Sea ports on Caucasian front to cut the rail from Stalingrad. Big battle raging in the Don bend to avert Gs mopping up Stalingrad and even worse the Volga area, with the great route, Volga to Moscow, from Caspian Sea. Russia has lost 50,000,000 men, one-third grain, half coal and iron. Will she now lose oil as well? Desert stalemate (too hot I suppose). RAF and American air force raiding heavily Tobruk, vehicle columns etc. Gs of course this side of Mersa Matruh. N landing in New Guinea not going very well. Threat to Port Moresby – they have lost some shipping here. Ns reached Darwin, headed off by Kittyhawks – loss of 30 planes.

2 August 1942

Sunday. Almost one year since 2/2 Australian CCS reached Palestine, so had a *Beit Jurja* Japan party (a garden party) on lawn outside my house with coffee, sandwiches of various sorts served on banana leaves on tables, cigarettes and talk. Over sixty of the unit were present and it was interesting to hear them talking of old times, back to Redbank even; 'Uncle Tom' and his brother 'Portugee' were actually helping Steve in the kitchen and beaming away out the window. Sgt Melsom and Cahill and one other in hospital so I sent some food to them.

A report on the diet is being prepared for presentation to the Ns, as after the deaths this may be a good time psychologically.

3 August 1942

The most interesting feature of the day was a late afternoon large-scale excursion of Nips led by a Lt-Col., some twenty officers, about same number W/Os, and some 50 soldiers – jack booted, sworded, clumping along from the hips down as usual. Went to Radio City; all present compelled to hold a super *keré* for what seemed minutes before *naoré*. Then 'The Band must Play' – it obligingly complied. Next the boxing ring, which was in readiness, so abracadabra! boxing. Starr and Monks obliged and Starr with a little loss of concentration really hit Monks in the mouth, absolutely messing up his lower lip on his teeth which came right through. Blood all over the place. Excellent! This produced the first sign of interest on the faces which were for the most part cast in the oriental mask. Really good show, so passed on to clump through a few barracks. Troops rather overawed and on best behaviour. During most of this time Nick and I had been lured to the *kebetei* by talk of tennis with Sato (via Jongehans); we heard Altmann wildly ringing the bell and came back. At *kebetei* warned that ?Chief of General Staff West Java to inspect tomorrow at 1400.

Boxing and wrestling in Radio City tonight. 'Babe Montana' (Simmonds) had some ribs stove in by his playful opponent jumping on him, so off to hospital. A bad day in the sporting line.

Mark Time, first edition, issued today with a rather horrid and heavy opening page by A/C Carter, today referred to me by Nick for insubordination – elected court martial. Told to think about it for a day and come back! BW* today being 'prepared' for acute dys. [dysentery] which may be a very cute idea. D co-operating; how they love intrigue.

4 August 1942

Inspection by full colonel with three rows of ribbons (or was it four?); attended by Sato and some three other officers, as usual bespectacled and impassive of face. No question, except one or two troops asked age and some comment on *beards*. I said we had no razors, no soap, no money – hence beards! It was intimated that there should be a little restraint in these things i.e. beards to be a little less voluptuous!

'Billy', Maj. W.W. Wearne AIF arrived in D hospital this evening, carried down with acute dysentery.† I saw him and 'arranged' that his temperature be high. He looks surprisingly fit but his eyes a little wild. His interrogation was conducted by 'Bird on the Bough' who showed his tough side at once by saying that we are now under the command of the Emperor and Imperial N army and it was necessary to co-operate or *die*. This was a bad psychological opening, since the ultimatum was too blunt to give a soldier much alternative. Result – instead of conceding some minor trifle – he refused to co-operate. He looked at it from the point of view where will this end if I start talking – there is perhaps no end to the sort of co-operation required. Serious threats were made without avail and then the interogator put a guard on the room and walked out.

From that day he has been locked up in solitary confinement without books etc., though some cigarettes, comforts of various sorts were got in and he was allowed to use a bath nearby. Lately the 'barber boy' [Japanese guard] has been to see him a few times and confided that he was in the wool business. 'I help you – after war you help me'! Sato did at last see that the chocs and cigarettes I

* Bill Wearne.
† This was rigged as an illness to get him out.

sent got in. Billy had some contact with Hamilton who was treated in exactly the same way: blunt threats at beginning causing him to shut down and say nothing, hence his similar imprisonment.

5 August 1942

Recall Bird on Bough's talk about *Hara kiri* to 'Skip' Glowry. All centres round Emperor. Emperor is apparently ubiquitous, e.g. the Emperor stormed Singapore – re Emperor recently took Dutch Harbour, Alaska! A real personal affair. It is, however, not possible for officers to see him. Thus, when they fail, they cannot go to him to make humble apologies. The only outlet for an impossible situation is in the spirit. *Hara kiri* is committed to free the soul from the incubus of the body so that soul may go to Emperor in humility to obtain forgiveness – en route, it is presumed, to some sort of happy hunting ground of the spirit.

There is considerable sports activity at present. Also much activity of arts and crafts doing portraits of camp celebrities. Christmas and I are going great guns in the bridge competition with 8 wins out of 9 contests. This largely due to John's excellent play.

6 August 1942

Inspection by CO [E.E.D.] – lousy show. UK group blasé. Had to go slow lest I walked past these men standing before the next in line rose to their feet! Australian group no signs of interest at all.

Warned of inspection some time today by high Nip officer on 15 minutes notice. Eventually he arrived at 1815 hours when troops should have been feeding. Yellow flag on car, big stuff (Brigadier General), Sato and Sekia in attendance, also several staff officers including 'sour face', who made a scene about our *keré* the day the Intelligence wallahs arrived. A polite Brigadier who removed his cap in our barracks and paid some attention to the courtesies – one of the few who bothered to turn and salute us on leaving the camp.

Gunsho Hoshina pointed out sourly to Mr Diesveldt (interpreter) that he should be addressed with the suffix *Dona*, meaning 'Most noble Lord'. This is an old classical thing recently revived by certain N officers at home in N. Good old 'Hog's eyes' most noble lord in his singlet and slippers and unshaven brutish face.

7 August 1942

P/O Glowry had 20 gulden given to him today by an Australian lady from herself and other well-wishers, also I believe Australians, for the troops' fund. Called to *kebetei* at 1200; there is to be black out exercise daily, 9th, 10th and 11th of this month. The try out tonight will effect the second night of a fine new show called *Hi Gang*.

Deficiency diseases in the camp are fairly numerous and include beriberi and a number of early pellagra cases, also many cases of accompanying scrotal dermatitis. Perhaps Vitamin C may come into this. Vitamin A cases have already cropped up: hemalopia or lack of dark adaption is the first sign, since

Vitamin A is concerned in the production of 'rod red' necessary for this purpose. It is formed from Vitamin A circulating in the blood. Next begin corneal ulceration, corneal opacity and affected sclerotics, loss of corneal tension etc. These are to be treated by placing cod liver oil or Vitamin A preparation in the conjuntival sac, since otherwise absorbed too slowly. In a well-fed European,the Vitamin A stored in the body will last a year to eighteen months, but it is easily understood why Ambons and Menados, who exist always on a diet of little reserve in protective factors, are the first affected. It is, however, a gloomy outlook for us all eventually; scrotal dermatitis, in particular, is very common in one camp.

About seventy arrived from Tjimahi Hospital today including some old friends. 'Denny' Love (quite fit), Lt Bowling, Beverly, and Tom the sailor who was burned with H_2SO_4 and skin grafted. Beverly was made a sitting patient and at the other end was made to walk to the hospital from the station. Naturally tore his skin graft to pieces and opened up his neck wound before he collapsed. Tom the sailor has his beard trimmed neatly and old horrid burns well healed. He is a very grateful patient. Beverly's wounds have healed very well, the main deformity being an asymetry of mouth on opening the jaws, due to facial nerve to mouth region being interupted. Bill Griffiths, the sightless and armless boy, now moves about cheerfully, also Gunner Archie Fletcher has had an operation on his smashed femur.

I made the evening *kebetei* report. There is a new horrid NCO named Corporal Watanabi who rudely ticked me off for folding my arms after *Yasumé*. It is announced that the year is now 2602, Nippon favouring somewhat different ideas of time counting.

8 August 1942

Saturday. *Hi Gang* attended by most of higher camp officials and the few Nips – no officers but Sgt Hoshina, who arrived rather late and seemed for once a little bit abashed. A most excellent show.

We are warned that tomorrow extensive air raid protection measures to begin as an exercise. Blackout to be effective from 2000 hours to 0800 and complete if alarm be given. Also we are to have runners at the *kebetei* to transmit necessary information.

9 August 1942

Sunday, runners arrived in afternoon and caught me sunbathing on the lawn nearly nude. Told me that the whole Australian group must tie a white rag around the left knee, hold their headgear in the right hand and be moved in columns of 8s to the street on the other side of the camp in D area facing to the east! English to do a similar move. Was cursing the Ns roundly when I became aware of Sgt Hoshina and did not know quite the etiquette of greeting him in my underpants. He suggested haste so I called in JDM whilst I had a shower and dressed in the approved style. The movement to the site took 40 minutes.

Full blackout tonight, all except N sentry post at entrance who got into trouble from Sato. Played bridge with Group Capt. Nicholetts and Sqn Ldr Schoppé and for the first time for ages had a drubbing.

10 August 1942

Blackout is very strict. Signals for 'alerts', warnings etc. are to be by siren and also by switching lights at central switch e.g. 5 times for complete extinction.

[My wireless] Large-scale Pacific offensive begun in SE Pacific by Macarthur directed at the Solomon Island group and intended, I suppose, eventually to crush Ns in New Guinea. N planes active at night during blackout. Some searchlight activity. N soldiers everywhere during exercise – piquet streets, and see that all lights out and hunt civilians indoors.

11 August 1942

Saw Sato today and presented petition re Wearne and Hamilton. It is reported W.W.W. is sick in hospital. It is feared Hamilton will soon get sick too. Please N army now return both to camp as an act of clemency and mercy as they have now been severely punished. S was very courteous and polite; Chief of General Staff has been away in Batavia but back tomorrow. Will pass my petition on and hope for good news soon!

Slapping and beating up of our soldiers is now almost a daily affair on *corvées*. In their impoverished state they cannot resist tobacco, which they are usually allowed to keep after wholesale smacking. Today saw about one dozen lined up and struck a heavy slap in the face with a slab of wood rather like a foot ruler. No gross damage done.

Have held up my medical protest re dietetic deficiency until Dutch finish theirs. I think their idea good re *katjang idjoe* beans as a source of vitamins B and C: 100g daily suggested. Further blackout tonight; I was nearly nabbed by two N sent in during a sparks session*

Near thing.

I am informed that my letter was read to Australia, with emphasis placed on my good report of facilities of the present camp and remark that I was being better treated than was Mr Churchill when he was a prisoner of the D! (I made the disgusted resolution never to say anything worth broadcasting again.)

* I was listening in and had just hurriedly turned down the blast of 'Hearts of Oak' on the BBC when I heard the stamp of feet at the door. I snatched the plug out of the overhead light socket, threw the warmed-up set into a box cupboard behind me and covered it with a shirt and turned back to the table, spreading my hands as though in meditation. The empty light reflector was still swinging above my head. Normally 'Blue' Butterworth guarded outside as I listened, but on this night he was not available and I took a serious risk, since I was on the sentry walk. Both sentries with fixed bayonets, one eyeing me off, as the other searched, beginning with my bedding. The thought was in my mind that if they uncovered the set I must kill them somehow, but what to do with the bodies. Desperately, I sought a diversion by offering cigerettes – a Dutch brand. One accepted. Then, to my horror, the other marched me to the door, leaving one to search. I was being questioned as to the occupants of nearby houses and feared discovery in the room behind me. To my relief, when we returned, the soldier was sitting on my bedding smoking the cigarette and the box cupboard had not been explored. It was curious that they had not heard the initial squeal of the set and thunder of 'Hearts of Oak', but perhaps they were not familiar with the sound. All other houses were searched thoroughly.

12 August 1942

Called on *kebetei* with Overste Willikens and delivered report on the diet. Willikens reports since 1 August (12 days) 303 cases of early forms of pellagra scaling affection of skin of face, cloasma and mouth affections, many scrotal dermatitis. Ten per cent of Menados and Ambons affected. We stressed that we wanted to see representatives of N medical staff and show them the cases, which are, however, responding rapidly to Vitamin B treatment.

Surge of D rumours, and Ns make following claims about Solomon Island battle: Americans have lost or have heavily damaged 1 battleship, 10 cruisers, 6 destroyers, 11 transports including *Astoria*, *Australia* and *Minneapolis*. America and Britain now '3rd rate naval powers'. No mention of N losses.

Our side silent. Royal navy have lost aircraft carrier *Eagle* in Mediterranean.

13 August 1942

A court martial will be held against Private Franklin for embezzlement of money in a money-changing swindle. He is a thorough dyed-in-the-wool young scoundrel, who is credited with a statement that if he is handed over to Ns (I don't know where that comes from) he will inform the Ns that Van is an 'SS officer' [Intelligence] and that I have X [wireless]. I am all for a very short sharp Field General Court Martial and would even consider the responsibility of summary action by Lt-Col. Lyneham, who has a written authority for a DCM or even GCM, so naturally, thinks one of those should be held. Good God, as if these things were designed for a prison camp. I am batting for F.G.C.M. but otherwise giving Lt-Col. Lyneham his head as convening authority.

14 August 1942

D clinical meeting re avitaminosis and opposition headed by Dr Simon, who says all the symptoms can be explained, that the report was hasty and will not impress Ns, who have no clinical acumen and will not be interested in an odd rash or two. Maj. Moon and I defended our point of view from the British angle that the strictly scientific attitude was not justified since we were dealing with our troops, not guinea pigs. If they take no action, we can later show the corpses to lend additional point to our argument! In any case, we are dealing not only with vitamins but an all-round report on the deficiences of the diet.

Sgt Hoshina announces we must begin at 1000 tomorrow to do *keré* exercises by platoons and sections, continuing all day! I am cross as I want the sports to be held tomorrow morning.

15 August 1942

Permission to hold sports. *Keré* practice in the afternoon. Needs, our star sprinter was unable to run owing to tinea of feet. I competed in three events for Aust. 1 and won each of them, with the best performance in each event for the day.

Hop Step and Jump	11 m 99 cm (uneven approach)
Discus	28 m approx.
Shot put 7.2 kilo	12 m 10 cm

Nevertheless, owing to losing most of the running events including relays, we only drew with Menados. Aust. 2 defeated D comfortably; Eng. were rather soundly licked by the Ambons (not much talent). These sports are very well run and kept moving. There is something doing all the time.

Air raid precautions continue with severe blackout restrictions, so that shows have to be put on early and tea very early. Lt Ronnie Daclos went to Tjimahi hospital yesterday with appendicitis, the first case for months. Can this be something to do with the diet or lack of it?

16 August 1942

Sunday. Church in Radio City with Fred talking about 'Waters of bitterness'. This Moses cured by introducing the right branch of a tree. I doubt if this could cure the bitterness of my water. The most marked one is in longing for movement to be 'in things' again, which is greater than any longing to go home.

17 August 1942

ARP continues. Lt-Col. Lyneham and Co. are proceeding with the court martial as though it were a Test cricket match. Such God damn bloody nonsense. Troops are selling clothing in a rather wholesale sort of way, I fear, and under present conditions we are avoiding forcing this issue.

20 August 1942

Lt-Col. Lyneham accompanied me on inspection and had a discussion afterwards concerning especially my position in the camp as regards discipline powers, in particular – and especially where affecting UK troops. Eventually we reached agreement as to the desirability of summary punishment if possible, if not FGCM, and he agreed that though I had nothing in writing my position probably sound.

21 August 1942

News at present is all about raid by British commandos and Canadians on Dieppe with big air force action. Our losses said to be 95 planes, enemy 88 shot down. 180 probably destroyed. Russians fighting grimly for Stalingrad and falling back in Caucasus. Mr Churchill has been to Egypt meeting all colonial troops – RAF etc. and then went to Moscow with a large staff for long conferences with 'Uncle Joe' – surely one of the strange meetings of history. Americans mopping up in Solomons. Raids on Timor and still guerilla action. What I dislike is big 'whoopee' celebrations of Ns here over sinking of almost all the American fleet! Local paper pictures dismaying state of American marines now marooned on these islands with no ships to help them!

22 August 1942

Evening *kebetei* told of an American sgt pilot imprisoned in the cellar of the *kebetei*. Sato said he was the chap who claimed to have made a parachute landing on the island but it was all leg pulling. I recall the sensation this story made two or three weeks ago. Sgt Geo. W. Hess (of all names), aged 22, radio operator,

Kansas City. Apparently he was 'out', protected by D living in a house in Bandoeng from capitulation until 19 July when it became obvious that the game was up. He made for the hills and a plantation, where natives gave him away. His story was that he had flown from Darwin in Yank plane on recce – engine giving trouble, parachuted – did not know where he was or where he landed – had walked a long way etc. A big capture for N, and all the big guns of N staff levelled at him for weeks failed to shake his story. He was taken to Batavia for further interrogation and by the time he came back apparently 2–3000 Javanese were looking for parachute and plane. He was then taken to the Homan Savoy Hotel to have his hair and beard disposed of and the boys gave him away as having stayed there before capitulation. Surprisingly enough, the Ns' treatment improved after this and some of those who had been interrogating him seemed to rather appreciate the joke on them (I too). He is still in durance vile. I had the luck to catch him being allowed to have a bath in Jongehan's house and gave him some cigarettes, chocolate etc. Hope he will now be OK.

23 August 1942

Sunday. We are commanded to put Hess on our strength but he is not to be released yet as he must be punished for doing 'bad things' (Sato told Jongehans that he lived with a D girl who is about to have a baby).

Evening notable for the Ambonese band and choir appearing before the brains trusts. Their music is rather characteristic with small range of tone but excellent harmony and rhythm. The Ambon is a rather loveable fellow like a happy child – and, like children, full of tricks and mischief. The Ambon CO, Capt. Tainu, came to see me the other day, as usual bright sparks of fun in his little dark cunning eyes, but more grave than usual: a knight riding the white palfrey of justice. Reported that his Sgt Major had caught a certain Cpl Tennison of the D camp coming from our camp with flour and rice obtained from a soldier in our 'shop' and this had been sold in the D camp! Enquiry revealed that the flour was *Ambon* flour left in our store by direction of the Ambon CQMS who had then sold it to the corporal. The rice was given away as sweepings from our floor. Both Ambons and D are incurably addicted to private rackets.

24 August 1942

Heavy rain last night – no general parade this morning. The pigs are to arrive – eight, I believe, for this camp. Billy W. was called upon by Sato, who seemed impressed with his illness. (He now has officially dysenteric arthritis of the right knee). Hamilton is still confined but is now allowed books and exercise. H has also been having twinges of dys., but unfortunately these do not seem to be severe enough to get him to hospital. S prophesies they will both be released next week anyway.

25 August 1942

Pigs arrived today – 8 fairly well-grown young white porkers. Van has fixed up a stye and there is a little swill to nourish them. *Kebetei* change-over today. Sato made a little speech to both adjutants and COs, saying that the command was changing but that he would not be going for the present and would be coming to the *kebetei* each day to give any help he could. (S is a fine looking little N with very dark complexion, an air of gentle, punctilious courtesy, finely chiselled features and the most elegant bow I have seen in the N army.) He is succeeded by three younger fellows, 2 2nd Lts and a 1st Lt, all seeming young and nervous and not very sure of themselves (particularly the one-pipper who, in a brand new uniform, stood stiffly and self-consciously at attention throughout).

I remarked on their seeming nervousness but Nick retorted that in the N army it is wonderful how nervous fellows pull themselves together if they have to give orders or be unpleasant. The impression of an inferiority sense is quite definite. One has the feeling that they envy us acutely our easy ability to enjoy life even under present conditions – the light-hearted way we play games, have shows, lectures etc.

The interpreter tells an interesting story of having some Ns along to the music the other night and of how they listened with growing sadness, finally all bursting into tears and leaving. Perhaps this brooding bitterness results in their occasional outbursts of bloody murderousness, a sort of *Götterdämmerung*. The Gs have this trait too.

N discipline, though excellent in its way, I think to be positively mediaeval or at least fifty years out of date. The harsh, severe regimentation produces automatons functioning jerkily as one man, the standard, of course, approximating that of the most inefficient man so that he can keep up. The mechanised nature of modern war must call for originality and a man in charge of a complex beast like a tank cannot be expected to behave like a chocolate soldier. They are definitely weak in all mechanised activity, witness the constant requests for the loan of all sorts of technical people such as telephone repairers, motor mechanics, bicycle repairers etc.

Sato, Orchida and another N officer (a propaganda chap) went to my office at about lunchtime and remained there most of the afternoon talking to Christmas, Nichols, John Morris, Russell and one or two other people. They were making preliminary enquiries with a view to radio broadcasts and I kept out of the way as I don't want to be involved in radio publicity or propaganda now that the letters have gone off to Australia. They wanted to know of professional actors (e.g. Bell), someone with a typical English voice (Lancaster) and an 'Oxford' voice (Gregory of Cambridge). The propaganda laddy spoke excellent English and discussed Batavia broadcast, saying that he let them speak directly to the mike – 'he trusted them'. It was indicated that the British were now to have the letter writing privilege.

There seems to be a marked swing to the left wing amongst our lads and socialist ideas are always heartily supported in debate.

There is a surprising rumour tonight that badges of rank are to be returned and pay will begin for all ranks. I will believe these when they arrive.

X [My wireless] Stalingrad in pretty bad way with Gs across Don. Tremendous tank action. Brazil is in the war with us now – a country of 50,000,000 (Nuts) – main activity to date is rounding up Gs and chasing one or two U-boats along the coast. Good egg! Churchill now back in England to riotous welcome.

26 August 1942

Butterworth's birthday. One of De Crespigny's lads ambitious to run a hamburger show along with the coffee stall as a private enterprise. I have advised that it must be a camp enterprise. Fuel is a likely difficulty. Have warned all ranks that camp HQ will not be responsible for swindles arising from private trading; all ranks advised to trade at the camp Trading Post.

The District Court Martial has gone on *over 3 days* (President, Allan Woods). I do not know the finding as yet. I am astonished to find that Allan Woods favours DCM, as he doubts very much if we can call ourselves on 'active service'! He is a shrewd, knowledgeable fellow too. 'Tinkle' Bell evacuated to hospital with severe dysentery today so 'Outward Bound' cannot start tomorrow.

28 August 1942

HMS *Anking*, which left Batavia on 3 March, was to pick up evacuees at Tjilatchap but were warned to put out to sea. Two hundred miles out, the *Anking* (a wireless depot ship), together with a sloop and a mine-sweeper, met with 3 cruisers and 22 destroyers which just shot them up as an exercise piece, completely smashing everything, including all the ships' boats but an RAF cutter and a lifeboat with a hole in the bottom. On these two boats clambered 26 men, with 3 gallons of water and a tin of biscuits. Whilst the few survivors were all struggling in the water, the N ships steamed close and they anticipated machine-gunning etc., but to their surprise all the Ns on deck solemnly stood to attention in their honour! Of course, no survivors were picked up! The two boats were three weeks making the Java coast, one boat rarely without about a foot of water. They ran out of food and water in about a week, but fortunately caught a little rain-water, killed three seabirds and shared them up raw. Of the 26 men, 18 were alive when they reached the coast, where there was a heavy sea running. Only twelve survived the struggle in the rough sea.

One exhausted man, who had clung to a raft all day, attempted to swim to shore but the sea was too strong and it swept him out. That night he found himself being swept between British warships and called for a rope. He received the astonishing reply, 'Keep quiet in the water there'. Next he found himself amongst Nip ships and was picked up by them!

[My wireless] Also N landing in SE New Guinea being heavily attacked by RAAF. Our planes seem to have acquired mastery over NG. Stalingrad is in great peril, Gs flattening it like Rotterdam.

29 August 1942

Sports today–Aust. 2 versus Aust. 1. Victory for latter 70–50. I won 3 events. Hop Skip & Jump, 12m 23; shot put approx. 12 metres; discus approx. 29m. Unfortunate exhibitionism in Hop Step & Jump loudly applauded! (I lost my pants.) Ramsay was only narrowly beaten by Holland with considerable improvement.

An exhibition of arts and crafts articles was held in the lecture room today. Some most excellent wood, aluminium work, needlework, sketches and painting. Handwork of all sorts, including British, Australian, Ambon, Dutch and Menado work.

Group Capt. Nicholetts dealt with A/C Leach summarily: 90 days detention for theft. Franklin's sentence announced as 6 months. Last night I lectured to the Dutch on 'Field Surgery in Modern War'.

30 August 1942

Sunday Called to *kebetei* where Lt Sato formally handed us over to our new commander, a Lt-Col. who will assume command of Tjimahi and Bandoeng prison camps with the three lieutenants working under him at this end. S thanked us for our co-operation in the difficult task of running a prison camp and was polite and sympathetic of mien as usual. The Lt-Col. inspected the camp and, amongst other things, asked three men if they had any money. Answer: 'No – none!' One of the lieutenants is a doctor, I believe. The Lt-Col. is a sallow little man with bushy eyebrows and a weather-beaten face which faintly recalls John Adey.* I fancy he will prove OK, since though not likely to be overflowing with the milk of human kindness he does not appear to have the persecutory zeal of certain young officers.

There is definite talk of pay in the air, though not official. I wonder. It is extraordinary that they have not made themselves generous hosts with a few turns of the printing press, thus reducing old war liabilities one day and creating a chivalrous atmosphere. Van and I think that though they have no morals, financial or otherwise, they are extraordinarily prudish.

31 August 1942

D *corvées* not permitted today. Our convoy officer P/O Glowry was treated very roughly by a warrant officer who, though saluted correctly and smartly, resented the fact that the party did not begin 'salutation' as soon as they caught sight of him! Result: a ruptured ear drum – a common accident these days. One wonders if there will be any ear drums left intact!

There is some prevailing nervousness outside which one rumour stages to be due to a N officer being assassinated or badly wounded. There is a rather remarkable change in the number of planes about, notably less Navy Os but also 96s. 'Outward Bound' play is a great success.

1 September 1942

Officers now forbidden to go out on *corvée* and Ns are arranging themselves to bring in the foodstuffs ordered through canteens to avoid any contact with Indonesians. Some Ambons arrested – tonight suspected of a conspiracy because they were having a church service. They were later released.

[My wireless] Stalingrad still holding but sore pressed. Australian success in Milne Bay area – now mopping up but heavy fighting at Kokoda. Americans holding Solomons.

Today, N medical officer starts to earn his grub: says we have more dysentery

* Col. John Adey, Psychiatrist, Australian Army.

than the D and native soldiers and must pull our socks up. Next, instructions to his grandmother as to how to apply the dear old oral orifice to a hole in an egg. Segregation, care with kitchens and so forth advised.

2 September 1942

Some N officers including our medical friend to inspect latrines. Further comments re dysentry. The new Lt-Col. 'boss', Kawamura, is at present working at *kebetei*. He is said to be keen on the *keré*, a cult not infrequent amongst the Nips. This sort of thing could perhaps be best indulged by special *keré* resorts, where true believers could indulge in ecstatic services of *keré*ing to their heart's content!

3 September 1942

Education: This is now a terrific programme in the camp, as the following figures will show. There has recently been a mid-term vacation and the latter half of term commences with a course of secondary studies: arithmetic, English, geography etc. The instructors are now to receive special consideration in allotment of duties.

Statistical report

Number of attending students	1207
Number of subjects taught	30
Number of instructors	40
Number of classes held weekly	144

Instructors

Sig. Fry	Lt Allen	A/C Longden
Sgt Wynne	F/Lt Boadman	Sqn Ldr Jardine
Sgt Wiseman	Sgt Baker	Lt Thode
Sgt Firby	Maj. De Crespigny	W/O1 Topping
A/C Gregory	L/Bdr Goulding	Pte Arnot
Lt Russell	Lt Miller	Sqn Ldr Roberts
P/O King	F/Lt Carr	Sgt Brady
P/O Bonaldson	Sgt Sheppard	Sqn Ldr MacGrath
F/Lt Phillips	Bdr Blake	Gnr Rees
F/Lt Rayment-Action	Sgt Griff	A/C German
Maj. Greiner	Lt Thirion	
Sgt Haddon	Maj. Moon (Medical Off.)	
Capt. Craig		
Lt Crisp		

Dutch

Dr Portman	Mr Binnendyk
Mr Cappers	Sgt van Klierden

Van, of course, senior educational officer, is a tower of strength, with an intellectual quality and depth of view beyond most of us. He is a most remarkable person and amongst the few really well-taught people on this island.

4 September 1942

Visited D dentist who is getting very low in amalgam etc. – I don't think the present diet is frightfully good for the teeth. Endeavoured to straighten out D troubles re the *kabaret* they are putting on and the request for more tickets to Outward Bound. Their affairs are fraught with the most dreadful misunderstandings owing to an utter lack or organisation and integration internally. Arranged that an extra night of Outward Bound be played to give them all tickets (when required) at the expense of Freddy Camroux's church service (hard battle that). Pointed out that church is on another plane altogether to other camp activities, but an occasional sacrifice was the sort of thing church represented! Orchida at evening *kebetei* and to my great delight promised almost immediate release of the two prisoners (Wearne and Hamilton), warning me they must not speak to the rest of camp about their experiences. I replied that they were 'sportsmen' who would play up, realising this would be the sort of thing sufficiently incomprehensible to get over. Also thanked him profusely for his great kindness to these unfortunates. Told Billy, who was of course delighted.

Also asked this morning for some hosing and a water cart to rig up an old pump as a 'fire engine'. Result: Ns all interested in fires and are doing an inspection soon. Rigid prohibition of peripatetic smoking (can only smoke outside near a special container).

5 September 1942

Sports in a.m. Asked Nick and Lyneham to put to their troops the principle of pooling *corvée* money and particularly mentioned the question of this being adverse to UK if it were a general pool. I hope they will be big enough to do it but it will need leadership to keep things on the right sort of uniform basis. Some sort of pooling will be required to retain our camp organisation and stop everything going to hell.

Great evening. Called to *kebetei* pm to receive *Hamilton*! He is fairly well but fat and white like something you find when you turn over a stone. He is definitely not so wild in the eye as Billy was and has stood his severe gruelling very well. He answered questions up to a point, sparring a bit until 'Bird on the Bough' asked him to draw maps of his particular locality which was first big refusal. Then things went from bad to worse. For a few days he felt shooting was very likely then gradually got confidence in situation. There was only the one interrogation with very nasty threats of death.

6 September 1942

Lt-Col. Lyndham in a great state because his Regimental Stretcher-bearers are not being included on a list of Red Cross Personnel the Ns asked for yesterday (name, rank, nationality, specialty, whether employed or not). I agree we should include them. The thing that emerges is that Ns are now recognising the Geneva Convention (or rather, saying that they will do so – quite another matter).

Prisoner Leach has achieved mild dysentery, was put in the hospital room with instructions to stay there and piquet posted. Promptly started breaking bounds all day. Yesterday he succeeded in getting a shirt from a comrade and exchanging it for cigarettes. His most notable stunt to date: selling portions of pencil lead to Ambons as flints.

Van has written a most lofty deed of trusteeship for the memoirs book and the camp commander is to determine all questions of major policy. A board of trustees is headed by the senior educational officer and Maj. de Crespigny is the Editor-in-Chief. I attended a meeting today and saw some of the material.

7 September 1942

At morning conference today, Ian Cameron was stating his troubles re kitchen when 'Nick' calmly announces that he wants Russell to look after his kitchens – poor Ian thus dropped in the most ungracious way imaginable, in spite of loyal, steady and devoted work with UK troops over a period of months of terrible difficulty. I intend finalising this question of camp control or getting out. I have poured out my troubles on Van, who is quite sympathetic and will, I think, support me.

8 September 1942

Have given notice of a special conference in the morning to evolve a new organisation of camp affairs. Nick, Lt-Col. Lyneham and Van as British Army representative will attend. The question of staff, including my own job, will be discussed. I wish to have some permanent system evolved; things are too labile for my liking. The instruction from the new command makes interesting reading.

'Now that I have become the Commander of this prisoner-of-war camp I inform you of the following. Recently the POW camps of Bandoeng area have become the first division of the combined Java Prisoners' Camps. Having become the commander of this division, it is my duty to supervise and control you. From now on you must obey the orders of myself and those appointed under me, follow the instructions and behave in an orderly manner. Also be careful to uphold the *honour of your own country* by not neglecting your duties as a prisoner of war.'

Lt-Col. Hideo Kawa Mura
Commander 1st Division, Java Prisoners' Camps
Sept 17th year of Syowa

With this, talk of *corvée* pay and of return of badges of rank, things are looking up. We now have new guards: Koreans who have not, I understand, had any real active service. They are rather brutal and most of those slapped down do not quite know why. I think it is due to new smoking regulation condemning 'peripatetic' smoking.

9 September 1942

Rain now almost every day, usually late afternoon, and the weather is hotter. Butterworth is intensifying the gardening. I have now given away most of my own money, so we will have to be very careful.

Meeting was held and I put all my cards on the table, giving an account of how my command had gradually developed and regretting that it had been more or less forced upon later comers. I frankly recounted my difficulties which were amongst others:

- a Only authority voluntarily ceded and sometimes withdrawn abruptly
- b No direct contact with officers or men of either group
- c No strong feeling by officers and NCOs that they must enforce the camp order – slackness of guards, piquets etc.
- d Difficulty in getting suitable men (poor support e.g. police etc.)
- e Discouragement of my staff by interference (e.g. Cameron and Willey)
- f Defeat of common weal principally through lack of prophets to preach it, e.g. *corvée* pay.

Did they want central administration or not? There are two separate problems: the first is the partly military one of maintenance of a force; the second is a body and mind problem. Central control was agreed to be necessary. I do not particularly want the job of commander, but I will carry on providing there is clearly defined authority and absolute support. The meeting agreed that there should be no change of command, but that the role of adjutant was now too great for John Morris to combine with his theatrical responsibilities. This principle I accepted, and he should choose which he was to be. A committee consisting of Capt. Lancaster, Maj. Beaney and three adjutants is to draft new orders acceptable to the three commanders.

During this meeting an altercation took place, Leach assaulting his two guards, who had taken from him a diary and library books. Japanese soldiers, who saw the affair finished up putting all three in the cage. John Morris intervened and told the Nips that Leach, a man with a grudge against authority, had assaulted these excellent fellows who were chosen to enforce the law. (No mention of the cell or theft.) The police were released with apologies and the diary (a most amazing affair of Leach's supposed experiences in Russia, Iceland and the Far East) was given back by Orchida. Leach was detailed in custody by the Ns.

We are now filling in two sets of records, one a card register of all prisoners with particulars of prisoner and relatives and a slip which records name, unit, place of capture etc., and also state of health (0 = good; △ = below usual; x = illness). Today the doctors are examining all ranks with a view to classifying everybody in those categories and getting statistics. I had a difficult conversation with Ns re *unit*, as they wanted unit as regiment and division. I said could not give as government forbade and would punish. They said, 'Nonsense! the Ns knew all these even before they came to Java – what was the good of making trouble now!' I said, 'Good. The Ns knew our units and divisions anyway, our government know if we merely give numbers, therefore there is no point in giving more and getting punished!' This line of reason did not please. I was told orders were orders and I must consider the N army, not my own government who now had nothing to do with it (old attitude). I then said but there *were* no Divisions; we were merely detached corps and service troops. This was acceptable; we are to give the unit and name of the expedition force

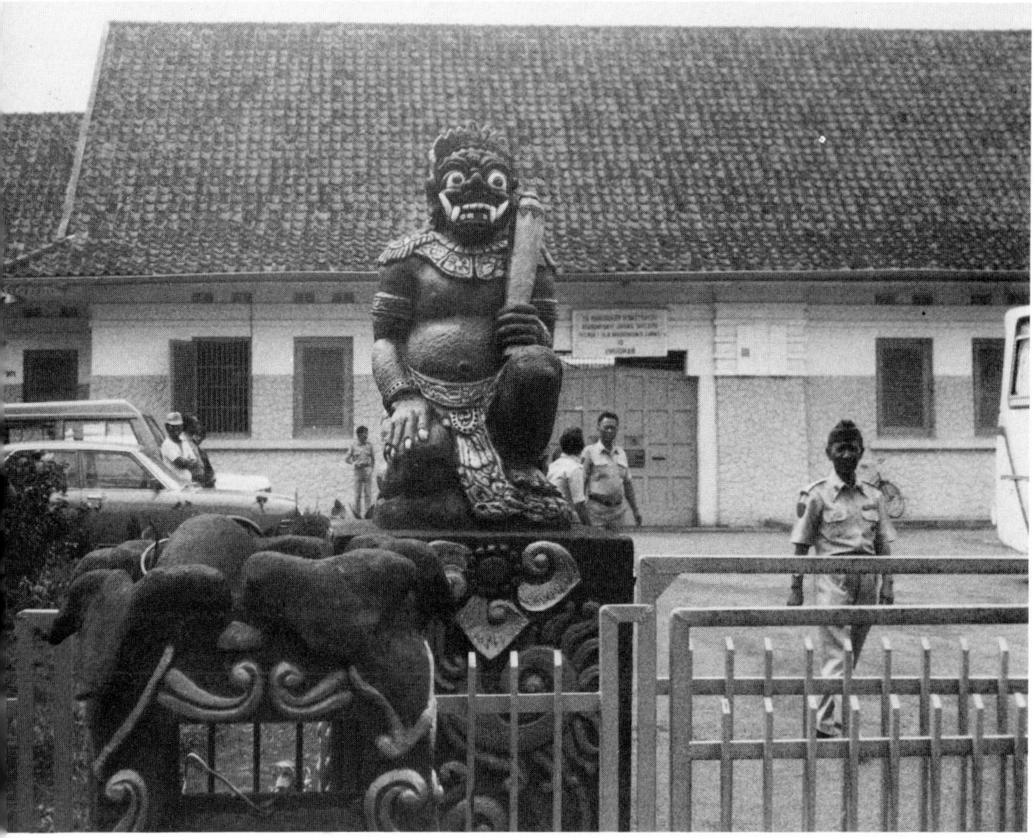

Entrance to Landsopvoedingsgesticht, 1985

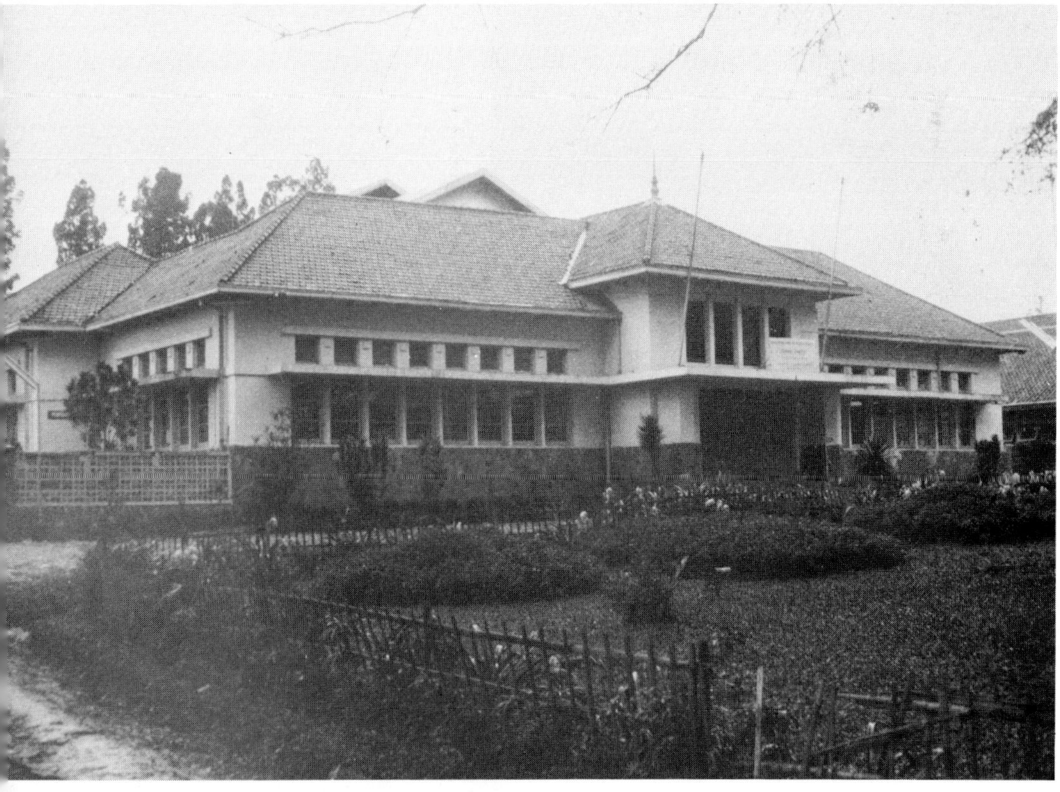

Christalijk Lyceum – the school which was converted to
Allied General Hospital

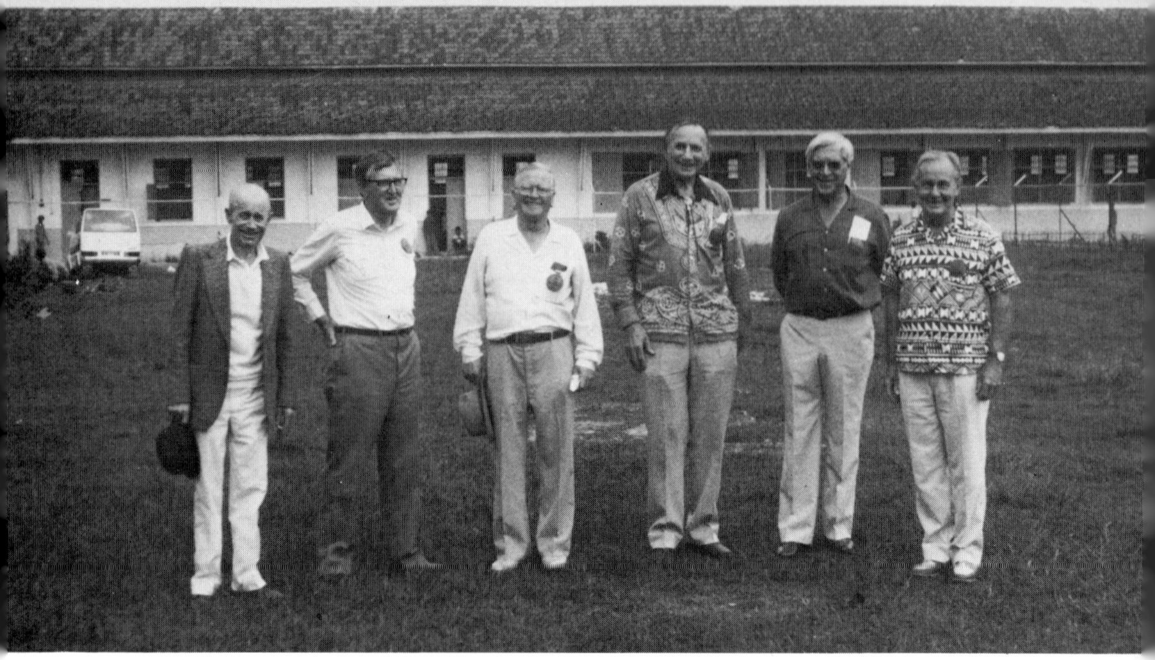

21 Old inmates of 'Landsop' revisiting in 1985. *Left to right*: Bill Garvie, D. Jackson, 'Blue' Butterworth, the author, J. Goodrick, L. Poidevin

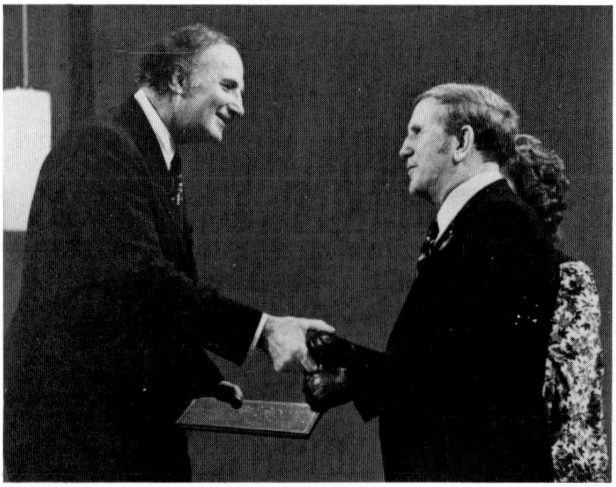

22 The author and heroic Bill Griffiths, my blind and handless Java patient, in *This is your Life*, 1979

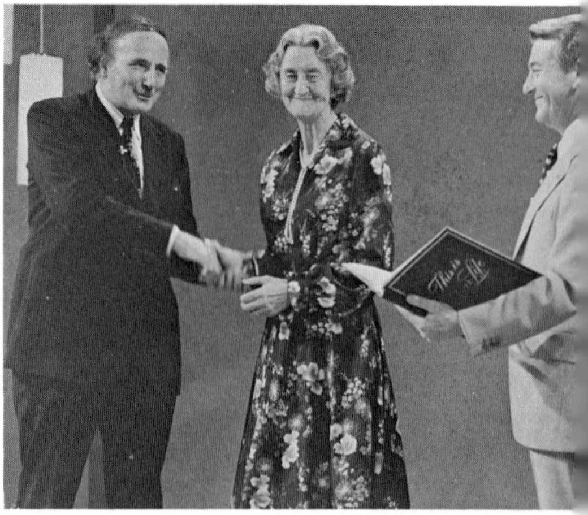

23 The author with Mevr. M.A. de Jonge OBE who was Matron, No. 1 Allied General Hospital, Bandoeng, Java, in *This is your Life*, 1979

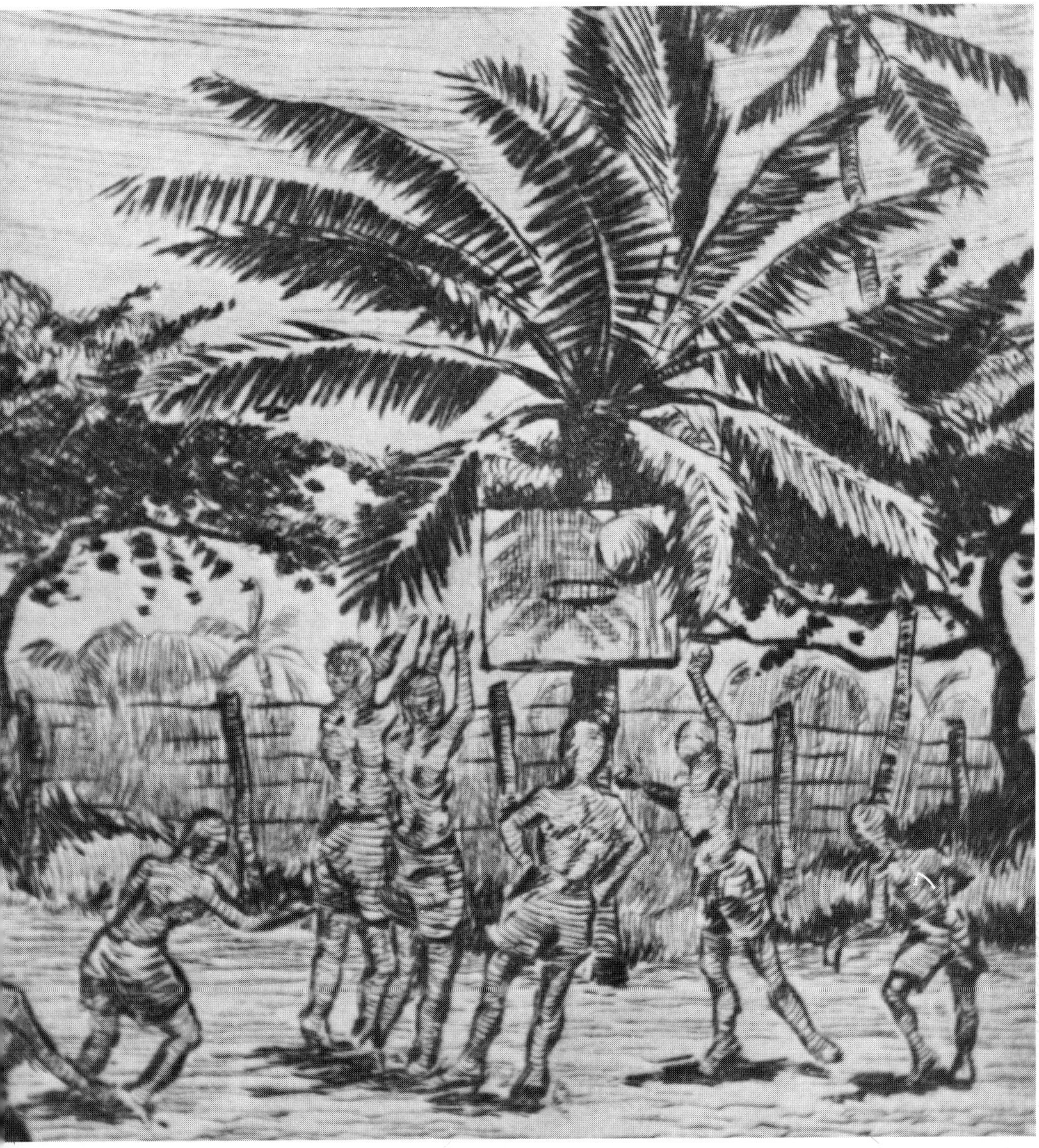

Basketball, Christmas Day 1942 (*Ray Parkin*)

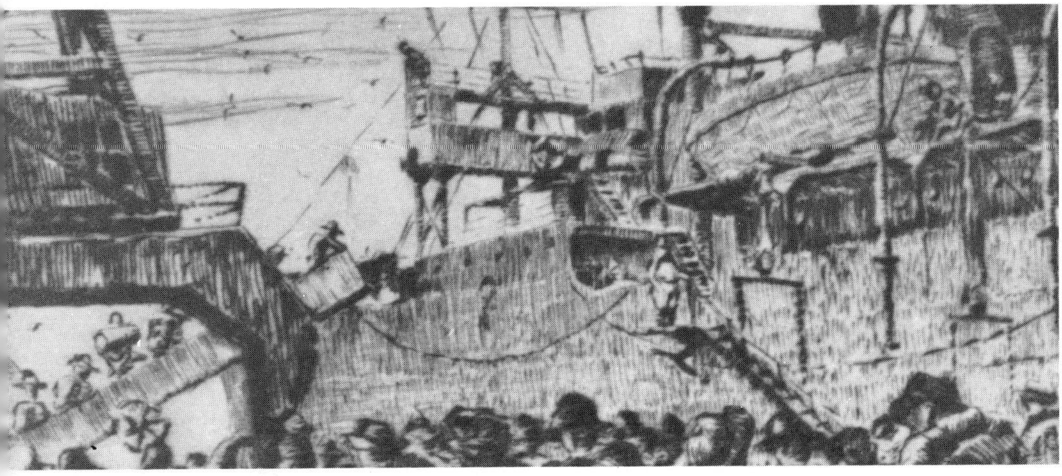

ıbarkation, *Usu Maru*, Tanjongpriok (*Ray Parkin*)

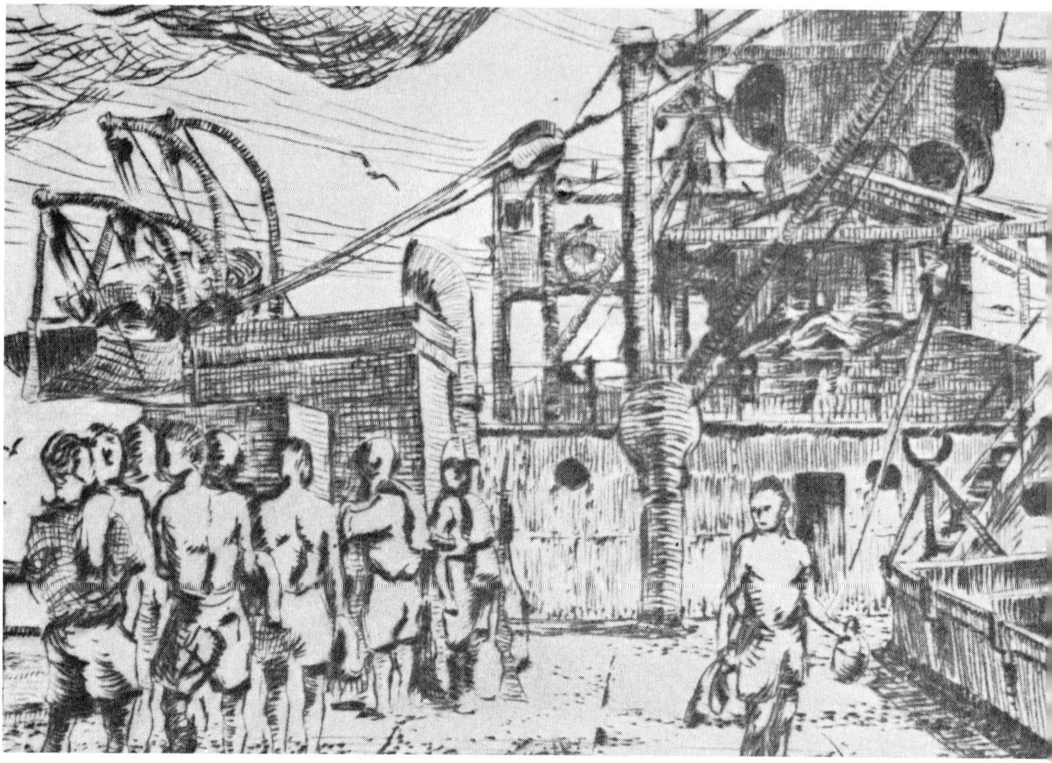

26 Water queue on deck, *Usu Maru*, once daily (*Ray Parkin*)

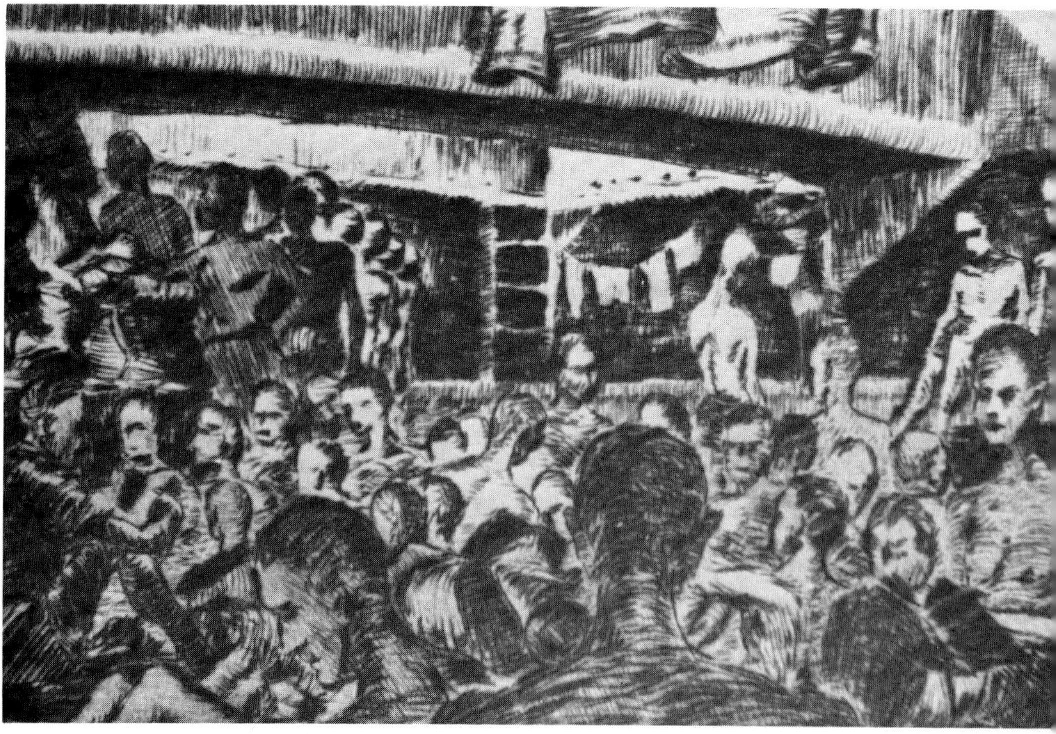

27 *Usu Maru* hold accommodation en route to Singapore (*Ray Parkin*)

'Blackforce', e.g. 1 Inf. Bn Blackforce, Westforce Java, RAF Far East Command, East Indies Squadron, Royal Navy etc.

10 September 1942

Vegetables increased to three times the amount. Promise of badges of rank soon. Great prospect of 5,000 gulden. Following document –

> Have received goods (foodstuffs) to the value of £1,000 from Mr K.J. Tan of Batavia. This amount being payable by the British and Australian Governments on demand.
> Brage Import Maatschappym
>
> Batavia e. 28 Feb. 1942
> *L.J. van der Post Lt-Col.*
> *G.E. Nichollets Group Capt.*
> *E.E. Dunlop Lt-Col.*

Leach is wandering about in camp today buying fountain pens for the poor Ns. Soon he will have the N treasury depleted! Warning given of inspection tomorrow and address by N. Lt-Col. in command. Microphone to be used.

11 September 1942

All troops on parade in column of eights, football ground, by 1930. N commander scheduled to arrive at 1000, but as usual about 1030 hours. 'Undergraduate' arrived shortly before 1000, made some minor adjustments of position and also gave us the drill for the *keré*. Commander arrived, flying his red flag on the car which drove up on the right. It was truly an odd scene: the squat, lighter skinned, plump Menadonese and the dark, woolly-headed, irrepressible Ambons (real chocolate soldiers with green uniforms), then UK and Australian, a sort of storm of confetti though of more impressive physique. Finally, the green of Dutch (Camp 5 medical, practically all *white*, 6 very mixed with ungainly bodies). A poor advertisement for racial mixture – led, however, by De Waal, who is a fine looking, grey-haired fellow with odd, clear hazel eyes which glint attractively. This mass of troops approximated 5,000.

The 'undergrad' took some photos. A few Nips riding about on bycycles with the inevitable sword. It is odd how a N officer looks quite at home on a bicycle, though in truth some of the soldiers with fixed bayonets remind me at times of Boadicea's chariot. The Lt-Col. first gave the address of the Major-general in charge of Java Prisoners-of-war, Batavia. Orchida – a new Orchida in smart uniform including cap and polished tan leggings (replacing golf socks), plus samurai sword and 5 green stars of air force on breast, star on arm – then interpreted first in Malayan, then English (Dutch neglected). The acoustics were peculiar, recalling someone bubbling underwater with fragmentary snatches being hurled over our heads like the staccato warbling of magpies! The same performance was then repeated with the Lt-Col's own instructions to POWs. Finally, the Chief having departed on a positive hail of *kashira nakas*, the commanding officers were hailed forth for some camera work by 'undergrad.' and old 'split the face smile'. Troops then dismissed.

12 September 1942

Evening soup with the Dutch doctors, a sumptous affair. Overste Willikens, Dr Lampa, Pruis, Simons and co. Table in garden outside recalled to me the last occasion I had sat down to a meal of that sort in Jericho! *Katjang idjoe* soup, a most thick nourishing affair with potatoes and even portions of a recently-killed pig. Vitamins of course ++. Soup (which had rather the aroma and flavour of pea soup) was followed by chocolates and cigars (definitely the doctors do well!). I left early with apologies and played bridge with Lt-Col. Lyneham and Tim Godlee. They bidding a grand slam and romping in with it.

13 September 1942

This afternoon Leach and Hess were released by Nips – the former of course returning to gaol (requesting his diary). It was announced that a new officer was in the N Guard room. US Army Air Corps Bomber Pilot 1st Lt Raymond George Teborek, 24, American, US Army Flying School, Kelly Field Texas. I managed to see him 'to fill in a form' but could manage very little conversation. He was rounded up from hills recently and has been with *kempi*. Says he feels very short of good food and looks pale and ill.

14 September 1942

Ramsay Rae* taking over duties today. Also Capt. Burdon (new adjutant) is on the job. Police question is under discussion as 20 policemen are badly needed. There are 7 prisoners and the cell is only advisable for three. Prisoners are giving endless trouble and only three of the present 12 policemen are efficient.

Returning from 1600 *kebetei* report today I was met by Cpl Zanetti (police) who said that Leach had been taken out of the cell to obtain watches by Nip guard. I went straight back and spilt the whole beans about our system of punishment to Orchida and expressed concern that the guard should have let the prisoner out – no doubt a mistake (I did not mention watches.) Orchida was most concerned and called the officer in charge of the guard who was very helpful, like Mr Moto speaking quite good English. They both seemed to feel that interfering with police and discipline was very serious. They were unquestionably anxious to atone by killing Leach and I back-pedalled hard. 'Leach was a man who gave much trouble?' Me – 'Yes, but he is only a foolish boy.' This point appreciated by both, who laughed. Officer in charge of guard went down to 'blow up' his guard who were terrified and denied knowledge of Leach. I had to take the officer and two sentries with fixed bayonets to show them the cell; both Japanese sentries pale, trembling and sweating.

Leach and other prisoners trembled still more when they arrived and Leach was pointed out. They then left with thanks and apologies. Later on in the night guard had apparently been getting a proper mauling, several showing signs of having been beaten up – all rushing around returning watches. It seems some Japanese had to return watches without getting money back.

* Wing Commander Ron Ramsay Rae: a fine athletic Australian serving with the RAF.

15 September 1942

It is now extremely wet in afternoons, usually about 1600 hours. Football ground is getting very wet and soon parades will not be possible there. This also affects sports badly. D are having one of their waves of incomprehensible optimism, expecting to be released in a day or two. This is said even to go so far as the women buying new evening dresses to receive their men when they go out. This, of course, is delightful nonsense for the most part.

16 September 1942

Innoculation commencing with typhoid, dysentery, cholera 'cocktail': we are to have three doses! Great stir in G.C.'s house by the birth of a duckling to Sqn Ldr Schoppé, the first of his icebox-electric incubator conversion. This triumph was duly written up in *Mark Time* daily news by the Officer I/C Pigs (Van) with cartoons showing Schoppé in bed with the duckling.

Education is flourishing mightily. The police are busy in a fever of activity converting new cells – these unfortunately on Nick's side and one of them quite hopelessly small. Today the N Lt-Col. accompanied by Orchida, came along to see a small exhibition of specimens of arts and crafts work with a view to arranging sales (mainly wood and aluminium work).

17 September 1942

Decided to arrange immediately at least one meal of *katjang idjoe* each week (cost approx 18 gulden for camp), also some salt to whole camp at least once a month (perhaps ¼ block each).

Our detention centre was shown to the Group COs with a view to stopping talk of brutality. Strange that as conditions improve there is more and more ill-considered criticism of everything and everybody, and of course camp admin. is always a fair target.

There appears to be a big N movement out of here and they are very busy. There were 400 D rifles approx on the floor of *kebetei*. D rumours now really prime: Ns leaving and the rifles are for their own police requirements; all Gs and D fascists warned by Ns to make their way to Singapore. They are about to be released etc!

Yesterday our troops had a big job shifting bombs locally; apparently most of the bombs were allied types. No one has complained about this as yet, the first really troublesome job for some time.

I approached Ns diplomatically for brooms and brushes required for hygiene purposes with suitable flowery remarks about the interest they were taking in our sanitation and the dysentery menace. 'Undergrad' told me that they were extremely busy, very busy indeed. They would first 'try to get us our fire-fighting requirements'. Later they might see about the brooms and brushes.

18 September 1942

Health of Camp: Report upon inspection 9/9/42. Normal health (0) 69%, Below Par (△) 27%, Definite Illness (+) 4%. (Bad illness.) Aust. 0:66, △:31.5, +:2.5, UK 0:72, △:22.5, +:5.5. Criteria for △ were mainly loss of weight, recent illness, feeling and appearance of patient. Malaria: many having relapses and very little plasmaquin available.

[My wireless] Stalingrad hard pressed with terrific fighting in streets on outskirts – looks like the end. Very heavy raiding RAF over Ruhr with loss of 39 bombers. New Guinea: tough fighting and enemy now 32 miles from Port Moresby.

Hand over of *kebetei* again, and our immediate commander to be 1st Lt Susuki, an obvious base wallah and a sort of officerial Hoshina with a big pot belly and great plump face with heavy growth of black beard. Three medals on the chest and a man who likes his beer, I should think. The guard are now absolute 'rookies' (most of them not even one star), brand new uniforms and Dutch rifles (which they have been shown how to load by Menadonese!). They do, however, take to drill smartly under the very critical eyes of the NCOs and look as if they will make soldiers all right.

Our camp police have been given armbands, and our stumpy Zanetti entering the *kebetei* was given a rousing *keré* from the guard – perhaps they thought he belonged to the *kempi*!

As his last act the 'undergrad' produced our badges of rank today – or at least the one or two bits and pieces left of them. We were told that if necessary we could wear D badges. Of course we said we could 'make them'. And that as some people at Tjimahi still did not have badges, we must only wear them on one side. Then what with the D raising questions of where they would wear them on their collars, it was ruled that we must all wear them *on the R. breast* as the Ns do when wearing a shirt. Nothing would persuade them to alter this except that commanding officers were to wear full badges (of course I still have mine). I am aiming at getting one full set of badges for everyone and then asking to be able to wear them on the shoulders. G.C., Lt-Col. Lyneham and adjutants are putting all their badges on.

19 September 1942

Ramsay Rae, a vigorous new broom with keen ideas, is actively on the job and nearly sacked my camp CQMS today when he asked 'Who would clean up the Q store if canteen products were sorted in there?'. Also questions the payment of 25c a head to D for hospital people. Sig. Wright fell from roof at *kebetei* where he was working this afternoon and broke his femur. Nips promptly called for doctor and stretcher and he will go to *kebetei* tomorrow. The new show, *In the Bag*, is excellent and includes 2 new song hits by JDM, one by Bernie Weller. Play (one act): *The Thread of Scarlet*. Excellent Ambon stringed instrument band (guitars for most part) and Ramsay Rae sings well – the usual sketches and gags.

The Group Captain and Sqn Ldr Schoppé are having bad luck at present with four of their fowls dead and only one duckling up to date. Their three rabbits, however, are does, and have all been left simply gasping after the attention of a large Flemish giant, who rolled them about in rapid succession. They are such hungry bunnies that they are even killing a large tree by eating the bark from the base.

20 September 1942

Sunday and a quiet day. We discussed the expansion of the accommodation in the education scheme. Ian Cameron is willing to change over from his big Q store to one of the canteen rooms. (Ian is always 100 per cent better than his Scottish façade leads you to believe.) Church with Chaplain Blakeway (always well attended). Billy Wearne is now co-operating with Van in the educational scheme and is full of life. Brains Trust tonight: Van and Nick and I – 'Believe it or not' has come into embarrassing popularity.

There is some beriberi amongst troops and a constant dysentery rate including some amoebic.

21 September 1942

Much trouble this afternoon owing to prisoner Franklin being reported out of his cell 1345. All prisoners have been reported to be getting out at night, another key is suspected, also connivance of the guards. New squad of police (Aust. and Brit.) are now detailed for police duty and take over today. Two of the kitchen staff positively identified, Franklin equally positively denied the charge, but under pressure confessed that he gets out through the back wire window barrier. A masterpiece involving the removal of the barbs from the wire with bare hands. Finally slid out like a snake as a demonstration. Punishment: 2 days solitary.

Franklin amazed me by referring to my wireless set and said he would tell the Japanese and have me killed if I did not do a deal. I told him, 'Tell them and be damned!, I will tell a few reliable men that you are a traitor and to kill you immedately anything happens to me.'

The new rookie guard are smacking people about in a most wholesale way and they often do not understand what for. Today those in trouble included Capt. Smith (who is about 6 ft 6 in.) and was amiably strolling along smoking a pipe and, to add to his crimes, he forgot to salute a N soldier. Grunts and roars; obliged by removing pipe and saluting, then replaced pipe. Fresh grunts and advance of Nip. Pipe finally removed and the good Capt. indicated his rank badges in vain. He was forced to *bend down* to be slapped. I am surprised that they have not invented a camel action of going down on one knee as a drill.

22 September 1942

This morning notified through Jongehans that we may wear full badges of rank. Following additions to be made to the diet from Public Fund. *Katjang idjoe* soup at least once a week, a little curry and monthly salt issue to each man. The D claim wonders from the *katjang idjoe* bean as a food. From the source of previous 1,500 gulden a further 500 gulden arrived and was handed to Mr Rintoul. Discussed this with John and suggest at present this be held separate from the fund. All other money held to be used on troops including old Allied General Hospital Fund.

Inspected the hospital where we have a number of cases, mostly dysentery and malaria relapses, one coronary thrombosis, one case of spinal haemorrhage with wasted legs and back (only able to stand with crutches). He is a relic of the ill-fated HMS *Anking*, one of the party of 26 who got in the two boats and of which finally only 11 Europeans and 1 Chinese are left. An officer, Gibson, has beriberi and amoebic dysentery. There are two cases of catarrhal jaundice. My old patient, Atherton, has early beriberi sys (the case shot through the chest, both pleural sacs); Bob Haddon is very thin and wasted and is in Dengue fever.

1530. Trouble! The new guard have just been playing hell like the little tin horn inferior sons of bitches they are – trying to get a little confidence I suppose. All camps are complaining. Their stock in trade today was walking into classes, kitchens etc. and smacking everyone about for reasons too obscure for us. This happened to a very large squad over at the Menado canteen this morning, including two officers of ours. Zanetti came running to me because Maj. Denman had been slapped in the drawing class. He was not smoking and did not notice anyone else smoking. He was struck by a *gunsho* after remarks he did not understand who then proceeded to take his name etc. I ascertained the facts and then deliberately became very angry and ticked them off (unfortunately in English), indicating I wished to report the matter to *kebetei*. I chose to be very truculent and ignored the two soldiers' bayonets which followed my back closely as I walked away in contempt, taking with me the battered Denman. Eventually decided to discuss the matter first with the guard, and Diesveldt arrived as interpreter. They seemed unsure of themselves and the *gunsho* concerned had left (I refused to allow him to use my bicycle). Soldiers looked a bit shaken but tried to brazen it out.

I then went to *kebetei* with Denman, and Nick and reported the whole thing and the unexplained orgy of slapping which I said we associated particularly with the new guard. He said that they were new, fresh from N, and no doubt are not very familiar with local orders and procedure. He would speak to them and make sure that no further soldiers were struck for 'things which they would not understand'. The Nippon Commander staggered me with the phrase 'They think that you are savages.' This had some confirmation when on my way back I saw the guard hurriedly erecting barbed wire baricades about the guard house. I later realised that they were largely Korean guards.

We are told that we must have plague innoculation tomorrow in the middle of our second typhoid, dysentery, cholera injection. Pestis vaccine is prepared at the local Pasteur Institute and lasts about three days (it is a live vaccine and requires expert care).

23 September 1942

There is constant patroling about the camp, whistles and alarms at night. It is a fearsome thing to see these fellows load their rifles which poke in all directions. At the *kebetei* recently, one got a round jammed in the spout and had to have assistance from his NCO.

24 September 1942

Slapping much improved but the extreme annoyance of constant patrols which expect the full compliments as for officers. Today a soldier went to the GC's house and was dissatisfied as to compliments paid. They merely stood at attention and bowed. (Apparently Wing Cdr Bell, who was nearest the door, should have called them up to the *keré* etc. He was marched to the *kebetei* where he was made to stand for a long period with knees at the half 'knees bend' position. Sgt Hoshina, the NCO concerned in yesterday's fracas, gave him a long impassioned harangue, his mean little pig's face shining with fury and veins prominent in the neck.

25 September 1942

VX25681 Pte Stephens G., 2/3 M.G. Bn, C. Company died suddenly in Barracks at 0845 hours immediately after breakfast. Diagnosis was difficult, but given as ac. hypentensive heart failure and beriberi.

Funeral service began at 1430 hours with escorting party of deceased's own company and one RAF party. Orchida arrived with wreaths and apologies at 1500 but no lorry, which did not turn up until 1610. Lt Susuki and Orchida came to the cemetery Algemene Affgraafplaats Pandoe – weg Bandoeng (8 bearers, company captain, Jongehans and I).

The Bandoeng General Cemetery is a lovely place, beautifully kept, sombre cypress trees, but many gay flowers and beautiful little birds. The native gravediggers quickly took over the coffin (after the long tramp our sweating bearers had to the graveside) and it was lowered into the grave in the rich red looking earth. Padre Blakeway then conducted a further simple little service and dropped some earth upon the coffin. It was all over very quickly and Orchida asked did we not all want to drop earth on the coffin. 'No.' Did we not want to mark the grave with wooden cross etc.? 'We are making stones – could we come out one day soon and lay all the stones?' This was agreed. Hoshina even expanded a little under the 'jovial atmosphere' of a funeral, at which Ns are at their best, and asked me conversationally if we were all Australians!

26 September 1942

Today, a *corvée* of 2 officers, 20 NCOs and 218 ORs left Camp around 0900 and marched to D ration store near Landsop (2 miles) to unload seven trucks of food (six to seven trips with carts over a rough track about 7 miles in all). No rests or smoke-oh. No lunch. Men frequently forced to double with the carts. One man collapsed completely, 6 were unable to continue, and several had to be brought back on the carts all in. The party returned to camp at 1515 hours. Butterworth was one of those who went out and he came back a tired and crestfallen man with no further interest in *corvées*.

Mock debate of Bandoeng Parish on a matter of a legacy of late Thos. Blogg. Propositions argued: Fox hunting pack (Ian Wynne); Home for fallen women (Gnr Rees); Cadet training ship (P/O Abbott – the Admiral!); or Home for illegitimate children (E.E.D.). The general tone of the debate was the reverse of lofty, with homosexual charges against the admiral! The Nips interrupted and inspected my 'Statistics' graphs of illegitimacy! Abbott romped home.

Today Red Cross cards being hurriedly sorted at *kebetei* with Horry Williams helping and being given cigarettes and plenty of good food.

27 September 1942

List of officers asked for today and Jongehans told Frank Burdon that this was on account of pay for officers as from 1 September at rate of 20c a day. I wonder!

Tinkle Bell taken out today by some Ns who wanted the 'Actor Bell'. They gave him an audition reading Huxley and said OK, then took him out to an hotel nearby. (I thought of Christ taken up on a high mountain and promised the earth.) They then said that he would be 'filled in' in a few days to broadcast British letters and he must not speak of it to anyone. Nick and I feel anxious for him, but can do nothing.

28 September

The prisoners Leach and Franklin continue to misbehave – stupid fellows. Maj. Moon compiling a medical report on troops' health and difficulties with working parties through low diet, the number with impaired health, lack of boots etc.

The sum of 500 gulden was distributed yesterday to needy officers (all who had less than 5 gulden). Lt-Col. Lyneham and Sqn Ldr Jardine arranged the distribution. It had been decided to make a canteen dividend of 50c a head to all troops tomorrow, paying by companies.

Nips decree now that all soldiers must be in barracks by 9 pm. This affects our lecture arrangements, which usually do not finish until a later hour, also entertainment.

29 Septembr 1942

Orchida invited to diplomatic afternoon tea with Russell and asked for the following: release of Teborek; some beds for officers; to have night classes carry on after 2100 if necessary; permission for Xmas arrangements; and given general facts about weakness of men and *corvées*. We gave him a picture by Parkin and an arts and crafts trinket box for the Colonel. He is a pleasant little fellow. Noted that he was suffering from a 'mallet' finger inflicted yesterday, and I offered treatment.

Burdon reports that Ns promise *corvée* pay from 1 October (10c a *corvée*) and pay for officers *at N rates*. Jesu! Horry Williams reports that Ns said Axis have things fixed. N to have Australia, Netherlands, Indies, China, India, Siberia, Italy and Africa; Germany is to have all Europe and South America. 'What are you going to do with us?' he asked. 'Of course we are going to kill you!' 'And Australia?' 'Kill them all!'

30 September 1942

American Teborek released (he was the officer out with Hess, I find). Orchida laid on the beds but could not fix classes after 2100.

Ns not quite so tough now – one pulled a cart today and gave Hillyard his rifle to carry on *corvée*. There is a story of a Menadonese who, when hit with rifle, to save his head, caught the rifle which came away in his hands. The N guard ran for the guard house for support and fresh arms. The terrified Menado ran after him trying to give the rifle back to avoid being killed but before he could catch him they ran into a N officer. He smacked down and beat the guard for losing his rifle and magnanimously pardoned the Menadonese.

1 October 1942

The following clothing requirement have been requested of Ns: *Australian camp*. Boots 734, Towels 550, Shirts 636, Shorts 520, Hats 108, Socks 900, Singlets 580, Drawers 560. Immediate minimal requirements indicated are smaller but this, of course, is the real requirement.

The pay question: it seems officers are to receive the pay of equivalent officers of N army, i.e. in my case 220 yen per month, but 60 yen per month is to be deducted for food, quarters, electric light, gas, water, etc. (*NB*: Our food = 10c daily!)

Also we are to be encouraged to save, so we have a savings account and even a dependents' sum (which will be paid after N captures Australia and defeats UK to establish new order). Meantime, the sum is ¥20 for those major and over, – ¥10 up to captain! *Corvées*: 10c ORs, 15c Sgts and S/Sgts, 25c W/Os each *corvée*.

What will our government have to say and will we pay the piper? In any case, much of the money will have to go to the troops and this should be done as a central camp scheme.

2 October 1942

No rain and oval and ground is very dusty. Group commanders are having some trouble over evasion of *corvées*.

3 October 1942

Trouble is brewing, since Nick is supporting a scheme to take from each officer all his pay except 2 gulden weekly. The rest is to be used for the troops and, it is hoped, one day will be repaid by H.M. Government. I support the idea but think that the method must be voluntary. However Lt-Col. Lyneham is entirely opposed, since it seems that the officers consider that certain troops are not worth being given officers' money and have not been grateful for previous money given to them. This is magnificent – it seems that an officer's duty is something which is only carried out if the troops are worth attention (i.e. those of 2/3 M.G. Bn)! The idea is that officers retain their money and help the worthy troops independently (buying gratitude).

4 October 1942

Ns today required a return of all educational activities and some other peculiar details: number of personnel in (1) Industry; (2) Mining; (3) Fishing, Cattle Breeding, Agriculture; (4) Commerce; (5) Officials and teachers; (6) Traffic and transport; (7) Building trade; (8) Public works (road etc); (9) Regular army; (10) Others.

5 October 1942

COs' parade – troops looking pretty rotten these days and more collapses going on (Page the trumpeter yesterday). Maj. Moon and I went to *kebetei* and presented his report to the doctor about the declining health of the men, deficiency diseases, low calorific value (2200 cals), low protein (60 grams). Doctor did not counter this very much, commented that dermatitis of scrotum not necessarily B2 deficiency – was told it responded marvellously to yeast. He also suggested that collapse might be sun stroke (No!).

At conference this morning raised Nick's argument re officers pay. Lt-Col. L. said he would never sign such a thing and his officers would object while I did not myself suport the manner of effecting the idea (which should be voluntary) we would have to go into question of proposed expenditure first to find out what was not necessary and. I asked R. Rae to do this. L. saw the Group Captain and represented the situation as his being requested to sign a ridiculous document to do with unauthorised seizing of officers' money; the latter said, 'It should be voluntary – you had best sound your officers out.' Result: a series of meetings in houses along 'officers' street' called by Beaney, who put the proposition that we now had sufficient money to look after the troops for 10 months (600 gulden a month – good God! as if 600 a month was a real contribution!) and therefore the officers were beautifully relieved of responsibility for an indefinite period. Amongst the people who were told the financial situation is Ramsay Rae who is engaged in working it out! I am livid and so is Van. I saw the GC, told him the truth of the affair and asked him to attend tomorrow's conference! He intimated that he would now like to command the camp – let him know when I would like to hand over.

There was quite a considerable explosion today in a nearby munition works south of Bandoeng.

[My wireless] In New Guinea, Australia have pushed N back to Owen Stanley gap. Much air activity in that region: our planes seem to be calling the tune. Americans now staging a counter attack in Aleutian Islands and have occupied some in the middle of the chain. Things almost wound up in Madagascar.

6 October 1942

Conference! Group Captain, Nick, Lt-Col. Lyneham, Ramsay Rae and I. I was in fighting mood and just gave L everything straight on the chin as to the state of the camp's finances and the troops' health and what I thought of the action in holding meetings yesterday. Particularly my disgust in his going to the GC without discussing the situation with me, which I said was not only a breach of military procedure but also of normal decent behaviour between human beings. The GC heard the facts and said of course the officers would have to contribute as a duty and sardonically remarked that it was not often that five colonels met to discuss such a matter.

7 October 1942

Helen's Birthday, God bless her wherever she is. Figures being prepared for expenditure on troops' diet and other essential camp expenses with a view to a meeting of officers and discussion as to pay etc. Meantime the balance of the 5,000 gulden is drifting in steadily. Arthur Moon is going carefully into the dietetic questions. The health of the troops is a source of considerable worry–

over a third of them now look quite ill, thin, pale and drawn. Nearly everyone is underweight with haggard, lined faces. Burning feet is one source of terrible discomfort, the feet being most exquistely sensitive, and sleep and rest are being lost. These cases are not responding to yeast, though the Bandoeng Balls, perlêche and stomatitis respond very well.* I saw a case today who had just developed absent knee jerks as well (presumably beriberi). The real source of worry is perhaps a combination of evils: diet only 2200 calories, protein only *60g*, with little range in protein and an absence of biological protein (meat, eggs etc.). Massive doses of Vitamin B1 by injection will now be tried for this lad. The acute syncopal attacks and one or two heart failure deaths are also a great worry. We intend to give a least two *katjang idjoe* meals a week and two eggs weekly to supplement the diet.

There is at present sustained and terrific clerical activity at the *kebetei* doing the Red Cross cards and making master rolls. Harrison-Lucas and Williams still work there like beavers all day and night. I am now becoming interested in French and my Dutch is wilting. I go to Rees for French and am reading a bit. A Sgt King speaks fluent French and he speaks to a small afternoon circle.†

8 October 1942

Ns taking great interest in our occupations which they are 'not satisfied with'. We have to fill in a new return classifying us into some 40 types of occupation (numbers only), also hefty master rolls in alphabetical order are to include occuptions. I discussed the limitations we intend to supply them (re technicians of value) with Nick and L who is quite cheery today. [We always concealed skills of value in war.]

The play *Journey's End* opened today.

9 October 1942

Ramsay Rae is starting a branch of canteen in officers' lines. F/O Charlton, who is conducting a technical works course, is to take over control of the works departments, retaining Ambrose Etherington on his staff. Beaney snooping round asking John Rintoul for his canteen books instead of approaching me in the correct way. Reason obvious: wants to examine the books in a critical accountant's fashion and there find faults and reason why he was 'misinformed' and misled. Fortunately, John Rintoul is a tough nut to crack. Discussed finance with Van today who expressed an outright desire for real 'communism' – all officers to put everything into the pool and live purely on the men's diet. This sounded rather like the New Testament; it has me in, but I fear it is impractical. ORs would not do the same thing themselves and would not understand, but that would not matter particularly.

Discussed plague injections with Overste Willikens and Arthur Moon. D army is not vaccinated against plague – unless they are doing some special job in

* Bandoeng Balls: a deficiency disease manifested by a raw, weeping scrotum. Perlêche was rawness and ulceration at the corners of the mouth.

† He was originally French – Le Roi.

the kampongs with Indonesians. Immunity from injection lasts six months. As a catastrophe might be terrible with live stuff, we decided to 'cook it'.*

Australian action in cremating with full N honours the bodies of certain N officers who died in the raid on Sydney harbour (where 3 submarines were lost) and returning remains to N in urns is regarded most favourably. Also learned of the sinking by a submarine of a N ship between Singapore and Philippines on which there were *1800 British and Australian prisoners*. Some were picked up by other ships of convoy, some swam to islands, but apparently loss was heavy. This clearly indicates shift of troops form Singapore to Nippon.

It is reported to me by Harrison-Lucas that all the medical cards relevant to officers have been put aside, also a certain number of medical personnel ORs. Question: does this mean a shift and, if so, what for?

10 October 1942

We are now informed that all the doctors and the two dentists (20) are required, also approx. 80 British ORs. This worries me since, if all these move, the camp will be cleaned out of MOs and dependant on the Dutch for a service. I went to see Overste Willikens who met me with the plump finality of a stone dropping into a well and at once said 'goodbye – good luck – pity we have all got on so well together here and come back to Bandoeng and stay with me some time!' Tentative arrangements were made with D to take over medical arrangements if we have to leave. They are shocked with the 1730 hours arrangement! [Later] It seems definite that the Australian medical officers are now out of the move though perhaps not indefinitely.

11 October 1942

Lazy day. In pm spoke to Arthur Moon about the old Dagoweg A and D book (Hospital Admissions and Discharges record), which I find to my horror is far from complete. They are going to try and complete it as far as possible before the UK fellows move. One of these days there is going to be a terrible struggle completing a report on the hospital activities. Records are terribly scattered and inadequate, thanks to Nippon.

12 October 1942

All British doctors and the dentist Frank Graham (14 officers in all and 15 sgts, 60 ORS, total 89) to move tomorrow with some Dutch and Ambonese, the whole making an obvious hospital unit, presumably to operate in some prison camp. The party includes amongst the ORs 'Nobby' Clarke, Clephan Bell, Sgt Baker, Cpl Nicholls, Cpl Burch and just about a clean sweep of 'Women' theatrical experts, including Radcliffe, Altmann etc. Theatricals are about the hardest hit, with about twelve foundation members. I arranged with Robbie Cummings to take with him 300 gulden on the basis of anticipated expenditure on troops in this camp for the next three months.

The Nips are showing a great interest in health and our rise in sickness rate.

* We boiled it to kill the living plague bacteria.

This results in a most extraordinary demand that UK Group provide on paper tomorrow for each person, 2 small specimens of faeces, the paper to be duly labelled with the serial number of soldiers and name (to be handed in tomorrow by 0900 hours). Everyone in the camp is most extraordinarily vitamin conscious – at Sunday Service Padre prayed specially for those suffering from food deficiences and I waited to hear of special prayers for those suffering from vitamin deficiences in sections A, B, C, D, E etc! This however did not eventuate.

Grass receives special mention in *Mark Time* daily news tonight as a great vitamin substance and I can see the troops taking to grass. The wily Ambons are great vitamin seekers and climb the highest trees to seek a few vitamins. Particularly do they seek them in the officers' lane.

2300 hours: a rather sad little gathering at my house for cocoa and a sandwich (Blue and Steve) with Robbie Cummings and his officers. How we will miss Robbie, Sqn Ldr MacGrath, Wiley, Peach and Co. They are a solid force for good in the place and so are the rest of the gang, including the ORs. I think their destination is Batavia. I said my farewells and wished them luck, observing that we were now experienced prisoners-of-war.

13 October 1942

Robbie Commings and men marched out at 0630 hours. Officers had during the night been *paid in full* for 2 months (less 60 gulden a month living deduction) so they were luckily well 'oiled' up. I went with them to the *kebetei*. S/Sgt Armstrong is the senior NCO and should be all right. I returned, watching the soft beautiful colour of a typical Java dawn breaking through the sombre clouds to the east, the dark drooping outline of Java trees, and a brooding quietness and a sense of transparency of air washed clean by rain. Java dawns and sunsets are often supremely beautiful. I then rolled up in my blanket and spent a luxurious hour thinking of Helen, who always comes to mind when I think of lovely things.

Morning conference discussed finance: Regimental Fund must be kept separate from the imprest account, certain sums to be transferred from imprest as needed. There was an existing mechanism for purchase through the Regimental Fund committee and PRI, guided by the doctors. We discussed how these transfers of money could be shown in the Regimental Fund without undersirable publicity of imprest money*, and decided to publish in *Mark Time* each week the additions to diet, and to publish for troops' information only a list of expenditure of canteen money. In view of the pay of departing officers last night, it was decided that a meeting of all officers should be held immediately to discuss policy of donating money to the imprest fund. This is only necessary because of the deplorable action taken by Lt-Col. Lyneham and Beaney in holding a series of 'indignation meetings of Aust. Officers' which have hopelessly prejudiced the whole system. I anticipate some difficulty still from that quarter.

* Imprest money was obtained largely from sympathetic Chinese traders, underground sources and officers' donations.

Meeting in Radio City. I in chair with Ramsay Rae; Arthur Moon ready with medical facts, Rintoul, and Capt. Burdon acting as secretary. I opened the meeting asking for absolute observance of confidence as wished to give frank information about financial matters involving dangerous negotiations. The following matters were out-lined

1 *Serious* decline in the troops' health now developing rapidly;

2 Iniquitous nature of the diet. Everything possible being done with Nips but we must help ourselves;

3 Origin of the Regimental Fund and its battles

Present Capital		
	x1256	Stock / Debtor / Cash
Imprest Fund	x3750	
	x5006	TOTAL

Total cash available for expenditure at present is 4024. Anticipated minumum expenditure from now on to be 1200 gulden monthly. Average to date has been only 560 gulden monthly; this must be greatly increased.

An outline was given of proposed expenditure, emphasising that only necessitous items were considered: food and medical including Sanitation requirements; boots if possible; little on Works dept.; Christmas effort (education, arts and crafts, sporting, theatrical if any crumbs to be spared). Every effort to raise outside money would be continued, but unfortunately this was most difficult and could not be counted on.

The situation was helped, however, by officers' pay totalling 1340 gulden a month on present strength. (Troops a negligible factor as far as *corvées* are concerned.) I recommended Wing Commander Nichols' proposal as a good basis for officers' voluntary contribution.

UK Field Rank	10	120	Aust	13	156
Under FR	44	88		44	88
Total:	54	f208		57	f244

This total is 452 gulden a month, each officer retaining only 2 gulden a week, and would enable the minimum necessary to be put into action with confidence of steady expenditure over three to four months to come.

Arthur Moon then outlined the gravity of the medical position, stressing that the expenditure of 1200 gulden a month was not necessarily the answer, but was the best that he could arrange with present resources. He accurately painted the picture of ill health. Ramsay Rae gave more detailed facts of financial interest and outlined what the expenditure would give. I then invited discussion, particularly from Group Commanders. Here, I said, you have heard the minimum required: let us do better than this and put in all September's pay. Lt-Col. L. unfortunately spoke first, and after an introductory admission that some help should be given, devoted the rest of his speech to statements about the poverty of his officers (particularly junior) and their own impaired health. First, he suggested pay back the 500 gulden recently distributed – this sufficient for September – then in later months officers could decide what they would do (voluntary).

Wing Cdr Nicholls was very curt and to point. What are we giving men? Little more than 2 handfuls of *katjang idjoe* and 2 eggs a week which will only keep men alive. Our duty is to put money in and we can't rely on outside money. Let us ensure that the monthly sum reaches 1600 gulden. Donate September's pay and all above 2 gulden a week. Some English officers think they should give more than suggested; it is our *duty* to give *at least* the sum suggested.

Major Beaney's deplorable effort consisted of unfavourable reference to the fact that the 89 men marching out last night were given 300 gulden, and a series of persistent attacks on the accuracy of the figures given, insinuating that the fund was adequate for six months without officers' aid. Ramsay Rae dealt with most of this. I was livid but said little.

Group Capt. Nicholetts completely bowled out Nick and I by deserting to the side of the angels, suggesting officers raise only 330 gulden a month (no reference to September pay). Meantime, keep trying to raise outside money. F/O Cadell was for officers giving 300 a month and all September pay. Van der Post supported Nick.

Capt. Macnamara then made a rousing speech about the plight of the men; were officers going to contribute, or did they want to lead out eventually a regiment of crippled and broken men? Billy Wearne believed we should put in all our pay for September and October; Lancaster supported Nick. I endeavoured to smooth things a little by saying that, as the administrative people responsible for the health of the troops, we must ask the maximum effort, agreeing that it was hard on officers who had suffered and some in worse circumstances will need special consideration.

My final statement was that it is a difficult job to run this camp with all the grave responsibilities entailed. I was prepared to make way at any time for any senior officer who could make a better job of it. If, however, I was to continue to discharge these responsibilities, I would not flinch from the task. I thank you therefore for expressing your views, but I shall now write to each of you personally requesting your donations at the level we have recommended.

I left this melancholy affair in almost the lowest frame of mind imaginable and disgusted at the light in which Australian officers had been shown. Imagine, after a clear statement of the miserable health of the troops and low finances, to hear a discussion by officers as to whether they would give the help required. Where is that principle 'my horse, my men, myself'? The leadership in this matter disgusting, and I feel I handled the meeting badly.

14 October 1942

Beaney at am conference. Ramsay Rae treated him like a draper's assistant and I should like to do the same. I drafted a memorandum to OC's Group asking that officers contribute pay on the basis of yesterday's request unless hardship is involved, particularly those recently loaned 5 gulden. I delivered this to L later.

He read my memo and said, 'Well, I suppose you are right. I will take the matter up privately with each officer and let you know.'

15 October 1942

Ns want daily particulars of men unable to walk to the station. This may be significant in view of careful information requested about various categories such as staff officers, technical officers. I somehow think moves are in the air.

Tinkle Bell was asked for after his move, so I suppose they must have chosen him for Batavia.* Spoke to Ns today re tools for various camp works. F/Lt Charlton is on the job and seems a first class chap. Have looked over CCS records and find there are painfully few left, even Routine Orders being lost. I will try and reduplicate assembled records – God knows if I will ever be able to make much of a report.

16 October 1942

I have seen during the last two days some excellent specimens of deficiency disease – pellagra type scrotal dermatitis (Bandoeng balls), perlêche – typical tongue. Rash on hands, ulnar border of forearms and elbows. A characteristic, though, is that great numbers of troops are troubled by *intense burning of the feet* and an exquisite sensitiveness which scarely enables them to walk and they cannot sleep or get any rest. I have seen one case who has also a slight burning of hand on ulnar side (one hand only). He is the only case that shows a tendency to the unilateral. In general, these cases show slight exaggeration of knee jerks, but one or two cases exhibiting the phenomenon have lost their ankle jerks. It is disconcerting how long it takes for improved food and yeast (of which we have great hopes) to do any good. We use a thick paste, black specimen of yeast (up to date we have only been able to afford about two teaspoonfuls per case daily). Some are having also injections or Bl, 1,000 units (300 units said to be curative). Some nicotine acid is also available.

The pellagra-like cases are not showing diarrhoea symptoms – which would seem to be late – and no marked mental sys. There are one or two alarming cases of failing vision (two soldiers have vision about 5/60 and can't see to read – there is a definite optic atrophy showing up). This is grave and would seem to be linked up with Vitamin B1 and neuritis. Capt Ifould AIF is amongst those with burning feet etc. in hosptial. A little *tempe* (a yeast product with a pleasant flavour) is to be added to troops' diet.

17 October 1942

Two Dutch officers (one the big fat interpreter) called in today with 50 gulden for Lt-Col. Lyneham from the PROVOS (this being almost certainly Douglas).

* The Japanese requested names of men suitable for broadcasting and expressed interest in Bell, Lancaster and one or two others. They had noted his booming theatrical 'Old Vic.' voice. He came to see me seeming rather exalted at the good he might do broadcasting news of prisoners to home. I said gravely '. . . remember when the pressures are on you and you are all alone, that you are really just an aircraftsman and can't . . . lose us the war'; also I heard later that when the intolerable pressures came, he had cut his throat with a razor blade.

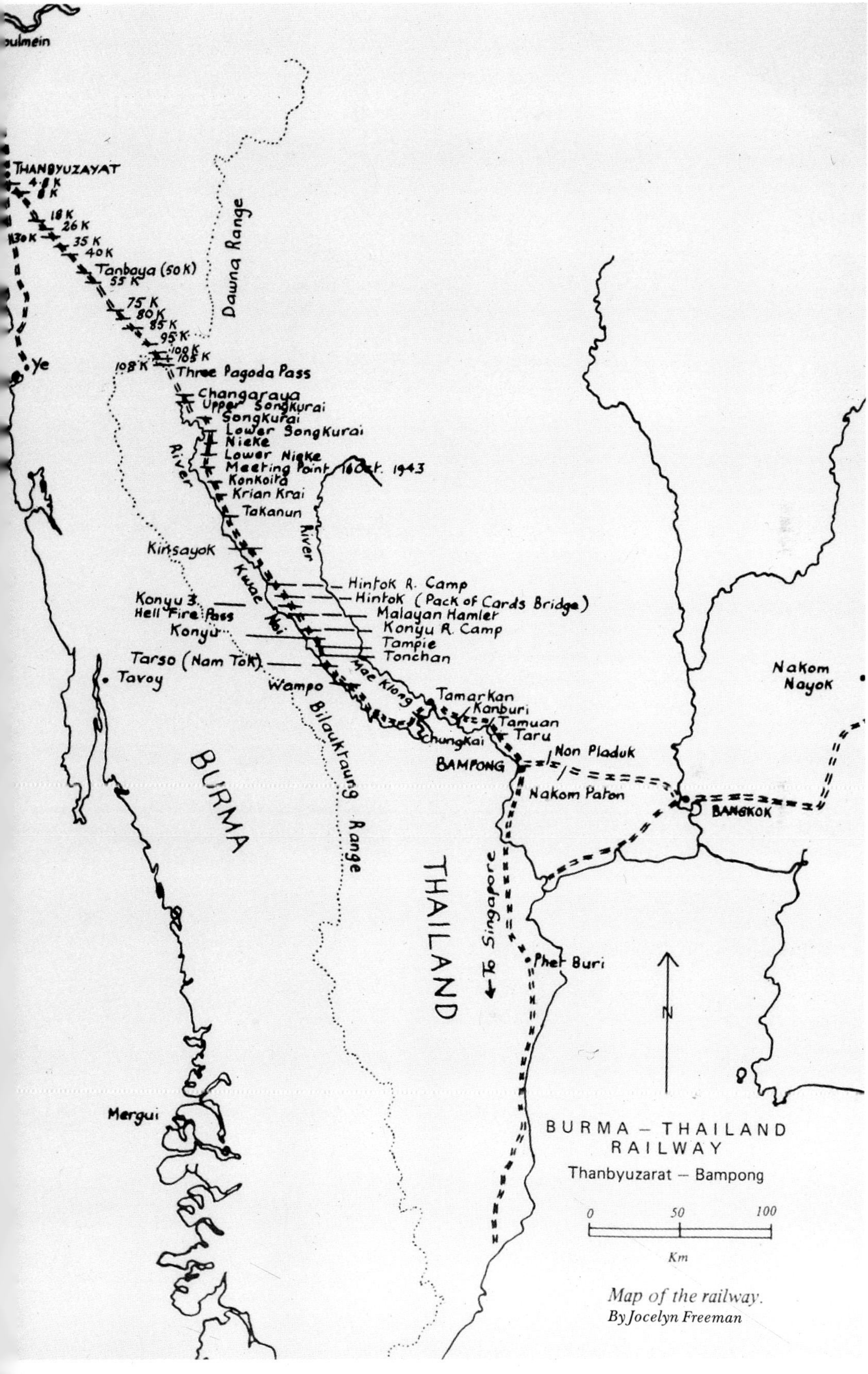

: Burma-Thailand Railway (From *Railway of Death* by E.R. [Bon] Hall)

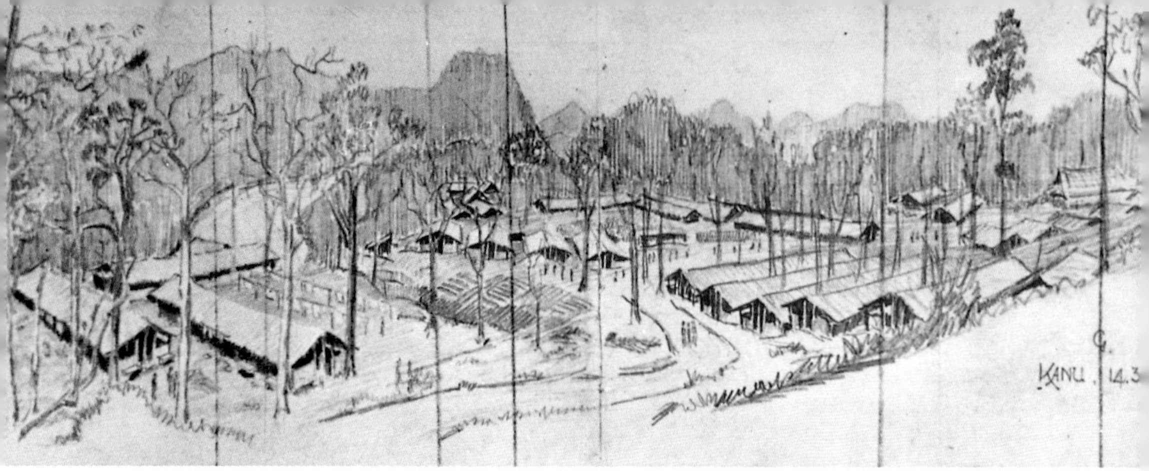

29 Konyu river camp, general view from the south, 14 March 1943 (*S. Gimson*)

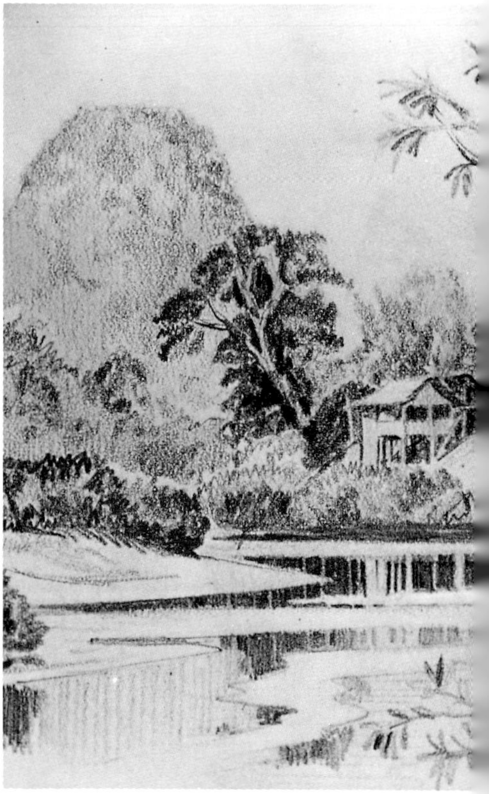

30 Konyu river camp, Commanding Officers' hut (*S. Gimson*)

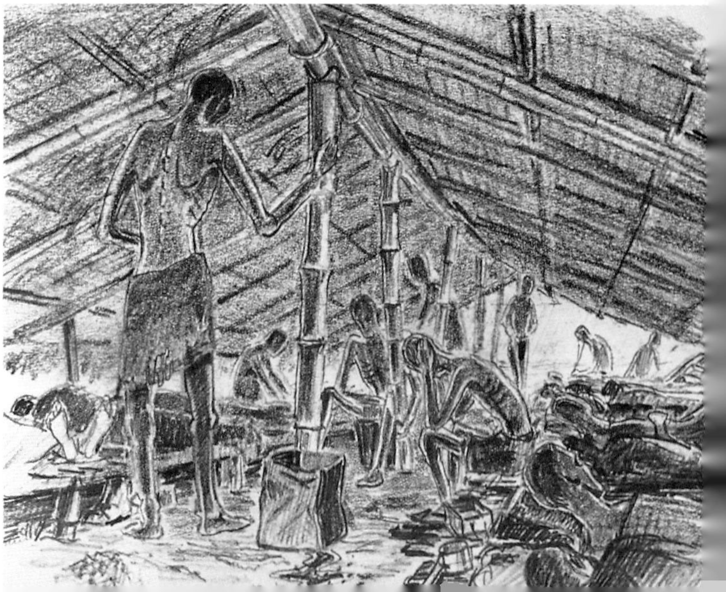

31 Dysentery ward, Konyu river camp (*S. Gimson*)

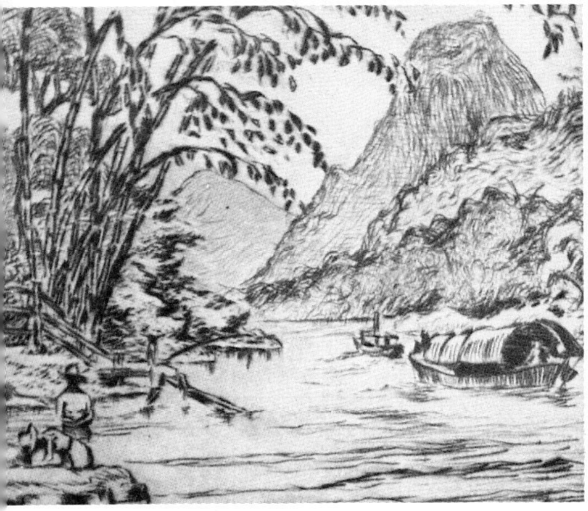

e river at Konyu

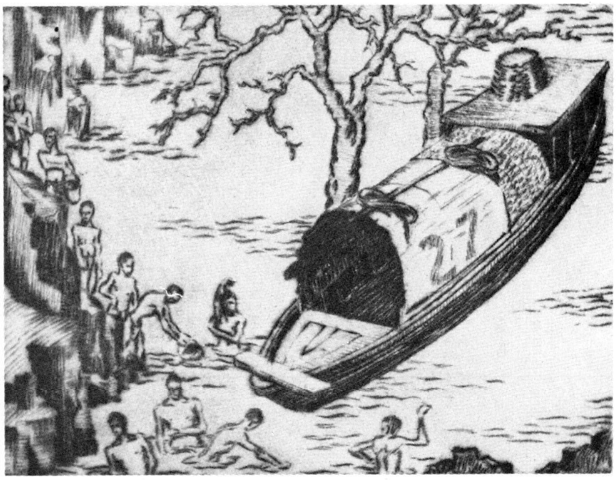

33 Water chain – drawing water for rice (*Ray Parkin*)

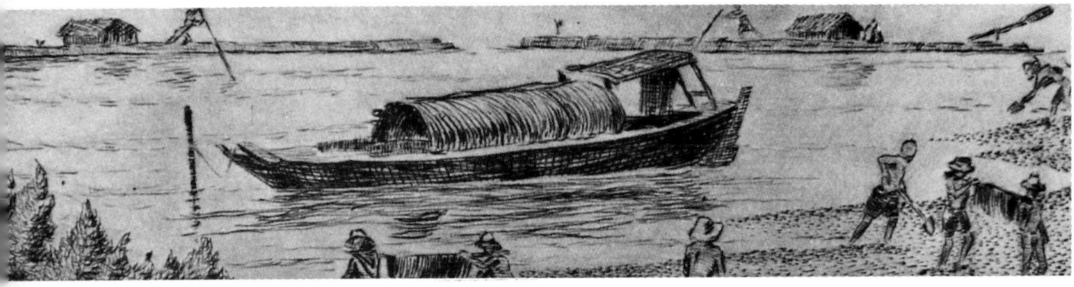

avel party and bamboo rafts (*Ray Parkin*)

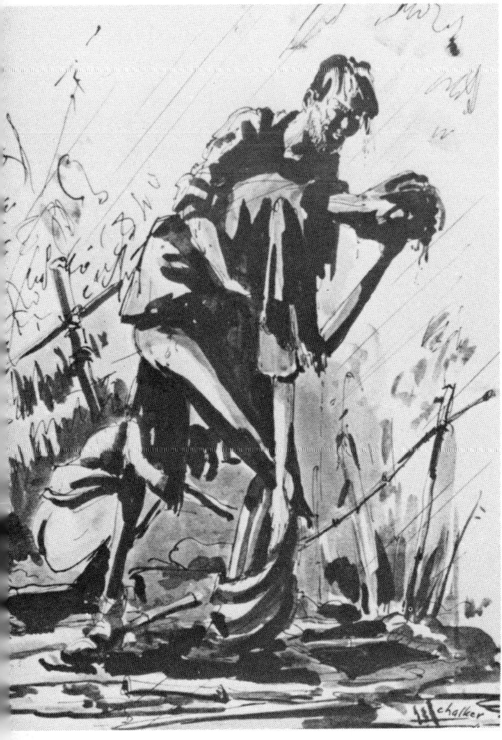

sentery latrines, Konyu river camp, 1942 (*Jack lker*)

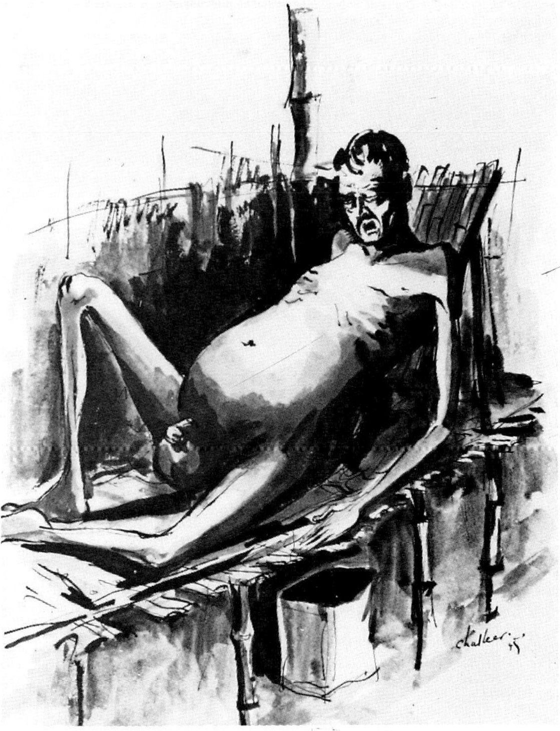

36 Beriberi case (*Jack Chalker*)

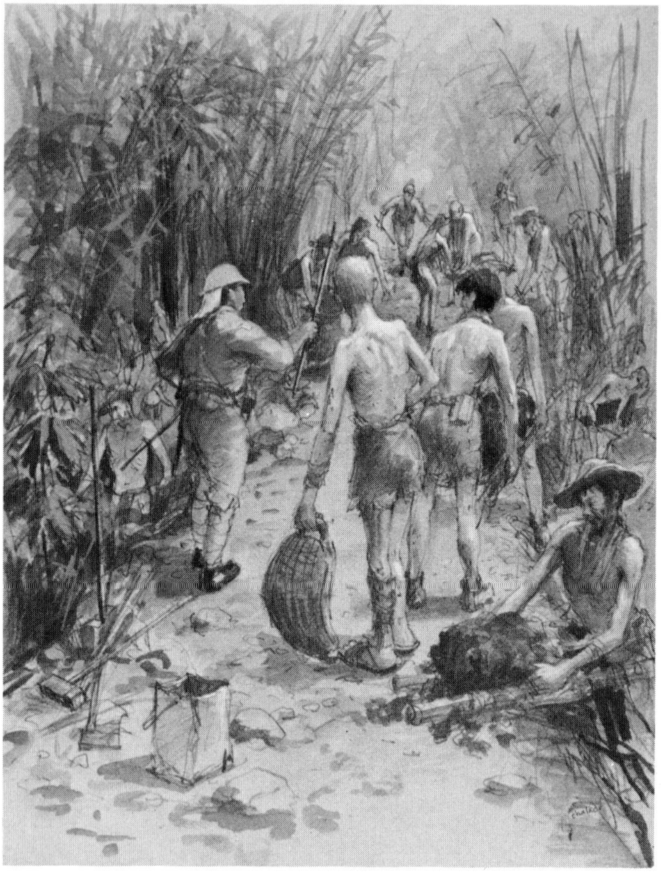

37 Building the *bund*, Konyu, 1942 (*Jack Cha*

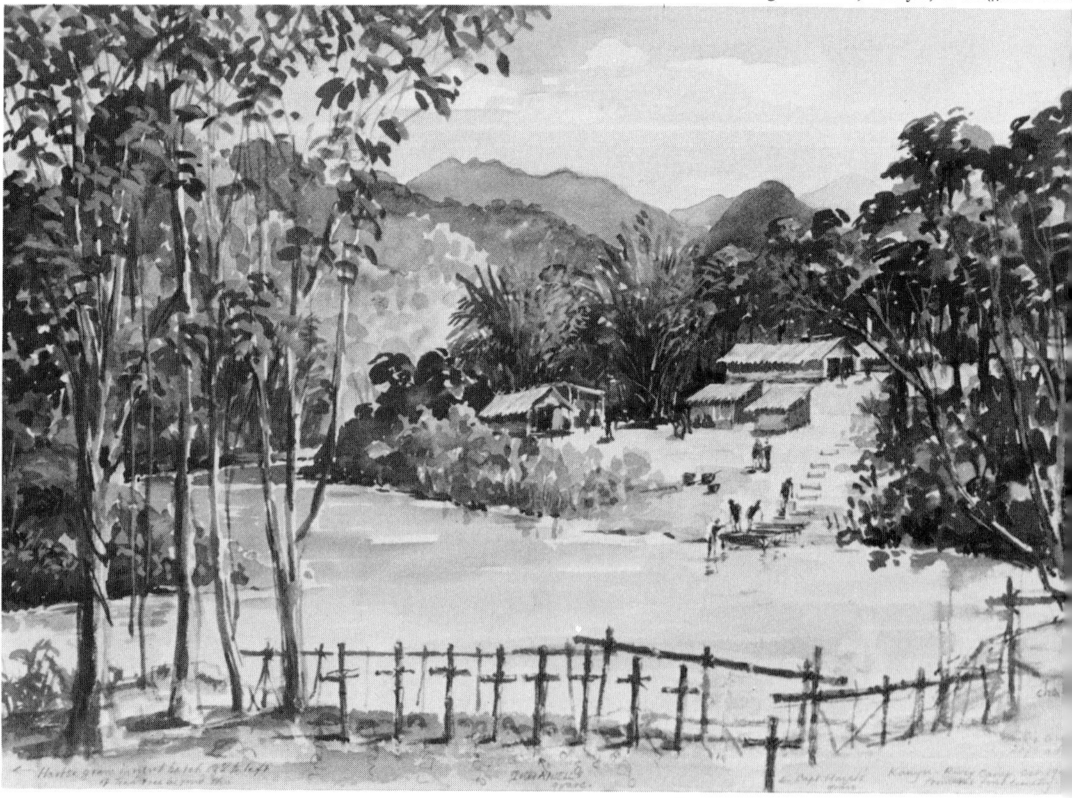

38 Konyu river camp, seen from the cemetery, October 1942. In Sgt Chalker's writing at the foot, he identifies three friend and notes: 'this area some 20 ft above river'. (*Jack Chalker*)

I took these men down to hand over the sum in question directly. An absolute surprise in the afternoon: all officers to the *kebetei* for pay, where we were paid the full amount for September and October less 60 gulden per month.

Thus nearly 1200 gulden has come into the camp in one pay – wealth beyond the dreams of avarice and all in new N paper money! This, in truth, costs little, but means a great deal to us. The only catch is that they made a statement that only the amounts previously suggested were to be spent – 10 gulden, 20 gulden per month respectively. The rest was only being paid to us as there was no channel of paying dependents or arranging our savings. All this must be rather galling to the people who opposed our financial proposals, since there is now no reason for any meanness.

Today is a N celebration day, a saint's day on which I gather they pray for the dead (which in this war *Tjahoha* fixes at 15,000). Tomorrow also. Certainly some N soldiers were very drunk today. Also today called to *kebetei* (Orchida) to discuss the form of a Geneva Convention postcard for mailing. God knows what it would mean to get some incoming mail! I outlined the system of correspondence (letters and parcels) as used in Europe and middle east, but they seemed to think letters were too dangerous and out of the question. They are anxious to design a postcard of the sort where you cross out things and do not write. Possibly a few personal lines will be allowed. We are to submit our ideas on Monday next. Perhaps we may get a line from home by Xmas!

[My wireless] Gs begin new offensive Stalingrad; hard fighting in Caucasus. Heavy air attack on Malta; Gs have lost over 100 planes. Ns have landed heavy force with artillery in Solomans. Our forces doing well in NG. Heavy RAF attacks.

18 October 1942

Saw 'Charlie Chan' at *kebetei* and explained that we had many sick and wished to help with extra food and preventive feeding. The provision for officers' spending was quite generous, but could we spend money on troops? He expressed sympathy with the idea but must refer to a higher authority.

S/Sgt Oliver told me today of his troubles as NCO in charge of ration *corvée* – Australian troops make trouble smoking and talking to civilians etc. He is then required by Ns to slap them himself which he has had to do three times. Slapping down is very rife still. Ns are dead nuts on matters of smoking and saluting. Some Ns adopt a rather nasty procedure of making you stand with bent knees – very tiring and exposes the scrotum to a well-placed kick.

19 October 1942

At conference, we decided that if Ns had not ruled on the pay question by 1600 hours report, we would collect as laid down in the original procedure with special exception of 1st Lts and P/Os. As no ruling was made by 1600, I asked Lt-Col. Lyneham to go ahead and make Major Beaney Australian accountant for the sums collected!

20 October 1942

Called at *kebetei* in an attempt to get a ruling on the money question but no luck.

21 October 1942

Visit to camp by Lt Susuki and Orchida; Russell and Bombs Charlton, also JDM to the fore. A real Father Christmas Tour – Orchida laid on coffee, etc. and discussed business. We were told we must turn much more land into gardens – even if all parade on the oval (this of course means more tools required). I am going to rule that permanent duties men share new money equally exempting, however, those who do not do a reasonable amount of work each day (3 hours). (Major B at conference began his usual opposition, but given no change.) Gave Van 6½ gulden for bookbinders and library and odd educationalists. And Chadwick 10 gulden for gardeners who missed on general duties distribution.

22 October 1942

Inspection of camp by Maj. Gen. Hiji Kata, a rather tall, soldierly-looking man – keen eyes but walked straight through one line of barracks and kitchen without looking to right or left or saying a word. He is said to be CGS West Java.

J. Morris's new show, *Fun in Tempo*, comes on tonight and he is distressed because the N sergeant major has taken away his only violin when it was prominently worked into the whole show.

Last night at 2205 hours N sentries very active about house and all houses nearby. Unfortunately, my light fused just as they appeared – perhaps fortunately, it was a keen search.*

23 October 1942

Rain everyday, in the afternoons for most part, and it is very wet under foot. 2000 gulden received and handled in to John Rintoul.

The 'secondary school' classes are now having term examinations. Blue has made certain changes in my 'wardrobe'.

24 October 1942

Permanent duties pay discussed; this is to be on the pool system and no option is to be given since, though a man may object, it is not necessary that I employ him on permanent duties. No difficulties in discussing this matter with Lt-Col. L. The CSMs were included in this group.

Today was the 50th performance of BTC (*Fun in Tempo*) and asked some Ns to tea. Lt Susuki wanted to come but Orchida came with Jongehans and Russell. Very polite as usual, and asked me one question about 'Roads across the desert in WA'. (No change!). Show was excellent with a simply first class band and everything going with a swing. O had to leave (with apologies) at 2030 hours. There was one further interruption in the middle of Jocelyn Cadell's excellent sketch of a white Russian Grand Duke but this did not put him out of his stride; O shook hands warmly with the Grand Duke on leaving, Russell

* This was contrived in a tense moment in which the wireless set, which was out of hiding, was tucked away.

making the introduction. I had to make a little speech re the fiftieth performance and asked them to welcome O amongst us as one who had done many 'kind things' for this camp. I waited expectantly for applause and none came. This rather put me off my stride! The evening finished up with several D doctors and Jongehans etc in *tête à tête* conversation over supper in my house.

15 October 1942

Wally Woolard, a CCS lad, has been very ill in hospital. Clinically looked like amoebic hepatitis, but did not respond after 5 days emetine injections so stopped, since Dr Smith (Dutch) had never seen a case of amoebic hep. with high continual fever which showed no response to emetine. Secondary infection would explain it, but there is no leucocytosis. He has been on M. and B.693 and suddenly crisised on the tenth day. It now seems quite positive that he was a case of right basil pneumonia with secondary (toxic) hepatitis. He seems to be getting better now.

I am very depressed to hear that my old patient, Piper Archie Fletcher, died at Tjimahi after an operation and reactionary haemorrhage following removal of his shattered patella. I suppose, poor devil, he was worn out by poor food and operations, broken bones etc.

Wing Commander Nichol's group are going to be further depleted I fear, by at least 150 (Works people, drivers etc.) that are – I imagine – going to Batavia to work for the Ns on the basis of 2/3 gulden per man per month. They received 300 gulden today (This is at present out of my N pay. I will reclaim from imprest.)

Later: They are definitely going in the early morning. Discussed the sum to be given to them with RRR and EL and fixed it at 450 gulden (NCOs to hold 300 gulden: rest given 1 gulden each). This was given to Nick to distribute and at 2300 hours I saw his Sgt George who has severe bronchitis and a high temperature. He is unfit to leave in the morning and I arranged this with Ns.

26 October 1942

Up at 400 hours. A dreary, wet morning. Departing troops were fairly cheerful and there was quite a crowd to see them off (can some of these have been interested in the beds etc. of the departing?). Number actually was 160, leaving only about 480 UK troops. Sgt Hough of *Mark Time* staff is one moving out and, as usual, John Morris loses his soloist.

Later in the afternoon EL gave me 500 gulden collected from Australian officers up to date and said that he had one or two to finish. I gave him 40 gulden from my pay. He does not seem to be carrying out the policy agreed upon in collecting the money. Also, English officers are deploring that while they are putting all theirs in, Australian officers who are not are buying a little gratitude from ORs instead, which puts the former in a poor light by comparison. Today I addressed the permanent duties (UK and Aust. groups) separately owing to a bungle in assembly) and thanked them for their excellent work. I warned them that everyone must make some sacrifice, including officers, and they were no exception because they were now being asked to share with all other PDs, who did at least 3 hours work daily, not paid by Ns. Rate of pay is approximately 1.5 gulden W/Os, 1 gulden sergeants, 50 cents ORs each 10 days. If there were objections I would listen, but I warned them that I would not employ those who objected – so consequently I did not anticipate any trouble! I am told my nickname rapidly firmed as 'Dictator Dunlop'. Pay was distributed today on that basis.

27 October 1942

EL asking for more accommodation and I have asked for this to be investigated on square yards per man basis. Dan Buckley 2/2 CCS, Crowley, Hughes, and Roberts have downed tools in the hygiene squad over my ruling yesterday. They are all Irishmen with strong trade union urges and their souls are offended by my dictating what the worker does with his hard-earned money! I succeeded into talking them into going back to work. I think they were a little influenced in that certain 2/3 M.G. Bn people they do not like had immediately seized their jobs. I was disgusted later to hear a camp rumour that I had promised them full pay and that was why they went back. Saw Dan Buckley who said he would deny it.

Nippon has today announced we must give back money over the proposed spending rate. Now there will be trouble, as I know some will have 'lost' some of it. Capt. R. Smith, for example, punted by giving 25 gulden to his gunners who marched out yesterday. One officer had 15 gulden stolen.

I am warned by Capt. Macnamara that EL did not make any attempt to carry out the money policy laid down and did, in fact, discourage certain officers in his immediate circle. De Crespigny, for example, tells me that he was definitely discouraged as to giving his full 32 gulden and when he did so was chipped as to having a lot of money.

An estimate of our future imprisonment must at present lie between six and eighteen months and it cannot but be expected things will get worse with less food, less money coming in and everything more expensive.

28 October 1942

Weather drier and ground fairly good underfoot except in the pig sty, where pigs almost sink from sight in the slush and flies are breeding badly. Tiles have been taken from in front of my house and Nick's to fix a dry corner for them.

Trouble. Yesterday afternoon one of the later additions to the Ambons who has given trouble informed the Nips of a hidden box of pineapples* and possibly other things. An obvious fifth column plant. Today I am required to certify that there are no such hidden materials in this camp. I did this, adding 'to my knowledge'. All camp commandants must do this and are then held responsible. This is bad for the head [i.e. risk of beheading] since God knows what the D could have hidden. Also members of our kitchen staff, Burdon and Cameron, were questioned today about food expenditure. They said they did not know the amounts. I have not been questioned but am ready now. This may be result of

* Hand grenades.

the same information. Ambons are informed that 1000 men must leave tomorrow.

Tjahaka is celebrating great naval victories in the Solomons again. Allied losses since 25 August are given as 63 warships sunk, 21 heavily damaged, 719 aircraft lost. USA admit in Santa Cruz battle the loss of destroyer *Porter* and heavy damage to an aircraft carrier.

X [my wireless] A push has been on in the western desert over last few days, mainly an infantry and artillery move over the whole front. RAF very active. During the week, heavy RAF raids on Milan by day.

29 October 1942

Departure of Ambonians (1000). Nice little fellows. Polite, well drilled, very honest, full of humour, good athletes and sportsmen. Happy fellows with excellent morale and last but not least a musical sense – witness the famed Ambonian band.

I have made it clear at conference that main expenditure on food will be directly through the imprest fund. I have informed Maj. Beaney that he may act as financial expert to advise Lt-Col. Lyneham and do any accounting that he considers necessary. All books etc. will be put at his disposal. It must, however, be emphasised that in this capacity he will act as an expert and not as 2 I/C Aust. Group or 2/3 M.G. Bn. Policy will be determined by three people only: OC Aust. Group, OC UK Group and myself (Ramsay Rae acts as my 2 I/C).

30 October 1942

Last night some Australian troops mimicked a N soldier of the guard and the guard could not then find the ones concerned so that there was an orgy of slapping and people were detained for hours (Burdon having much hard work). This sort of stupidity is most unfortunate in its results. The Ns are enraged and claim also that the As pretending to throw stones at dogs go suspiciously close to them. Therefore, no more dogs and no throwing stones. What with this silly affair last night and a suspected escape of an Ambon recently, even going out for a leak at night is fraught with danger. Sudden yells and flourishes of bayonets, also many smacks.

L says that the collection from the rest of the officers is complete: 438 contributed, 320 returned from loan, to make total of 758. This compares with 880 raised by the UK from fewer officers and they have only 500 in all. I told L that I hoped there would not be this discrepancy in future months, and he agreed.

The thought of the day is that all men *en masse* are shites (or super shites) and it behoves the more intelligent to do their best with full realisation of their limitations. I would dearly have loved to see a few people with socialist convictions watching the conduct of this camp and knowing the inner story. If socialism won't work amongst a few men under these conditions, it surely is utterly impractical on a national basis.

A clinic today discussed the burning feet syndrome and the grave worry about the 16 cases of retrobulbar neuritis detected. Eighteen per cent of the camp are under treatment (200+). Maj. Moon has observed that the first men to suffer in a big way were the Australians, particularly the big burly athletic outdoors types (but not particularly those who played much sport in the camp). English then followed and have nearly caught up. Ambons, Menados and D have practically no burning feet trouble. He thinks it is due to more than one factor and that the absence of protein, particularly of biological type, is important. The Australians and the English are much bigger meat eaters usually than other camp members. The salient feature is that Vitamin B1 and nicotinic acid, even in a dose of 500 units daily, do not touch them. Combination of yeast and the increased feeding of 1 duck egg daily +35 grams *katjang idjoe* bean is doing great work. This brings the diet to approx 2800 calories and over 80 grams of protein. (Mens' morale is greatly improved and they all say they feel better on the new diet.)

Nicotinic acid has no effect. Recovery of feet and eyes seems to go together and yeast and extra protein feeding have been effective in making great improvement in ten days.

This clinic reminded me of the fact that *my* feet have been itching a bit lately, particularly in bed at night. Joked about this with Ewen Corlette and Co., when I happened to notice that I had quite marked oedema of the legs and no knee jerks could be elicited. My diet is not bad at all really, but I suppose during the last six months I have gone very short of proteins for a fellow of my size.

31 October 1942

Camp now working fairly smoothly. Skip Glowry's birthday – heralded by steak and eggs – delicious.

1 November 1942

Sunday. All 'excess' officers' money was to be handed back to Ns today, but later this decision was reversed. (Rae Smith in trouble owing to having given 25 gulden to some departed gunners.) Church service Padre Blakeway.

2 November 1942

Momentous day opened casually with CO's inspection of barracks and morning conference, at which were Group Capt. Nicholetts, Van, Nick, Lt-Col. Lyneham, Capt. Burdon, Arthur Moon and I. Each group commander given 100 gulden private impress. Capt. Burdon reported that Sgt Hoshina had told him that all Australians were to move to Tanjongpriok (less 1 officer and 5 senior NCOs and sick – largely those unable to walk to the station). Party to be approx. 1000. We believe this is a big movement; we are to take all office documents. Officers all to retain the money paid to them and were advised to wind up our canteen assets to UK group.

Officer to stay: obviously to be medical since to look after sick. Fixed as Macnamara by cutting cards with Ewen Corlette.

* I subsequently found I had suffered visual loss in my left eye to 6/60.

Money: officers' contribution – loan to be repaid to fund, return rest – then settle on a *proportionate* basis troops departing and staying.
Canteen: decide on what assets are realisable or can be distributed after next two days big buying, then settle on same basis.
Q: share out tinned stuff on a proportionate basis to companies.
Library: call in all books; set aside those belonging to Dutch, distribute rest proportionately.
Education: some certificates handed out.
Memorial book: several copies taken, artists to carry own stuff.
Records: carry what we can; each take a list of other camps' personnel. Medical records. Arthur Moon to do all possible.
Sports material: take a little.
Tools: take a few.
Pigs: Nips said we might kill 3 out of 8 – half a pig to go to *kebetei* for officers.
Grave Stones Bandoeng Cementery: Nips agreed we could send a party at 900 hours tomorrow to lay the gravestones. Padres 'Fred' and Tom to go with party of six, including Malayan interpreter.

Blue and Steven are settling the question of our packs for the road – 'Blue' is taking a merciless line with me this time as to how much I should carry. We are trying to lay in a little ration reserve.

3 November 1942

Gravestones fixed. At the morning conference, finance settlement was postponed until tomorrow. Heads of departments asked to give me a short final report of their activities to date – education, theatre etc. I wrote to all Bandoeng camps and thanked them for their fine co-operation and neighbourly help, also to especially the medical group camp 5, who looked after our sick and to the interpreters Diesveldt and Jongehans. Wrote message to troops upon relinquishment of command.

Somehow terribly busy all day and haven't got my own affairs into shape at all. Dr De Raadt – very nice fellow – called to take an affectionate farewell.

Evening. British Theatricals Ltd had a delightful little wind-up ceremony with several stage skits: Sgt Wynne and P/O Abbott both dressed as whores and looking the part; Berny Weller and his band. Some very pleasant Nip soldiers gave money to players, tried the instruments and eventually came back loaded with cakes! They overlooked the lateness of the hour.

[My wireless] Our attack in western desert going well. We have pushed forward and taken a number of prisoners. Big tank battle now on. Nineteen planes shot down; we hit 2 destroyers and one merchant ship at least on fire. Stalingrad: Rs improving position. In central Caucasus Gs are meeting some success. Australians have taken Kukoda (New Guinea) and pushed further on. Convoy off Buna driven away, 5 planes shot down and 2 merchant vessels hit and on fire.

Battle of Stewart? Island resulted in loss of 100 N planes. 2 aircraft carriers badly damaged, 2 battle-ships hit plus 3 cruisers and 7 vessels sunk in Buni

Harbour. Altogether 200,000 tons N shipping sunk or badly damaged in 9 days. Our air force on the top anyway and Yanks improving.

Gear has been sorted out as follows for all ORs (all extra clothing in these items are returned yesterday):

1 suit clothing (shorts and shirt)	1 water bottle
1 pair footwear	1 mosquito net
1 pair puttees	1 pack
1 cap	2 blankets
1 sun hat	1 belt
1 mess tin and cutlery	1 sleeping mat

Will be glad to see the last of these guards as very sadistic.

Camps 2/4 Funds Accounts
Balance Sheet as at 4 November 1942

Liabilities			*Assets*		
Public fund account schedule I			Cash		
Camp 3	f2375.31		Camp command	6108.47½	
Camp 4	4093.00		Main canteen	1062.12½	
		6468.31	Officers' canteen	5.00	
					7175.60
Regimental Funds A/C Schedule II *Nil*					
Creditors and credit Balance 389.83(?)			Debtors + Debit Balances		464.35
Officers' Subscription A/C			Stocks		
Camp 3	f760		Camp 3	506.54	
Camp 4	433		Less reserve	93.35	
		1193.00			411.19
		f8051.14	Camp 4	164.30	
			Less reserve	164.30	
					8051.14

Received the sum of f4526 being total public funds held by Lt-Col. E.E. Dunlop AAMC on behalf of Aust. troops

E.D. Lyneham Lt-Col.

Prepared by John Rintoul Lieut.

Audited by Robt Haddon AIF

Received from Lt-Col. E.E. Dunlop proportion of camp funds the property of camp 3 in accordance with audited balance sheet dated 4th November 1942.

Nichols
W/C RAF

4 November 1942

Movement considered unlikely tomorrow. Overste Willikens called to take a very affectionate farewell on behalf of Dutch. Spirit in the camp is splendid. I am very busy packing up and going through the files – much appreciate the extra day.

The following special things came out today: special issue of *Mark Time* with messages from Nick on one hand and Lt-Col. Lyneham and I on the other.

Education: a special conferring ceremony – at which Van made me distribute certificates and diplomas! He then made a most excellent and lofty speech, finally leaving me in possession of the platform so that I had to make one too. I am strongly impressed with the spirit of a university that we have built up here. Same sort of atmosphere as in a college, with young people constantly exchanging ideas on all sorts of subjects and vastly improving their knowledge of life and their understanding. It is most noticeable that the men who have really made their mark here are all those first in the field of intellect.

Kicked off in a match English and Aust. *vs* combined Menados, Ambons and D. From the kick off sent the ball spinning about a yard over the centre of the goal, going hard. Goalie was anxious for a moment! Told those lined up how much we had enjoyed the football and that no matter where we were going we would stand more chance of winning a match than here.

Nick gave a very charming little farewell dinner party with L and I, John Morris, Frank Burdon, Christmas, Ramsay Rae (administrative staffs). It was the nearest thing to home conditions I have seen, with little table markers and a bare table with a nice centre and flowers! We drunk much sergeant-brewed beer – peculiar taste like mild ginger beer.

5 November 1942

We are definitely off tomorrow. Paraded this morning as a check for entraining. Saw Laurens about my X [wireless] who advised me to try and take it. Finally, after the conference with Phillips (expert) also Roberts (super expert) decided to carry pieces and hope to reassemble. I carried her over, smartly saluting as I walked past the N guard.

Kebetei Report: movement fixed. Returned and put out following order:

From: Camp Administration
To: Aust. Group UK Group 5 Nov. '42
Subject: Movement Aust. POW to Batavia

1 Strength	The Australian Group less 89 men will move from Bandoeng to Batavia on Friday 6 Nov. 1942		
2 Routine	Reveille	0315 hours	
	Breakfast Pde	0340 hours	
	Breakfast	0345 hours	
	Fall in	0430 hours	
3 Formation	Sections of 50 will form up in columns of fours on road near the guard-house.		
4 Casualties	Any casualties will be notified immediately so substitute can be arranged.		

5 Entraining	At station there will be one train of 20 carriages. Troops will entrain on false platform in order of march sections 1–20.
6 Baggage	One handcart will be available to carry office records. The camp commandant has kindly detailed 3 UK ORs to take this cart to the station. These troops will report to camp orderly room at 0430 hours and take up a position at rear of the officers' section nearest main entrance. Other ranks will carry only pack and haversack with bedding disposed around the pack.
7 Command	Lt-Col. E.E. Dunlop will be in charge of the party until entraining and command will then be handed over to Lt-Col. E.D. Lyneham.
8 Rations	Each man will carry one f packet portion of the day's rations.

E.E. Dunlop Lt-Col. Commanding British

Wound up all financial matters as shown above, with clearance for everything from E.L. and Nick (L asked me to carry 300 gulden for him as part of the distribution) when handing over requested change of command at *kebetei* for following reasons: I am medical; I am not the most senior officer; and I have only retained command so long because it is such a pleasure to deal with the Nips!

Many visitors in the evening – called at hospital to say goodbye to Woolard and dropped into Van's farewell supper party. News frightfully good: great success in desert 9,000 prisoners, including 2 G generals 1 Italian; over 300 heavy G tanks destroyed and 600 planes, 300 in the air, 300 on ground. G in retreat being heavily strafed. Aust. have Kokoda and moving on; and so to lie down at 0030 hours.

6 November 1942

Reveille 0315. Fell in 0430 marched out at 0550 reached station 0625. Large crowd up to see us off included Van, Horobin and Nick. A little confusion at station owing to train not completely coupled up. Most of officers in a 4th class carriage. Lyneham, Beaney, Burdon and I in 'luxury' 3rd class. Sgt Okomura and N officer (Lt Susuki) came to see us off, also Hoshina, who cheered us up by saying that we were being shipped first to Surabaja then Australia which was now in Nippon hands! Train departed 0740 hours with our compliment of 1,000 and 54 officers. I have given my armband to Lt-Col. Lyneham.

It was a magnificant sight to see the green jungle valleys full of mist and the verdant mountain tops striking up on all sides, as the train weaved a tortuous course amongst them. Java is almost terrifyingly green and verdant (a green succulent death); everywhere kampongs and Javanese in their primitive houses of attap.

It was almost cold in the morning, but as we descended to the low-lying country approaching Batavia, steaming hot. Little check-boards of paddy-fields on all sides. I feel perfectly cheerful and don't give a tinker's damn what happens – become a prisoner of war and see the world. But oh, for better company than B's!

Meester Cornelius station at 1520 hours and disentrained. Nips first said that we must carry luggage then, later, that officers could put it in lorry. As I had so many XXXX parts, I decided to send only my pack and valise and medical haversack, carrying suitcase with records and two haversacks. Butterworth as usual in luck and given a lift with luggage as guard. The march was about six miles along the Buitenzorg road south of Batavia – it rained like hell and this diary got sopping wet. Troops stuck it well – pathetic to see poor old Sgt King ahead of me, staggering under his pack. Men began to drop out about 4 miles on, but by this time N lorry was picking them up (Butterworth on this). It was a sorry sight to see some of these emaciated forms and haggard faces as they fell out. The pace set was rapid and instead of slowing down in front, always the back flogged on. (Incidently, the guard on the train was 40 N soldiers.) Some Javanese police in blue-grey uniforms with sabre and revolver formed up this end. (Sods!)

Finally arrived at camp No. 5 Makasura, a low-lying plot of land amid coconut palms. The huts are thatched attap with a little rough brickwork just in the centre. Continuous row of bamboo bedding down the sides with about 1 metre per person.

Officers have the same accomodation as men. Latrines are a primitive open drain straddle system leading to seepage pits, and overflow goes to adjacent paddy-fields. Rubbish is buried, of course. Showers are taps 2 ft 6 in. from floor and the whole camp is a sea of tenacious red-brown mud. It was an incredible sight to see the guard doing a *hotio tutoré* with one or two kilos of this on their boots. There was the usual wearisome period of waiting about in the rain and mud until the local old prisoner grandee – a bearded, elderly fine featured N (Maj. Anami) made us give the usual compliments. *Kashira naka* etc. Of course some asses saluted British fashion and we had it over again.

L is in charge with B as 2 I/C. Wing Commander Alexander RAF is in charge of the camp (nice fellow); have met before and, joy of joys! Sqn Ldr MacGrath is here with Capt. Rees and some of the British ORs – and of course has been doing wonders with the primitive hygiene. He has been begging and pleading with the Ns to make some provision for the new troops coming in by allowing one extra latrines and ablutions hut to be put up, but he says they are just absolute idiots in this. The 'hospital unit' which left Bandoeng is scattered all over the place, some in staging camps, some in the military hospital in Batavia. Frank Graham's dental personnel were sent elsewhere. Sqn Ldr MacGrath has been in the same camp as A.V.M. Maltby, Sitwell and Brig. Blackburn. The latter is in charge of the 'staging' camp near Princess Juliana School; he is the only one of the officer group allowed to enter the troops' area, except one officer and W/O who administer the camp. It seems that mostly D have been through the camp. John Disse is said to have had a beating up and to have been taken to hospital off a vessel after having been told they were off to Siam!

It is terribly wet and miserable tonight – and I'm still soaking wet but I can't be bothered changing until 'Bed'. Tea: rice and tea only. Had got my hip placed nicely on the bamboo frame when N soldier did an inspection – everyone has to get out and *keré*. Lights out 2200. This is pretty poor but better than *Landsop*. Sqn Ldr MacGrath is looking after the sick; only 2 admitted to hospital tonight.

4 Batavia

November 1942

7 November 1942

A very muddy vista and my clothes still very wet – but don't care. I feel fit and cheerful enough, though my ankles are puffed up.

Sick parade postponed till pm on account of a special parade for Major Anami. We paraded at 1000 and he did not arrive, then again shortly after 1200 and waited about half an hour. Inspection finally over by 1320 as Nip W/O clad in a tennis shirt, no socks and tennis shoes gave us a little *keré* practice himself in role of officer. He said the Aust. group were a bit slow. Discussed with Lt-Col. Lyneham his organisation, requesting that all medical personnel including all CCS personnel (plus Fred Smedley's lads) be put in one company with all CCS officers. I will be detached as SMO, Arthur Moon taking charge and John Morris for administration. Also suggested all RAAF men be similarly separated under Ramsay Rae, and W. Wearne to take over the Pioneer Company. This was all agreed. Sqn Ldr MacGrath and I arranged medical programme. We are providing a hygiene squad – Jock Clarke and 15 ORs to help them – and will make our own arrangements for sick parades 1015 hours daily. He says there has been very little sickness in this camp.

We are going to try and get *katjang idjoe* and 1 egg daily for each man as before. I am very pleased with the way they stood the march yesterday. Many, however, have blistered feet. Discussed with L the question of other inmates of camp and extra rations; the share-and-share-alike policy to be adopted if possible. Sqn Ldr MacGrath has been buying a few medical stores when possible. L is agreeable to put up 100 gulden from our side for this purpose.

[My wireless] Number of G prisoners in WD is now 13,000. Heavy concentration leaving Mersa Matruh being heavily bombed at low level.

John Morris is already teeing up some entertainment and Billy Wearne preparing some education scheme. As all the barracks are full this will have to be either in barracks or out of doors. Much less rain today.

8 November 1942

L seems to be playing up well on every point now and is of course happy as a sandboy to have the command. Inspection by a general today and everything to be in inspection order by 1000. Saw Sqn Ldr MacGrath and discussed hygiene difficulties. There is too much sewage with 1400 men, so some effluent has to be drained away by an open drum system after passing through the reservoir.

N. General: we went On parade by 1130 hours; everything over by 1300 and went off well. He was the portly, rather jolly-faced Maj. Gen. who did our first inspection in Bandoeng. He was accompanied by Maj. Anami and the party was in all 9 officers, 3 under officers (most of the officers very old indeed). The general wore 4 rows of ribbon (including general service and Victory British!), Major Anami 2½ rows.

Billy Wearne, Alan Woods and Ron and I have discussed financial matters and will only contribute in future if the others will come out into a common pool scheme with no more holding out. I think L will play now.

9 November 1942

Camp is drier now. We rise at 0700 N time and parade by companies at 0720 in long double line between huts. N W/O is supposed to appear at 0730 when all called to *kiotské*, *kashira migi*, *naoré*. Finally after parade state given *yasumé* and dismissed. Some mornings the sky is filled with light clouds of cumulo-stratus ilk – the rising sun fills the sky with pale gold and the beautiful coconut fronds catch the glinting gold and silver with enchanting effects. Most intriguing little animals, the coconut squirrels, make the most amazing runs and leaps from tree to tree, buzzing merrily around the inner circle. They jump unerringly some 3 feet or so from swaying frond to frond at heights of up to 60 feet or more. With their furry little tails they silhouette very clearly against the sky.

Our company parades and P.T. will be at 0900 hours as before but have not yet begun. Breakfast 0800 lunch 1300. Evening 'roll call' at 1900, tea 1930. Lights out 2200.

God, these sloping 'bamboo beds' are hard. I have a little slab of rubber sponge that I use for a pillow and am now using this for my hip and my coat for a pillow. This is fairly good but requires good balance and one keeps sliding down till the feet stick out a foot over the end. Also apparently all night carts with hexagon wheels roll down and up the Buitenzorg Road.

10 November 1942

Several men have failing vision; I have seen 4 today. One considers that his vision failed even before his feet began to burn and, despite the fact his feet are now much better, he cannot read at all and could not recognise me. I think he will be permanently affected.

We have another opportunity to write a letter home today and we were given a letter instructing us to express in our letters three points of propaganda, one of which was that Japan was obeying the international convention. Lt-Col. Lyneham, Wing Cdr Alexander and I discussed this and we agreed not to write letters under these terms. I pointed out that we could say 'To what convention do you refer? If it is the Geneva convention it is obviously not heavily observed, or we should write letters once a month without being required to say these things.'

When this was referred to the local commander he advised us to write the letters leaving out the propaganda points and including any complaints so that the higher officers would get to hear them. So I wrote mine to Helen, a stiff, unnatural letter designed to air my grievances about food, overcrowding and lack of any distinction between officers and men. I do not expect the letter to get home. Only officers wrote this type of letter, ORs writing the usual censored 'we are being very well treated' type.

In the evening about 12 of the higher officers went over to *kebetei* to see some films shown by a N officer. Many Ns in the audience were quite pleasant looking types. Some of the films were war films – Battle of France, Oran etc and a lot of 'Mickey Mouse' stuff. One of the news films revealed that an early American call-up was of 16,000,000 men!

11 November 1942

Education scheme floated again today after N permission obtained. Instructors and classes sorted out; many new pupils.

Three cases evacuated to hospital in Batavia, to a D school which acts as a clearing station. Cases requiring operations are said to go to the military hospital and are operated on by Nips. Two of the cases are of the burning feet *optic neuritis* type. Case of Sgt Page: complete collapse, weakness in legs and arms; would seem to be definitely a neurosis or hysteria. Treatment: massage and encouragement. From today we take over our own sick in hospital (Sqn Ldr MacGrath Maj. Moon and I). I was given 500 units Vitamin B1 today by injection for my ankle oedema and absent knee jerks.

Financial arrangements as laid on with Lt-Col. Lyneham. The following amounts to be held for him from their savings allowance:

Captain	55 gulden
Major	130 gulden
Lt-Col.	230 gulden

Thus I retain 50 gulden out of 320 and all ranks should have about this sum out of their total pay. Monthly expenditure on the whole camp is to be 2232 gulden approx.; medical supplies and hospital fund extra. I have also collected 100 gulden from the CCS officers and Fred Smedley for the Theatrical Company, this to be distributed over 91 men. My contribution 30 gulden. Fred Smedley 20 gulden. Officers are now actually receiving a special ration from the Nips three times a week.

Cigarettes	10	Tea	30 g	
Butter	20 g	Coffee	70 g	
Sugar	100 g	Banana	150 g	three times a week
Pepper	20 g			

I presume this is out of our 60 gulden a week for food and lodgings. At any rate, it is the first special recognition of officers.

[My wireless] Fighting now in vicinity of Halfaya; American triple landing effected in North Africa – Algiers, Casablanca, Oran – announced intention of advancing to Tripoli. Fighting at Dakar. Large activity NG airborne troops between Kokoda and Buna, Solomons. China: Hankow captured.

12 November 1942

Letter written to Ns addressed to Chief of the Java Prisoners Camps, I.J.A., Batavia, complaining of inadequacy of the diet and deficiency diseases in troops.

13 November 1942

Friday the 13th – quiet enough. I am asking for a special diet for all the hospital patients including bread, milk, sugar, banana + 1 egg. This has not begun yet. I have a few patients in the hospital, none very sick. It is interesting that following Sgt Page, several other soldiers complained of sudden loss of all strength in limbs and trunk, unable to walk etc. I 'jollied' these fellows and asked one of them if he had had bad news from home! Their improvement is very rapid indeed.

14 November 1942

Arthur and I making a big drive on the deficiency cases avitaminosis and had a parade to compile special pro formas for them. We were working hard from 1100 to 1800 hours and saw some 80. In the typical case, 'Bandoeng balls' is the first complaint, often some months before possible mouth trouble, and the sensation of burning feet, first in toes and ball of foot, finally extending up the leg. There is a deep ache as well as burn and the loss of sleep is considerable, some roaming about at night and putting feet in cold water. Some show well-marked rashes on elbows, knees, etc. and very distressing degrees of loss of vision.

Three persons sent to hospital today: one of these, *Low*, an avitaminosis case with loss of vision; one chronic malaria BT and MT; and a chronic dysentery.

There is now P.T. every morning by companies. Special officers' P.T. 1000. Otherwise, recreation is walking round a small enclosure. I introduce a little variety by running with a coconut football for rugger passes.

Education is now fairly well established and we will have first aid classes included next week.

15 November 1942

Sunday. Church services under the coconut palms.

I think a great deal of Helen these days. Poor darling I don't know how she can stand these long dreary years of waiting at home. If she packs up and marries an American or something I suppose it would be best for her, but I don't know what I would do with my life then. She is the only stable thing left in life – the only thing which enables me to see anything to look forward to in peace. Somehow, peace has been spoiled for me; I crave movement, adventure, new countries, variety – the strangeness of things, and shun the old life of solid endeavour amongst people who haven't suffered or been unsettled. Apart from longing terribly to see Helen, my one desire is not to be home but to be back in the war somewhere.

16 November 1942

When we go on parade in the morning 0720 N time it is just before dawn and it is a lovely sight to watch the ceremony of 'gilding the coconuts'. In the hushed stillness the palm fronds droop more quietly, darkly and delicately than usual – and a golden radiance can be seen through the mass of fronds and hutments away to the east. Suddenly the ripe coconuts on the tall trees grow a lovely orange red and *de zon gaat op*.

At present my day is like this. Reveille 0700, Parade 0730. Shave then breakfast by 0800. Clean up my bed space, smoke and read until 0930 then see my sick in hospital. Arthur does infectious, I do the ordinary sick; 1000 P.T. under Bill Aldag, Sergeant P.T. instructor. 1045 tea; 1100 French lesson or conversation. Perhaps a little more hospital work; 1400–1600 see avitaminosis cases, fill in pro formas and do examinations; 1400 exercise such as volley ball, or sometimes more French (I have now stopped Dutch); then a run or exercise; 1800–1900 Chess or reading; 1900–2000 tea and chatter; 2000–2200 (Lights out) reading or chess etc.

17 November 1942

Still having Vitamin B1 injections 500 units (3 a week); have just had the 4th (still no knee jerks). Possibly oedema a little less – anyway, feel extremely well.

18 November 1942

All troops have now been having *katjang idjoe* soup and egg a day for about a week. No yeast and no oven, therefore flour is just cooked as a dumpling. Officers, however, are getting good additions to the diet: tinned food, fruit, eggs, bread, jam. Hospital patients are being given similar additions. I have one interesting patient named Dennis, who at first appeared to be a case of dengue fever (rash on body fifth day etc.) though pulse rapid. Temperature has not settled down, remains a continuous fever rising in afternoon to as high as 104. We think he is a case of *tropical typhus*. Of course a Weil Felix reaction would give the answer.

19 November 1942

Yesterday narrowly escaped a face slapping by going into a blissful dose *dans le soleil pendant une tour d'inspection par une sentienelle*.

[My wireless] Tobruk has fallen. We have also occupied Tunis taking over two equipped aerodromes. 30,000 *Leg. Étrangière* have come over to us. Dakar expected to cave in any time. Ns have now only one airfield left in New Guinea and recently our bombers shot down 18 N fighters.

20 November 1942

Continuing with the investigation of all the deficiency diseases group. Trying hard to get some yeast: Ns have been approached from several angles, but in vain. Seem to be interested only in infectious disease which might spread to them. Indian supply agent with monopoly here is a greasy, shifty, avaricious blob named Seth – a Hindu. Of course there is a N racket here, too; they fix the exorbitant prices and the one or two local price contacts made have shown us how excessive this is. I was told that he couldn't get yeast since all controlled and not for sale.

21 November 1942

Lovely weather continues. Ns actually laid on 5½ bags of *katjang idjoe* today. There is a catch as usual: these beans are not *katjang idjoe*, but a larger, worm-eaten variety, white in colour and with a bitter, rather unpleasant taste. 1000 kilos – the 5½ bags delivered – is our issue for a month, and according to the lump of grease that supplies us, they have now controlled all supplies of *katjang idjoe* so that we will not be able to go on buying our usual 80 grams a day per man. Also, today we get our medical supplies (for the month presumably): approx. 500 creosote tablets, quinine tablets and some yellow tablets said to be wonderful for typhoid – acriflavine. They seem to think they have done wonders in supplying these and that we ought to be very happy, though of course they bore no relationship to our requirements or requests.

22 November 1942

The Ns are setting the whole camp chasing flies and are said to have stated that anyone who cannot produce 4 tonight will be in for trouble. Soldiers are anxiously at work with improvised swotter. One who was anxiously watching the ground was asked by an officer, 'What are you doing?' Answer, 'Catching flies.' 'But you haven't a swotter!' 'Yes, but I have one fly. I took it away from an ant.' The parade was rather amusing; most of we officers did not bother about flies and there were anxious moments as to whether we would get into trouble. '*Shoko* no catch flies?'.

23 November 1942

One of the patients recently sent to Batavia reported on conditions today: bloody. Sleep on the floor. N issue ration badly cooked and apparently damn all in the way of drugs and treatment.

24 November 1942

Bed bugs are rampant, rats rattle about and eat anything exposed and the only decent bedmates are multiple lizards who croak '*yasumé*'. With all the mosquito nets up, each touching the adjacent one, the heat and oppression is most troublesome.

Of course, upper respiratory tract infection is prevalent. Insensibly, the squalor and oppression of this life stirs a streak of bitter perversity in one and you hear arguments being waged interminably about stupid little things. It is indeed difficult in these cramped quarters to find much intellectual escape, and of course there are few books available.

There are 120 men of our 1000 suffering from degrees of deficiency disease.

25 November 1942

A typical display of propaganda today from a superior nation. A N air force Lt-Col. and some other air force officers asked to see some officers of the RAF. Thereupon his lordship said a few chivalrous things!

1 That he failed to understand why they had not committed *hara kiri*. That they would be miserably in prison 'for ever' doing nothing since it seemed unlikely that the war would ever end. As for him, his children would grow up during the war (had they any children he enquired?).

2 That he had known England was a weak nation, but that even so he had not

guessed just how deplorably weak (some incompatibility here). Further insulting nonsense of this sort. A noble nation!

26 November 1942

Twice a day these wearying parades, waiting interminably for two minor NCOs to appear (usually in singlets and wearing tennis shoes – dreadful slovenliness of dress on parade is characteristic). The Australian troops are now prepared for a movement, as our cards are out and typing of rolls going on. Sqn Ldr MacGrath and the Bandoeng crowd of orderlies with him are said to be included in our group. I hope so.

27 November 1942

Endless fine days. A conference of all camp medical officers with two N *orderlies* because they think we make errors in the returns (dysentenes *not* put on infectious list etc.), this owing to fact that they are kept not yet diagnosed until such time as case is established as true dysentery. We are told not to evacuate cases unless very urgent ones as Batavia Hospital is very full–yet we have no drugs or dressings. Medical stores here are marvellous – portions of torn-up flour sacks used for dressings. There are a number of rather severe tropical-style ulcers of the legs.

28 November 1942

Last night an absolute stinger, terribly hot and airless, sounded like a Chinese joss-house. People tossing, moaning, cursing and muttering in sleep: a sort of febrile delirium.

Persistent signs of impending movement including the usual batteries of people typing out Nominal rolls – it seems that 1000 Australians are affected. Information has also been requested re equipment of officers (clothing etc.). Some N guards have announced that they are returning to Nippon in a day or so.

29–30 November 1942

Uneventful hot days under the coconut palms. I have a fine book, *Ghenghis Khan*, written by one Lamb and am greatly enjoying it. History will always be a passion with me.

[My wireless] Advancing 14 miles from Tunis; 365 planes shot down over Tripoli. But stationary some 80 miles south of Benghazi. Bitter fighting in NG. 15th Aust. M.G. Bn said to have ambushed a N battalion wiping out all except 50 taken prisoner. When Gs entered Toulon there was a certain amount of resistance and units of fleet in port were scuttled, the captain of the *Dunkerque* going down with his ship.

1 December 1942

Prospect of movement seems to be receding. Sidelight on N equipping of POWs – having collected deficiency in clothing, boots etc. for all this camp of 1400 men indents may be submitted to HQ but not more than *30* articles to be requested in any one item! Nevertheless, though nobody has a respirator, seeing that these were on the list we must ask for 30!

Lights out extended to 2230 hours for officers, who may sit outside until 2300 hours. N guard have moved outside of camp.

2 December 1942

Ns carrying out some most badly needed improvements to camp: cookhouse floor being cemented over and ovens of a sort being built using native labour.

Hygiene arrangements being improved by the introduction of additional larger seepage pits for 'septic tank' system.

There has recently been some confirmation of a report that 370 crew members of *Perth* (apart from our batch) are on the island. It is very hard to be really sure whether our troops have been shifted from the island or not.

3 December 1942

Difficulties in the hospital are really the limit. Resources rapidly diminishing to practically just tablets for above the diaphragm (acriflavine) and below the diaphragm (N creosote). No vaseline, no plaster, no Whitfield's ointment (nearly everyone has tinea), no mag. sulph, no ointments – yet many tropical-type ulcers. We have fortunately held grimly on to a few quinine tablets and a few M & Bs, but these will be gone soon. Patients lie on the universal bamboo 'bed' – the bug-ridden, iron-hard, slippery structure common to all huts. A primitive disinfector has been constructed and we manage to disinfect and 'debug' the bamboo of these beds by 'companies'.

4 December 1942

Asia Raya is rather interesting of late, drawing attention to the futility of American resistance in the Philippines and that American guerillas have not accomplished anything in the last three months up to October. Stalingrad area (southern) and a grand counter-attack is in progress. This they attribute to an act of desperation designed to raise the waning morale!

5 December 1942

Suffering from a large boil and cellulitis of the left forearm, and have had four sleepless nights with burning pain. Have been through a phase of 'rice poultice; now just hot foments 4-hourly' and glycerine dressings. (Luminal, 1 grain, to be taken tonight, S/Sgt Gibson having unearthed it on my behalf.) I hope this doesn't mean another break-out of the boil-ridden misery I enjoyed in the middle east. It is quite likely with this change to the humid tropical belt. In order to encourage our soldiers, the Japanese commander of this camp has said that 800 prisoners from this island who went by boats have arrived at their destination. Asked 'Where is this destination?', he replied, 'It's not possible to say but at that place it snows a lot.' Naturally that is not difficult to understand.

6 December 1942

Arm and forearm frightfully swollen and feel a bit toxic but the pain is easier, being reduced to a dull ache, and I slept on my bamboo horror much better last night. Our number showing malnutrition changes amongst the 1000 is now 160+.

On the 4th of this month an 'arts and crafts' exhibition was held. Numerous RAF exhibits included a number of articles cleverly made out of the plastic used for the windscreens of cockpits etc., a transparent, glass-like material with perfect finish and polish, also a number of paintings and drawings. A Dr Dawson has some excellent stuff in his sketch diary – a pictorial record of prison life. Some of this work touches me deeply – not only the faithful work of the craftsman scraping with the blunt penknife, but the sketches and paintings which depict the vivid beauty of sky and earth and tropical vegetation about us, all so easy to overlook when your heart is bitter and squalor and oppression crowd the mind.

[My wireless] Soloman Is losses of N in the various battles 250 ships; men lost: ¼ million and for the month up to and including October, 450 to 500 planes. Also during November planes lost in Solomans and New Guinea: 250, not including last 3 days when losses 60, 40, 23. This due to desperate efforts to supply troops by plane since they are splitting up into bands in NG.

7 December 1942

No further talk of a move and perhaps we will now be here until after Xmas anyway. Too much to hope that we will be saved by the gong I think. I had an argument today with Sgt Le Roi and was silly enough to bet that the attack in Burma will begin in the next month this causing a wager of £5. *Asia Raya* has had yet another desperate and bloody battle in the Solomons on 30/11 with great destruction to American Fleet for loss of only one N cruiser. It is amazing how the US navy keeps going!

8 December 1942

A year ago this very day N entered the war: in other words, today is 'Pearl Harbor Day'. As this is likely to be the last year that Japan will be in a position to celebrate the triumph of that fateful decision you may be sure that it is not being neglected.

As our camp is beside the main road from Batavia to Buitenzorg, we have seen something of the celebration and I was gratified and wholly amused by the excellent representation of N grotesqueness by groups of Javanese schoolchildren, many with a primitive band showing a most deplorable lack of 'Brasso' in all cases. First, I saw a large party of small Javanese children all carrying the N flag and nearly peeing themselves with laughter at the sight of the prisoners behind the barbed wire who in truth were hardly less amused; then a band; then a large party of children dressed as miniature N soldiers and carrying rifles and bayonets of wood. These goosestepped and showed the highest morale and fierce demeanour. Among other notable sights a tank, an armoured vehicle mounted on a lorry (perhaps it could even have been a battleship!) but out of the turret appeared a martial head and shoulders of one who stared ever ahead into the distant spaces through 'field glasses', whilst another stood alongside for ever rigidly at the N salute. Followed a fine Navy O in wood and paper on a lorry accompanied by intrepid aviators, more lorries and more flags. One still more amusing sight: picture of cringing white captives (Javanese youth whose faces were plastered with flour) slouching along before a couple of resolute N soldiers also with rifle and bayonet of wood.

A most noticeable thing was the absence of evidence of N might. Not a tank or armoured vehicle passed and not a plane to be seen or heard overhead and this would seem very significant, *n'est-ce pas?* It is a long way to Batavia. I hope that the decent thing was done and the kids given a drink of ginger pop when they arrived to help them with the long and more dreary tramp home.

9 December 1942

N up to old tricks – requires of Jock Clarke (dentist) nominal rolls of people requiring dental attention labelled urgent, very urgent, very very urgent, very urgent urgent, but as they did not envisage any arrangements for men *without teeth at all* he was advised not to include any of these. The first list was regarded as *too big* (79); the next was *lost*; and the next he was instructed must not be bigger than 35 names! Irrespective of whether urgent or not! The engagement continues. Meantime, Jock continues to pull any really bad teeth and does temporary fillings with zinc oxide and oil of cloves. So of course the only very urgent cases are those poor fellows who have no teeth (broken plates etc.).

We have actually had a little in the way of medical stores for the next two months – this would constitute normally a nightmare supply for a RMO for say one week. Still it is something. It includes 2 bottles of 'Ebios' powdered yeast (about 1 lb in each: even this amount a godsend), and a little in the way of dressings, plus some salicylic acid (also godsend). The two little N orderlies here are not unhelpful but that does not help in combatting the system of supply for the prisoners.

Private circular for officers from CO re leakage of XXXX [wireless news] which has been most annoying.

10 December 1942

Today we had in the hospital hutment a meeting to sell the idea of the Memorial Book. Read many of the contributions and there was an impressive display of artistic exhibits (Dawson will be a great help there and of course Parkin's work is excellent).

11 December 1942

Dreams, nearly always of home, often come these nights and in consequence the dawn is heavy-lidded misery. There is such a complete detachment in a dream and such a gloomy chasm which lies between the dream state and normal contentment or semi-contentment. Nevertheless, to have dreamed of someone you love brings a lovely unreality into the day.

Previous fears appear to be realised; the supply of *katjang idjoe* beans has stopped, being no longer available after N requisition. Heavy evening rain at present, and the thatching over my bunk leaks like hell, though everyone else in this hut seems to be dry. When it is raining heavily parades are called off.

12 December 1942

Bandoeng Theatrical Company, local branch, are working on a new Xmas open air show, but otherwise I think this Xmas will be one of those which just slip into the limbo of forgotten things almost unnoted. The best present I could possibly receive would be a strictly private note from Helen saying, 'I am quite well. I am still in love with you and I will bear this waiting somehow.' I am not a jealous person and I am sure I could take any sort of blow to my engagement like a sportsman, but this complete separation and sensation of being dead as far as relatives or loved ones are concerned brings a cold fear to my heart sometimes. For at home people will be so much alive, there will be the keen bustle and romance of a country close to war – young men going to war, young men pathetically and romantically wounded and everything combining to underline the importance of the present tense.

The UK medical officers have started working on their avitaminosis cases on the basis of our pro formas and seem to be having rather startlingly different ideas about the sensory findings. They consider most cases show sensory loss on dorsum of feet to pin point. I think this is tripe and so do Arthur and Ewen; it is due to a lack of appreciation of normal sensation in parts where there is no hair.

13 December 1942

Rain at 0700 hours today – a rather exceptional time – parade cancelled. This is a poor spot for leather. Even if you do not wear the shoes they go mouldy.

14 December 1942

It is interesting that we have not seen any N planes in this area for at least two weeks – a highly significant fact.

15 December 1942

Jock Clarke has received some dental equipment which, in itself, would be almost useless, but when used with what he has already enables him to do some work. There is no amalgam for fillings, no facilities for denture work (Ns are not interested in dentures) and (if he did not have some himself) no local anaesthetic. A company competition at deck tennis is in progress: Arthur Moon and I won our first game today. A grand cricket match (under local conditions using a baseball bat) took place: English *vs* Australians. Aust. won by an innings and 6 runs.

Another short letter to go off today to home and I find writing very difficult, especially in view of the fact that the wireless propaganda is no doubt in use. Also, writing one letter means writing to the family and Helen all in one, not very satisfactory altogether, and I find it impossible to say anything significant or sentimental or real and feel rather like one trying to speak from the dead.

16 December 1942

Everything going smoothly. It is almost impossible to keep count of time and the writing of this diary lags steadily behind. The blackout regulations lasted only four days and things are now the same as previously. I have an awful fear that I am going to seed as regards efficiency and that after the war I will be able to do just damn-all in a day. At present there are about twenty Australian patients in hospital, mostly avitaminosis and a few ulcers of the leg which are very difficult to treat under present conditions.

17 December 1942

Have begun the first review of the avitaminosis gang and find that a great number of them have improved. Many fellows receiving an extra egg are going in for a great deal of sport (basketball, volley ball, cricket). This is absolutely anomalous and I have asked the CO to forbid the practice.

18 December 1942

A revival of bashing (N officers away). Four RAF officers struck for not paying compliments to N NCO *outside* the fence (no orderly armband). As a result, orders have been issued that all ranks will pay compliments to N soldiers at all times, including those outside the fence who are posted on duties (sentries).

Sqn Ldr MacGrath suggests we combine medical administration, which has previously been on the basis of Australian group (temporary) tacked onto RAF (permanent), and that I act as SMO. At present, hospital is in two halves and orderlies function independently. I agree with this policy, subject to Sqn Ldr MacGrath agreeing to carry on with supply arrangements, which he understands well; Sgt Wiseman (Aust.) to take over any 'dispensing' and control and issue of drugs (subject to Sqn Ldr MacGrath); S/Sgt Gibson and present acting British Sgt to confer in picking a team common for all hospital duties (S/Sgt Gibson to take charge); and a roster of all suitable orderlies to operate with change of duties each week. Sixteen NCOs and orderlies on duty each day. Those on duty for one week to share the N pay (which is for 2 sergeants and 6 N orderlies). I have suggested segregation of orderlies living in the hospital hutment as much as possible (a partition), if not, to get their bunks into inspection order and then get right out during medical activities in the morning.

Some attempt must be made to sterilise dressings and maintain an antiseptic technique. Sick parades to be changed from present 1100 to 0910 so as to synchronise dressing work of British and Australian campments and reduce orderlies.

19 December 1942

Feeling on top of the world because I managed to avert my next boil with phenol cautery method. Feet still moderate oedema.

Reading *My Country and My People* by Lin Yutang, a most interesting book. The Chinese character is a subject of universal interest these days. The western world is 'sick' without doubt; and perhaps we are not as happy as the Chinese. It is a striking error to assume that the comforts and amenities of western society necessarily bring happiness. *Au contraire*, possibly most happiness of this world is that of simple people living close to the soil. Even my present squalid conditions with the terrible limitations do not make me really unhappy. Happiness is something rather individual and internal. Not even the precarious prospects of the immediate future disturb one very much. Supposing our Java adventure ends in death somewhere, somehow, in this sullen soil, or under these eastern seas, there is something in the thought that perhaps my love was a thing which soared so wondrously above other things life which in turn have suffered the 'corrosion of the world's slow stain'. Already it has been the most beautiful and real thing in life for over five years. Is this the real reason why Helen and I have not managed to break down space and time to be together? Some deep subconscious instinct not to risk something very precious in the ordinary commerce between humanity? The old have your cake and eat it controversy.

20 December 1942

Sunday. Last night rather trying as I found the top of my mosquito net alive with some hundreds of bugs in various stages of development, which no doubt have been accumulating for weeks. Scrapped my net to await disinfection in the morning and spent a rather poor night with bug phobia and constant attacks from mosquitoes. John Morris works out our present accommodation as 11s 0d per square foot/month: 'Living at 11 bob a foot'.

The band have been given permission to play on Sunday, yet today they were broken up and slapped. When a protest was made Ns said today was not Sunday, could not be Sunday in fact, because look at everybody working, *corvées* out etc! Later, face saved by saying new regulation now – band may play on Wednesday and Saturday of the Christians' week!

[My wireless] The attack in Burma has begun around Akyab. The English are between Benghazi and Tripoli – my wager is won!

21 December 1942

Quite a few soldiers have an external otitis of 'the Singapore ear' type which is not very easy to treat under present circumstances.

22 December 1942

Momentous day: received per radio by means by the Batavia station and the ABC the following message from Helen: 'Delighted to get your message. Splendid efforts commanding your hospital. Am happy, well and not worrying. Keep cheerful. Our future holds so much. Love Fawn.'

This is the very best sort of Xmas present and makes imprisonment just possible to put up with. Also the Ns have supplied us with little pro formas for *lettres* home (every two months in the case of officers). These are a series of semi-propaganda statements, of which one may select three, but it is possible to send 20 words of a personal nature. I have written mine to Helen today, it being more or less a reply to her message, informing her of the receipt of hers to me at Christmas.

23 December 1942

Ns have supplied pestis vaccine: injections of ½ cc per person given (excepting some 80 men for whom there was insufficient). Went very smoothly with four doctors, Moon, Corlette, Godlee and I, injecting over 700 in 2 hours. Commenced today a series of lectures on the stock exchange in Australia by Dick Allen (Altmann, London Stock Exchange, will also talk at a later date and there is a separate series on economics).

One of the CCS lads, *Quinn* (a good fellow), has been in hospital for two months with suspected TB. Most of the signs are in right lower lung lobe.

24 December 1942

Christmas eve, and in spite of prevailing conditions there is a Xmas feeling in the place. The troops have been surprisingly happy in this camp, since they have not had enough to quarrel about. I have been very surprised to find that many ORs under present conditions convey all the appearances of complete happiness. This no doubt is due to the fact that their lives are completely ordered for them and there is no possibility of any advancement, hence no place for jealousy or competition. The troops know that they have no rights whatever as far as the Ns are concerned and, when all is said and done, man does not need very much excuse to do sweet nothing all day indulging in conversation with his fellows.

Two sources of 'belly aching' always remain: the distribution of food and 'the officers' (never the N officers).

Games are being enthusiastically followed, especially cricket, basketball, 'circlos' volley ball and 'golf'. Balls are canvas affairs made out of insulator tape and things of that sort and the courses are miniature. Sticks 1, 2, 3 'bamboo' – or 'palm' – some of them now improving vastly with a genuine 'iron' blade made of petrol or garbage tin material curved round the end and finishing in a suitable blade. This game is enthusiastically supported. The courses are many and various in the rough red-brown cracking earth under the palms, the holes being simple little excavations in the ground.

Local N soldiers recently on day leave in Batavia came back *un peu gris**. The N sergeant-major took a poor view and paraded them for a piece of his mind. They were then sent on a *run* to Batavia (17 kilometres) with ordinary equipment, side haversack, water bottle, rifle and bayonet.

Christmas eve show *Xmas Krackers* produced by Ian Wynne (JDM in the background); quite good slapstick. John Morris produced two new songs of his own, a slow fox trot 'In Every Song', and 'Happy New Year' chorus:

> Happy New Year to you – good cheer to everyone
> Put on your brightest smile and let's have lots of fun
> LEAVE ALL YOUR CARES behind for bright days are in view
> LIFE UP YOUR VOICE IN SONG – There's a happy New Year for you

A windfall arrived this evening in the form of presents sent in from outside (presumably the generous Dutch women again). Cigarettes, cigars, sweets,

* A little drunk.

peanuts, biscuits, clothing, few boots and shoes, some sporting material – something for everyone in camp. Our company and some of the others are giving the whole of this to the men. It will be a wonderful thing for the lads to all have something to smoke for Xmas.

25 December 1942

A cheery Xmas spirit prevails in spite of everything. *Happy Xmas to you Helen dear*

Menu for the day

Breakfast	Lunch	Tea
Rice as usual	Rice with meat	Vegetable stew with
a bun per man	*Katjang idioe*	sweet potatoes and
	Egg 1	50 chickens added
	Roly Poly Pudding	Tea
	1 banana per man	
	coffee	

As officers also we achieved two superlative additions. Lunch: *FRUIT SALAD*; Tea: *a chicken between John, Arthur and me*. What luxury!

An impressive combined service at 0930 of some 1400 men in the form of a hollow square in the recreation ground, with a choir at the eastern end. All the old Xmas hymns, and the choir sang some carols very well, accompanied by Page of the silver trumpet and 'Curly' with the baritone. 'Silent Night' was very well done. The rest of the morning was spent in hospital work, calls and playing 'circlos', Arthur and I beating up Jock Clarke and JDM 3 sets to one. Some games in the afternoon but much post-prandial torpor (perhaps a little of this due to half a mug of crude white wine given me by Lt-Col. Lyneham).

Rain only in the evening and the good news that the Ns had procured for us a piano for the day. The evening was positively hearty, beginning with open-air carols and singing round the piano. I visited the RAF mess with Ron Ramsay Rae and Lt-Col. Lyneham – much fun, all officers contributing songs, monologues and horse play e.g. 'Hit me Here'! A few pitched battles with pawpaw skins, even.

Quite a few of the Ns had passed on bottles of beer, one or two officers having even donated 3 bottles! I achieved a whole mug of beer! Strolling entertainers kept calling in to entertain, clothed in odd costumes e.g. Salome's dance of the veils and many strange affairs. At one stage Wing Commander King, replying to an attack from Rex (NZ) in the form of a banana in the face, leapt like a stag upon his victim seated on the bamboo bed. Rex somehow slipped out with an equally rapid leap and Winky landed in a 4-point crash with supreme astonishment on his face. And so on, with uproarious tomfoolery and merry chatter until about 0130 hours when we moved out to the group round the piano.

Major Anami himself puffed into the camp earlier and was in jovial mood, even shooting off a specially learned phrase 'I send you happy Xmas'. He decreed that lights might stay on all night and all night revels permitted if we were on parade on time in the morning.

Huge crowds around the piano, faces vividly lit up by the cookhouse lights, all animated and very happy.

A lovely night with a splendid moon flitting amid banks of clouds and the dark palms showing delicate silvery fronds. The pianist (Williams) is one of those people who can really get emotion out of a piano, and many of the songs were filled with that lovely old melancholy that endures. Everyone singing lustily, happy but with that warming, intimate, inner sadness. Artists appeared endlessly as they drifted along, some old, some quite new, even grand opera. Ron Ramsay Rae sang 'The Singing Soldier', some RAF lads have fine voices. A few in much lighter vein. To bed about 0400, but the singing was still going on when I entered 'the land of Nod'.

26 December 1942

Tremendous sporting enthusiasm prevails. I find myself running against Ron Ramsay Rae, playing basketball and so on. Relay Race. The senior officers' team was Fred Camroux, Hec Greiner, Billy Wearne and I. 440 laps each on a terrible track with hazards of drains, wires etc. and real tropical heat and humidity – assorted footwear. My team won their heat: time: 2.47. But the best time of the day was put up by an RAF team: 2.41. My time was the best individual run of the day, 53 secs, which surprises me in view of the fact I never run or train. Some of the interstate basketball was very good, especially a very fast match between WA and SA and a final between Vic.and WA (21 all). My team was eliminated by the NZ All Blacks 16–6.

Bosch. Two or three buses stopped just outside our camp area today, with N soldiers saluting and paying compliments freely. Some of the passengers were wearing naval caps, but most of them were in white sun helmets. As they were white European types, some blond and 'Aryan' in appearance, the conclusion above was drawn.

27 December 1942

Sunday. All the screening is being removed from the barbed wire round the camp, exposing the road and the rather squalid buildings opposite. This particular point is a sentry post and all vehicles stop here. Strong rumours arising today as to movements and conflicting rumours as to movement of senior officers, as usual some claiming that Brig. Blackburn had left already. A Nip walked into G camp barracks and confided to all, 'You go Nippon'. Nippon propaganda circular handed in today, much after the style of thing we use but very exaggerated with practically all old news – staggering success Solomons, New Guinea and much talk of Pearl Harbor and Philippines.

28 December 1942

Clear and fine. We were ordered to supply the names of all those men unfit to march apart from those in hospital.

Ns asked for a return of medical personnel today requesting medical and dental officers, medial orderlies and dental orderlies. Specimens of stools are required from all dysentery and diarrhoea cases, and return of all deficiency diseases, beriberi etc. is to be made. This confirms the prospective movement and now, in the evening, the usual battery of typists is at work on our cards and a return is required by 0900 tomorrow of troops without a blanket, footwear or eating utensils.

Nip commander (Lt Tanaka) had a parade of all troops marked unfit to march. He inspected them all sympathetically and marked his movement rolls without comment. He is a very intelligent fellow who speaks a little English and has always behaved well to prisoners here.

All troops are to parade at 0930 in morning with a specimen of faeces on a bit of paper, a somewhat dextrous and maladorous feat.

'Mac' came in tonight with 'Gin'; our cards are marked 'S', or should I say T; on the whole, a better destination than N.* What is the reaction to all this? Very philosophic and fatalistic, almost to the point of apathy. Those who are sick and likely to be left behind, however, all want to come and that is easily understood: it is good to keep old friends around in times of trouble and the unit spirit remains. God knows what lies ahead in the way of hardship, short rations, disease and death before the end of the road, but the mind does not speculate much about these things. As for me, I am perhaps a *vrai voyageur* and hanker for new countries and new experiences that we sum up as 'adventure'. My attitude is that I should like to stay in Java if there is a hope of relief and getting back into the war effort again, but otherwise I should prefer to be moving on, even to Nippon itself. I think I am right in saying that the experiences of the last three years have left me with a nervous system as strong as an ox. I am not one of those who do not know fear, but I have learned that fear is easily trampled underfoot by self-discipline and a resolute and steadfast way of living. Also, despite the all too rapid march of the years, I am lucky in my constitutional toughness. Life really hasn't been too bad, even under the squalid circumstances of this camp. There have been a few good books and some good fellowships.

30 December 1942

Everyone on parade this morning with the jolly old faeces in hand – but worse to come in the form of rectal 'swabbing'. N officer arrived with his team and a previously prepared list of 972, consisting of groups of 50 (haphazard apparently) with no relation to our companies, one subaltern officer or CSM to each group and other officers left over in one group until last. They were most efficient: our adjutant called the men up by numbers from the roll. He then passed on to the rectal swabbers (2) who inserted a glass rod and transferred a drop to the culture in the petri dish. This was in turn passed to two further technicians, who smeared the culture with platinum loops. All attendents were gowned and the swabbers etc. were masked and gloved. It appeared to be a very thorough and efficiently organised affair.

It now appears that certainly a few CCS people will be left behind; W/O Etherington, who has infected tinea of feet, J.C. Brown who joined the unit

* Interpreted as Singapore/Thailand.

rather recently and is NBG (discharged dysentery recently), Roberts, general duties, quite a good chap, also Anderson 'Pluto' otherwise Henry, who is in hospital with malaria and Quinn (Sapper) with TB. None of these were swabbed this morning, but a number of NZs and quite a few RAF Australians were. Probably some of these will be going along with us.

General parade 1400 hours to show specimens of faeces on papers; N doctor was late – a damned hot and smelly spectacle. Eventually, as it began to pour, troops dismissed to barracks where inspection was carried out by the beds. Arthur Moon accompanied N doctor, sergeant and 2 orderlies plus MacDonald as interpreter and Sqn Ldr MacGrath. Doctor seemed a decent sort. He looked at each revolting specimen and then hard at the face of the prisoners. Three or four sick men were smoothly knocked off, also one or two whose motions showed diarrhoea. He then inspected the men labelled too sick to walk and knocked most of these off the draft.

Many moans now, both from those on draft and those not permitted to go 'who want to go with their cobbers'.

At 8 pm Ns ordered injection of typhold/cholera/dysentery, ½cc to be given to all those on draft. As there was now no daylight, we rigged up two tables just outside the cookhouse and using the cookhouse fire for sterilisation started at 9.15 pm, finishing in 1½ hours. It was heavy going in the half-light, wind and shadows but all went off fairly well. The cooks then kindly laid on some tea for the workers. We crawled into bed tired enough at 2315, after another of these dreadful faeces parades was announced for tomorrow.

31 December 1942

A day of rain, mud, parades and surprising reclassification in groups. Usual parade 0730 but no PT at 0900 owing to sore arms. At 1 pm faeces parade but dismissed because N doctor did not arrive. Reassembled 20 minutes later and English Dr Dawson (RAF) did it assisted by a N orderly.

General parade at 1600 hours: all Australian troops on the recreation area, British troops on the ground just inside the barbed wire fence between. N commander and sergeant orderly and interpreter 'Mac' had the Australians called out in groups of 50, these commanded either by an officer or CSM, the highest officer being De Crespigny (major) captains Allen, Piper and Hands, lieutenants Smedley and Airey, the rest CSMs. Eighteen groups of 50, one extra consisting of majors Wearne, Woods, Greiner, Moon and Corlette, Capt. Godlee and me as senior officer. This complete disruption of our organisation included even 2/3 M.G. Bn! Notables not going apparently include Lt-Col. Lyneham, Ramsay Rae, John Morris, Fred Camroux and Tom Elliott, Ian Cameron and Bill Clarke.

I was required to find some replacements of men rejected and falling out sick from the already rejected sick, plus 8 RAAF men from the UK side. I then approached the Nips re two padres, but was told I could only have them at the expense of other officers and reluctantly decided not to replace them owing to the shortage of the latter. We will miss Fred Camroux and Tom Elliott no end.

Nip doctors later came to take rectal swabs of 8 cases of dysentery for whom we had supplied specimens of faeces. They are faeces crazy and at 9 pm we were again issued with cellophane for another parade (faeces in hand) at 0900 hours tomorrow!

This is a 'shocker' to me. Billy Wearne will be the next senior officer in my party and I think of Smedley as adjutant. I have spoken to Lt-Col. Lyneham re distribution of money on a *per capita* basis.

Good Lord! This miserable travesty of an evening is really New Year's Eve – no celebration this time. Lights out as usual at 2000 hours N time. We may even move tomorrow.

1 January 1943

Fine but wet underfoot – feel rather murderous towards any one who talks about Happy New Year. Mass and church services held. Early sick parade and then injections TCD 1 cc. Move now probably not for a day or two. Some signs of Happy New Year about in the form of intoxicated Nips, one in particular upending a native girl by the road outside *en plein air*. Much singing, *kiotskéing* and beer flowing. Many sore arms.

Faeces parade on sports ground in sections. I wrote a letter to Helen and left it with JDM*; also wrote a recommendation for award for him covering his services with 1 Allied General Hospital and as 'camp adjutant' in various camps and 'for distinguished services'. JDM is fixing our marching hard rations, chocolate and tinned food. (I have one tin of bully beef, 3 tins salmon still.)

2 January 1943

Total for move at present is 895, made up of 15 officers, 12 WOs and 868 ORs.

Orders and cellophane for a new faeces parade tomorrow.

I was called to the *kebetei* and told that the move was tomorrow night – 'too hot for march by day'. The following stores are to be drawn by 0830 hours tomorrow:

Coats 173	Mosquito nets 885
Shorts 173	Underpants 173
Shirts 173	Plates 430
Singlets 173	Forks 430
Caps 173	Buckets 36
Rubber boots 862	Ladles 36

1 Mosquito nets to be issued (all men in camp who have not got one were issued);
2 20 men to collect at 0830 stores;
3 Parade at 0900 hours without baggage;
4 A previous issue made of a few stores. My signature now required for these.

Unfortunately the rubber boots are the N horrors for the most part with bifed toe piece and lace up the back. Also all sizes are small.

Had an appalling affair with a large rat which got inside my mosquito net and chewed my hair, finally running over my face and becoming tangled in the net.

* Poor John Morris; he was torpedoed and died at sea.

A short, horrid struggle while striking it with my torch which kept going out. Finally the rat escaped – he bit my chest twice; damn him and his family.

3 January 1943

Stores collected 0830. Parade; faeces inspection; officers were then given an account of their 'savings' to check and keep. Mine now amounting to 280 gulden (440–120–40). Then the cards for personnel were checked.

After the parade we were given more TCD, 1½cc each for injection (all these at two-daily intervals, and our men moving tonight. You can guess where these injections went!). Parade at 1800 hours on the recreation ground, wearing our numbers, in full marching order and kit. Movement on 4 January to occur as follows: Groups 1 to 9 are to assemble on recreation ground by 0130 hours, I/C Maj. De Crespigny; Groups 10 to 18 at 0230 hours, I/C Lt-Col. Dunlop. Parties said to meet again at 0700 hours in morning. No rations to be supplied tomorrow until evening, so we are to take what we can with us. Each man has 4 eggs and, if he has kept them, will have 2 buns. In addition I have arranged with Lt Tanaka to collect potatoes to cook and take in our buckets in bulk for later issue. It was agreed that Maj. Moon and four elderly soldiers will accompany baggage on the lorry.

The orders for movement were then issued to Group OCs and arrangements made. Each man is to have a full water bottle and as much additional rice as he can carry.

We had at 0800 hours a sad little farewell gathering of 2/2 Aust CCS and 1 Java Amb. Car Unit to say goodbyes. All officers and NCOs made speeches. I then visited the hospital, the RAF medical orderlies and the RAF mess to say my 'ta tas'. F/O Young very decently gave me a tin of pipe tobacco.

5 Singapore

January 1943

4 January 1943

A day like an incredible nightmare or an old-time yellow-back fiction. First parade assembled under 'Crep'* at 0100 hours, parade state made and N officer arrived punctually at 0130. Party finally moved off at 0200 hours towards Batavia. My parade was then assembled and also checked. The parade states are as follows:

Group	*Off*	*W/O*	*ORs*	*Tot*	*Group*	*Off*	*W/O*	*ORs*	*Tot*
1	1	–	49	50	10	–	1	49	50
2	1	–	47	48	11	–	1	49	50
3	1	–	49	50	12	–	1	49	50
4	1	–	48	49	13	–	1	48	49
5	1	–	49	50	14	–	1	49	50
6	1	–	47	48	15	–	1	48	49
7	1	–	49	50	16	–	1	49	50
8	0	1	49	50	17	–	1	49	50
9	0	1	49	50	18	8	1	26	35
	7	2	436	445		8	9	417	433

Parade states moved off in 4s, No 10 'platoon' leading, myself in rear with officers.

We reached the station (Meester Cornelius) after a continuous march 8 kilometres through the warm starry night. The moon was not up so it was very dark, which slowed the pace a bit at times. No traffic was on the road except cars of accompanying N officers. We reached the station 0445 and entrained 0610, reaching Tanjongpriok Station at 0630. From there, we marched to the wharf by 0700 (no sleep of course last night) and as we marched up to position on the wharf, we passed a party of approximately a thousand Australians, though I did not recognise them in the half light. A party of about a hundred Dutch immediately began to give us the 'gen' – same old 'bull', with a little truth here and there and a few optimistic opinions thrown in.

My wordly possessions are contained in my pack, haversack and respirator

* Major J. Champion De Crespigney.

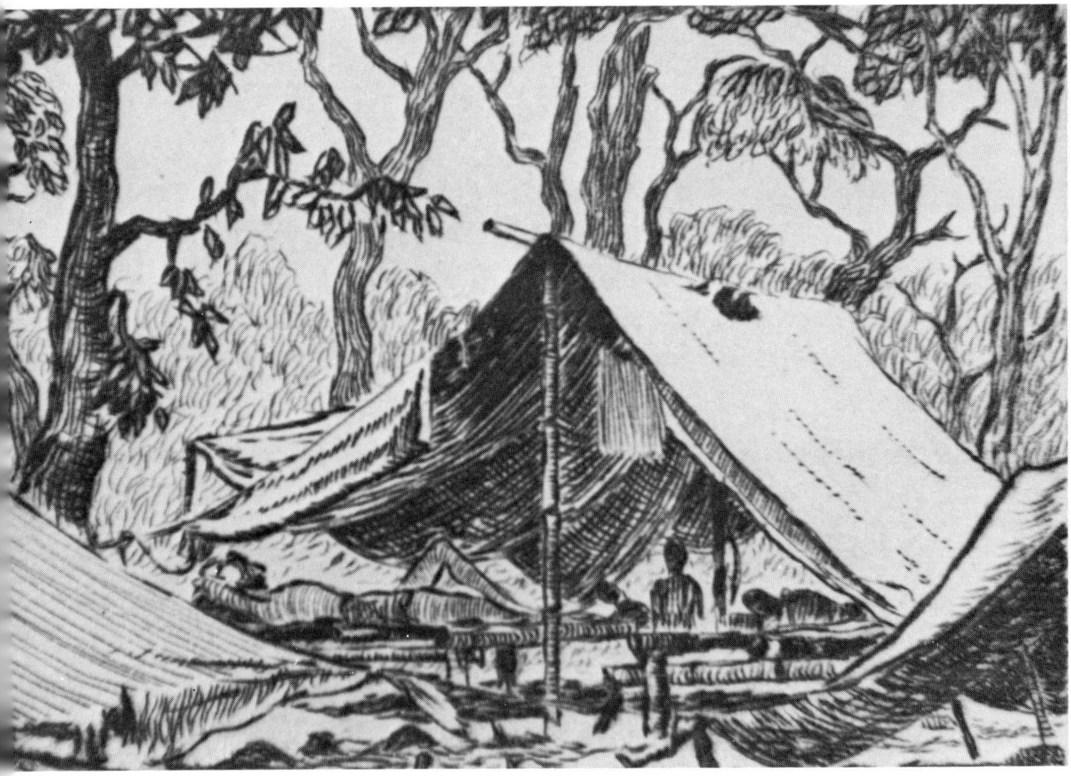

ts at Hintok (*Ray Parkin*)

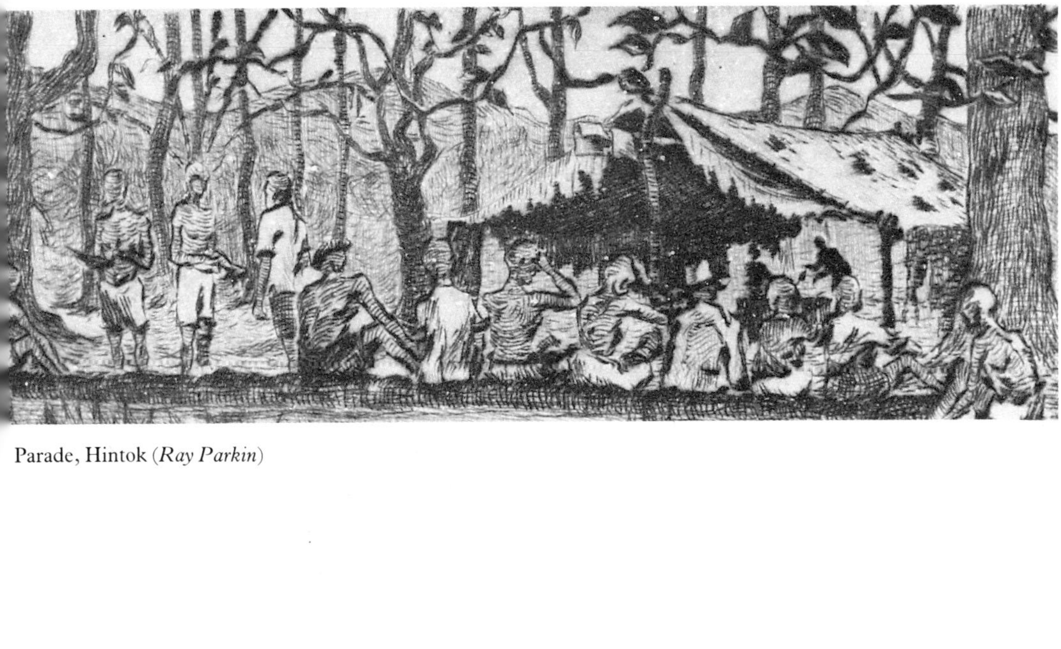

Parade, Hintok (*Ray Parkin*)

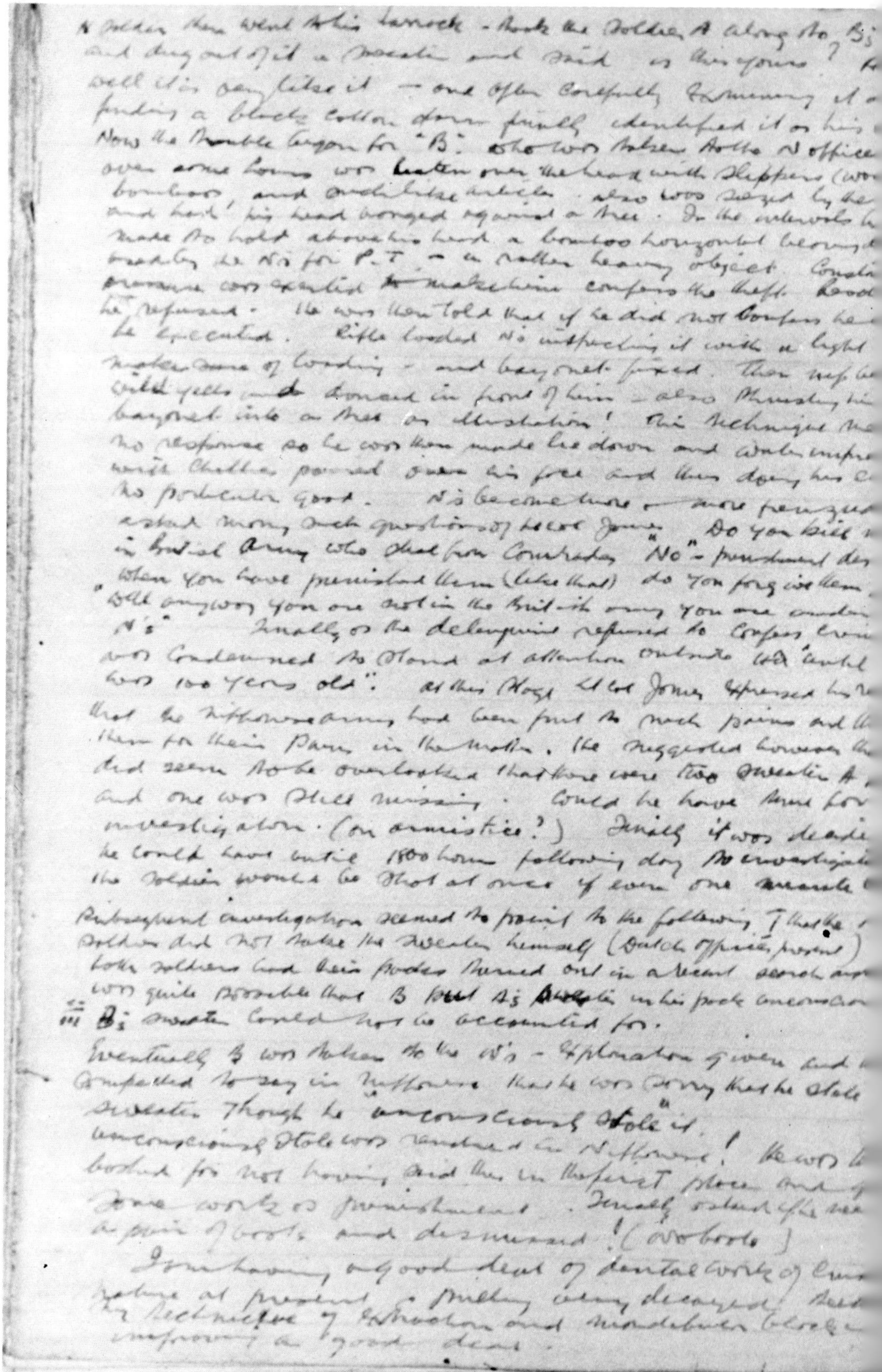
A soldier then went to his barrack — took the soldier A along to B's
and dug out of it a sweater and said is this yours? ...
well it is very like it — and after carefully examining it a[nd]
finding a black cotton darn finally identified it as his.
Now the trouble began for "B" who was taken to the N office
over some hours was beaten over the head with slippers (wo...)
bamboos, and such like article. Also was seized by the...
and had his head banged against a tree. In the intervals he
made to hold above his head a bamboo horizontal bearing...
probably the N's for P.T. — a rather heavy object. Consid[erable]
pressure was exerted to make him confess the theft. Needl[ess]
he refused. He was then told that if he did not confess he...
be executed. Rifle loaded N inspecting it with a light
make sure of loading — and bayonet fixed. Then N...
with yells and danced in front of him — also thrusting his
bayonet into a tree as illustration! This technique ...
no response so he was then made lie down and water impr...
with chatties poured over his face and thus doing his ...
no particular good. N's became more — more persuasi[ve]
asked many such questions of Lt Col Jones. "Do you kill ...
in British Army who steal from comrades" "No" — punishment des...
When you have punished them (like that) do you forgive them...
"Well anyway you are not in the British army you are under
N's". Finally as the delinquent refused to confess ...
was condemned to stand at attention outside "till" until [he]
was 100 years old". At this stage Lt Col Jones expressed his re[gret]
that the Nipponese army had been put to such pains and th[anked]
them for their pains in the matter. He suggested however th[at it]
did seem to be overlooked that there were two sweaters A...
and one was still missing. Could he have time for
investigation. (an armistice?) Finally it was decide[d]
he could have until 1800 hours following day to investigate...
the soldier would be shot at once if even one sweater...
Subsequent investigation seemed to point to the following: i that the ...
soldier did not take the sweater himself (Dutch officer present)
both soldiers had their packs turned out in a recent search an[d it]
ii was quite possible that B put A's sweater in his pack unconscio[usly]
iii B's sweater could not be accounted for.
Eventually B was taken to the N's — explanation given and ...
compelled to say in Nipponese that he was sorry that he stole
sweater though he "unconsciously stole" it.
unconsciously stole was rendered in Nipponese! He was ...
booked for not having said this in the first place and ...
some works as punishment. Finally asked if he ...
a pair of boots and dismissed! (no boots)
I am having a good deal of dental work of ...
nature at present — fillings many decayed ...
my technique of extraction and mandibular block ...
improving a good deal.

41 Diary pages, Thailand, 1943

O P S T
Sept. 22 11 20 17 = 70

Okada now knows it the own discretion as to how many
"heavy sick" are turned out – so long as not supplied enough!
The Lombok Wooly was very popular with Nips as a go to work song.
Today Lt Col Nagatomo turned a soldier over to the Nip for
striking a Sergeant Major. He was given a long lingering time undressing
and kneeling in the sun – sitting back on the heels splashing like which
buckets of water poured over the face – followed by blows & kicks and
few bouts of jiu jitsu as a means of beating up. No gross bodily damage
inflicted. The Col & Sergeant Major were formally called to
see that latter part of punishment. Finally both parties lectured
by Yamaka. The soldier not to be so impetuous & heed story
next time punishment would not be so light (and indications
of possible hanging invoked). Then to Lt Col & RSMs – must remember
that young soldiers required careful handling and tact. Discipline
must be enforced but must make allowances for youth etc and
must. Heart tactic.. In this case the soldier had been punished
must now be careful not to victimise and make it clear that
incident was now forgotten – admirable!
Into bitter boy soldier came to me to have a R upper molar
extracted. Novocaine ½%. Tooth broke leaving 2 roots embedded
and could not get them. He gave me $3 as he had no
cigarettes. I asked him if I could spend it on the sick.
Agreed very politely. A tough boy.
A party from Konkoita staged here on the way through
to ? Kami Tin. Arrived in darkness through...

Sept. Cholera Vaccine 1 C.C. injected

O_{22} P_{12} S_{24} T_{17} = 75. AIF.

Total Hosp and laid down figures for the camp range from
approx 250 – 300 depending on energies of Okada.
The latter is most frank at times and does a preliminary
inspection of the real figures and at times of Lt Col
Is Osuki etc may ask that the figures be
"adjusted" to "acceptable level". This proposal
is certainly dangerous as O might well then insist
on us and hold us to our figures. And also
requires considerable mathematical ability in keeping
our true & false figures in "gymnastic" style.

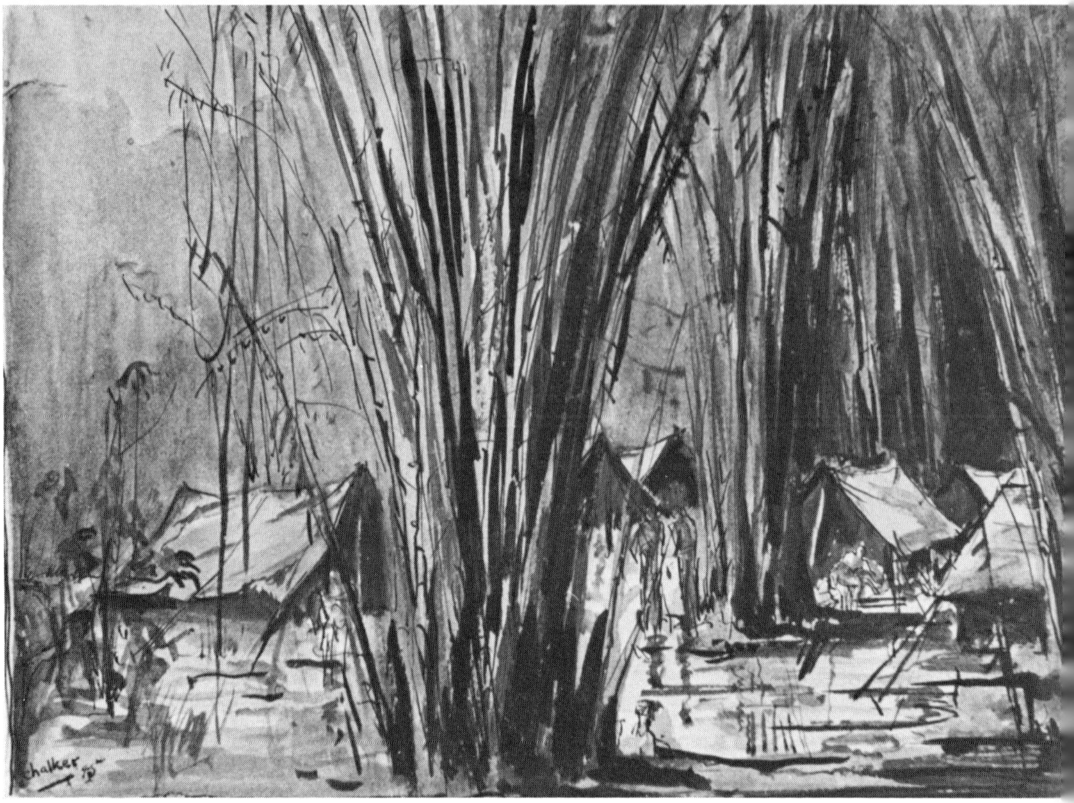

42 Cholera isolation area, Hintok (*Jack Chalker*)

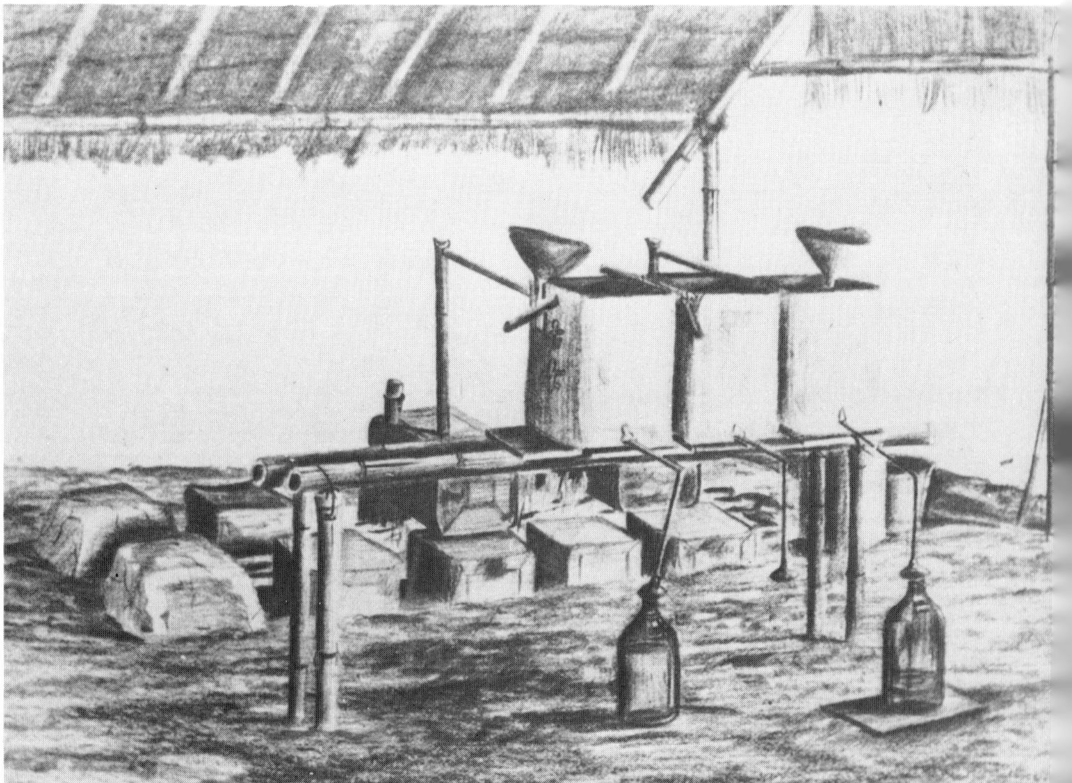

43 Still for distilled water, saline manufacture – petrol cans and bamboo. In the Hintok cholera epidemic we projected ste
a stolen petrol pipe through a water circulated bamboo jacket (*Jack Chalker*)

haversack, which I am carrying. I have a small suitcase (borrowed from John Morris) for my records and papers and everything else, including a leather medical haversack, is in my valise. Thus, with this arangement, if we fail to get transport, I am properly in the cart. On this move Arthur is baggage officer but he has been placed on the train at Meester Cornelius without knowledge of what the Nips are doing with it.

The embarkation. We were allowed to sit on the quay and debated who would be first aboard, because they would go to the very bowels of the ship. We were allowed to eat our breakfast meanwhile. The loading of troops was done with one gangway only, though another was available for the coming and going of ship's personnel.

The other Australian party began loading first and as they reached the gangway, carrying their baggage, they were dealt with by a gowned and gloved disinfecting party who lustily sprayed carbolic solution over them and their baggage with two sprayers. This gesture is like trying to combat filthy conditions with perfume. It is interesting that though our troops must presumably have all sorts of bowel infections nobody was knocked off the list after the rectal swab parade. Another gesture?

Embarkation of our party began last at approximately 0930, commencing with 10 group → 18 group, then 1–9, these parties of 433 and 445 to go into separate holds. Loading time for our party (878): approx. 1 hour. We had by this time got our baggage and had spread the food buckets, so that some went with each group. Maj. Moon stayed to distribute these and to get all baggage aboard. I managed to carry all mine aboard with me.

There were two small gangways to our hold for 433 men and all were drafted like sheep to these, duly stumbling down to a scene which surely is some figment of the imagination when one ponders over the black hole of Calcutta. A typical hold of a rusty old tramp, a square vent above practically covered with heavy planks, rust and cobwebs everywhere. Every square inch of space is occupied by a man or his baggage, which at present is in a hopeless pile in the centre. Rats and cockroaches aplenty. The ship, of 6–7000 tons according to P/O Abbott, has 1 funnel and is a coal-burning, very old hulk lightly loaded so that the Plimsoll was right up above the quay.

Our two groups are in two separate holds aft. Ours is formed by one deck only, an area 30 yards by 16 in all. Along the complete length on either side there are crude stagings to form 'bunks' – just a continuous stage throughout, of course, covered with rush mats, and going back 12 feet so that two men can lie head to foot. So this gives two layers, one at approximately deck level, one 3 ft 6 in. above. The central area is partly open to the sky – the loading hatches – and the floor is the planked-over hatch to the deck below which is filled with empty oil drums to give ballast.

A few Nipponese are sleeping at the aft end of our hold and these have much more space than our fellows. The guard can watch us through the open loading hatch and will allow only one man at a time up to latrines etc. There is a crude cooking galley with rice steamers etc. on either side of our 'quarters'. The aft quarters, in which Arthur and Crep are incarcerated, are even worse than ours, since the deck below is used as well and they are packed in the vertical as well as horizontal sense – though the net result is a little more space but less air.

The only Nip who has been down to see us is a *keicho* (L/Cpl), a funny little man with a hairy face and cap pulled right down to his eyebrows who has very little to say but is anxious apparently to help. I have found a Sgt Cameron who speaks a little Nipponese. Billy Wearne is undertaking to sort out troops into areas. After a little angry persuasion, the group W/Os were induced to make the troops take their kits up into the crowded bunks and the kit of the remainder was then sorted out in lines in the centre. The troops are all tired out after no sleep all night, marching some 10 kilometres with all equipment and the foul air down here.

Latrines are crude little rows of dog kennel size (which I can just get into), very foul and smelly wooden boxes. Excreta is passed into a central trench of sheet tin so that they can be flushed out with sea water. Washing is not allowed until late afternoon, when we could go out one or two at a time under supervision and use a little fresh water to wash face and arms. Soap not permitted (too much water required to lather up I suppose).

My cobber the *keicho* required a complete account of troops in this hold and as I did not know, he said we must have a roll call parade in 4s! This was tried but owing to the terrible congestion when men got off their bunks it was simply impossible. By calling group rolls it was proved that the only man missing was Arthur Moon (in the opposite hold). We were then told that we would be given tea at 1800. That we could 'have music' (that is, we were allowed to sing) until 2000 and smoke until 2100, then 'lights out'.

Roll call parade at 1730 and 2000. Tea was brought in about 1300 and the evening meal was a very thin vegetable soup and rice. They then let up a bit by saying that four men at once could go out to wash the face. I have paid one or two visits to Arthur and Crep to exchange information. At evening roll call several officers came through wearing staff bands. Usual *kiotské keré* regime. I then had a talk to N Lt about medical arrangements (no stores, though we were instructed that we must not take any from camp and that we would be given plenty on the ship). He vaguely promised to get some and said to put all the sick together in the morning so that he could see them. I also asked for some men to take exercise a few at a time. He could not allow this, but said that we would be at sea for only two days *until Singapore was reached.*

Later we were allowed to go up in twos for a breather and I stayed up talking to Crep and the Nipponese guards for an hour or two then found my way back to my sleeping area with difficulty. I am under the central opening with 6 officers.

Having just got a portion of my frame under the canvas cover of my valise, the rain poured down on us in torrents so that my feet were awash and water was getting in everywhere. I just refused to move. After about half an hour they closed up the hole above with planks with an awful clatter and began to pull tarpaulins over. In the process gallons more water poured down. Having not been dislodged by all this I was disgusted to have to get up to see young Watson who was complaining hysterically of pain in his calf and thigh. Cramp, poor chap.

5 January 1943

Slept like a top in spite of the wet, but I suppose the atmosphere would drug anybody. It makes the old cave in Tobruk seem like fresh air.

Troops were allowed out to wash this morning 20 at a time and a few at a time are also allowed to have a hose bath of sea water on deck. Only one other vessel in sight: a small steamer which was berthed behind us in Tanjongpriok. No escort. Land in sight both sides. 'Food' to be laid on (rice for breakfast and tea). Troops on board are *Australian* besides ourselves (40th Bn from Timor, no senior officer), about 20 2/2 Pioneers, some 3rd M.T., some engineers. Also a Dutch party. All other troops are in forward holds and number approx 570. I was amused that in the early hours of the morning a message was sent down from the sentry asking whether the *shoko* would like to come up for some more air – I sent Fred Smedley for a change.

Much more freedom being allowed on deck than hitherto. In fact, by getting hold of a lad carrying a bucket I managed to make my way right forward (through the N officers' quarters). There I found Lt Happy Houston of 2/2 Pioneers whom I did not recognise at first; he has had malaria and dysentery, losing some 5 stones in weight and had three months in hospital with arthritis following the dysentery. He told me much of events in Batavia, including some particulars of the torture of Pioneer officers to gain information. Naturally without results. He thought that some 14 men had died from various causes but that the health of the Australians had been better than the British. All Pioneers except the sick and one or two officers left the island three months ago and about a week ago the higher officers of N.E.I Army, British, Australian and American details left. This included Blackburn, Maltby etc. They left with all baggage, camp beds etc. and were said to be going to Formosa. Even ceremonial swords were returned. I estimate from this conversation that about 500 Australians, the sick and a few officers, remain in Java.

I returned safely by the same device of following a soldier with a bucket, as though detailed to supervise an official task. There are no senior officers with the 40th Bn party.

6 January 1943

Islands visible practically all the time. We will not be disembarking today, though we may make Singapore by evening. By various dodges, such as long queues for washing and latrines, most of us get 'upstairs' a good deal. Blue Maher has been looking after me very well in Blue Butterworth's absence. Arranged with Blue today to take my sea-kit bag with some books and instruments when we leave the ship. In the late evening we anchored off the east side of Singapore and are to disembark tomorrow.

7 January 1943

It is now rumoured that we will not be off until after lunch. It is much hotter here at anchor and we are eager to be off the ship. Meals as we know them have been good: rice and soup for each with tea, and the soup is often a good thick vegetable soup – also sometimes even with meat in evidence.

Later: we moved inshore in the afternoon, then moved south again down the coast so that the main buildings of Raffles Square showed up very clearly. Finally we rounded the southern part of the island and went into Keppel Harbour. We had a good view of all the main buildings from the sea. The much talked of destruction of everything was not very evident and it was a more or less orderly scene, though many of the buildings had obviously been renewed. There is an island for oil storage just off Keppel Harbour and the big oil tanks seemed to be all in order as before.

Presumably much of our careful manoeuvring has been through the enemy mine-fields. We have been without an escort during the voyage and no life-belts were issued. There were no special signs of vigilance on the ship though no doubt most of the lookout is kept forward. Only the sentries on duty have worn lifebelts. Very little shipping was seen until we actually got into harbour, but there we saw a number of ships ranging up to around 10,000 tons, including one rather new ship with good lines and a cruiser type of bow. Dock facilities seemed to be fairly normal.

'George', perhaps remembering his *keré*, made Billy Wearne and I enter the galley and eat a couple of large steaks streaming with sauce – this under the eyes of several troops, which made us feel fearful worms. Nevertheless, the gustatory satisfaction was unmistakeable.

Disembarkation finally occurred at 1700–1800 hours, going off in groups. We assembled outside about a hundred yards from the quay. There I found to my delight that the whole party was to be transported. At 1800 hours we were instructed to have *makan* [food]. By this time all parties were off the ship including the 2/40 Bn, Dutch etc.

As we entered the harbour Billy Wearne said to me irritably, 'What a place to lose!' and that, I suppose, is what we all felt.

Loading of N transport is a revelation. For example, on one 30 cwt lorry, 35 men of 18 group and one N sentry ('George' in body of lorry, two or three Nips in the cabin in front). This 35 included 8 officers with all their gear and some stores, practically everyone standing up massed together and swaying about. About forty is the usual load. Our Cook's tour then began in the evening light through the heart of the city. We had an excellent view since there was no cover on the back of the lorry. (N lorries never have covers.) Many of the buildings were bomb or shell-splattered but few showed any real wreckage. (I suppose that would have been cleared by now.) The central portions of the city, the city hall, post office, banks and fine buildings about Raffles Square, seemed to be quite undamaged. Raffles' statue had been removed. Many Malayan and Chinese civilians were about and some gave friendly signs.

Business seemed to be much as usual, although British banks have now become Yokohama Bank of Nippon etc. We moved on briskly until we were out of the city, past coconut and rubber plantations, until we reached the East Coast road. It was now evident that we were going to the Changi area and the burning question was Changi Gaol or the barracks? There was a bad moment when we stopped outside a large, forbidding structure with high walls (Changi Gaol) and cheers when we started again. Actually we have since found out that this gaol contains British civilians including women and children, who have all been there for months. As we moved on we noticed splendid stone buildings in a beautiful part of the island filled with British and Australian troops and – an astonishing sight – diggers *on guard* controlling traffic at points! All these troops are well dressed, very spick and span, officers with sticks and ever so much saluting. It was a clean and beautiful sight, with the sea sparkling away to the north across the Straits of Johore. The camp sites are hilly areas close to the shore and ideal for this part of the world, so our troops are singing and very cheerful.

The whole drive was about 24 kilometres. Finally we were set down in a large square (parade-ground) and, to my astonishment, neatly-dressed officers came up carrying canes, blowing out puffy little moustaches and talking in an 'old chappy' way. Aghast, I looked at their arm brassards, which were the red and black of army HQ (Malayan Command!). Much fuss about 'better get moving' and guides and chatter about our baggage which they said they would lock up and send on under Malayan Command. Movement control arrangements! Hurriedly and determinedly I grabbed my entire baggage and refused to be separated from it again!*

After about a mile of marching we reached our destination in southern area presided over by a Major Denaro MC who is in charge of 'the Reception Unit'. Nothing is simple now! A portion of southern area is given over to 'units in transit' and it was soon apparent that, so far as this area was concerned, this is not a good thing to be. Malayan Command arrangements proceeded merrily on during the early part of the night, resulting in my party being split into three groups as far as arrival into this area was concerned and Capt. Hands and 49 ORs were shunted over to 18 Div. area camp; in exchange, some similar number arrived here with Lt Primrose 40th Bn. The magnificent stone barracks of three storeys with red-tiled roofs occupy a lovely bluff overlooking the sea. They will take 200 troops to each floor with ease, using also the spacious balconies.

No lights on in this area except in the *kebetei* building, so the successive parties had to find their way into quarters in the dark. A meal was then provided (rice and tea), our cooks taking over immediately, releasing the Dutch.

I called over with Maj. Wearne to visit Brig. Blackburn who was in a nearby building with the D General staff, Governor-General, General Taporton, Air Vice-Marshal Maltby, Maj.-Gen. Sitwell etc. (These are to go on to Formosa on 10/1/43.) Brig.Blackburn was in bed but tumbled out and was very delighted to see Billy and me. He said he would be over in the morning to talk and to see his 'boys'. He is extremely thin and wasted, but his skin remains clear and eye keen.

8 January 1943

Surprisingly cool last night, had to get up for my rain coat as extra cover. I am sleeping hard with just a folded blanket between me and the cement floor. This is my only blanket but my canvas covers most of me. [For several years later, sleeping on slithering bamboo and rough, uneven surfaces, my mind turned to that lovely concrete in Singapore and its snug, matt surface. The nights not too

* I recalled the ghastly debacle of movement control arrangements for Australian Corps M.E.-Java.

hot or too cold, soft moonlight, no bugs or insects and the waft of hibiscus and frangipani – Malaysia heavenly comfort!]

Parade this morning to sort out all troops into the companies we used in Bandoeng. A.A. Moon has G company again; Billy Wearne is now my 2 I/C and Lt F. Smedley is adjutant. Sgt Barbett called in to say that he was running a Bureau of Records and Enquiry and requested a nominal roll with *Reg., Number, Name, Unit, next of kin*. This was promised. Brig. Blackburn VC came over very early and was soon plunged in conversation with 2/3 M.G. Bn lads.

Troops this morning are in 3 blocks: H, D and White House (latter is mixed Dutch and us). Dutch are everywhere here. Attended routine Reception Unit conference at 1015 but special newcomers' conference at noon. Some of the Reception Unit are O/C Maj. Denaro MC; Maj. May 2 I/C; Adj. Capt. Bailey; Q. Lt Wraight MBE; Hygiene Lt Jones; MO Capt. Diver my old voluble colleague of the Woolwich Memorial Hospital, long haired and irrepressible.* Still a useful contact, who at once promised to put us right medically. Lt Houston is in my area with 78. Capt. Trevena with his 2nd 40th Bn are over in 17th Div. area.

Conference: Denaro (bushy moustach and bristling with his own importance) has terrific organisation but no real 'low down'. Points:

1 All personnel White Block, H Block, so now to be in two adjacent blocks.

2 Orderly rooms to be established and reported to his HQ, where tables and chairs laid on (we have one little typewriter).

3 Conference 1015 each day adjutant or CO.

4 Adjutant to contact Fatigues officer (Lt Stamforth) each day (only fatigues paid are heavy fatigues at light duty pay).

5 Notified of acute shortage furniture, paper, firewood (former not to be used for latter purpose).

6 Areas of the camps: AIF 11 Div., 18 Div., Hospital area, Southern area (still Changi).

7 Passes: movement to be restricted to a minimum only on duty; pass to be signed by me or adjutant.

Camp Orders

1 No one allowed outside wire without a flag or armband.

2 No conversation with or buying and selling from natives permitted.

3 All cars with flags, Jap. patrols or sentries must be saluted when seen (safest to salute all N).

4 All ranks must be in quarters by lights out 2245 each night.

5 No fruit or vegetables to be taken from gardens or coconut trees.

6 No Java party personnel (ORs) are allowed inside the wire of southern area before 1300 hours each day except Sunday.

7 Only wood as issued from wood dump to be used.

8 No 'black marketing' allowed i.e. no trading for profit, though personal sales permitted.

9 All officers will be saluted by all ranks. All British officers will salute D

* Poor Diver, of St Mary's Hospital, is remembered by a memorial library. I last saw him before his death when we were in a *kempi* prison in Thailand.

officers of whatever rank. All officers here wear only one pip. By local arrangement in the case of field officers a red cloth background is introduced.
10 Nip roll call every day except Wednesday and Saturday at 1930 hours. Morning roll call is our own affair – 0815 each day, 0730 reveille, 0830 breakfast. For evening roll call we submit Parade States (Blocks) and also each evening Strength Return (Parties).

It is now arranged that Capt. Hands and his party return at once from 18th Div. and they are being replaced by Lt Primrose and his men.

Normal rolls in duplicate of all personnel to go to the Reception Unit. *Number*, *Rank*, *Initials*, *Name*. Money is to be handed in and changed for equivalent amounts of this island's N currency gulden for dollar. As far as the canteen is concerned, there is practically no food obtainable and prices are like skyrockets. A few odds and ends like peanuts seem to be the main articles! To my amusement, officers' baggage is still proceeding under Malayan Command arrangements! We are forming an officers' mess; De Crep is busy getting things together. Typically, the Reception Unit made no arrangements for officers and we had to ask, being then given good quarters M Block.

The commander of AIF details on the island is Lt-Col. Gallaghan DSO (Black Jack). He insists on a proper dress and smart turn out and has lashed verbally all Australian troops into smartness and saluting – a praiseworthy achievement! Much 5 and 28 days in detention barracks!

Troops all busy and shifting in today when a party of fellows with red arm bands arrived (a formal call by an expanded Divisional Staff without warning). I was suddenly faced with Lt-Col. Glynn White OBE (same voice too). I saluted on principle, though no badges of rank of course. Unfortunately, I did not catch the fact that one of the party was Commander AIF (Lt-Col. Gallaghan) and spent my time in reminiscences with Glynn White and Bruce Anderson asking many questions. Glynn promised to lay on medical stores for wherever we go. Unfortunately, the troops did not pay compliments as the party entered and it was only when, on leaving, Command AIF asked if he could do something for me that I caught on. I said we were badly off for clothing and he promised help, though there was little on the island. I was to consider what our requirements were and tackle him later, Billy and I are to dine with him on Sunday evening. Exit a flock of red armbands!

I then called on the hospital (Lt-Col. Hedly Summons) and he and his registrar spoke to me for some time. He told me of a message picked up here. No date. 'All's well, Love, Helen Ferguson' and I told him of a message for Wally Summons that I had seen in Java giving some particulars of the family.

Charles Osborne, Jock Frew, Howard Eddy, Orr (eye specialist) and many others I knew well were working at the hospital. The hospital, half Australian and half British, is housed in very large and excellently equipped buildings. They carry on much as usual and have plenty of work. They have exactly the same vitamin trouble here as we had in Java; scrotum, mouth, burning feet, some cases *spastic* paraplegia and amblyopia. With all their facilities they do not seem to be much ahead of us. They also are firmly convinced that it is a B_2 deficiency and they introduced rice polishings. Cases treated with marmite. Some cases even developed burning feet when under treatment – there seems to be a big lag there, both in onset and in recovery. They seem to have not had much luck with yeast and they have not used beans such as *katjang idjoe*. This trouble and beriberi was becoming acute before the hospital ship arrived in September, but since then they have had few cases.

9 January 1943

A.V.M Maltby seemed very pleased to see me and was grateful for information about the hospital (Java). He wished me to give him some names for recommendations etc. and particularly asked about Matron Borgmann Brouwer. I gave him my recommendation in respect of the following: Robby Cummings, Squadron Leader RAF Medical Services; Fl/Lt Willy, RAF Medical Service; 930618 Cpl E.J.S. Grove, A/Sgt-in-charge Medical Wards; 920405 Cpt J. Gibbs, Theatre Orderly. I also gave him notes on 1079384 A/Cl Griffiths W. and 977872 A/Cl Gannon J.D., the two lads with the eye injuries etc.

Group Capt. Nicholetts, who left Bandoeng on Xmas day, told me that 'Tinkle Bell' had cut his throat, so that great voice will now be silent forever. Poor Tinkle – the devil that took him up into high places and showed him the earth got him quickly enough. I suppose he just could not go on with their propaganda line.

Surprise of the day was a missive from Command AIF Lt-Col. Gallaghan, which ran as follows:

> To Lt-Col. Dunlop I/C AIF S. Area
> From HQ AIF Q.3250 9/1
> Com. AIF desires following information:
> Name of senior combatant officer with party
> Suggest changing O.C. party to combatant officer
> Is there any reason for not making change?
> 1600 *Alex Thompson Maj.*

My reply to Comd HQ AIF:

> From Lt-Col. E.E. Dunlop I/C AIF Sub area 9
> Ref your Q3250 9 Jan. 43. Senior combatant officer with party is Major W. Wearne. Your suggestion welcomed. Present arrangement result of Nip policy in Java of not recognising non-combatant personnel. As senior officer Lt-Col. E.E. Dunlop was instructed to command the party in transit. Before making any change your further advice would therefore be appreciated. Could this matter be discussed with Comd AIF tomorrow 10 Jan. 43?
>
> *E.E. Dunlop Lt-Col. 1730*

In the evening, Brig. Blackburn came in to say farewell and I brought the matter up. He was annoyed and wrote the following memo:

> I have considered this matter and desire Lt-Col. Dunlop to retain command for administrative and disciplinary purposes so long as the troops brought over by him remain together as one body.
>
> *Arthur S. Blackburn Brig.*

I discussed money, whereupon he gave me full support, both in the policy of levying officers hard and raising any money I could from any source, and in disciplinary matters. He says that he has insured the safety of all promotions by careful burial of records and dispersal.

10 January 1943

Called over very early and saw Brig. Blackburn giving him the recommendations for awards in Java which I had made. None of these were for specific awards (just a statement of circumstances etc) and they included John Morris. The generals and Governor-General reported in two lorries nearly as packed as the ones we came out here in, but their ship is reported to be a new transport, probably the one we saw coming into port. All their heavy baggage is already abroad.

I have asked company commanders to stress to all troops the importance of smartness, saluting and order in movements about the camp areas. We are sadly handicapped by our 'scratch' clothing. We seasoned veterans of three services suffer the term 'Java rabble'.

Dinner tonight at AIF HQ: Lt-Col. Gallaghan, Maj. Thompson acting A.Q., Capt. MacCauley, Maj. Anderson (Bruce) and Lt-Col. Glynn White. Capt. Peach. 'Black Jack' said that my position was quite incorrect and that as a non-combatant I had no authority whatever to give commands to or punish combatant soldiers. It was laid down by the book etc. (This is nonsense I know, as I have already had plenty of combatant soldiers under my command in units, and, anyway, note the case of a large Convalescence Depot [these are commanded by Medical Officers] and that sort of thing. However I could not be bothered arguing; I simply agreed with everything and said coldly, 'You are the Commander of Australian troops here, so take appropriate action.'

After a while I produced Brig. Blackburn's note very casually and he read that. He then asked what he could do for us and I spoke about: Leave parties (100 daily); clothing and boots (we are to submit requirements tomorrow); transfers (nothing doing); entertainment sports and education (Peach and other appropriate officers directed to give any help possible); and general matters of troops' health, discipline etc.

It was a pleasant dinner, anyway, with me devoting most of my attention thereafter to Glynn White and Bruce Anderson.

During this time, Billy had been dragged off by 'Black Jack' and interrogated *à propos* of the previous conversation. Billy is staunchly loyal; disagreed most entirely with BJ and told him that if he thought he was neglecting his responsibilities in not taking command he was prepared to give his reasons against it in writing. Billy intimated that no other officers in my party would accept the assignment. As a result BJ then saw me again and said he was now satisfied, but that in order to regularise things he would now give me a formal authority to command the troops. I remained bland and friendly and assured him I bore him no resentment (for meddling in my affairs) and that it was nice of him to go to all these pains on my behalf!

11 January 1943

Arranged with Jock Clarke to push on with dental arrangements, getting fillings done and plates under way immediately by direct negotiation with the hospital. Kit sort-out going on today. Glynn White fixing up medical stores to go along with us.

12 January 1943

Called at clothing depot (Capt. Carthew, Sgt Emmett, Sgt Ross). My stuff all ready, but very little for the troops: 6 pairs of boots size 11,150 pairs of socks, 20 Glengarry caps. Boots are the worst problem, as we have 189 fellows without them. Back to AIF HQ where I saw Black Jack, who talked to me about movement of my lads – straggling on the march, irregular movements etc. In truth I think they look pretty dreadful, but it is hard to put up a good show in rags. We then discussed our clothing problem and he sent Capt. Bennett off with me to pull every string possible re boots. No luck. It seems the real difficulty is that the Dutch passing through this area share equally in things and have to have full information [therefore] must avoid any suggestion of favouritism.

Called at depot Medical Stores. The stores as supplied for train parties of 650 are rather meagre (even though riches as compared with N supply); probably we will get one lot for 650, one for 350. I am giving Glynn White particulars of extra essentials.

13 January 1943

An irritating day. I can't help feeling disgust at all the well-shod and clothed people here when contrasted with our ragged mob, and the story about equipment at 'the other end' does not wash with me.

W/O 1 Mackenzie 2 Echelon Records AIF then called in and it seems that there is an opportunity to bury records securely here; he advises unloading all essentials. I must have some copies of essentials just in case, so I urgently want typewriters and help with typing. I passed on the information re records to reps of 2/3 M.G. Bn and Pioneers etc.

14 January 1943

Troops now organised and domestic routine is satisfactory. Parades, however, are a great worry to me, as the troops fidget continuously and move about with a constant buzz of conversation.

The weather is simply lovely and the nights cool enough to require a raincoat in addition to my canvas. This is a delightful spot with the sparkling sea of the straits stretching across to the green jungle of the mainland and the perfume of frangipanni and hibiscus, both of which abound here. The one thing missing is enough food: all the time one feels ravenously hungry and rice is very inadequate. There are quite a few admissions to hospital and we are getting rid of all cases that might prove a burden. I am very busy trotting about the camps making all useful contacts possible. Java records are to be 'put down' in a special container; W/O MacKenzie 2 Echelon will take mine. I will leave A and D books etc and take extracts. I hope to carry essential things with me, but it is a relief to have another 'saver'. Typing and paper is a great trouble.

In a recent conversation with Black Jack, the subject of finance came up in connection with the necessity of troops working to earn money: if any of the officers were short he would dig up 5 gulden per officer, he said. I did not want to make it an officers' issue as it should be a matter of troops, and the officers, if necessary, could have an advance from my public funds. On hearing that this was nearly 2000 gulden, however he said that was more than he had himself in all the area and that I certainly could not expect any help with anything. This I know to be absolute tripe – given that I am told his canteen runs to some 5000 gulden capital, and that there are very large numbers of officers contributing to his funds. More blustering nonsense.

15 January 1943

All troops are to contribute a third of their Nipponese pay to a fund to purchase food for the kitchens for all. Remainder for money is go to those who earn it. A higher levy may yet be necessary. This will be well received by troops because they can't purchase much in the area anyway.

A somewhat bitter letter was written to HQ southern area (admin. channel to Malayan command) re boots.

Position is: no boots – 178, and situation is rapidly deteriorating. Unserviceable boots: 204; urgently needing repair: 304. I took this along to CO Southern command personally.

17 January 1943

I am frightfully annoyed to learn from Glynn White that Black Jack turned down his offer re rice polishings because we had 2000 gulden and said we must buy it (approx. 90 gulden). He had his own 10,000 to look after. I wrote a rather dirty letter pointing out the difference in the lot of my transit party and his command and their correspondingly lighter rate of sickness, expressing the trite hope that these things would receive consideration in future. Also pointed out that the sum was raised by a sacrifice of officers' pay not regarded as expedient in this area.

Early movement seems to be certain according to Maj. Denaro, who anticipates our first party to go off in three days time.

18 January 1943

Went to hospital early on and told ADMS, who seemed uneasy about my rice polishings letter, that we would need less, as Maj. Denaro told us at the conference this morning that we were all to leave on the 22nd and 23rd. I asked him to lay on one or two odds and ends of stores, anti-dip. serum, ATS, and he went to the stores to do his best. Earlier in the morning Billy and I received the pay of officers in our party: full pay less board in respect of November and December (mine was 280 gulden): total 2125, paid in Java money. (Also 780 gulden for Trevena, 60 gulden for Houston, for which we enquired. This is a windfall.)

Just after lunch we were notified that movement time changed to 20th.

19 January 1943

All finance pooled in kitty and divided on a *per capita* basis, including details staying behind and in hospital and Capt. Hamilton's party. At an officers' conference at breakfast yesterday details of the movement were given. Transport is to pick up the parties on the road opposite our barracks.

Maj. Greiner OC of this party; Capt. Brettingham- Moore and 2nd party to assemble in the same area at 0915. Details are shown in the movement order. Troops are to carry a full water bottle and will be issued this evening with two meals for tomorrow (fried rice in dixies).

In respect of yesterday's pay, officers were again asked to put in all the latest 'extraordinary months' pay apart from 50 gulden which is to be retained. The rear party is joining up with 2/40 Bn AIF and will come on in a 625 party tomorrow. Each of our parties (325, 300, 225) will have its own MO, and 1 NCO + 4 ORs (medical). Tim Godlee will be with Brian Harrison-Lucas and as Sgt Cameron is in hospital we will have no real interpreter.

Stores were collected in the hospital area for two parties of 625, Maj. Moon taking charge of one and Capt. Godlee the other. Lt-Col. Glynn White arranged for us to take on 2 bags (220 lb) of rice polishings and a couple of pots of marmite for the trip, plus a little extra NAB, Atebrin and anti-dip. serum (very scarce).

Hard at work finishing off medical records, most of which given to W/O Mackenzie at 1000 hours. One nominal roll of British personnel I left with Brian Harrison-Lucas for typing.

6 Konyu

January 1943

20 January 1943

Reveille 0430. I saw Greiner's party on the mark at 0715; they were collected by N lorries at 0800. Our party assembled on road at 0915 in ranks of 5; split into 13 embussing parties of 25 with one extra lorry for baggage. It was then arranged that the Ns hand over some clothing – 100 garments of each NEI type. Officers travelled in the baggage lorry with some of the same Nipponese with whom we came over on the boat. Embussed at 1000 hours, reached Singapore Station at roughly 1100. Then sorted out into 22 freight cars of box type as follows: the first three to have 29 in each, the remainder 28 in each (an officer or senior NCO to each 'car'). Six officers, Commander, 2 I/C, adjutant, Maj. Moon, Maj. Clarke and Maj. Woods were at first to travel in special car No. 13 with Nipponese but this was changed, and we were redistributed to other trucks.

The interpreter, an immaculate and very polite Nipponese, delivered the following instructions after introducing the Commander: we must obey all the Commander's orders and those of the N army; disobedience would be punished on the spot (commanders in the trucks were to be responsible); we must take great care with the natives and neither buy from them nor change money because they are thieves and will take us down, even to stealing our boots off our feet! The guards are not here to watch you, because you are gentlemen. They are on the train to take care of natives! This applies particularly to the natives in Thailand. We were also cautioned about the danger of fire, and of allowing our limbs to project from the carriages because the bridges are narrow and accidents have occurred (four Tommies are said to have lost their legs recently). The box cars are of the sliding door type and we are advised to keep them open unless the natives become troublesome, but we should tie a wire or something of that sort across the opening. We must not leave the cars for food or latrines except with the permission of the guards. Two buckets were issued to each carriage to carry water, rations and so forth.

We pulled out off Singapore Station at 1255 hours, a portly Nipponese officer advising us to take care of our health and that peace would come soon. We crossed the causeway in about an hour and were quickly in the rubber and jungle country with endless dense green walls of tangled green twenty to forty feet high or the depressing grey-green and shadow of the rubber plantations. Apart from many typical Malayans in skull cap and sarong I was surprised to note the number of Chinese and Indians. One of the sights of the country are the

Chinese coolie women, either in gaily coloured cloth headgear or in great straw hats with a peak in the centre like a pagoda, showing like mushrooms above the rice in the fields.

The routine at these long stops is that everyone is to be in the train 10 minutes before movement, the whistle is blown etc. and off we go. The Nipponese seem to have plenty of our rolling stock, as we are passing many trains each day. The populace watch us with interest, but only occasionally wave. The old English station names remain and there are Nipponese newspapers in English freely available for 5 cents. These naturally portray a dim picture of the Anglo-American war efforts everywhere but especially the hopelessness of recovery in the Far East.

Later in the day I noticed that the country approaching Ipoh was more open, with much signs of dredging and large sheets of dirty water. Ipoh was reached at 2100 hours for the evening meal of good rice and soup. Arthur Moon and six other fellows suffered nasty injuries to their legs from hanging them out of the train and hitting a sleeper just on pulling into Ipoh. I had two severe cracks on the foot early in the day and slightly sprained the left knee, such is the desire for fresh air!

No sign of planes or aerodromes though presumably these are a little off the beaten track. On the way by 2200 with prodigious crashing. Somehow we 'bedded' down a little more comfortably and I even got my legs down some of the time, with several layers of legs on top, of course.

Jungle, jungle, all the way to Gemas, where we arrived at 2300 hours and were given just a light issue of rice, nothing to drink. A short halt and we were off again, trying to sleep on the way during a night to be remembered. Filthy-dirty and smelly humanity massed approximately thirty to a box about 3 m × 6.5 m with all equipment. No room for everyone to lie down, so we must try to sleep in a squatting position with a horrible aching in the bent knees. As people get uncontrollably sleepy, their legs and arms tumble onto other forms. To add to the trouble, the floor of wood and metal has no springs to speak of, and there is continually the most diabolical stopping and starting with a ringing, crashing of trucks, and finally a most teeth-shattering crash of your own truck.

21 January 1943

Morning – an almost incredible effort of the spine required to get up – about the third convulsion achieved an aching vertical – and everyone is black with soot and looking like chimney sweeps. The sun rose over endless jungle the same as yesterday and finally we reached Kuala Lumpur at about 0845. All troops out to latrines and for a wash under a tap. Breakfast of rice and a soup distinctly hot with curry (but thin withall) was soon available. KL seems fairly intact now with not much sign of damage visible from the rail. Almost all the bridges we crossed (very slowly) during the first two days of travel in Malaya, however, were being repaired. New bridges were massive girder affairs equal to the previous at least. 'George' (our new sturdy corporal) and Co. are quite considerate.

22 January 1943

On the estuary of a river at 0615 brilliant moonlight. Turned out for breakfast but hunted back on board train before it was all in the buckets. Rice with a soup containing some lumps of pork – this to do for lunch as well and rather 'light on'. Then began a terrible endless crashing of trucks while we manoeuvred from point to point and eventually we came to a rest back at the same station and then had some breakfast. The train pulled out with engine at the opposite end and an illusion of going south. We now entered paddy field country with fully-grown rice being threshed in the fields into little structures of attap. Occasional giant outcrops of rock occurred on the plain and there were some mountains evident at first, but towards Alor Star the terrain was much flatter and the first signs of an aerodrome were evident. Closer to the Thai border the country became more rugged, with sparse jungle growth. There were frequent stops, during which we could stretch our legs, until Padang Besar, the border town, was reached at 1515 hours. Here, we were able to make tea from the engine. The weather is hot and fine and the troops are so dirty and suntanned that if they were to get hold of a bunch of pisangs no one could distinguish them from the local inhabitants! At 1730 we left Padang Besar to travel through sparsely populated, fairly flat, country with the same sudden outcroppings of rocky mountains until Hadyai Junction was reached at 1920 hours for the evening meal.

This was our first real sight of the Siamese, whose dress is more European than in Malaya – most seem to be wearing trousers rather than sarongs and hats of a European type. They did not come near the train but gave us an occasional wave. The local script used for the station names is quite unfamiliar and the English equivalent, which was previously underneath, has been painted out and replaced by Katakana. The Thai flag is still flying. Several officers and NCOs (apparently Thai Army) were acting as police about the station as well as the Nipponese military police and movement officials. The pistol-carrying Thai officials were dressed in showy uniforms with forage caps and European-type khaki drill. Badges of rank are apparently very like our own. They paid compliments as the Thai flag came down but the Nipponese took no notice. The women are dark and buxom, with raven black hair, good teeth and a rather pleasant smile; the children mostly wore ragged European-type dress. We pulled out through the paddy fields in the late evening and Billy remarked that he felt a little more cheerful now we were in Thailand. I am not so sure!

23 January 1943

Last night was rather hellish, what with fidgetting, movements, cramped position, legs and arms exploring your body in a horrid way, weight of other people's legs and bodies. It was cold for the first time, with resultant shivering and irritability of contracted bladders. In spite of the shortage of water, I and some of the officers shave almost every day to avoid that going-to-seed appearance.

After Hadyai Junction the countryside became rapidly very primitive with attap and bamboo house. Thai cattle with great spreading horns and elephants were doing various types of work. It is rough, primitive country with much jungle, little evidence of roads and many quite big rivers. Arrived Chumphon 1510, departed 1600.

Of all the rum goes: when I started this war I hardly expected to find myself a POW seated on the border of a railway in the depths of Siam. Last night was bitterly cold in the early morning with Billy and I having a silent controversy over the covering afforded by our groundsheet. Lord it is cold. All gear packed up to be off the train at Bampong at 0730 hours. Nipponese time is utterly unsuited to Thailand and the local time is well behind the one we follow; thus, sunrise is about 0900 N time and 0730 at present is night (with bright moonlight fortunately).

24 January 1943

Off train and almost immediately embussed about 200 yards away, 25 per truck (God, my gear is frightful – just about as much as I can lift and carry). Unfortunately, heavy gear (clothing, buckets, bags of rice polishings, heavy articles in general) was all seized by N movement control officers who said it would be sent up five days later. I am pessimistic about this. It includes our typewriter. My gear comprises a pack, haversack, side haversack, Dutch medical companion, water bottle, small suitcase (records), instruments and books (terribly heavy). No water last night as our water bottles are only partly filled. Breakfast consisted of a few bananas placed on the cab of the lorries.

On the road at about 0915; a bitterly cold sun was just rising. Bampong shops appear to contain plenty of goods, such as tins of condensed milk, and there are cattle in the fields. Several British POW camps were seen containing crude attap huts. The condition of the men in these camps appeared to be fair.

The road took us through wild, hilly country with terrible dirt roads and choking dust so that everyone was soon practically black in the face and khaki could scarcely be distinguished from green. The jolting was severe and jungle branches kept brushing us. Bridges are terribly primitive affairs of wood and bamboo.

Arrived at Wandon bridge at 1400 hours and then had a nasty trip carrying baggage across the bridge and on for half a mile through very thick dust and under a sun now hot as hell. To complete the picture, the sole came off my shoe. I looked so like a pack camel that one of the troops actually offered to carry my suitcase (gratefully accepted); even so, my legs were trembling a bit at the end.

The two-hour halt was near a tommy camp and we got some water in our bottles (no food). A British Officer said that the food situation is bad. Occasionally a friendly Nipponese allowed an officer to shoot a buffalo. They were eager for news since the only source was passengers coming up the line. He said we were going right on to the jungle to build our own camp close to the Burmese border.

Embussed again at 1600. Wild jungle country with vultures much in evidence – bamboos, some enormously thick and forty to fifty feet in height, are interspersed with trees, tangled undergrowth and tough vines winding python-like about great stout trees rather like ironbarks. It would be frightful country to find one's way about in by day and impossible by night!

Arrived at Tarsau around 1800 hours and went into a small bamboo-fenced compound where we have just sufficient space to sleep on the ground and in some shelters. Trench latrines (filthy) are already in use. We were instructed to stay in the compound and not to speak to the British. N interpreter, a long-haired, larrikinish type (a Bombay dentist), Nipponese guard and NCO checked each party as it came in – officers, W/Os, NCOs, ORs – till numbers complete. I

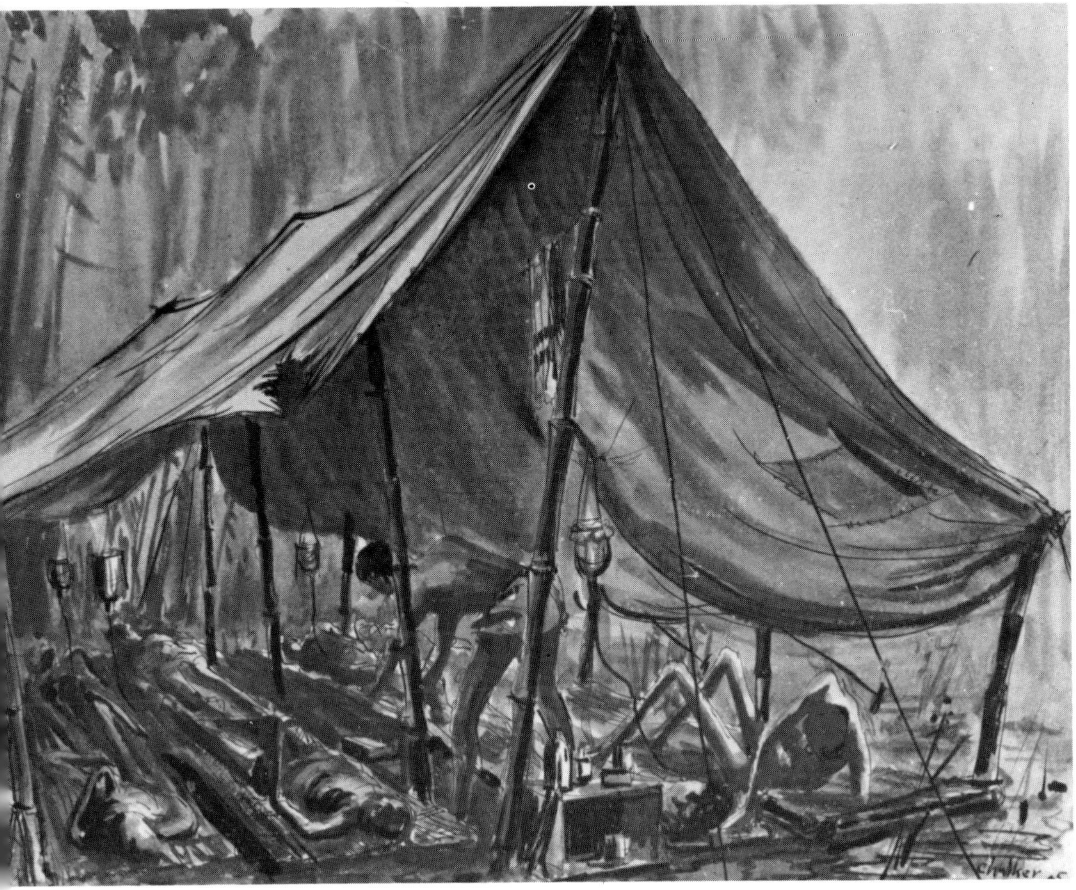

e author attending cholera patients, Hintok (*Jack Chalker*)

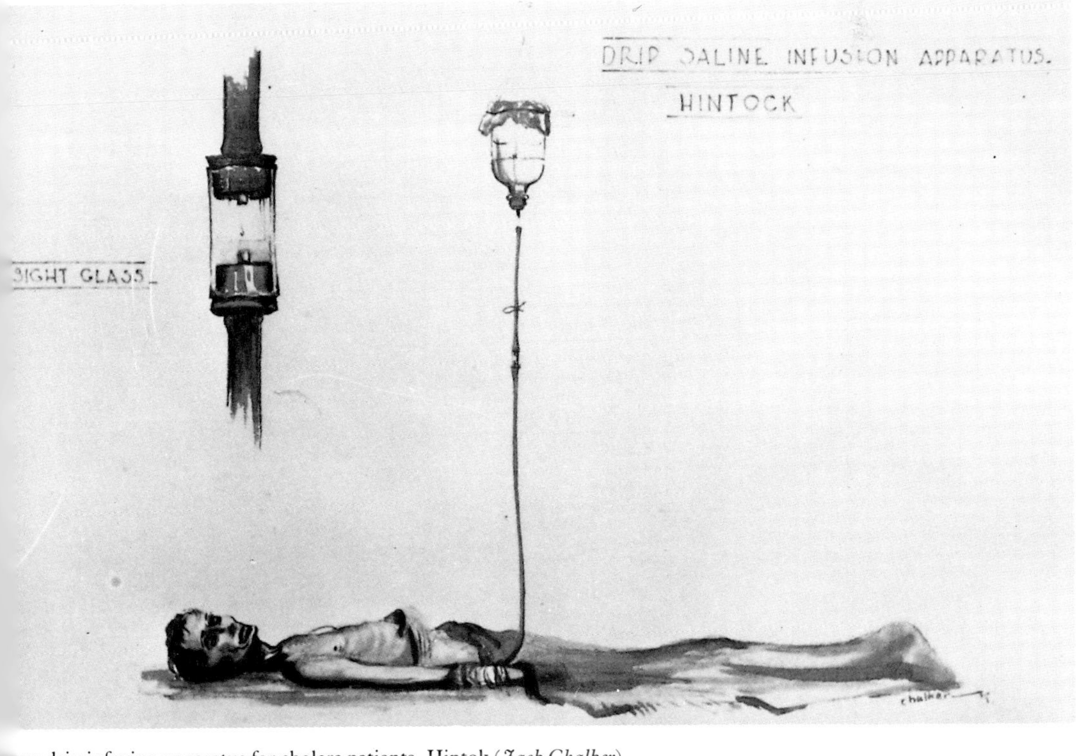

ne drip infusion apparatus for cholera patients, Hintok (*Jack Chalker*)

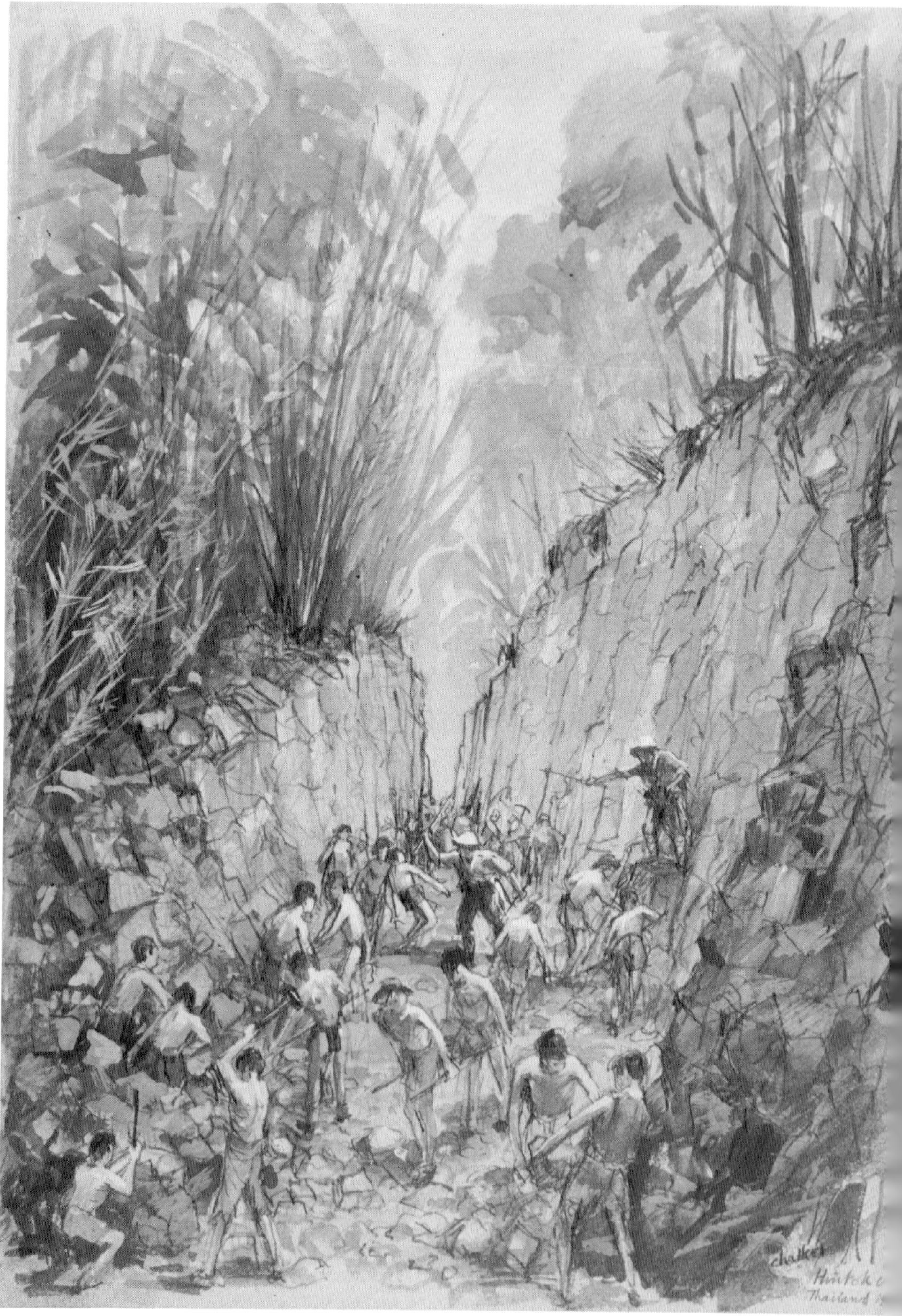

46 Hintok cutting (note two men lower left – 'hammer and tap' (*Jack Chalker*)

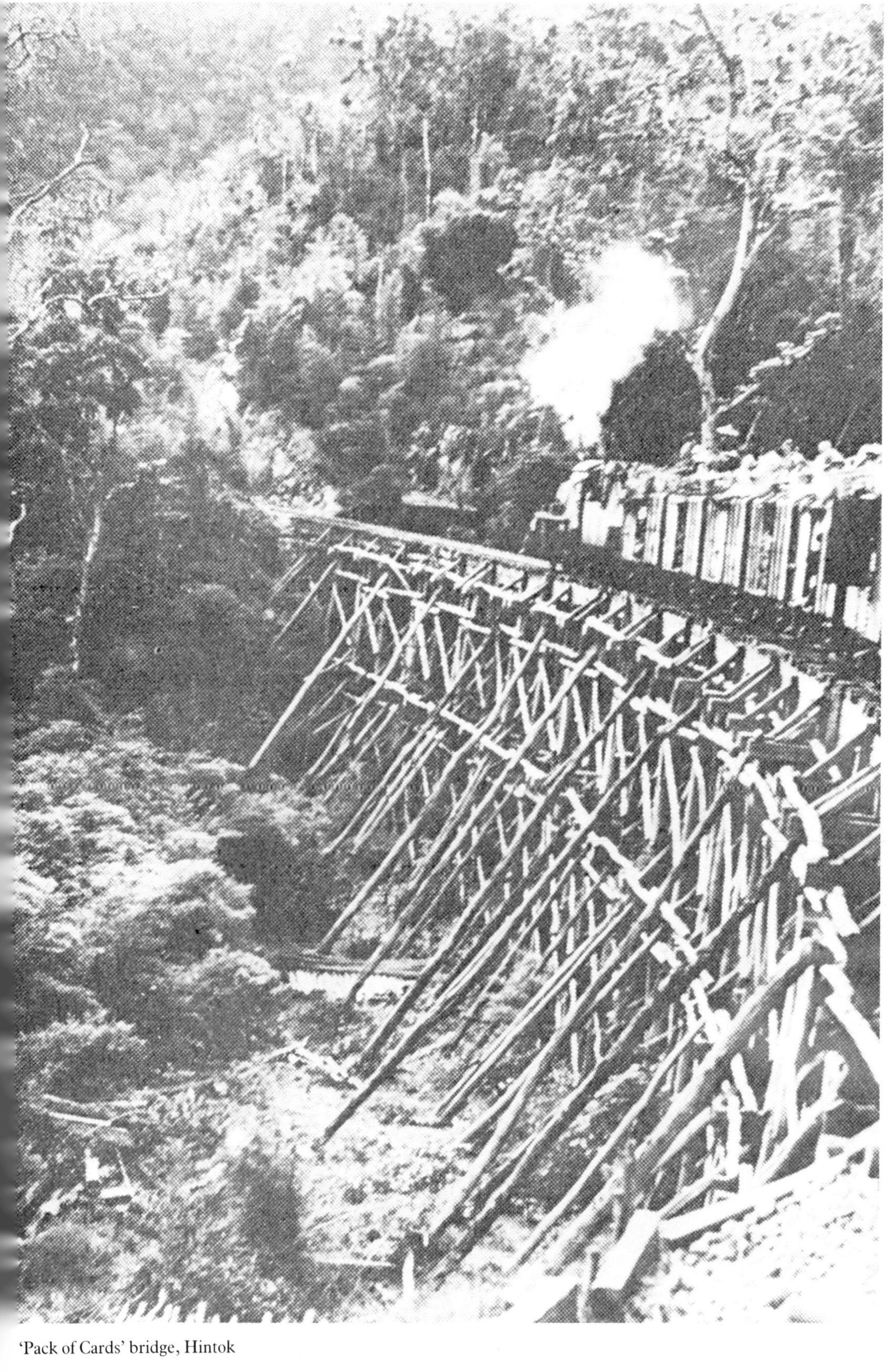

'Pack of Cards' bridge, Hintok

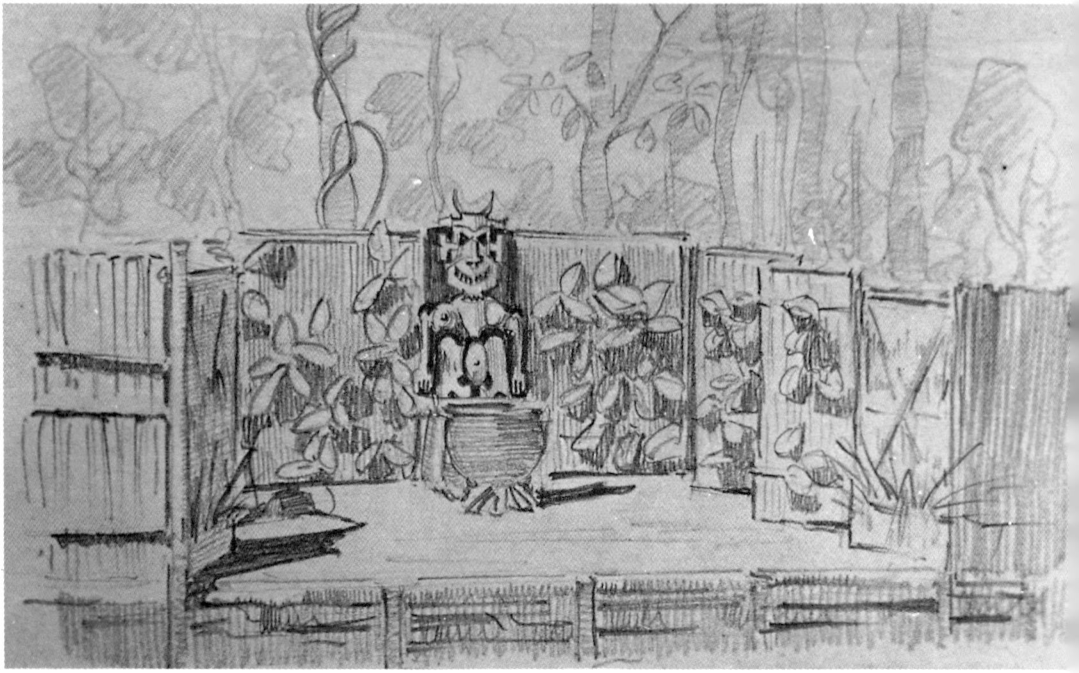

48 Stage setting, 'Kannibal Kapers', Hintok river camp (*Ray Parkin*)

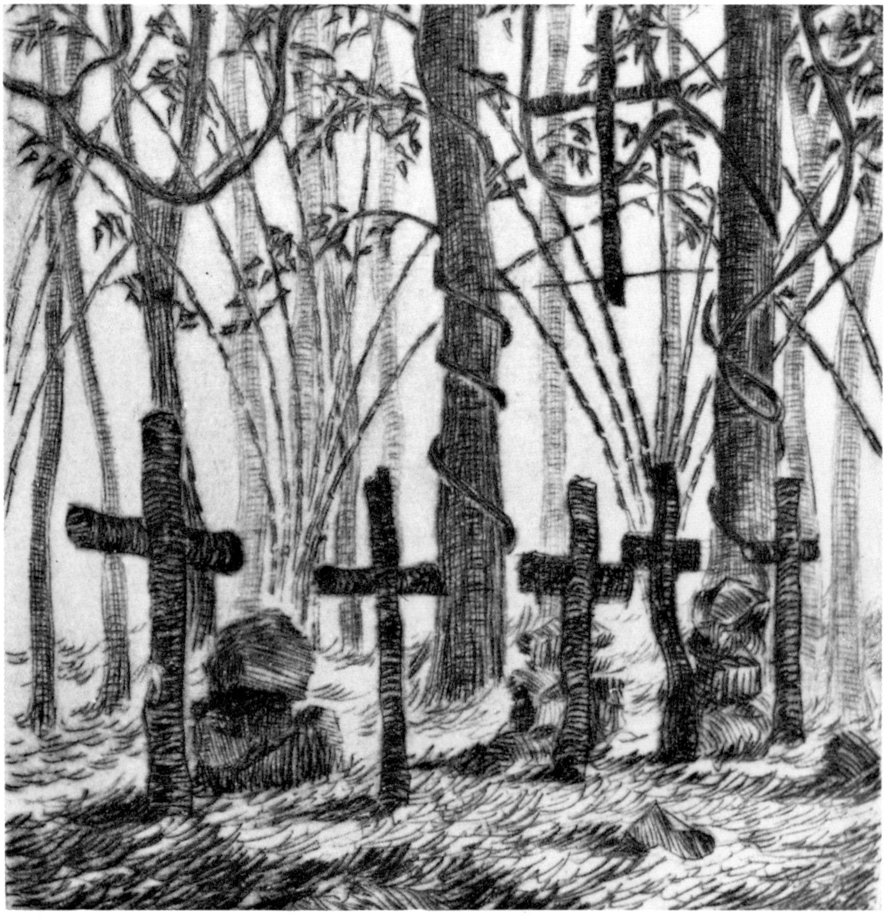

49 Graves in the English cemetery, Hintok (*Ray Parkin*)

was required to help and was asked many questions. A tow-haired, fresh, beefy-faced, brainless type of Englishman with no particular thought for the tiredness and dirtiness of the troops was present. I asked that water bottles be refilled and that some extra water be provided for washing, but he insisted that there was only enough water for bottles. Lt-Col. Harvey, who runs the local hospital, seemed far more interested in the news than the sick and irritatingly talked awful 'flap' when I wanted precise information about stores, medical arrangements, evacuation, dysentery, incidence of malaria etc. Both these chaps stressed that we must not expect much: they had had just as bad a time but in addition had had to walk up from Bampong, and when they arrived here they had to build a camp. There was very little food and much illness – malaria and dysentery – but the real cause of sickness was malnutrition. At first, food would only come up river by barge, but road transport had improved matters. About 300 troops had died in the area over the last 3 months. They were unhelpful when we told them we had only Java money, though no doubt it could easily have been arranged to exchange a little money locally. Apparently it takes many weeks to exchange money through the Nips, so I suppose we will have purchasing difficulties for a time.

After these five days of appalling travel and sleeplessness I was shocked to see my face in a shaving mirror – just a pair of haggard eyes looking out of caked dust and sweat. I shaved and washed in my shaving water (about 2 fl. oz), had rice and a half cup of tea then went to bed on the ground under the stars. This felt like heaven after the last four nights and I slept like a top in spite of the bitter cold, which got nearly everyone out of bed to dress themselves. Thank the Lord for my policy of tenaciously holding on to my valise and greatcoat. Big fires lit everywhere.

25 January 1943

Reveille 0600. Moon shining brightly. Breakfast and parties organised in 25s for lorries by 0800 and on the road about 0830, the sun rising beautifully on the way with striking effects on the jungle and mountains about us. Air very keen and cool, road terribly rough. The distance was only about 25 kilometres, but there were many delays when we had to get out and push the lorries uphill. Finally assembled in 5s at a place called the road junction ready for march about 1130 hours. Blue Maher took my little suitcase, Butterworth my raincoat, leaving me a pack, two haversacks, the medical companion and my terrific weight of valise, roll of books, and instruments etc. The way wound for about a mile down a steep mountain-side in which some rough steps had been cut. Unfortunately, the pace had to be terribly slow in places, so that we took about an hour in all to reach Konyu Camp (English). I could feel my legs trembling and my shoulders were like hell. Our new camp site is about another half mile along a jungle track. Everyone seemed to get down with his kit somehow. The N commander of Konyu Camp, Osuki, then got me to parade the troops in 5s for counting; this was difficult amongst the semi-cut jungle, but the check was OK. The Commander then dressed the troops through his pidgin English interpreter, Susuki, and me. He said he spoke for the Commander of the area, Commander Tanaka (Capt.). Name of camp: Konyu. First he was glad that the troops had come such a long way to come under his command! He would do his best to help. Please accept apologies no camp and very little food at present. Must build camp and things then perhaps improve. Very important to work hard. We must obey all orders of Nipponese implicitly; all Nipponese officers, NCOs and soldiers are to be saluted; CO of party and 2 I/C to report to central office for detailed orders at 1500 hours; there was to be a water and rations party of 100 men at 1500, tent-carrying party of 50 men at 1500.

Maj. Wearne and I went to the office at 1500 hours with N soldier who let us have tea in the English cookhouse on the way. Reported to Lt Osuki (The 'Boy *Shoko*') and S. The former is a one-pip beardless little youngster (few hairs on chin) with a face like a spoiled boy and much laughter but hard as flint. Perhaps an alcoholic. S is a long-haired businessman type of Nipponese with a hook nose – egregious, smart, pidgin English and instincts of a snake. O would pass with us as a tough little larrikin; he mixes rather vulgarly with his men and drinks like a fish, I believe. Anyway, both were very polite to me, 'Take seat', offered me cigarettes all the time and plenty of tea to drink (actually with milk, too).

He then proceeded to lay out the organisation. I as senior officer to be in charge, Maj. Wearne 2 I/C; we were to constitute HQ personnel, so to speak. All the others were being organised into two works battalions each with a CO and 2 I/C and composed of sections 1–9, each of 40 men, and section 10, the remainder. It was terribly difficult to make out the precise organisation. All the Nips were simultaneously drawing 'family trees' and none agreeing for the next three hours or so. Each battalion must have a doctor and, if possible, the following: works officer, accounting officer, general officer (adjutant) sanitary officer, QM, liaison officer. They heard of the 'tooth doctor'* with much amusement and enquired if there were chaplains. There was obviously a little confusion in the conception of HQ of a camp and battalion organisation. The following camp duties were fixed:

Daily routine

Reveille	0800	Work begins	1500
Roll call	0830	Work finishes	1800
Breakfast	0830	Dinner	1900
Work begins	0930	Roll call	2000
Work finishes	1230	Lights out	2200
Lunch	1300		

1 *Present organisation* suggested is perhaps as follows:

No 1 Bn officers	8	*No 2 Bn* Officers	7
Cooks	13	Cooks	12
Duty	27	Duty	22
Sections 1–9 each	40	Section 1–9	40
Section 10	30	Section 10	34
TOTAL 438		TOTAL 435	

* This was Maj. Jock Clarke.

2 *Building Construction*

Officers	1	
Barracks	9 (1 barrack per 100)	
Cookhouse	1	
Rations	1	
Hospital	1	
Benjos (W.C.)	Deep trench type with covers	
Ration Store	1	

Barracks: To be 3 metres to ridge pole; dimensions 50 m × 6.5 m. (This is said to be larger scale than that allowed Ns, but all N huts in this area are much higher and larger).

Officers: Also 3 metres to ridge pole; dimensions 13 m × 6.5 m includes 3 m for office.

Beds in Barracks to be bamboo platforms running length of building and 2.5 m deep.

It is said that 100 men can make 2 houses a day approximately.

Hospital is to be 50 metres long, 8 metres wide, 4 metres high and building to include administration.

3 *Work*: work inside camp is construction at present and almost all the men are required. Later, only maintenance (duty section) will be necessary. Outside work will comprise clearing the jungle for the railway.

4 *Returns rendered*: This gave rise to an appalling 'explanation' session going on for hours which could have been fixed by simply giving me a copy of the forms and the times at which they were to be rendered. We are to furnish a Nominal roll (Rank, Name, Initial, Former Occupation) and an Officers' roll (as before, stating whether 1st or 2nd Battalion). Daily we must supply: 1 Camp work analysis; 2 Roll call reports; 3 Works reports (battalions); 4 Sick report (Hospital, No duty, Light duty); and 5 Sick analysis – systems etc.

I then raised the question of how we were to recover our heavy baggage from Bampong; the importance of keeping clean and in good health by swimming in the river; and the prospect of evacuating the very sick to Tarsau. The last was approved for those 'very, very sick' and swimming would be allowed, providing it was well policed and men didn't drown!

I was also anxious to discover how quickly Java and Singapore money could be changed in order to buy stores and organise the canteen. All stores come up by barge, and we must make all food and money-changing arrangements through the Nipponese since security considerations forbade any contact with Thai people. Money is also an area for personal 'perks', although the official explanation is that the Thais are 'very unscrupulous', the exchange rate is bad and food prices very high!

The most sinister feature of the whole talk was the insistence that if many men are sick we will draw less food! After these *pour parler*, the Nipponese commander accompanied me on a tour of inspection of the British camp so that I could note some of the hut-building construction details. I was very pleased with the deep trench latrines, urinals and kitchen soakage pits, which go down about twenty feet below a bamboo and earth superstructure with little sliding covers of bamboo. These seem to be fly proof.*

The deep trench latrines are about 1 metre across and 5 metres long. In the kitchens, ovens are dug out of solid earth with rice bowls (or *cwalis*) resting over them. The whole range is dug out in one block; approximately 22 ovens per 1000 men are allowed. The quality of the metal used for the *cwalis* is poor and they crack easily when dropped or when the heat of the fire is excessive. Lord knows what happens to everything when the rains come. Sections of attap roofing should not overlap by more than 3 inches and the roof should slope at least 30 degrees.

After a rapid look around the English camp, we came across to this camp site, where the commander had a look around. An area was appointed for shallow trench latrines, which are to be dug at once; water is to obtained for troops bottles; company areas have been established in the jungle close to the clearing where work is proceeding; and five tents have been erected, one for the Nipponese guard, one orderly room, two hospital tents and one medical inspection room.

Temporary cooking trenches have been dug for *cwalis* with wood fires and we asked for drums for water containers, chlorine for chlorination, buckets in greatly increased numbers and boots for the men. Only a little footwear in small sizes suitable for Nipponese troops is available, unfortunately. The troops were warned to rig mosquito nets and practise strict hygiene discipline. Nets have been rigged with bamboo fences in company area with a maze of streets and lanes, 'Weary' Lane etc. Huge fires were lit to give warmth and, as Nips emphasised, to keep the wild animals away. I think they like to have these to give light in patrolling, although the reason advanced was leopards etc. Roll call was delayed until 2030 tonight (nearly dark), after which Major Wearne and I managed to have that so much needed swim and evening rice before finishing some admin. work. To bed in the open air, sleeping on the ground. The nights are extremely cold but I had a magnificent sleep, most other people getting up continually to put on more clothes.

26 January 1943

Reveille 0800, Parade 0830. Maj. Greiner was organising all parties for the heavy work of clearing the area when the Nipponese arrived and began bagging parties here and there, converting a well-ordered scheme to a crazy sort of muddle. The W/O (Socho) is an amusing N who either calls himself (or has been dubbed) No. 1 George and wears a 'tiger tamer' sort of tropical sun helmet. He is very dark with a head shaped like an egg, long teeth, drooping sparse moustache and a long melancholy face but humorous eyes. He talks a little pidgin English and has keen wits; always very generous with cigarettes.

Today a pig supplied for rations escaped and swam across the river, getting into the jungle. A great hunt by dismayed British tommies and N soldier with rifle failed to round it up. An amusing conversation went on between RAMC officer and No. 1 George, the former accusing Ns of responsibility for loss of

* Alas, this did not prove to be the case. They were always full of maggots.

pig and the latter insisting that the tommies had been 'too tardy', which word he had just looked up in the dictionary. Have had Ron Lum and another lad surveying the area and working out the sites for huts. The existing cleared area is much too narrow for a reasonable disposal of huts. These two lads are also inspecting British latrines, cookhouses etc., so that similar plans can be made.

At 1400 hours Maj. De Crespigny's party arrived. Capt. Hands and Tim Godlee had gone to other camp in charge of the detail of 375 all ranks AIF. He was split off with this party at the road junction; only 3 of the Changi group of AIF (my own party) going with him. This left a party of 250 to come here including 3 2/40 Bn officers (Primrose, Williams and Groom) and 20+ details of Timor party. This group also had much trouble getting water for the last couple of days and were walking like men in a dream, 15 being practically right out to it including De Crespigny, who was bathed in sweat, glazed of eye and talking wildly. However, everyone got in, and only two men had to be admitted to hospital after they were all given a rest.

They were duly numbered off and checked. Finally, all were speedily fixed up and given tea, bath and so on. The removal of six days growth of beard and soot and dust made a big difference to their appearance.

We are now working on the organisation of the two works' battalions and Maj. Greiner and Maj. Woods will command them. Very fine work has been done already by the troops in clearing the area and the glade rings continuously with the swing of axes, crash of timber and thud of picks and shovels. Called on Commander of the English camp Lt-Col. (Mackie) More (a gunner) and Lt-Col. (Hookey) Hill. They were in a group of officers at CO's house near the river and their appearance shocked me – all dressed in pyjamas and sarongs, unshaven or bearded, sallow and dull of eye, full of a sort of hopeless depression. They told me a doleful tale of the dreadful march, underfeeding and illness with malaria, dysentery etc. – over 30 men out of their 1500 have died in the last three months. Canteen arrangements impossible – can't change money quickly – when you do can't get stores; these previously came all the way up river, now perhaps by road as far as Tarsau but difficult to get any up here. At this stage Lt-Col. Hill, who had been giving me a bit of aside information, said something about 70,000 eggs since beginning January. I murmured that I thought 1 egg a day and a handful of beans might keep our fellows fit. Hill advised me to approach the Nips for a purchasing officer of ours to go down to Tarsau with their two and to pay and buy on the same basis. Their purchasing officer, Lt-Col. Warren, is down there at present but December order has still not arrived. Their working strength has become so low that even the officers (of which they have over 300) are now working on camp duties. They listened in gloom to the news as I had heard it last and after hearing that it was probably not true that Akyab had fallen or that the Burma offensive was very big at present, they seemed to have little interest in other parts of the world.

At this stage Fred Smedley and Arthur Moon rushed in: it seems they had got hold of a barge which came up with attap and could get 900 eggs or thereabouts but were short 15 ticals for the purchase–could this be borrowed. Lt-Col. Hill loaned the sum right away; apparently they had tried to stop the barge but it had got past to us. I said to Fred: 'Have the grace to send the Colonel a few eggs.'

In the evening Maj. Wearne and I were told by the commander that a party of 625 would arrive tomorrow to go to a nearby camp *which we must administer*. The strength of the new camp will be 1000 and ours is 875: thus the total will be 1875!

The Dutch party coming in is known to have seven officers and two doctors in the 625. A clear cold night with bright stars; moisture dripping from jungle all round in the morning. This due to the dew. Not many mosquitoes seen.

27 January 1943

Reveille 0800 is well before dawn (we worked on Tokyo time). Both sunrise and sunset are very fine spectacles, with the surrounding hills and dense jungle traced against the gold and rosy colours. Sgt Page's trumpet is now in action.

Reported to N commander at 0930 and went up the hill by that tortuous path to the road junction (very heavy going), he sweating a great deal and clumping along in his top boots. When we reached the top, D party getting out of lorries with great confusion of baggage and men. Capt. Smits and Lt Toets party. Nips required Billy and I to help sort them out into officers, NCOs and soldiers. They have a tremendous percentage of NCOs, many of these Eurasians and a lot very old.

After they were sorted out and the commander had addressed them I told him it was an impossible arrangement to make the Australian commander administer the Dutch in a mixed camp. Much better to transfer all Australians to one camp. He listened to all the arguments but said he could not alter things since it was a high N order. He then gave me a clout on the shoulder, as much as to say 'Buck up'. So much for all that. After much delay the party again fell in; officers were addressed by N commander and Capt. Smits, then marched five km to the camp, Billy and I each carrying suitcases for D. Arrived camp site about 1300 hours. Australians were busy clearing a space big enough for D to bivouac in. Only one tent available and to be used for the officers. Right alongside the area is a surveyors' camp. The water supply is not good: a little trickle down the mountain with some shallow, rather stagnant pools near the camp. I would regard the area as probably malarious and the creek needs work done on it urgently. Jack Hands is very busy.

The Dutch are an ill-disciplined mob with a tendency to wander all over the place in search of this and that, Smits meantime waving his hands like King Canute and using his voice weakly.

I informed them that Capt. Hands would be regarded as camp commander and consolidate returns etc. I arranged for Ns to transfer two Timor officers, Lt Williams and Lt Groom, who already have their troops in the area. After a brief inspection of the camp, Maj. Wearne and I outlined the organisation to Hands, Smits and adjutants, also the returns required and some outline of canteen and food responsibilities, assuring them that we would share all foodstuffs on a *per capita* basis.

Maj. Wearne and I were then given a meal in the guard tent with Commander O and the interpreters and sundry Ns waving chopsticks and making gustatory noises: rice, bean soup and tea and cigarettes ++. It seems that to keep up the

Organisation

BAMPONG GHQ
Six areas

1 2 3 4 5 6

TARSAU

1 2 3 KONYU

We were part of 4 Group, based on Tarsau, and one of the Konyu camps. There were two hospitals:

1 Bampong
2 Tarsau

KONYU CAMP ORGANISATION

Works battalions Konyu area

English	Aust.	Aust./Dutch
E.J.W.	O.P.	Q.R.

Dunlop controls O.P.Q.R. group (4 battalions)

Q (Aust.) Bn		*R (Dutch) Bn*	
Officers	7	Officers	7
W/O	4	W/O	41
NCO	53	NCO	212
Ptes	313	Ptes	363
TOTAL	377	TOTAL	623

Allotment of Officers

Commander Q	1	Hands	Smits	1
Adjutant	1	Thyne	Weber	1
Doctor	1	Godlee		2
Liaison	1	Williams		0
Works	1	Groom		1
QM	1	Trevena		0
General duties	1	Padre Kennedy		1
Sanitation	0		Toets	1
TOTAL	7		TOTAL	7

Duty Personnel

Duty	Q	R	*Duty*	Q	R
Cooks	15*	25*	Medical orderly	6	8
Wood & Water	8	12	Clerks	5	5
Batmen	2	2	Military police	3	4
Barber	1	1	Bugler	1	1
			Batman to J.J.A.	1	1
			TOTAL	41	60

* These were increased at my request to Q, 26 + cooks; R, 35 + cooks.

percentage working rate we are also to help in a little swindle of having no 'no duty' men except those in hospital. These are all to be ranked 'light duty' and they will receive pay. There was again much emphasis on commander's policy of 'much work, much food, much pay; little work, little food, little pay. We must encourage much work!' This went on for three or four hours.

I saw Tim Godlee for a while – he with a cold and rather knocked out. Practically all the Timor crowd are in bad shape having had malaria etc. followed by many relapses (say twenty). Some eighty of these have deficiency diseases, bad mouths, scrotums etc. – much worse than ours. He is treating his sick in the lines at present.

A lorry passed just as O and S, Billy and I were leaving the evening meal and we tore away to get a ride back as far as the road junction. An anti-malarial squad is working round about the road on the way up, draining stagnant pools. I saw the officer-in-charge this morning and he said there is plenty of stagnant water and malarial mosquitoes up in the hills about us. Also some 350 cases of malaria in the British camp. He considers that his work will show no results for two or three months as adult mosquitoes can live for that time. The river is fairly safe from the mosquito point of view since the water flows very rapidly.

On the way back, I emphasised the boot question to O who has very few boots indeed and those only in small sizes. Arrived at 1930 hours and addressed the troops on parade about mosquitoes, emphasising the importance of malarial precautions and bodily cleanliness, washing etc. in relation to jungle sores and dysentery.

I congratulated them all on the grit they had shown on the move and the fine work put in over the last two days. During the evening I made the following appointments in the camp for O and P battalions:

O AND P BATTALIONS

Appointment	O	P
Officer-in-charge	Maj. Greiner	Maj. Woods
2 I/C	Capt. Piper	Lt Primrose
MO	Maj. Corlette	Maj. Moon
Works	–	Maj. De Crespigny
Accounting	–	Capt. Allen
QM	Lt Airey	–
General officer	Lt Brettingham-Moore	Lt Smedley
Sanitation	–	Maj. Clarke
Liaison officer	–	Lt Houston

We discussed the batman issue and policy is to be that older ones are to be used in N appointments and the others, if possible, are to be given camp appointments so that we retain their services to some extent. Dick Allen will also act as purchasing officer and canteen officer. Airey is a good type and is pitching into the kitchen, stopping a lot of nonsense. He does not get on well with W/O Exton.

28 January 1943

To see Nipponese and informed that battalions are now designated O, P, Q and R and are all part of Konyu Camp No. 3. We were given N letter cards and told that we would be allowed three a year. This one is to be sent tomorrow; a few simple words might be added at the bottom. Some paper was issued for sanitary use in the camp. Nipponese require two men at their HQ: a batman and an interpreter/batman.

An Australian Red Cross message via Geneva and Tokyo was read to the troops wishing us a happy Christmas! Estimates of money for changing reveal to date, Q Bn: 1163.16 and R Bn: 3375 (Dutch, with typical foolishness, have mostly NEI currency and Straits Settlement dollars).

Padrés services are to be in common with British: Father Kennedy from Q Bn will come down from English camp and our troops march over there.

Lt-Col. More and Lt-Col. Hill agreed to give us further credit to a total of 1000 ticals which they said was their limit. Hence more eggs were purchased.

Fights in our lines rather common, probably due to tobacco shortage. Two or three Nips had a terrific and bloody struggle down by the river, using boots etc. and semi-drowning. [They were actually Koreans. When they rolled into the river they beat each other's heads with clogs.]. Yet No. 1 George called me in when he caught two Australians fighting and read a fatherly lecture: all *tomadachi*, no fighting allowed; Australians shake hands etc. As a deterrent I ordered extra work for one day.

Discipline: punishment is to be field punishment, e.g. chopping wood for wood and water carriers under supervision of MPs of which Maj. De Crespigny is O/C. Nip pay to be forfeited to fund for the period of punishment. A lock-up to be built as soon as possible. Bn O/Cs to exercise powers of commanders.

31 January 1943

Sunday. Inspections from Nips. Work to begin at 0800 and continue until 0930 then roll call and breakfast. Rest of day to be holiday. (There is no lightening of the dawn at 0800 – just pitch dark) W/O Exton relieved of Q responsibilities last night by Lt Airey. Sgt Cory to be the new RQMS. The morning meal was naturally after 0930 – everyone very hungry – then parades were assembled for church. I did an inspection of hospital, was about to go to church when Capt. Smits arrived, so I showed him over the camp instead. Kitchens and ovens now complete and one hut except for 'beds'; two others building. Capt. Smits seems happy with arrangement.

Finance and Canteens: each camp is separate but to be organised on the same lines.

1 All pay: Officers and ORs: one-third to be contributed to a regimental fund for purchase of food in kitchens and sick

2 Canteen articles to be sold to all ranks in a controlled manner to give fair distribution. Profit 10 per cent to nearest cent to go to fund. (Present funds to be set aside in a special reserve, Australian and Dutch separately.)

Troops spent an amusing day on the river ranging far and wide, swimming, fishing with improvised gear and diving for giant clams, of which there are plenty. Very few fish caught. Attempts by Maj. Greiner to net small fish with a mosquito net unsuccessful. The great shortage of tobacco is a trial. I try to take out my 60 dollars 'board and lodging' by smoking N cigarettes whenever I can get near them. The guard commander is a 2-star soldier and looks like a little frog but is OK. (We now have a retreat ritual on each night's parade.)

1 February 1943

A year since leaving the middle east (and what a year). Conference after breakfast – morning reveille now 0845, roll call 0900. HQ organisation now slightly altered. De Crespigny to act as works officer and adjutant, Lt Smedley to act only as adjutant P Bn. Houston L.O. to understudy De Cresp, and liaison between camps and N HQ.

Much cheer over the arrival of 1½ 'bullocks' and the prospect of steaks. It seems that two died on the way up from Tarsau. So I suppose none for some days after these corpses are eaten.

Practically all hands working hard on camp building and jungle clearing. Tadano Socho has gone to Tarsau and we are hopeful about the advance on our money so necessary for purchases. Lt-Col. Hill today suggested that we should send a representative over for all buying and share through the camps according to strength. Advised that we have someone over to see all goods come in so that we will be satisfied as to a fair deal. Meantime, Billy was having a good talk with Lt-Col. Warren [exchanging wireless news].

2 February 1943

I paid a visit to the mountain with Houston. The jungle is full of birds of every sort and game. Ns are always warning us against 'panthers and tigers'! I noted today some wild pigeons and wild-fowl. There is a constant flurry of life going on in the undergrowth. I saw some banana trees off the road and did a recce but no fruit.

Capt. Hands is in good fettle but his camp is not progressing so rapidly because many of his men are taken out to work all day (0800–2000 hours at times), leaving fewer men for 'inside work' Kitchen ovens are finished, but the only buildings finished are the Nip guard room and the ration store – also a pigsty! The D area looks like China-town, almost everyone having built a crazy hut of some sort with interesting leaves, bamboo etc.

The stagnant creek is a problem. They are draining it and will carry the water across in a bamboo pipe to the ablution area where they are building 'showers'. Latrines and pits give trouble down near the creek because water starts to seep in about 18 inches down. Permanent latrines will be dug on the high ground across the road. Both elements of camp have a good number of sick: a number of Australians have sore mouths and scrotum etc. and one or two are complaining of burning feet. Tim Godlee is looking these over with a view to special feeding. D have built a temporary bamboo hospital which is cooler than a tent. They have a few dysentery cases and have evacuated two men to Tarsau (regarded as tuberculosis).

The D are having discipline problems (some insubordination and minor thieving from the kitchen etc.); I told them of our decision re Nip pay and field punishment. I also discussed canteen arrangements and the money question. They agree with the policy laid down. Eventually walked home by the jungle road.

Arrived to find that the troops had killed a very large cobra. Typical hooded snake about 5 feet in length, dark green back, mottled whitish belly and very thick. This the boys roasted and ate (I was given a small 'steak' myself which was rather stringy but with quite a nice flavour).

Confusion exists owing to soldiers wandering off to gather clams etc. in middle of parades to bathe. I now have ordered that swimming parades are restricted to a defined area and that special permission must be got to go off and gather clams. Very few fish have been caught and no very satisfactory drum nets (being made from bamboo fibre) are working yet. Everything here is *à la* Swiss Family Robinson – there are practically no resources, not even the odd tin or petrol can or pieces of wire. Fish hooks have to be made from safety pins, bone etc., containers for food and water out of bamboo. Baskets are being prepared from bamboo and fibre. It is an interesting life.

Tadano Socho has returned and we are told that Osuki will collect our advance from Tarsau. This sounds hopeful but I hope that he does not go on the 'aboriginal jag' down there. The nights are not so cold and I sleep like a top on the ground.

3 February 1943

Disturbed sleep last night owing to being called out of bed over a squabble arising from the sale of clothing and valuables by a soldier. He went over to the other camp apparently by permission of the guard but was later charged with having taken a fountain pen from the Ns earlier in the day. The whole thing is an annoying affair from both sides. It arises mostly from intense jealousy and cupidity of N guards who try to keep the camp to themselves for trading exploitation. Hence make a terrible scene if they catch soldiers trading with outside Nips. The system works like this. N commander fixes prices of tobacco, cigarettes and foodstuffs coming in. Will not allow us to pay more, for example, than 25 cents per packet of cigarettes. N troops then buy up all the valuables of the camp – watches, pens and trinkets for a small percentage of their real value, then offer to sell cigarettes etc. for twice their value at least, e.g. cigarettes 50 cents. Shortly they have both the valuables and most of their money back again. (They, of course, have no restrictions on buying.)

Called to see N commander and received a 4000 advance on our money.

Saluting: we must salute all N soldiers except when working, when only the NCO I/C party salutes. When a soldier is without a hat, he salutes by bowing in the N position. I protested to S about the beating up and slapping and he said he would look into these matters. Food situation: S called in English camp canteen representatives and told them we must share 50/50 on all foodstuffs etc. coming up the river. This is good for them, really, as our strengths are 1600/1875. He gave the following official prices:

Eggs	7c
Dry fish small tin	25c
cigarettes Red Bull for 20	25c
Tobacco roll	1.40 or 1.50
cigars small	1c @
large	45–50c for 8
Peanut toffee small	10–15c
medium	15–20c
large	20–25c
Fried banana 10c	4 pieces
Sheaves of rice	25c
Cigarette papers	90c box 100
Pig fat	$24 4 gal. tin
Sugar, Malacca	$14–17 4 gal. tin
Brown cane sugar	60c kilo bag
Salt (bag)	$8
Chilli sauce small	25c
large	50c
Soap, cake	22c
Dry fish:	
Blakina	60–80c kg
Bla Too (Dried herring)	50c kg
Bla Chon	$1.40 kg
Bananas, small	1c
Limes	$9 1000
Peanuts	$69, 107 kg bag
Small Calos	3/4c

Dahl difficult to get a quote
Rice polishings, bag $15 dollars (This is a very high price. Ns say they are going to deliver rice polishings as part of deal soon.)

Twenty thousand eggs are available which the British camp wish us to take, also some onions, peanut toffee, a few rolls of tobacco and oddments.

I then went to see the English commander who took me to see the cemetery after a lot of preparation as though setting off for an all-day journey. It is about 150 yards! Along the line of construction of the new road and right on the river bank. There he seemed to come into his own and dilated on the whole show with the pride of a sexton in a village churchyard. The 'cemetery' is just off the 'church', both marked by a cross down by the river and walled in by a bamboo fence. The graves, 26 in number, are each surrounded by stones and marked by a bamboo cross and name plate (ten other camp members died at Tarsau.

The colonel showed great enthusiasm (for him) and wished to know if we desired to share in the cemetery (Yes); if so, did we want a separate part made as an extension? Not if it would not take up too much of the accommodation. Then he waxed keen again and said 'Oh no, I want to fill up this part first – but there is plenty of room here.

He ran on in this way quite pathetically. A wistful silence brooded over the scene, the pathetic newly-turned earth, the stones and bamboo crosses, the stark simplicity of the bamboo fence, the soft murmuring of the River (Menam) Kwa Noi and the rustle of bamboos in the tall surrounding jungle. Then parties returning from work on the new road came wearily by, sallow, haggard, bearded, gaunt and pitifully thin. Amid their chatter we returned; I thinking, 'I wonder how many more will eventually find peace there beside the Menam Kwa Noi and how long it will be before the relentless jungle obliterates all trace of their coming and their departure.'

4 February 1943

Conversation with Maj. Moon about the 312 men with sore mouths etc. at present. These are improving with eggs. All cases are divided into mild and severe. Each of these is to buy one egg a day at cost (= 49 cents week), thus covering all pay less 21 cents to fund. Mild cases to be given one extra egg; severe cases to receive two extra eggs.

Jungle clearing is going on at a great pace, but further hut construction is stopped owing to absence of ties. Huts are, of course, built without nails – simply bound together with jungle fibre. Only about 12–15 in hospital each day, largely due to the complete efficacy of M & B 693* as a cure for dysentery which has them out of hospital in two to three days. Regrettably our stocks will soon be finished and probably we will get no more.

Something is terribly wrong with the British camp; all the barracks have a terrible sick smell and it is appalling to see the mess of dirty, gaunt bodies and unmade beds all hours of the day.

5 February 1943

I have a septic scratch on the back of my right leg – retribution for not taking care and going gathering clams in the mud last night. Mild cellulitis; inflamed glands and great pain walking. Capt. Hands and Capt. Smits to visit today. Talk again of canteen arrangements. Some at least of Jack Hands' fellows are all for complete socialism – all men put in all money. This, it seems, comes from the W/Os.

We spend these days in medieval conditions, rising in almost complete pitch darkness at 0800 and at evening roll-call, 2000 hours, can just make out the troops. Can't see the officers at other end of parade. After that retire to the camp-fires – no lights, so usually in bed by 2200!

One of our lads (Denny) killed a plump wild-fowl with a stone the other day, much to the delight of his intimates. There are traces of game about here including pig, elephant, buffalo and panther. The cigarette shortage is acute – borrowed a few off S/Sgt Gibson today, he having sold a Rolex Oyster watch for about 12 ticals!

* M and B 693: the May and Baker 'Sulpha' drug.

6 February 1943

Leg rather painful so keeping very quiet. Over to see Ns twice today – 'Pushface' in one of his terribly dilatory moods, fussing for hours over his returns and every now and then saying 'Why'! It is suggested now that we have the *shoko*'s [officers'] house up at river end of camp and church at the previous site of the *shoko*'s house. Caught tonight to give medical attention to the N QM's toe and to one other N for a pain in the belly. Retainer: one packet of cigarettes. Paraded all W/Os and Sgts and told them that I was not satisfied with their control of the men, drawing attention to the prevalence of insubordination and of fidgetting and talking from the ranks. All NCOs were asked to squash insubordination on the spot, and if necessary to put men on the peg. All measures taken in the camp were for the men's own good. There was at present no other objective than to return everyone to their own country morally and physically fit. Every man would have his own serious problems to solve as a citizen after the war and it is doubtful if being a 'returned soldier' would help him very much. Therefore anti-social and anti-authority ideas were not going to be much help. It is hoped that this pep talk will bear some fruit.

7 February 1943

Sunday and *Yasumé* day. Reveille in pitched darknesses at 0730 and work until parade at 0930. My leg now improving greatly. Church of England service in the little riverside church at 1130 (no padre–just the form of service). Padre then taking communion as he was not regarded as fit to take two services). There is beauty in this spot with the quietness of the river and the large stone of the altar with the simple bamboo table and cross built over it. Alongside is the little cemetery with some great trees. The altar rail and seats are provided by bamboo (two trunks) and these rise up the bank theatre-wise. All around the green life of the jungle and the challenge of a little cross down by the river.

N HQ Bampong are concerned about rations and propose to do something about them. Present ration scale – if you can get – it is:

Rice	650 g	× 873	=	567.45 kg
Veg	500 g	"	=	436.5 kg
Tea	3 g	"	=	2.619 kg
Sugar	20 g	"	=	17.46 kg
Salt	5 g	"	=	4.365 kg
Fat	5 g	"	=	4.365 kg
Meat	100 g	"	=	87.3 kg

The only item anything like up to scale at present is rice. All the others have been extremely short.

Money: final figures were

O and P Bns	6822.07
Q and R	4387.99
	11210.06

Received advance 4000 ticals on 3 February 1943.

Finally checked personnel strength as follows:

Bn	Officers	W/Os	S/Sgts	Sgts	Cpls	Pts	Total
O	7	8	4	37	37	353	446
P	8	5	9	51	56	298	427
Q	7	4	5	22	27	312	377
R	7	43	–	165	43	365	623

Medical supplies are a cause of grave concern. The British camp have some 300 men in hospital and some hundreds more sick. The total number of men in the camps is nearly 4000, yet the much vaunted supplies that have arrived are as follows (for the whole of Konyu):

Scotts Emulsion Bots	12	Iodine	2/3
Quinine tabs 300 tins	35	Plasmoquine	1250
Sulphur lye		Tab Aspirin	300
Past Atebrin	1200	Tinea lotion	3 fl. oz
Meth spirit		Morph Amp	8
Bandages	10	Ungt Sulphides	1 lb
Vit B1 Tabs	50	Tab sulphonomides	30

8 February 1943

Site for *shoko*'s hut now definitely down by the river on opposite side to hospital and cookhouse. Officers to build the hut themselves with some help in clearing the site and with the plans (Cpl Heywood and Ron Lum).

9 February 1943

Worked on site for officers' hut and most foully blistered my hands which are very soft. My leg healing very slowly. I am ashamed at how little energy one has in this climate. The nights are not quite so cold which is a good thing as I have given my great coat temporarily to Bob Haddon (who has pleurisy). It's worth at least two blankets. Bamboo beds are diabolical, owing to their hardness, smoothness and irritating irregularities.

Kempi are known to be here. All N soldiers having their kit checked etc.

10 February 1943

Notified last night that nobody must go to British camp all day today. Also heard Lt-Col. More was not allowed to go to Tarsau and Capt. Hands not allowed to come to this camp. Wonder why? Answer: *Kempi* warrant officers and another NCO arrived approx. 1200 and I, Billy and Crep summoned to guard tent where we saw them with P., F., and S. All men were summoned out to continue working and the rest of the officers were summoned, also permanent duties. This I misunderstood deliberately. The search then began officers accompanying the search party and *kempi* W/O obviously in charge.

Sentries were first placed to guard all areas and then quite a large party did the searchings with considerable efficiency at first, gradually becoming less careful. I gradually edged my way clear and visited officers' quarters which were not searched with the same thoroughness – everything OK*. Three excellent prismatic compasses, several cameras and binoculars taken, also numerous tools of various sorts, several troops were found to have vegetables, even pumpkin and cabbage. (It is known that the Ns ration vegetables and give the ration-bearing party one or two sweet potatoes each, but this is too much. There will be a few please explains! Meantime, I issued an order on tonight's parade absolutely forbidding any man to be in possession of vegetables without permission of QM.)

This evening was Ewen Corlette's birthday (35 years) and I donated a tin of salmon to make a salmon omelette. (This solves a problem, as that damn tin has been gnawing at me for days to go off quietly and eat it by myself.) We toasted Ewen over the evening coffee. It is astonishing how primitive life is here, bamboo being almost our only resource. I have a bamboo water carrier, bamboo wash basin, bamboo bed and will soon have a bamboo house and bamboo furniture I suppose. There is no such thing as wire or nails – just jungle fibre for ties – and a few axes, picks, saws, shovels and knives. It is an unimaginably primitive life which begins an hour before the dawn and finishes by the light of the campfire and brilliant stars. I'm very familiar with the gentle rustle of bamboo. Wood – teak logs burn very slowly of course. The second row of huts has now been begun, 400 troops having moved into the four already built.

10 February 1943

Yasumé day. Roll call at 0900 hours. Went to Nippon commander and waited two hours while he played majong, then asked that 8 chronic sick be sent Kanburi base hospital. (In the morning noticed that a lorry had actually reached the camp, by *road*, with vegetables – a new thing.) After much discussion about the sick and being told permission must be got from company HQ, suddenly told 'quickly quickly get sick'! Rush departure – each man was paid his credit and 5 ticals from fund. Included Cpl Gill and Cpl Woodley, otherwise sickness rate is most satisfactory: only 10–12 men in hospital each day.

Curious evidence of efficiency of N Guard today. I wished to tell them of the party going over to English camp – sick and Sato and baggage party. All N guards, however, absolutely fast asleep with rifles outside and calling out to them failed to wake them. This is a daily occurrence. Ns in a state of drunken revelry today, which I believe is connected with the commencement of the year 2603. The soldier who acts as QM put up an outstanding spectacle staggering round hanging onto the arm of the English CQMS (Muir) and taking a smack meantime at every British soldier he saw. Finally he collapsed on a British soldier's bed in one of their barrack huts where he was in a state of coma until the morning, making a horrible mess of the blankets with urine etc.

11 February 1943

Friday. Framework of all huts now finished except hospital and officers' hut. Five men's huts are completed except for beds and side walls. There is another

* I removed some wireless articles and other contraband.

surge of innoculation and we have to start all over again with dysentery, cholera, plague and typhus. Today all received dysentery vaccine ½cc. Dick Allen got another 2000 ticals out of Ns today just when the situation looked very bad and our credit practically finished. This they just produced nonchalantly out of a drawer, so it seems they are up to some hanky panky.

[My wireless] Tripoli fallen but Tunis not yet, though some transports sunk there. No real news of Burma except bombing, but talk of Mandalay-Maymo sector. NG area: six transports sunk.

12 February 1943

Visited mountain camp with Hec Greiner – very hot and going tough. We were given a lift about halfway up by N lorry–we squatting on top of the marrows, pumpkins, sweet potatoes etc. Considerable work is being done on the road up. Engineers in charge of Australian and Dutch working parties. Capt. Hands in good form. Many Dutch, however, sick in temporary hospital (approx. 50 including commandant, Capt. Smits). Dutch sanitation is pretty grim and I am told that soldiers take their mess tins into the latrine areas (instead of the ubiquitous bottle); also they use the same tin for washing hands and face. Their lines are slovenly (like Chinatown), egg shells lying about and of course every man has a separate fire and messes around with his own cooking. One D doctor is naval, the other Indonesian. Neither seem very bright and of course they have no stores. I suggested that they draw up very strict rules re sanitation, kitchen, food, latrines etc. and that these be strictly enforced. They should immediately site deep latrines (permanent) and press for medicines and come up to see me. I will go to Nips with him. They have the framework of the hospital and one other hut up and have done some engineering work on the creeks, damming and delivering water to 'showers' by bamboo pipes. Latrines are of a temporary nature and all are troublesome owing to water seepage. They have done some good work with basket-making (both Australians and Dutch) and are tanning cow hides (with hot ashes) for boot laces, 'leather' etc. Had an excellent lunch (a four-egg omelette! and a little fish with the rice). On my return to camp I saw 'Pushface' and spoke to him re dysentery, to which he only replied 'Why?' To which I could say little more than 'No medicines' and talk about latrines. I am having a vague shivery day today with dysentery injection and at one stage wondered about malaria.

Excellent lecture this evening by a Royal Marine officer on 'the *Prince of Wales*' covering the sinking of the *Bismarck*, Churchill's meeting with Roosevelt, convoy to Malta and her final sinking in the Far East.

13 February 1943

Sunday *Yasumé* day with only a little work in morning and anti-cholera injections, ½cc, producing no reactions, but a few people have stir-up of malaria. Many men fishing today. Herb Latcham conducted a service this evening with some very well-known hymns. Much swimming, which is a great blessing.

14 February 1943

A perimeter area cleared in the jungle round the camp and a peripheral bamboo fence being built. English camp practically complete. Also lorries are now getting down the new road to the British camp fairly regularly with vegetables etc. We have a party working on the road between this camp and the British. Bridges are being built. Eggs are coming up by barge in almost embarassing quantities and a few other things are also available at times! Salt, pepper, sugar, coffee, tea, occasionally small calves, peanut toffee, limes. Pig fat, coconut oil. A little Black Market also opening up; viz., tonight bought a little fish and had this with some awfully good rissoles (rice). Very few of the lads catch many fish and these very small.

15 February 1943

All the vegetable kings have been on the spot with summaries of evidence being taken but none of them seem due to catch it this time, as they all claim to have bought or been given vegetables from sources that could 'possibly' have been honest sources–though of course, setting aside technicalities of the law, they are a pack of bastards. There's evidence of dirty trading between camps of cigarettes for vegetables.

Visited mountain camp with Billy Wearne. Dutch dysentery now about 60+ and Smits still ill. Everything much the same. I did a round of the camp with Hands, Godlee, Toets and Dutch officers and had a long talk with Smits, advising him to have a central camp comand for domestic matters which I wanted Hands to run on the grounds that he has fewer troops and more time and also has a senior man to help him in Capt. Trevena 2/40th. He seemed a bit dubious about this, so I pressed the urgency of immediately drawing up rules and standing orders and the importance of co-ordinated activities of the two camps. Eventually I gave a letter to Hands covering his appointment.

I spoke to Toets about the importance of improved sanitation measures and got a list from the doctor of drugs and other materials desired. These include (of course) mag. sulph and M and B 693, also lime for latrine lids and boiling vessels for clothes etc. I promised to see Nip commander tomorrow and spoke to guard commander re benjos.

In the jungle here birds seem very shy. Often one hears the monstrous cacophony of monkeys loudly calling, but they are rarely seen. Squirrels are rather common but deer and pigs etc. are very shy. There are all sorts of birds, large and small, including parrots, plovers, doves, pigeons, wild-fowl and others that I fail to recognise. (Vultures were amongst the first birds I saw in Thailand.) Jock Clarke is now anti-malarial officer, in addition to his other tasks, so he has an extra armband and with his squad is allowed to go at least 1 kilometre from camp over the river.

16 February 1943

All men's huts are now finished as regards the framework but owing to the shortage of attap only five roofs done out of nine. Officers' house is well under way and now the hospital. Bedding rows complete in two men's huts. 'Pushface' seemed very cheerful after a big 'bender' last night. He came to see how the huts were getting on and I tackled him about the Dutch dysentery: 'Yesterday I go mountain camp. Many Hollanders hospital, very sick. Many, *many* men. *Roku ju mei*. No good I speak. No medicines. No good. Benjos not built yet. No wire for covers. No good. Also must boil clothes. No drums or boilers. No good. Very, *very* urgent. Soon all men sick. Hollander, Australian Nippon soldier *sama*, *sama* all go sick, quickly die, finish. No good. Must have medicines – very, *very* urgent. Also wire and boilers. Medicine from Tarsau 3 days. No good – quickly, quickly. *Mushi*, *mushi* Tarsau. Otherwise all men die – quickly finish!' (All this at least induced him to give the indent to the medical corporal!)

He took me to the English camp and new road to see the 'Springs'. I heard of these two days ago. We walked down by the new road and bridges on which our men have been working and he amused me by his great interest in 'No 1 Build Bridge', a certain Cpl Doherty who has been doing yeoman work with the teams of men working the huge logs across the water course with ropes, runners and crowbars etc. He is very skilled in handling timber. We wandered down past the cemetery where he made the most profound and prolonged bow I have ever seen, removing his cap – so long that I nearly bumped into him and I had to stand for ages at the salute waiting. Then we pushed down through the bushes where 'path make' opens out into an area of Thai garden containing the crude remains of a house amid the fast-encroaching jungle. Here there is a good wide stretch of river running very quickly over stones. The quiet waters of the Menan Kwa Noi, green and impassive, sweeping down a few more sands of time. Arising from the gravel on this side of the river there are hot springs. A large log has been felled to wall off a little rectangular area roughly where the water is rather more than comfortably hot, and a big square is being cut out of the bank with the idea of extending the area for baths. Pushface enthusiastically examined the water and asked about its treatment possibilities for various illnesses. Dysentery? No good. Malaria? Good. These – indicating my jungle sores on leg. OK. er-er, er-er-suck-er, diph-er-er diph-ther-ia? No good!

Returned by the cemetery with the same profound, meaningless bow and told to come back to the office at 1230 with Corporal Doherty (No. 1 Build Bridge). This I did, when to my astonishment he was given a *presento*: package of 200 cigarettes with the following 'Honorary Certificate' (typed neatly).

'An Honorary Certificate' 17th Feb 1943

COP DOHERTY.

We hereby certified that the above mentioned person have been worked earnestly during working time and also followed good example to command of his soldiers.

The Commander of Konyu Camp

18 February 1943

Last night a Nip soldier was going around with Lt Smedley trying to buy a watch strap 'for No 1'. It was dark and not easy to see him; nevertheless, he became incensed and went in for an orgy of face slapping and also much *Keréing* practice. Today the same soldier, Takayama, is making a great deal of trouble about our permanent duties and insists that everything be changed: no wood and water duties (this done by Ration Party); sanitation squad 10 only; doctors must see sick in evening not morning; and all people for light duties to report direct to him etc. etc. He summoned me, Maj. De Cresp and Maj. Moon to discuss all this at 1200. Kewpie, the commander of the guard, did not seem very enthusiastically behind him. I said that No. 1 required me to see him with my officers at that hour and perhaps he did not know he was keeping me late for No. 1. Then went over to No. 1 full of wrath and 'complained' in the laconic, smiling, dawdling pidgin-English style as affected in his office. 'You No. 1 speak–fix duty section–I arrange–all men work, all men happy, very good. N soldier speak, change duty section, change wood and water, change hygiene men, change medical arrangements, change-change-no good. You speak good, soldier speak bad. No good. I commander *hara kari* – perhaps! Also same soldier last night try buy watch – soldiers no see dark – Nippon soldier smack face, many face, No good.

Much interest about this. 'What, hit face?' 'Yes, hit face!' When? Where? How many? Which soldier etc. and guard commander was sent for. Of course then every soldier was produced or discussed except the one in question. After much face saving assured that they would 'examine'. In such cases always bring all soldiers whose faces were slapped to office so that they could 'examine'. Meantime sorry.

New rates of pay announced as from 1 Feb. 42: all men 25 cents a day, NCOs 30 cents, W/Os 40 cents. This is a marvellous improvement. There are to be new canteen arrangements run by a Nip civilian and 2 Chinese (? contractors). They arrange for stores to be brought up and sell to us – both prices and range are said to be better.

A long-expected emergency cropped up tonight in the form of an abdominal emergency. I have been carrying a surgical kit for some time and we have a little chloroform and ether, but no other facilities whatever for operating, sterilising etc. To make things worse, the emergency arose at night when there were no lights. At 2200 hours I was called to see SX Pte Jones who has had epigastric pains off and on since in Bandoeng. This evening at 2130 hours he had sudden agonising pain in the abdomen whilst lying down on his bunk. Rapidly became collapsed and was carried to RAP. When seen, pulse 50 (strong), T. subnormal. Patient realised he was very ill and for the most part remained on his stretcher in a sitting position, very rigid, and trying ineffectively at times to vomit.

A conference was held between Maj. Moon, Maj. Corlette and I and full deference was given to the 'difficulties' of trying to operate at night in the Siam jungle. At the same time, the diagnosis of perforated peptic ulcer represented a sentence of death without an operation. Eventually it was agreed that if we still upheld the diagnosis by a further examination at 2400 hours then all would support my contention of immediate operation somehow. Meantime we would try to get ready for it. A circular white tent, 12 feet in diameter, containing dysentery patients, was picked out as being the best for feeble illumination (reflective qualities). Accordingly the patients were shifted out into the open and an 'operating table' constructed out of bamboo by Fred Smedley and Fred

Airey, assisted by the CCS orderlies who were now all up and very interested. Brian Harrison-Lucas went over to the N office to borrow lamps and although the Ns were very interested and the medical corporal at once got up and came over, only two hurricanes could be obtained and a torch. (This made two torches and a few candles) Some extra light was given by big fires lit round the tent and these also helped to warm the tent.

Cyril Cahill made a bamboo mask for anaesthesia. Bert Lawrence carefully laid the dust by sprinkling water over the tent floor. A stretcher was borrowed from Fred Smedley for an instrument table and many towels, which were sterilised by boiling for use as packs, towels etc. Most of the officers were up and helping in every way. The CCS lads got straight on with the sterilising, boiling the set of instruments I picked out, together with towels and three pairs of gloves. All the Nip guard and the medical corporal were in full cry, with all sorts of queries and comments and, of course, resolved to see the operation. After a cup of coffee at midnight we saw the patient again and operation was regarded as definitely indicated. Further preliminaries of shaving, skin preparation etc. took until 0225. During the skin prep. the Nip corporal became excited about the patient being exposed and began calling to cover him with a blanket. He was restrained! Maj. Corlette gave a chloroform anaesthetic (about 4 fl. oz in all), Maj. Moon assisting most capably. Bert Lawrence scrubbed up; the instruments were laid out on sterile towels (boiled).

This was one of the strangest operations I have ever been at: the fitful light of weak hurricane lamps and the large fires, the beam of a torch and, on one side of the tent, a fantastic audience of mixed Nip soldiers, our officers and the CCS laddies who were up (of course one doesn't notice spectators when operating any more than the crowd surrounding the football oval). The exposure went very well and the puff of gas on opening the peritonea resolved all doubts as to diagnosis. The perforation was at the first part duodenum anteriorly, and the ulcer was large with much stenosis, fibrosis and adherence, so that it was not easy to infold. A Z-pursestring was introduced then transverse matress stitches, finally bringing one omentum across the area, also liver margin in *à la* Grey Turner. This seemed air-tight and water-tight (and the rice stopped oozing out – to the delight of the Ns, one of whom had meantime been out to vomit). The great difficulty of the operation was closing the posterior sheath of the rectus and peritonea with everything tight as a drum and deplorable needles for the job. This took ages comparatively, so that with various difficulties inherent in our scratch organisation, the job took over two hours. Hot bottles were then produced and he was wrapped in blankets but left in the same place on the 'table'. Condition very good. All hands then had coffee and the CCS boys had some rice too. They were all in great fettle and had done a marvellous job in organising the theatre. I finally left the patient at 0530. He had had some morphia and was sleeping (Thomas in charge). He should have a good chance. Nips astonishingly impressed. Me 'No. 1'!

19 February 1943

Hec Greiner's birthday. Everyone who was at the operation naturally a bit tired, so that when on the 0800 parade I called the parade up to attention the second time, nothing happened except a sort of click of well-nigh dislocated joints. Some pillows requested for Jones who is in good spirits and good condition. No vomiting after the anesthetic.

Ron Lum and Heywood doing great work on the officers' house which looks quite a magnificent framework now. Billy does a great deal of work too.

Decided today to change the pay contribution to one-fifth of all pay, all ranks, in view of new rates. N Corporal brought over two tins of condensed milk for the sick man and fortunately some medical stores from Tarsau arriving today include a few more tins so that patient is already on some milk and water. Tomorrow he will have egg and milk flips.

20 February 1943

Avitaminosis parade

O	P
73 mild	50 mild
39 severe	24 severe
1 very severe	
113	74 Total

Men improving and numbers lower. Jones very well – comfortable.

English entertainers came over to our camp tonight for a concert and put on a very good show – singing and light comedy. Meantime I had gone to the British camp to lecture on the Greece campaign. This lecture presaged by an excellent dinner with the English colonels. Asparagus and egg, soup, meat stew and rice, peanut toffee, cigars etc. Lecturing and concert difficulties were, however, almost insurpassable: first a howling dust-gale, then rain for the first time in months when I had half-finished my lecture, getting wet, by which time audience had nearly vanished. Concert party did a little better. All troops however rushing to cover up bedding. Butterworth saved mine from the worst ravages of the rain by a ground sheet. Anyway, I find wet blankets surprisingly warm as they break the wind.

21 February 1943

Sunday. *Yasumé*. Unexpectedly Padre Parr (C. of E.) and Padre Bourke (RC) turned up. (No *yasumé* English lines today.) C. of E. turn-out was very small (20+) Padre Parr ran a very good conventional C. of E. service with trumpet (table for altar). His robes and communion kit battered, travel-stained and with water stains. Above this a gaunt, bearded, spiritual face (at times I caught a distinct resemblance to a bedraggled and ill J.C.), below a gaunt thin pair of legs and army boots. Up on the hill near the *shoko*'s incomplete house a scintillating brilliant spectacle in scarlet and gold: Padre Bourke presenting the colour, dignity, purple pomp and power of the church temporal. Afterwards tea.

Evening: much diving and swimming for clams. Lost the whole 24 trying to

* He died shortly after.

swim with them in a rice sack (heavy as lead) so it was them or me after about 40 yards.

22 February 1943

My patient Jones: temp. rising to 105° today; I think and hope chest but Maj. Corlette is rather fearful re subphrenic, so I am a bit gloomy about him. Changed his sulphonilamide to M and B 693 Tab 0/4 Ads.

Hospital state now rising and primary malaria now coming in (Damn). Information reveals that malaria is highly endemic in Siam especially *in the hills*; not much in the low-lying coastal areas, particularly about Bangkok. *A. minimus* breeds especially in slow-running streams with grassy edges, also in barrow pits, rice fields and seepages. The work of anti-malaria squad is going on but it is greatly handicapped, like most other camp work , by shortage of tools. They are doing good work burning back jungle and tracking down water requiring drainage. Another curse of this site is the frequency of very painful scorpion bites – usually several men daily. I have tried mild cauterisation with Phenol though I doubt if it is very effective. Frequently people come in in the dark with severe bites and I suspect snakes etc. There are many huge tarantulas and centipedes, not to mention multitudinous ants (many of these in dreadnought class) and every type of fly, sandflies etc. Mosquitoes are not plentiful but sufficiently evident after dusk. I never see them in the cold hour before dawn.

Reveille is well before any trace of dawn; shortly after parade there is a slight lightening in the sky to the east and then eventually there is usually seen pale rose streamers, apparently an effect of the light mist and cloud. This strongly reminds me always of Homer's metaphor – 'The rosy fingers of dawn showed through the mists'. Later, there are the same effects on the towering crags and the dense jungle comes to life. The fronds of bamboo look especially delicate in the morning light and the chatter of monkeys is at its height.

23 February 1943

Jones much better. T. rising 102° then fell to normal today. Is definitely a chest. Tincture Benz co, menthol inhalation. He is also having ascorbic acid 2-hourly feed still (no antacid available). His progress is a great relief to me, as I should hate to lose a case at present when the whole inspirational life of the camp seems to depend on such things.

Malaria still coming in and all troops given solemn warning re mosquito net drill, clothes and going to river after nightfall (cooks and others near the river were first affected).

Socho Tadano came in to see me today about his tonsils. He accepted a gargle but would not take sulphonilomide tablets as we had so little medicines to treat our own sick. Said he would take them tomorrow if he were more sick. Good work! The curse of my successful major abdominal op. is that all the Ns now look at me with bated breath as No. 1 doctor and are chasing me for advice. They are like a lot of frightened children about their health: worry re chest, stomach etc. etc. Much fuss about any scratches. N medical service locally is a corporal (a rascal and trader-in-chief). He gave Arthur some Vicks vaporub the other day, indicating at the time 'Eyedrops – Nippon soldier no like'! Suffering cats!

The practise of eating snakes continues. One soldier found one in his bed the other night and succeeded in killing it, whereupon his mate remarked: 'Some people have all the luck with *makan* crawling into their bed.'

Fantastic rumours e.g. the war in Europe is finished; and protests in Geneva about the treatment of British POWs in Siam, quoting the extremely high death rates. More English have died in our camp and the Dutch total is three, two more having died recently. About 130+ now sick. The Ns, of course, show a callous disregard and dismiss all requests for drugs with 'go Tarsau tomorrow – tomorrow' etc. The state of health in these camps can only be regarded as an everlasting appalling disgrace and a perfectly natural result of the administration and general treatment. One gem of a rumour is that the Siamese have been told that they will be held responsible and that they are taking over admin!

24 February 1943

Malaria 29, Dys. 17, Op. Case 1; 8 Malarias admitted today.

Flies are terribly hard to fight here. Jock Clarke and his benjo squad have skilfully split and cut trees into timber to make fly-proof seats. This is terribly hard work and beautifully done. Jock is energetic and capable. Notice served on the troops of an absolute blitz on malaria, and since the general attitude has continued to be deplorably careless, definite orders will be issued tomorrow and failure to carry them out will lead to disciplinary action. (Men persist in going to the river after dark and in going about without shirts after dark.) A campaign of lectures and so on will be conducted with officers in conference this evening. More hospital accommodation is now required and hospital is held up for want of attap.

25 February 1943

No. 1 George came over to camp this evening most opportunely with tonsillitis (improving) so I asked him about hospital tents. He said collect 3 tents immediately. Hospital held up on account of attap like all other hutments. A perimeter fence is now complete but the officers still live in the jungle outside, sleeping in the open.

I also asked No. 1 George for more boots for the anti-malarial work. Not much luck there. Sgt King in an altercation with a N today which began over his carrying bamboo when the N disagreed, King shaking a tomahawk finally and saying if he was hit he would knock the f____g Nip down. (The Ns do not like this word which is a point in favour of their taste.) After marching the party as far down to the camp as the cemetery! the N walked up with a heavy bit of wood and asked for the f____g, f____g soldier. He then swung the stick at his head. King saved his head by his forearm which is greatly swollen, the skin broken (narrow shave from a break I should think). The N then beat him up on the ground. I took King over to No. 1 who was entrenched behind a wall of our Thai money which had arrived (NEI money [Dutch] and Straits Settlements money not changed). After the usual quarter hour of English speak-pidgin patter I produced King with the story 'Sergeant speak Nippon soldier, say "f_____g". No Good. Nippon order Sergeant speak back No good, very bad. Nippon soldier hit Sergeant with big stick very hard No good, very bad. Please see. (King made an impressive sight and played up, I saying 'perhaps bone break'). The soldier was at once called and 'dressed down' by No. 1 and finally left at attention for about ten minutes before me. Soldier Susuki stand at attention absolutely see. Then Tadano had a go at him and he finally bowed his way out with tail between his legs. Later he came over and asked King to accept his apology and offered him cigs but old King angrily waved him off (wrong).

Dick Allen arranged money collection today and all ranks may have the sums lodged as credit or cash if they require them.

Anti-malaria orders were announced on parade. Rostov fell on the 10th; battle raging NW of Kharkov biggest of Russian battles; Gs counter-attacking at Tunis and repulsed. Channel ports bombed day and night. Goebels has made a 'backs to the wall' speech: 'This is Germany's darkest hour'. Men, women and children must man frontiers etc.

26 February 1943

Disgusted with my ankles which remain ulcerated five weeks. Went fishing with rice for tiddlers and slipped on the bank breaking my precious Dunhill pipe; Jack Ross is going to try to make a temporary repair – a bad day. Caught 2 tiddlers. Ns now say there is a cholera outbreak up the river and we must not swim in river or clean teeth etc. with the water though we can bathe and wash our clothes. Cholera would be the final touch!

27 February 1943

Nights grow bitterly cold again and one's whole body aches if once one wakes up on this damn bamboo. Yesterday Maj. Moon collected from the N corporal (medical) 1 sack of rice polishings (134 lb) and soya beans (20 lb). Ns have been promising supply of rice polishings in view of poor quality rice. This supply will be given to hospital cases and avitaminosis cases. Rice polishings at 1 oz a day will last 8–10 days. Soya beans for hospital cases. 70 lb of fresh meat (cow) today. Three new hospital tents received (2 put up) RD American type C, mosquito gauze lining. Malaria cases respond rapidly to treatment. Vegetables very light of late. Some smoked fish has been available but this is often blown and maggotty, needing much washing and removal of guts. Conference of Maj. Moon, Maj. Wearne, Ron Lum and I re hospital buildings, which are shockingly jerry built with no roof as yet in the most deplorably low and uneven areas of the ground available. The smaller of the two huts nearest river will be used for admin. and sick parades, also dressing and operating room and accommodation of orderlies; rest of space is for ordinary sick. The sloping ground is to be floored and there will be four rows of beds 1 metre wide × 2 metres long allotted to each patient.

Following questions were handed to me to be answered by three people, officers or ORs: impression of camp; impression as to future progress of war; impression as to Nipponese Army; impression as to camp sanitation and accommodations; impression of Australians as regards Dutch Army.

This seems to be a prelude to a conference of camp commanders in Bampong where apparently the general will see commanders instead of coming to see us. Questionaires: Maj. Moon to do one, Brian Harrison-Lucas and I the others. It was decided to put our case fairly strongly. The following strong criticisms were made:

i unhealthy site – malaria and dysentery – hence sickness
ii *Food* – inadequacy of rations supplied
iii Hospital arrangements-medical supplies, evacuation arrangements
iv Clothing and boot situation
v Letters and home communication

We had no comments on 2 and 3, except that N army maintained good discipline in the camp. We commented on the shortages of containers for boiling water; No chloride of lime or containers for chlorination; No disinfectants and the shortage of tools which was delaying the construction of latrines, the anti-malaria work etc. As to 5, the Dutch have co-operated well in camp and relations are good.

Blitz being carried out on dysentery precautions, care re washing of hands etc and deploring certain men who have accidents before reaching the latrine and do not clean up. There seems to be a growing tendency in some to become 'benjo happy' and to be always hanging round latrines or rushing to them during parades. This is being discouraged.

Seventy-one men in hospital today: 15 out of 30 cooks have been down with malaria. One latrine innovation Clarke's hygiene squad have made is in the form of tall air vents of long bamboo pipes; still, a latrine is a smelly thing whatever is done and I am glad we insisted on fifty metres away.

28 February 1943

RC redemptive mission continues. I attended one night to 'hear about death' and retired with my tail between my legs. Let one not console himself that we were much more fit in this camp than others. Death always comes like a thief in the night when you are not expecting it and are in a complacent state of mind! In a sense, I am perhaps less a Christian even than I was before the war, but I have been taught very soundly that one must believe in some religion, or sink into the terrible mire of utter selfishness and materialism, so I will always hesitate to say anything against any religion. Man seems to be still far too unintelligent an animal to realise that happiness comes from harmonious relationships with one's fellows and service to mankind rather than in a dirty, unprincipled self-seeking existence.

N rations: these a constant battle. QM of QR Bns say that they have only had 640 lb meat for 1,000 men in 1 month. Our sugar supply is only two-thirds of normal ration, 6 g/man per day.

Dutch deaths now 6, including one lad of 19 years, and these are mainly Europeans.

1 March 1943

Hospital: 65; light duties: 73. Sgt Honeyman and the anti-malaria squad have been doing great work burning undergrowth, clearing the riverfront, searching for and dealing with pools etc. He ranges the jungles over the river like Dr Livingstone. Recently he was furiously lighting fires when he turned to face three angry Thais, all with knives, apparently resenting the firing of their bamboos. Advance with peaceful gestures was rejected with a flourish of knives, so he dived back into the jungle and crossed the river near the English camp, very scratched and somewhat upset at having lost his belt and towel in the crossing. One breeding source to be watched is the stumps of bamboo cut about the camp.

We are warned today that soon we are expected to supply 500 men a day for outside work on road and rail. This will be very difficult because of the number of men sick or suffering from post-malarial or post-dysenteric debility.

There have been great lines of fires on the hills round here of nights, particularly north-east and south-east, these making an impressive sight. During the day the sun rises blood-red in a mist of smoke and the hills are frequently purple in the slanting rays of the sun. It is queerly hard to place the season, as many of the trees – especially the teak – are shedding their leaves, giving an austere autumn appearance; yet I suppose if it is any season it is spring. Bamboos are forever moulting their light yellow leaves which mount up in our encampment and in the forest.

Most remarkable ingenuity is being shown in camp works, exemplified by the hygiene men in their carpenter's shop. They have not only split and squared good timber out of trees (using wooden wedges) but improvise nails out of wire to nail them together. Practically all the Nips have given us here for camp construction are bad tools – 'folding shovels' etc. – and we have to keep these in order. The ties for bamboo construction are either jungle vines or the inside bark of trees which we cut (better).

The basket makers are interesting and mainly naval personnel who work down on the river. They first cut out long slivers of bamboo to make the side vertical struts which are then softened by soaking in the river. The horizontal winding is done either with vine or further bamboo, which is woven in and out of the radiating rays forming the vertical supports. Excellent twine is also made from bark and fibre, an interesting sight. These brown, thin, bearded naval fellows are the heroes of many hard battles in the Mediterranean and the Java Seas – the other day one was sitting on the sand with the eventual base of the basket poised on his head and the radiating spider-web rays of bamboo struts projecting all about him like some bizarre, giant headgear. One dextrous sailor walked around the web, winding vine alternately over and under while yet another manipulated the strands close and tight. The slanting sun made a grotesque picture on the sands as though two giant figures were dancing on the N naval flag, the central figure being obliterated in the round shadow of the bottom of the basket. P/O Abbott and P/O Parkin have both had dysentery and are particularly thin, the former having lost about four stone.

Cookhouse experiments are being made with bamboo structures supported with well-plastered mud to make chimneys etc. Also an Aldershot oven, the door being made of bamboo heavily plastered over with mud. These are very successful. If we have fractures I think I will try making splints of bamboo and mud.

2 March 1943

Hospital: 59; light duties 77. For the last two days I have resumed some 'medical' work with one tent of patients, almost all malarias. These are not very sick and most of them get into hospital before having much in the way of rigors etc. Very quickly they develop a large spleen, which seems to almost always be present. I have one case of relapse within a fortnight.

Egg Parade: new routine owing to new pay rates. All avitaminosis cases to receive three eggs (or nil) and they pay for two themselves at 7 cents each. A review today showed great all-round improvement and many cases were struck off. Some debilitated cases of post-malaria/dysentery were added. It can be deduced that eggs do the trick but at least 3 a day are required. The little bit of rice polishings available will also help.

Maj. Wearne and I then set off to the mountain camp, calling in on No. 1 N on the way. It was early on a fine morning and on the way up the mountain we saw some big monkeys leaping magnificently (drops of 15–20 feet) then swinging off amongst the bamboos. There are magnificent birds, including the great hornbills which wing their way over usually in the morning or evening with a great whirring of wings. We made good time to Dutch camp where Hands and Co. in fine fettle.

The Dutch: 204 in hospital last night, mostly dysentery. Smits is out, but is quite hopeless as a leader. He says that when the Javanese leave Java they lose heart and it is no good trying to drive them. Also 'we have too many old men; we cannot work like the Australians – we cannot dig the deep latrines – it is too hard for us'. They have been messing about for days to get down 2–3 feet and even the Ns have been going stone mad at them about it. There is the same hopelessness about anything one speaks about. 'The work is too hard. We cannot do it.'

[Smits] himself and a party of W/Os are thinking of escaping and he has damn all in the way of a plan. I did all I could to discourage such foolishness.

The Dutch hospital has very few orderlies as the Javanese are frightened and will not help. The patients are not well cared for, in my opinion. There is a most inordinate amount of bed soiling and fouling, necessitating continuous boiling of clothes – 'but there are not enough containers!' And then 'the friends of the patients are supposed to wash their clothes but do not come'.

I saw one case lying in delirium and semi-coma regarded as a meningitis but no lumbar puncture had been done and when I asked about intravenous quinine, Dr Brouwer said no, as he had no adrenalin. After asking Tim to give him some I heard that he had been promised some whenever he wanted it! What most upsets me is the sight of the dysentery latrine, over which *shallow* trench is rigged a sort of rough garden seat. All men then clean themselves with water, using their hand and go through the process of sticking their hand down into the one disinfectant container, a single, long and narrow, hollow stick of bamboo. No thought of soap and water, even. Jack tells me that even the dead men are hardly below the surface owing to the difficulty of old men digging graves!

Tim Godlee has opened a new tented hospital of his own and runs it very well, right away from the Dutch. He is going to give all rice polishings to about 40 men 3 oz/man/day concentrating on those with mouth or scrotum trouble and will try to get these OK quickly. He has very few *burning feet* patients but now three *corneal ulcers*; these coming very quickly.

Cod liver oil is not available: he is giving pumpkin on account of the yellow colour. I do not know if any night blindness was noticed.

As I was returning, I ran into N medical corporal outside hospital. He seized upon me and said 'Oh No. 1 – much dysentery. You speak Hollander – fix!' This very dramatically. I reminded him that the D must have more medical stores and containers for boiling. I am glad to see that they at least have mag. sulph. now to carry them on for a week or two.

Hygeine matters: Maj. Clarke has introduced disinfectant 'bottles' of soap and cresol antiseptic (made out of bamboo) available for each benjo (Castellani bottle idea).

In spite of much ashes from fires being tipped into benjos, they are regrettably smelly.

The Ns are making great fuss about their benjo which has to be completely walled in so they are not seen, despite the fact that they publically pee all over the place about their hut and foul the scrub about without covering the mess. They never use our latrine.

Apparently the Ns are upset about our letters of 'impressions as to camp' and now say we must write further on 'attitude of mind as to camp' Can this be an attempt to get a face saver for No. 1?

3 March 1943

Hospital: 62; light duties: 78; egg parade: 139.

'Attitude of mind' answered by all three in much more round terms than before and must be only said to be extremely 'bloody minded'.

Mine: 'My attitude is one of gross disquiet and fear for the lives and health of the troops placed in my care...

'The following matters worry and perplex me.

'Although I have found that our soldiers do not remain healthy with the full Nippon ration only a fraction of the promised scale of vegetables and meat has been supplied.

O & P Battalions period 25 Jan–2 March 43

Meat	*Entitlement* (100 grams/man/day)	*Supplied*
	3212 kilograms	300 kilograms
Vegetable	18,000 kilograms	4500 kilograms

'As no attap. is available after many weeks many of the soldiers have no house and most sleep in the open, though some have almost no clothes and blankets.

'Supplies of medical stores and hospital and sanitation arrangements are not satisfactory.

'Out of a total of 873 men I consider that only 350 are suitable for heavy work outside the camp.

'It causes grave alarm that other troops I see in the area should look like living skeletons. As I have always been informed that the Nippon army has an honorable tradition I cannot understand why prisoners-of-war should have been shifted to such an unhealthy place, or that conditions should be so inhumane and discreditable to the detaining powers.'

E. Dunlop Lt-Col.
Konyu No. 3 Camp

Called on N No. 1 with our letters and had an unsatisfactory discussion with Osuki about camp matters, in particular that there is to be no more attap to complete hospital, 4½ huts, officers' house and other buildings. ('All transport now use to shift food for rainy season. Must make roof bamboo etc.') We said bamboo roof no good – anyway would need about 1000 perfectly straight bamboos for each hut – so more than 100 men must work all the time to finish before rainy season. Therefore outside work must finish! Following position put up to Ns.

Analysis of work 3/3/43

Cooks	30	Sick in hospital	70
Wood & water carriers	20	Light duty	115
RSM and clerks	10	Sanitation	30
Medical orderlies	15	Canteen	8
Police	5	Ration party	21
Batmen	3	Guard house orderly	1
Anti-malaria	5	Basket & repairs	10
Orderly I.J.A. HQ	1	Officers	15
Barber	2ea	TOTAL:	363
Duty Section:	93		

(approximate number still requiring footwear: 120)

Capt. Allan back from Tarsau and reports that the canteen under Ns is most unsatisfactory; goods not available in quantity required, terrific queues, exorbitant prices (e.g. 30 cents two egg omelette; 20 cents large cup of coffee).

Work is being done on the floor of *shoko's* house (the verandah is already finished) and on flooring the hospital. Today we decided to try reed thatching as a roof.

4 March 1943

A Nip major is said to have inspected our camp today and to be satisfied that the food was very good and cooking satisfactory, in fact everything good. No camp official was called or saw them.

We recently bought some chickens (4) on the black market (one for Jones, the perforated duodenal ulcer who is now out of bed with perfectly healed wound, all sutures out. He should do very well now.) Ron Lum has been keeping him supplied in fish and he has much milk and about 8 eggs a day!

The medical team are doing a great job and I am certain that the low mortality up to date has been due to the medical care of all these troops. Arthur Moon is always one of the busiest men in the camp and Jock Clarke is one of the best.

5 March 1943

Evening: many troubles.

1 We may not wash ourselves in river because of cholera. Must boil water carried from the river in bamboos (impossible).

2 Must number our sections in Nipponese language.

3 Bugle calls to be Nipponese.

4 May not shift hospital into jungle further from benjo (offensive); must shift into cleared area of camp. This would be hot as hell and very difficult.

Chaplain Gerard Bourke, in trouble, was arraigned before blotch-faced Osaki, sword in hand.

O: Why do you disobey the orders of Japanese Army?

B: I take my orders from a much higher authority than Japanese Army.

O: (More angry) Nunda! Nunda! Higher authority – where?

B: (Pointing to sky) My orders are from up there!

O: (Perplexed, then explosive) Bugero! (raising sword)

B: (Face happy at prospect of martyrdom)

I intervened, tapping my head. 'Kistian priests very eccentric men!'

O: (Mollified) Ah, 'eccentric' man.

6 March 1943

Up betimes and took over new tent of patients, mostly malaria, then off to British camp where much X [exchange of wireless news].

Called upon Padre Webb. He is having service tomorrow, 'sacrament of Lord's supper' to which we all are invited and he wants me to dig up some Elders of the Kirk from my men. I have none, but since Arthur Moon looks like one, I have recommended him and he will function (much to his protests about this).

Evening concert which I had to open. Sgt Wynne was to have been compère but has recently twice fallen into the benjo with injuries to his arms, hence P/O Abbott (who is always a great favorite with the lads). I opened with reference to his having got himself in a hole or two but that at the next concert he would give us one or two 'banjo' items. Artists involved here including Herbert Smith ('the singing soldier'), Ivor Jones, Jack Rourke. Scotty Starr, Allan Woods (bush ballads) and George Page (trumpet). Ivor combines excellently in duets with either Smith or Rourke and they sang delightfully. Great fires lit the scene and the crackling of bamboo with showers of sparks drifting up to mingle with the stars so multitudinous and bright. The surrounding jungle was black and mysterious and forgotten.

7 March 1943

Saw Tadano (who has tonsillitis again) and asked him re rumour of movement; he said 'don't know' and possibly Australians move to Kinsayok.

Church: Padre Webb officiated at sacrament of the Lord's supper – a very simple and effective Scottish service with Arthur and other elders round the table and taking round the 'bread' (made from rice) and 'wine' (Some sort of synthetic produce of the padre's). One of the chalices was a bamboo cup. Somehow my thoughts were racing all over the world in a crazy kaleidoscopic way. I thought of Helen often, and of many, few were holy I'm afraid.

8 March 1943

Of tragic memory. Amusing confirmation of yesterday's X [wireless news] by Thai people: almost the same, even figures. Also some amusing stories of Ns slain by blowpipes! Again 'confirmation' of the fact that we are going to move to Kinsayok. Thai people know apparently. To British camp, and had morning coffee with Lt-Col. Hill, Lt-Col. Moore and Warren etc who are very interested in our fate. Hospital shifted today inside fence taking over No. 1 barracks O Bn and 2 tents.

Quinine given to us today: Tabs sulphate 3 grams and Bi-hydrochloride 4 grain, to be taken by *all* troops on *tenko* parade each night – *suppressive*. I do not entirely agreement with the principle seeing that our stay in the area may be long and the dose not very effective, but so many men have already had malaria it may be a good idea.

9 March 1943

To N No. 1 for complaints and enquiries. Apparently we move. Bampong HQ will say when and how. Thirty-four bags of appalling rice – musty, broken and full of dirt and filth with a sour smell – obtained for this month. No. 1 says he will change it.

We were warned again against the river and its 'cholera' and given times for the use of the 'hot springs' as from tomorrow, *yasumé* for 'Memorial Day' (what memories for us).

One soldier came up the other day with a large skinned goanna in his mess tin; very white, tender-looking meat rather like rabbit and much yellow fat. He reported very good eating. Price of Red Bull cigarettes remains 50 cents a packet. Meeting of officers' mess decided that expenditure on mess to be 50 cents a day for all officers and to share all money (four officers get 25 ticals a month and four 30 tickals – this pay after the one-fifth deduction has been 20 and 23 respectively.

Since our arrival, the average meat per day has been 7⅓ g and vegetables 3 oz per man/day (dreadful).

10 March 1943

Hospital: 64 (0 29; P 55); light duties: 49.

Yasumé Day – Nippon Russian Memorial Day. Total men unable to march if we are moved is at present 95. Boot situation since arrival: 155 canvas and rubber boots supplied and 19 pairs canvas shoes – all poor stuff for jungle.

My patient, Jones, now eats 15 eggs a day and milk and 2–3 fish (from Ron Lum).

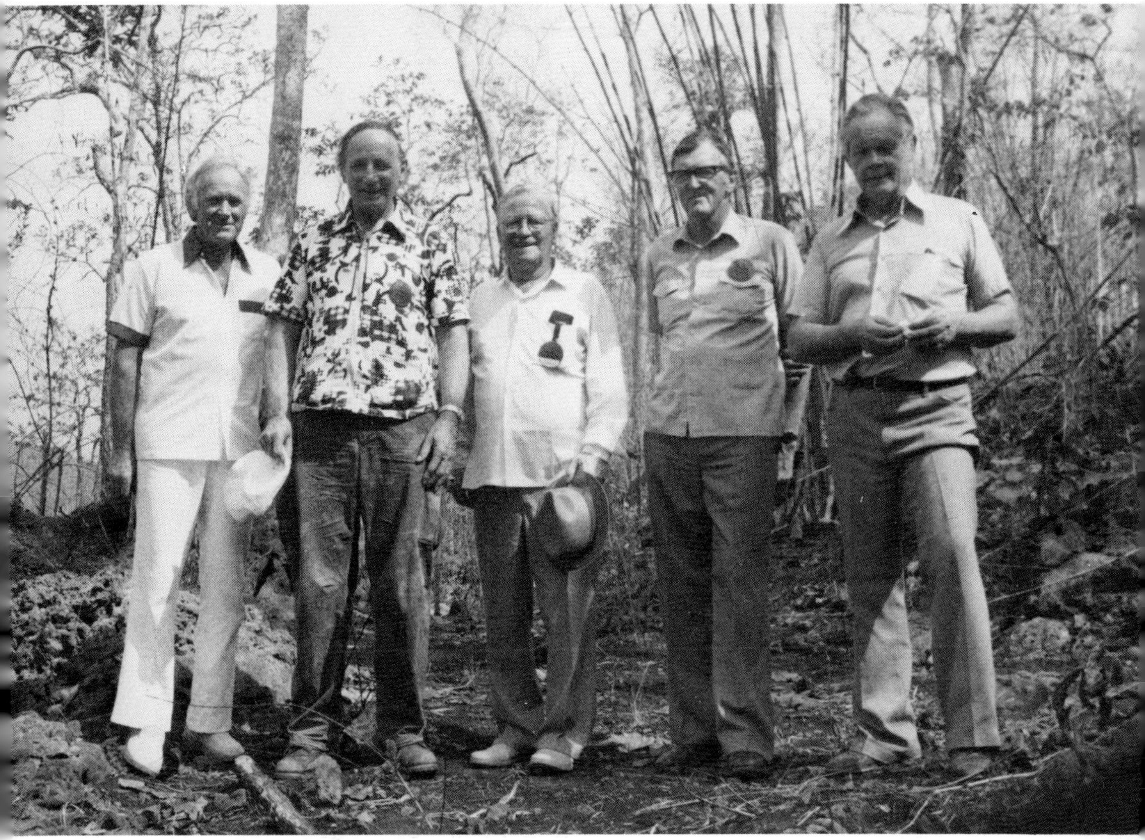

er railway workers revisiting the track at Hintok, 1985. *Left to right*: J. Chalker, the author, 'Blue' Butterworth, ckson, Keith Flanagan

51 'Blue' Butterworth, a 'hammer and tap' man, in the Hintok rock cutting, 'Hellfire Pass', 1985

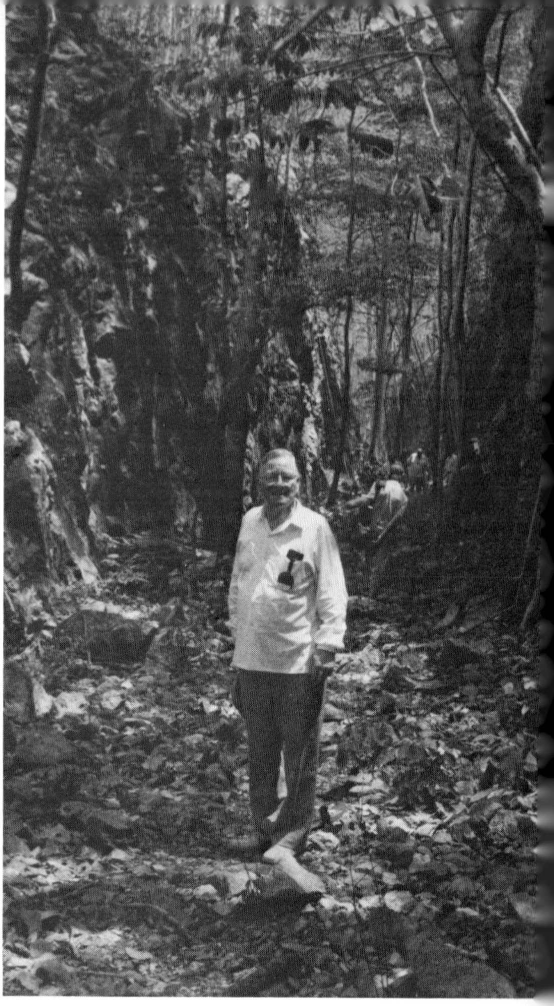

52 View from the railway track, Hintok, 1985. The jungle of teak and bamboo has largely been cleared

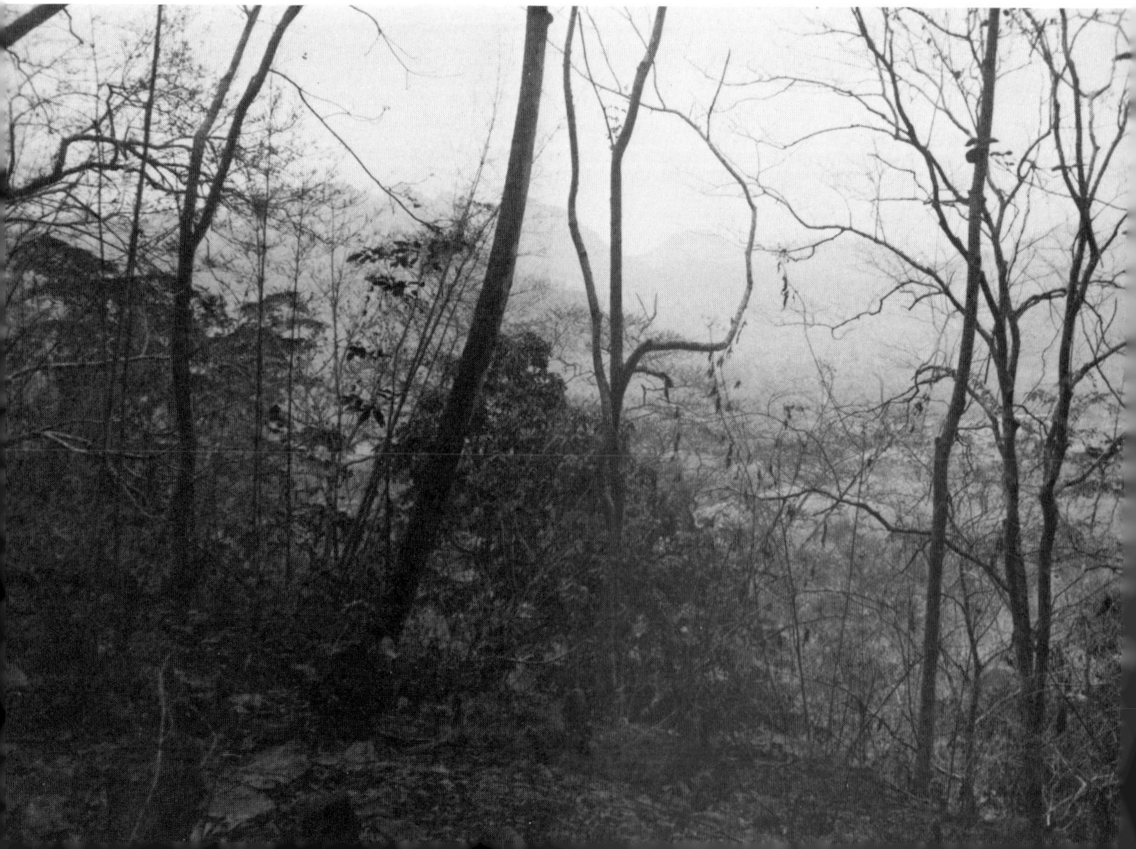

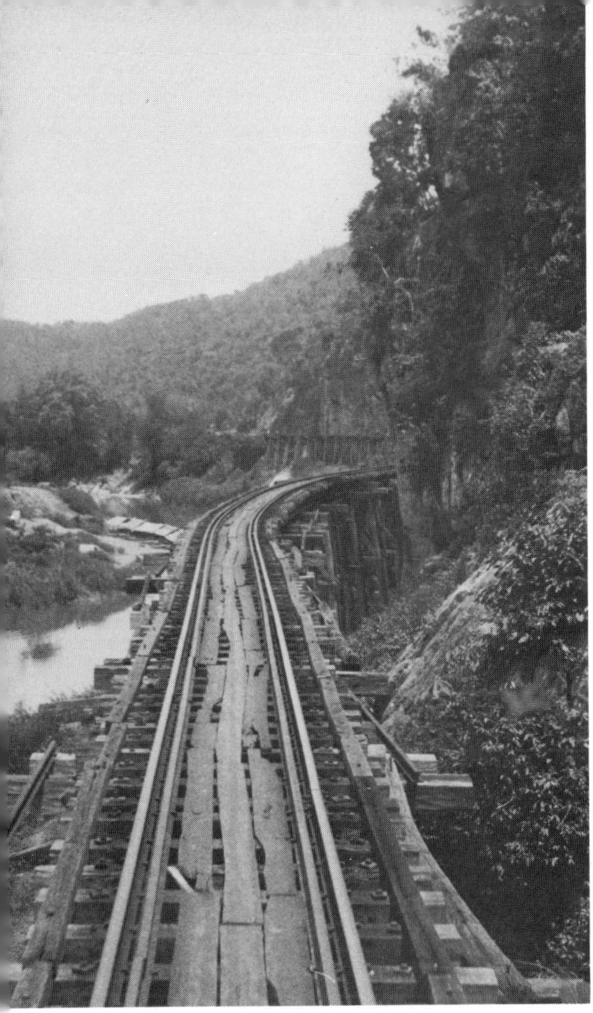

53 The Wampo viaduct skirting the Kwai Noi River, Thailand, 1985

54 Tamarkan bridge – the 'Bridge over the River Kwai' – as it is today

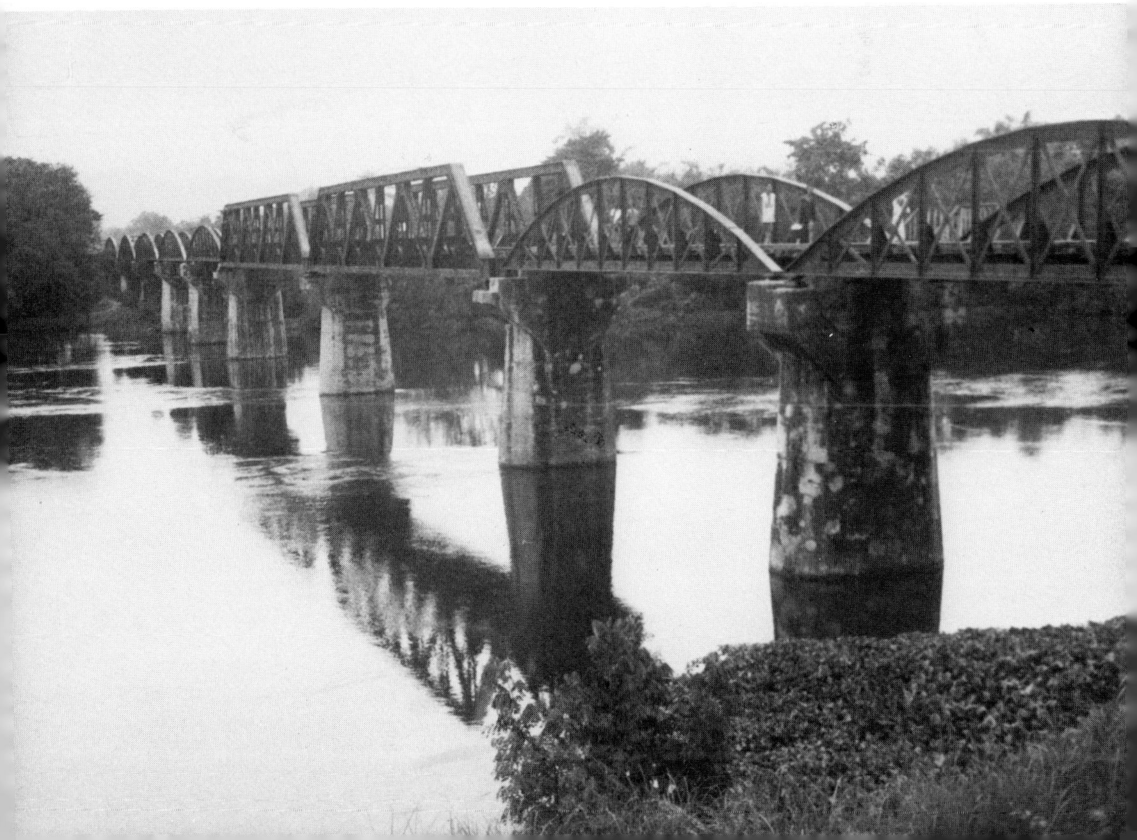

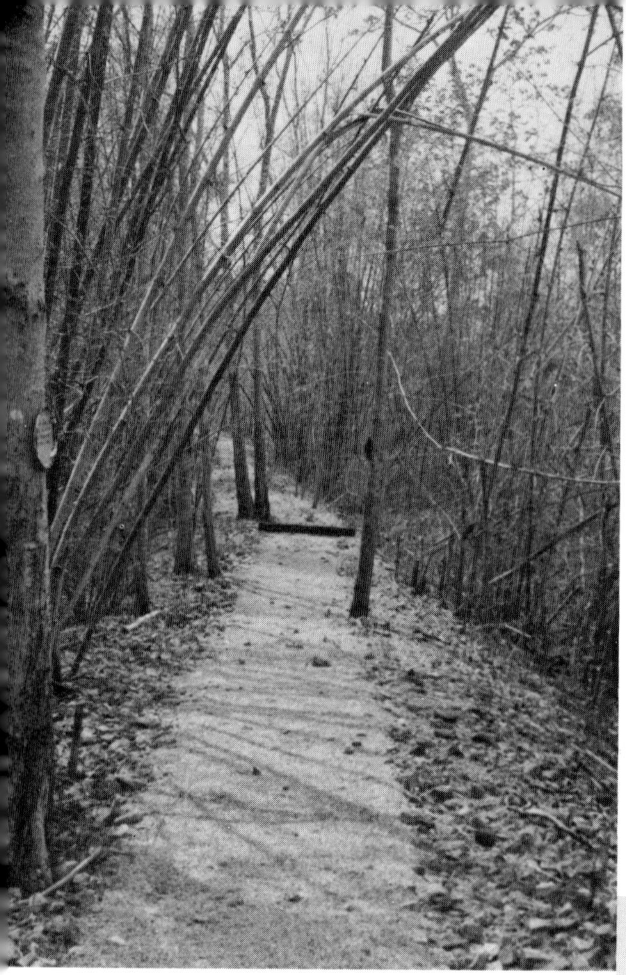

55 Desolate railway track, Hintok embankment, 1985

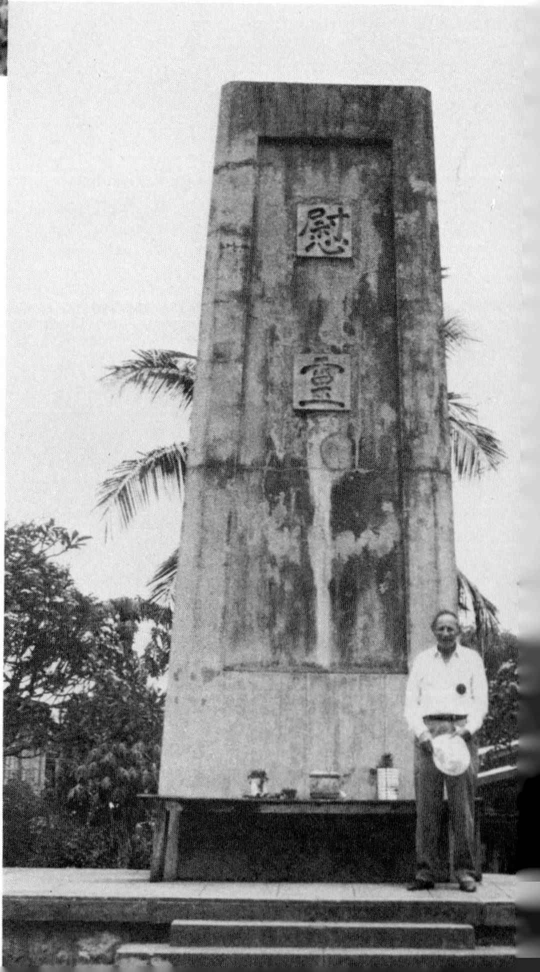

56 The author revisiting the Japanese Memorial at Tamarkan dedicated to the railway builders.

11 March 1943

To English camp where S warned me of movement tomorrow to 'mountain camp'. Capt. Hands' group meantime to move to Kinsayok (actually Capt. Hands called earlier in the morning with this news gleaned from the Engineer officer). This news is as bloody as could be received, in view of the fact that the river here is the life-line and to be away from it in wet weather is too unpleasant to contemplate. Also we have done a great deal of work here on construction and sanitation – hospital, benjo, shokos' house etc., all of very superior design.

Capt. Hands' camp is a bad site – a 'waterless bog'. The construction (such as is finished) is bloody awful. The Dutch have fouled the whole area and some are bound to remain. Tadano gave Billy and I a glass of local brew, a slightly opalescent, clear fluid looking rather like ginger beer but with a very pungent nip which made our motors race (Billy's face flaming rosy red immediately – can this be Thai whisky?). We visited Lt-Col. More and were perhaps a little bit talkative, so much so that with the dangerous outspokenness of small children and such-like I suggested that the only really good thing the English would be leaving behind if they shift would be the cemetery and the view from the officers' hut, so why not take the cemtery with them? (A sensitive spot that.) Much joking about handing over our magnificently built and floored shokos' hut and the great table and chairs etc. I felt rather like one at a late afternoon sherry party and in great form.

In the afternoon, I went out on a malarial recce with Sgt Honeyman and Jock Clarke. The former set a terrible raking stride up the rough rocky ravine to the north. The sun beat down intolerably and I could feel it concentrated as from a burning glass, so that streams of hot sweat poured down my face and blinded my eyes as though pressed against one of those irrigated plate glass butchers' windows. Eventually Jock was asking quarter, and it was only pride that kept me from yelling for mercy too. I don't know where old Honeyman gets it. We found many intensive breeding places for mosquitoes.

The railway track still being cleared is an astonishing affair. It seems to run without much regard to the landscape as though someone had drawn a line on the map! In this particular area it runs along the precipitous slope of a hill instead of the ridge. Terrible gaps and boulders and descents.

Tommies were at work, tree felling, and the course was littered with broken axe handles–those trees felled, as Jock put it, showing signs of having been gnawed down by inferior false teeth! The Ns appeared to take no notice of us wandering about the country even though Honeyman was the only one of us wearing an armband (our shirts off). The rocky mountain-sides are covered with sharp flints and a fall would be very dangerous. Back to camp in evening for about two pints of coffee (Billy this evening making visit to X [wireless]).

At approximately 2100 hours I received orders for 'Transition of Troops' commencing tomorrow; Hands' camp to Kinsayok and we go to Hands' camp. Movement said to be by lorry: 2 lorries daily at 1030 and 1530 hours (same lorry back and forth) with approximately 50 troops per lorry load. Baggage is to go in afternoon with each day's move; morning troops are to carry only water bottle and eating gear; sick are to remain, also duty section and camp HQ details (those sick unfit to move should be sent to Tarsau soon). Nevertheless, it seems probable that we will not be moving entirely, as some details are remaining here.

I protested against sending troops without packs on back, since trouble always crops up with these moves separate from baggage (to no avail of course). It rather looks as if each camp chases the next one; one further up the river whilst possibly some Singapore details move up into the comfortable base areas. Perhaps we are regarded as jungle shock troops! The leap frog principle would seem to be much better, sparing unnecessary movement, but this is (as always) the N method of combining inefficient behaviour with 'hurry', 'hurry', 'speedo', 'speedo'. Hec Greiner and Bret. Moore to move tomorrow and No. 1 and 2 Section O Bn.

Heavy rain in the evening soaking the beds and clothing of most who were still out of doors but 'Blue' did me magnificently – I returned to find a borrowed canvas cover rigged over my bedding and everything dry, so just went to bed. Very hot now.

12 March 1943

Most disconcerting changes of plans. Fifty men ready for move as arranged when at approx 1100 hours N runner arrives saying 'Now 200 men marchy, marchy, hurry, hurry.' 'Lunch?' 'Don't need.' Six cooks to go also.

13 March 1943

Further 200 men to mountain camp including Ewan Corlette and Reg Piper. No lorry for their baggage and they were instructed to take bedding rolls. This makes total 400 ORs and 5 officers transferred. Capt. Hands came up and position in that camp is as follows: some to Kinsayok – D. 130, Aust. 10. Tomorrow no move but 15th and 16th 100 each day.

Hut position; 2 built, framework of 8 (no beds). Rations at this camp are said to be considerably better; rice and other rations are to be left behind with all other kitchen stuff. Agreed on complete settlement of the canteen money.

Of our men who arrived yesterday 155 are working today. Saw Susuki today and he agreed to send eggs to other camp. Told me 'going Bangkok soon'.

Seven elephants are now in English camp as part of 80 going up for railway construction work. S told me dramatically of an incident at Tarsau when an English soldier aggravated an elephant. Elephant very, very, angry; soldier climb tree (pantomine); too late. Trunk sieze. Hospital! No good! Mackie More's convoy silent [no wireless news from that source].

Rain, rain, with a vengeance. What a night – muggy and terribly hot, then severe thunderstorm which turned the whole area into a lake. All our troops here under attap cover but huts swimming in water; nevertheless fairly snug. Officers of course still in open and got a thorough drenching.

My canvas stood it off for a little bit and then water began pouring in. Alan Woods and I stayed on soaking wet until 0200 hours when the water rose above my bed bamboo and our backs were in the water. All the officers had a most bloody night recalling the Somme.

14 March 1943

A surprising amount of water drained away but benjos in trouble – one over-filled and ran all over surrounding area. I suppose the 400 who went to the mountain camp were in the open last night, so I went to see Osuki to ask that no more troops be sent up until present troops move on in corresponding numbers. He said if lorry can get down must go, as it is order of Nippon HQ.

Eventually, in the afternoon, a lorry did come down, we ignored this as regards troops. Nothing being said (we begin to understand procrastination and face-saving).

N soldier tonight says Nippon bomb bomb Darwin, bomb bomb Brisbane, bomb bomb Sydney, bomb bomb Newcastle. Australian soldier: 'Bullshit!' Nippon: 'Yes, Bullshit bomb!'

15 March 1943

Maj. Wearne to mountain camp with Jock Clarke plus 100 men. Mountain camp report by Maj. Greiner:

1 Tents: O Bn completely under canvas today

2 Movement yesterday 14th: 105 Dutch Kinsayok

Today ready: 100 (which will make some tents available to P Bn)

3 Cookhouse. Fred Airey has taken over.

4 P Bn directed by N Engineer officer to go into unfinished hut area north of hospital.

5 Deaths. Another Dutchman yesterday, another expected to die today.

6 Requested to forward any tents possible as half the men (200 approx.) were out in the storm last night.

7 Canteen party being sent to collect stores.

8 Camp cleaning: Shinbone Alley, the old Dutch area, is being cleaned up. Some of it will be a parade ground.

I have mild dysentery, a little blood and mucus. Damn.

16 March 1943

Still feeling rather poor with a tongue like a birdcage. Early morning Ns said no movement today. I went off to mountain camp and walked into a Dutch funeral, the fourteenth in 28 days. The body was wrapped in a mosquito net and on a rough litter with a small D flag and a large wreath made of jungle flowers and leaves.

Railway course work is very hard. Men yesterday went out at around 0915 hours, had 50 minutes for lunch then worked until 1825 continuously. There is a four-mile walk each way and they arrived back after *tenko* – 2000 hours. One man was beaten up. Engineer soldiers lay down a figure for the men they want, and insist on getting it, so all men not in hospital usually have to work – light duty is no security.

There was an accident out on the course today. RAAF Sgt Pilot Geof Dewey was cutting a tree when the axe slipped and cut his foot, breaking metacarpals near heads and severing all the tendons on extensor aspect of 4 small toes. Bones not displaced. He was brought down here on a litter and lorry. Fortunately

Tadano was here and I indicated Dewey must go to Konyu for an anaesthetic. We got a lorry in half and hour and went down the rather terrific new road to the camp. Made a right-angled splint out of a kerosene tin and wire and borrowed two plaster bandages from the English. Maj. Moon was the anaesthetist $ChCL_3$ and ether, Ken Walker assisting. The tendons were sutured with parachute silk.*

* The wound healed perfectly, with good function.

7 Hintok Mountain March 1943

17 March 1943

Left at English camp hospital. Staff: Maj. Moon and 5 ORs: Sgt Harrison-Lucas, Cpl Walker, Thomas, Tarron, Simpson.

Hospital cases:	37	Dysentery	12
		Malaria	16
		Injuries etc.	9
Stretcher cases	3		
Convalescent	14	Dysentery	6
		Malaria	4
		Trauma	4

TOTAL: 51 plus 1 officer and 5 staff plus canteen staff, Capt. Allen, Sgt Reed and Don Blakeney = 60.

After breakfast the rest of the troops began portering all kit including the officers' kit to the top of the hill. The movement of hospital patients was to occur after lunch.

I called over to the English camp where I saw Maj. Marsden and informed him of arrangements and remaining staff. I also told him that I would be glad to help with a team and equipment in any real surgical emergency. Lt-Col. Moore expects a bill soon for the expenses of O, P, Q and R Bn patients sent to Kanburi, the arrangement being that Tarsau look after all sick expenses, but that the camps contribute 10c per man per day to Kanburi expenses. We will meet this sum, but from today Q and R Bns must be the responsibility of Kinsayok.

Movement began shortly after 1600 and we straggled in to the mountain camp after about an hour and three-quarters. Things up there are just so-so; Hands and Godlee have gone on today – Maj. Wearne and Hec Greiner negotiating with the N engineer No. 1 to ease down a bit, particularly on railway embankment work, where they expect one man to do 2 metres a day (terrific). It is temporarily agreed that men only work until 1700 hours. There is much jealously between arrangements in our camp and the engineer's camp, and Maj. Wearne had his face slapped for going to see the latter without permission. Very stormy affair. No. 2 of this camp, 'the Lizard', who does all the returns, is a proper little bastard. No. 1 is a reasonable sort of private.

Lt-Col. Ishi, the new commander of Tarsau, was here today with Osuki and made a scene about the state of the huts and camp generally. There is talk of putting 2000 troops from Singapore into this little hole in addition to us! Maj. Wearne raised much oposition to this on the grounds of an inadequate water supply, sanitation etc. Osuki said later, perhaps only 600 men.

Canteen supplies were maintained. It has been a fairly smooth move up to date according to Nip standards – nothing at all that some hundreds had a night out in drenching rain, and sick just do not enter into calculations.

Back to camp where Crep., Bret. Moore, Blue Phillips and Smedley in awful grips with 'the Lizard', who was cheerfully transferring men from battalion to battalion and doing ghastly sums interminably with his abacus. He bitches all common sense camp arrangements. This little sod fixes reveille in the morning now at 0730; roll call parade 0815; falling in for work 0830. To hell and all for the cooks and breakfast arrangements, since men have to eat and draw lunch as well. Water is drawn from our miserable little spring stream and passed through a Nip pressure filter pump of some sort and sent out by elephants to the workers. May not be safe for drinking, but we cannot arrange boiling.

18 March 1943

Arthur Moon arrived about 1200 with medical corporal Okada. All is well at Konyu. Dewey has no temp, pulse good. Orders here today are that Q and R personnel not in hospital are to go on to Kinsayok as soon as possible. I objected that most of them were recommended for evacuation to Tarsau/Kanburi, but Okada says that it is full up and there is no chance of evacuation for some time: Kinsayok will be at least as good as here.

I spoke to Okada re the necessity for a benjo party of 30 to dig new, deep-*benjos*, also anti-malarial squad of 10 as before. He supported this with our No. 1, Ikimoto. Okada said Maj. Moon must correlate the medical returns: all men from O and P battalions and remnant of Q and R battalions are now to be put on one form.

Took No. 1 today for approval of new benjo sites south-west of road, since those on north-west side up against the mountain are very poor and could not be made much deeper owing to rocks. These are uncovered and crawling with fly larvae and are to be fired. Ikimoto approved the new site if it is well covered. The Woods water conservation scheme was also shown to him and he said he would try to help; it will greatly improve the water supply. No. 1 spoke at length about soon all friends, Australia, Nippon, very good *tomadachi*. I laid a trap by saying, 'OK. You speak Tojo, I speak Churchill.'* He did not argue, so presumably the latter is not dead. Much talk of Nippon never surrender, a *hara kiri* gesture across abdomen and disparaging references to others including Engishmen – to which we checked by saying 'Good – *sama sama* Australian.'

19 March 1943

Resting up with mostly septic sores and cellulitis of left leg. Intended to march to Konyu to see Osuki about overworking of men, lack of consideration of sick

* The Japanese said that Churchill was dead.

and the boot situation, not to mention the rations. Position is No boots, 224; beyond repair, 184. Condition of men on outside work 17 March:

O Bn		R Bn	
Fit	170	Fit	110
Bootless	35	Bootless	70
Avitaminosis	45	Avitaminosis	20
TOTAL	250	TOTAL	200

If the Ns do not supply boots, 400 men is about the maximum we can reasonably supply.

Lt Thyne (Q Bn) and Lt Schroeder (R Bn) moved into the mess. Woods water scheme party of twenty men working well and the new benjos going down. This time they will make box seats which will be more fly-proof.

Dreadful news in the evening: Engineer officer Hiroda has been over tearing strips off the 'Lizard' and tomorrow 600 men are required for the railway. An work on benjos, anti-malaria and 'improve water' schemes must cease; worst of all, light duty and no duty men and all men without boots to go just the same. This is the next thing to murder. Obviously the Ns have a great reserve of manpower here and at Singapore and they are showing every intention of just breaking men on this job, with not the faintest consideration for either life or health. This can only be regarded as a cold-blooded, merciless crime against mankind, obviously premeditated. I am told that conditions are pretty frightful in Kinsayok and that the Dutch have had six deaths in six days. We will start going the same way soon at this rate. I will have a showdown about this tomorrow with somebody.

20 March 1943

After parade I asked battalion commanders to fall out all light duty or no duty men detailed for railway work. O Bn had avoided the issue by changing these men to camp duty, but P Bn had 32. Of these I reluctantly decided to let 12 go. Saw 'the Lizard' and angrily told him that 20 were unfit to go out. To my surprise he said 'OK, OK,' meekly and the Engineer Nip who collected the men accepted the position. Then I felt I had been a bit of a sucker not to stick out about all the other ND and LD men. Total number for railway work: 577.

I then had a conference with battalion commanders, Crep. and Billy, and fixed the following points of policy: after consideration of duty section (144) it was decided that it would carry about 42 light duty men, these being replaced so that a corresponding number can do railway work. We will try to stick on this number.

Footwear is also a matter for a fight; it is murderous working on rocks as hot as hell and covered with knife-like edges with no boots to protect the feet. (O Bn have many light duties and no-boot men in duty section; P have only 2 LD men, 14 no-boots).

Ration position: no vegetables, meat or fish for five days, just rice, and no man available to go to Konyu for canteen stores. (Canteen eggs are the only thing keeping the men going. N commander talks of giving eggs 2/man/day in lieu of bread etc., but this is obviously poppycock.

Tools: none are available for sanitary squad or anti-malaria or water supply scheme even if men were available. Ns say Q and R Bn semi-sick must do this work.

Strength in camp: 796. There are 566 fit men, of which 224 have no boots.

The road to the railway course is a branch from the Konyu road running towards the river, distance about four kilometres to the nearest point, which is the blacksmith's forge. There we found Lt Hiroda and gave him the figures, explaining that it would be useless for Nippon to send out sick and bootless men to work as they would only crack up and soon be a bad economic proposition like R Bn. (The humanitarian point of view is quite useless with Ns.) He is a pug-faced, fit-looking fellow with a charming, show-the-teeth expression which does not conceal the fact that he is a vicious, spoilt child at heart. He noted the figures without comment. A party of N engineers arrived on an inspection round and went off to view the work. Next to arrive were some Thai elephants (about seven working out here); their chief duty is to carry bamboo water containers out to the troops on the course.

They put on a bit of a turn, shorting, tramping and swishing their trunks, and Ns scattered in all directions. One of the elephant's tricks is to insert his trunk in his unpleasant triangular mouth and squirt water over himself and the surroundings.

We then inspected the blasting party working up on an outcropping of rock where a siding is being cut. This involved many of our 2/2 CCS boys with Dave Topping in charge of section. They drill with the crudest of hand drills like a short crowbar with slight annular rings on the side and a hammer. White rock dust flies in all directions so that the men are plastered with rocks and sweat like bakers or plasterers. The heat is infernal: hotter than in the camp where recently the temperature at midday was 130°F. and 108° in a tent.

The course runs for four kilometres in a horseshoe with the open side to the river. Two great sidings are to be cut in the rocky mountain side and a great deal of embanking to be done in between (up to eleven metres). The site is hot and airless, with the containing hills rock-jungle. The jungle view is rather ghostly with the prevalent grey/brown; almost all the tree and bamboo leaves have fallen at this time so that the vista is gaunt and cheerless, like a woodheap without end. Work in general is of three types: drilling and blasting; work on the embankment; and jungle clearing.

Work on the embankment is done with picks, shovels and baskets as mentioned above. If lucky, the troops get 10 minutes *yasumé* an hour – often, however, only one rest in the morning and one in the afternoon. Embankment work is hard in that the ground is very stony and the brick red soil has to be picked and shovelled out from between rocks. NCOs in charge work on the principle of endless 'Bullo', playing one battalion against another, and section against section. A particularly obnoxious trick is to set a task for a body of men for the day. Then when they finish, 'Changy, Changy' plans and do a lot more work. There is not a great deal of bashing. One NCO recently was made to stand at attention with a basket of earth held over his head, Atlas-like.

In general, the drillers have to do a maximum of 80 cm per day ready for the blasters (Nips).* Their blasting work is most inefficient as they lay charges stupidly with superficial types of bore holes and do not tamp the charges. As a result, only a little superficial rock is blasted into the air, much of the force of the charge going upwards. The tools are terribly shoddy, the drills in particular, which cause many injuries with splinters flying from the head of the drills.

Lt Hiroda by way of oiling the troubled waters, asked me to go to the pictures at Kinsayok that evening. I accepted for reasons of propaganda and recce, though feeling very much a severe cellulitis of my left leg with two ulcers on my shins.

'The lizard' then said no, but I overbore him with a wave-of-the-hand reference to No. 1 and he finally gave way. No. 1 rode in the front of the lorry with a W/O (beautiful N courtesy). The road does not rise very much and is locked in by the mountain and very thick jungle. Arrived at Kinsayok and saw many long huts (at least twelve) of the attap type about a hundred metres long. We pulled up directly against the screen, and I found myself in front of some hundreds of Ns seated on mats or earth. I also enjoyed this luxury, feeling all sorts of crawling pests on the skin (presumably lice bugs). The films were super productions: the first, a sort of news review, showing Nippon tearing Asia up into strips by the employment of every conceivable arm of the service, mostly all together, planes, ships, tanks, guns, artillery, tractor-drawn and horse-drawn guns and waves of N infantry charging endlessly through shot and shell – even a cavalry charge! Nippon planes roared overhead straffing and bombing everything to hell. Great show, sir! Presumably China for the most part.

Next, a fantasy and lastly a propaganda film about a N naval officer in the fleet air arm, a superman who takes part in the bombing of Pearl Harbor and the sinking of HMS *Prince of Wales* and *Repulse*. The unpreparedness of the US is stressed in the film. Of course, they showed all hell being knocked out of the place: ships keeling over with aerial torpedoes, bombs and fires stem to stern, then systematic bombing of harbour installations, oil tanks etc. The *Prince of Wales* and *Repulse* affair was not very well filmed and could well have been the real thing. I was the only European and placed right in front of the screen with thousands of Japanese behind me better placed. They reacted to the massive destruction of Pearl Harbor and the triumphant sinking of the ships by screaming '*Banzai!*' in great excitement. I jumped to my feet under the screen and roared '*Banzai!*' Perplexed soldiers said, 'You think good? Nippon bomb-bomb, sink American and British ships.' 'Yes,' I roared, 'Old ships no good – *taksan* [many] new ships now build – better!'

After the film home to bed, so a failure as regards contacting Jack or Smits and propaganda a failure too.

21 March 1943

To Konyu, where I met Arthur Moon and Dick Allen. Okada in a flattering mood. I asked him to get me some ether and plaster of paris. He asked for particulars of medical personnel and considers that they are going to start a new

* Later this became 1 metre and up to 2 metres.

hospital (like Tarsau) at Konyu. He also says that some 3000 men from Singapore are coming into the area in the next few days, some of whom are presumably going to our mountain camp. He then gave me lunch, both of us sitting cross-legged in the N hut with a small table between. Disadvantage: seen by the majors of English battalion, who looked at me with dropped jaws, so that in consequence I felt a woggy guilt and tried to laugh it off.

Interview with No. 1 was quite appalling. I told him of the horrid position yesterday – all men, including light sick, working; no boots; no veg. or meat for five days; no tools for work; no men for canteen or carrying; and just bad rice to eat. To all of which O smiled in his nasty little bad urchin way and said, 'OK, you speak to No. 1 engineer.' To which I replied, 'No good. He is an even harder wretch than you and it would be useless.'

Only new things he had to offer were:

1 150 men without boots to come to Konyu tomorrow.

2 A 'cow cart' (indicating horns on his beastly little head) might take certain stuff up in a day or two.

3 Men are coming down to work on the new road replacing the defective bit near Konyu camp (rail is to be through to Konyu by end of month).

4 Q and R details to go to Kinsayok soon, but meanwhile they are to stay with us. Dutch doctor is also to stay for the present.

5 No. 1 (general) from Bampong is to inspect the camp tomorrow.

6 There is a new interpreter – a bespectacled, nasty specimen with poor English.

Capt. Allan has the pay and will go to Kinsayok to pay Q & R and battalions and also come to our camp tomorrow. Dick is to concentrate on bread and butter lines for the canteen in future, as we have been exceeding our means a bit. Eggs, fat, onions, sugar, coffee or tea, fish, tobacco and soup are OK but he is to cut down severely on cakes, coffee, guala, arrowroot, rice flour, pepper and cigarettes.

I saw Col. More, Lt-Col. Hill, Lt-Col. James and Lt-Col. Warren with whom there was much coffee, cheroots and chatter. [Wireless news.] Gs making counter-offensive in Donetsk basin, Rs fighting very hard (particularly west and north of Kharkov), inflicting heavy losses. N position rather static. Burma: a little activity only, with a good deal of bombing. N convoy destroyed near New Guinea. Not very much afoot. How slowly this damn war moves. Privately I don't think this year will see the end and how my men will suffer by then. Left rather late after talking with Warren and a merchant seaman officer, Jock Muir. On the road I met the first party of 150 moving with Fred Smedley (all no boots) and also Tadano, who had been to the mountain camp. Just for variety he said all Q and R battalions stay with us!

22 March 1943

A frightful day. Ns fixed for all light duty men to go out to work and terrific beat up of all available labour, with none left for sanitation and anti-malaria work. I ruled no light duty or no duty men to go and we fell them out (46 in all). Then began a terrific row: I attacked Kanamoto furiously, saying that the men were sick and must not go. Engineer said march them over. I went too. No. 1 came out, his nasty face now set like a ham and lower lip stuck out (the spoilt child touch), and scarcely spoke to me but tore strips off Kanamoto, who seemed to be battling on our side. He was white in the face, sweating and saying 'I don't understand.' I was furious, too, and angrily told Hiroda that I objected strongly to his sending sick men to work, adding a few comments on the rations, camp sanitation, bad medical arrangements and the general bloodyness of N.

I invited him to make good his threat to shoot me (rifles were trained on me). 'You can shoot me, but then my 2 I/C is as tough a man as me, and after him you will have to shoot them all. Then you will have no workmen. In any case, I have taken steps to one day have you hanged, for you are a black-hearted bastard!

Hiroda: 'You can stay here as long as you like. You will get no food or water and the sick will do the work!'

He retaliated by getting out the Lizard, who siezed upon 46 men from Q and R battalions doing light duties and marched these off without water or food, turning the tables on us by saying that the others must carry rice and water out to them.

The Lizard and I had a real hate then, with S/Sgt Oliver as interpreter, I telling him exactly what I thought of the arrangements. He looked at the troops and said that they were fit to work and must work tomorrow. I told him that after making us administrative officers they did not accept our decisions on the men's health etc. and therefore they could go to hell and run the camp themselves. They were a lot of murderers and (indicating a cross on the ground) that was the fate for us. I finally swung the bomb at him that if sick men driven to work all would 'down shovels'. This threw him into a severe rage and he raved at the men as if working himself into a passion to hit me (but I bet he never could if I was looking at him). He went on talking until he ran down and finally said, 'Send the troops off to work in camp.' This was done.

Then a pocket edition of a N general arrived in a lorry and we all turned out again in a furious temper. He did nothing but walk through the hospital and go down to see the water (filthy) and the kitchen (did not look at rice). Asked that sweating little pup Osuki a few questions and then drove off with a salute from N and our parade.

Maj. Wearne and I plus a few of the light duties men carried water out to the railway course and returned for lunch at 4 pm. Some of the light duties had collapsed and returned (Dutch), the others all working away. On the embankment is perhaps the hardest work of all. N Engineer No. 1 was in a sulky mood and we both pointedly ignored each other. There are many injuries from flying drill fragments.

The Australian resilience is startling; the men are extremely cheerful and emphatic that the Ns will never get them down and that they will be square one day. Their morale under terribly trying conditions is excellent.

23 March 1943

N demands today quite moderate: there must be a catch. No sick men required to go out today. Capt. Hands arrived from Kinsayok and reports that his duty section has become so reduced that the work has become terrific and all officers are required to do normal heavy work. Even Tim Godlee compelled by Ns to do pick and shovel work. Benjo work and wood and water carrying now almost entirely thrown on the officers, who have become normal labourers. The hospital patients are repeatedly paraded and kicked out to work; there are no canteen arrangements, the food is bloody and Lt Tanaka is an awful bit of work, full of military arrogance. The quarters the troops marched into were one attap hut 100 metres long (all Q Bn). This was in a supremely filthy condition having been occupied by the Dutch who even dug holes in the floor for defecation. The last ounce is being got out of the men without any consideration for their health or the future – evidently there is a terrific 'blitz' on the railway work with a view to an early finish before rains. In one English camp recently, men worked 62 hours out of 72. Two more Dutch from R Bn died at Tarsau (total now 18).

Kinsayok
English 34 deaths. Total now about 400 (was 600) men
Dutch 31 deaths. Total now 1000 men
Rin Tin
84 deaths, presumably Dutch

Railway is now at 40 kilometres mark and is expected to reach Konyu by the end of this month.

The blow now falls. Duty section reduced from 144 to 80, all officers to work and no consideration at all shown to sanitation. A council of war was held and arrangements were made to keep cookhouse, anti-malaria, wood and water squads duties etc. operational.

24 March 1943

All men other than duty section out at work. The rest of us, including officers, doing camp work. Wearne, Clarke and I firing maggotty benjos all morning, others were gathering wood, working on water supply etc. In the afternoon I dug furiously in a big benjo, with the Lizard having exquisite revenge by watching me.

About 10 lorries went through in forenoon from up river, presumably with sick from Kinsayok-Tarsau. About 20 in each lorry. Movement is absolutely crazy at present, some of our fellows moving to Konyu one day and back the next. Simultaneously, men go to Kinsayok and then back to Tarsau. A party of men arrived from Konyu this evening, including some of those whom we sent down yesterday.

This evening a heavy storm worked up, rain falling heavily just after we got to bed. Thank the Lord for these tents. We are in a complete hollow of the mountain and the wind could be heard howling in tornado fashion in the hills about with an almost continuous thunder of heaven's artillery and lightning lighting the camp like day. The crashing of timber in the jungle could scracely be heard.

25 March 1943

The effect of the storm was very evident today in fallen trees about the camp. Some details of Q Bn sleeping in a 'humpy' moved yesterday and last night a large tree fell right across the area – a lucky escape. Ten more N lorries with Kinsayok sick bound for Tarsau went through today but had to return because a tornado had swept through between our camp and Konyu, hurling great trees and debris right across the road and hopelessly blocking it. A belt of destruction was cut through the jungle, clumps of bamboo and trees having been cleared like straw. The camp this morning is full of Thai bullock carts, each pulled by two strange water buffalo beasts with great curving horns shooting back at such an acute angle that it is hard to envisage them pointing forward at the 'charge'.

The carts are queer, crazy things built almost entirely of wood. The wheels are about six feet in height with wooden rims and spokes (though there is apparently a steel axle). These two great wheels are set extremely close together – thus the body of the cart would take about two kerosene cases end on! – and curving longitudinally on either side of the wheel are two great 'outriggers' looking also like buffalo horns. Numerous similar, smaller struts along the cart make the whole thing look rather like buffalo horns on wheels. The Thais in general have masses of jet black hair tumbling into their eyes.

Included in the lorries from up river were four tommies roped together who had escaped and been caught. They had run away with a lorry until the petrol gave out. Then the Thais who were guiding them gave them away after the payment of money. They have been told that they are going down for execution.

Nipponese presents are to be given to encourage work. Prizes of 1 tical approximately – 32 presentos for working parties and 8 for inside work including three officers, Crep, Bret. Moore, Jock Clarke who will of course hand it over.

O says all men O and P quickly come back to previous camp – Singapore men arriving will go to mountain camp to take our place. I hope this is correct. Evacuations from British POW camp hospital Konyu to Tarsau arranged by Arthur Moon are as follows: P Bn 12 (includes Geof Dewey); O Bn, 2 (includes Jones); Q Bn, 13; R Bn, 21. Total 25/3/43 1400 hours: 48. Lt Thyne has been worrying hell out of me by in addition to other troubles getting a severe infection of his small wound.

26 March 1943

Apparently Nips have been discussing No. 1 working in benjo: 'No. 1 not work benjo. No good.' Therefore today I was given some six men for benjo work but *no tools*! When we requested them, Ns funnily say 'Use hands!' Apart from these few, all other men work on the railway course.

27 March 1943

Tanaka brought our officers' pay for which I signed ($430). This includes the Konyu officers. Dick Allen came up today and tells me that Arthur and Maj. Marsden got about 190 sick up to the top of hill yesterday 'speedo speedo' only to find when they got there that the only transport to be provided was any vehicles which happened to pass empty, i.e. 'hitch-hiking' arrangements for the sick! Lt-Col. More and 'Hooky' Hill departed with the sick, both apparently having had enough of it (Lt-Col. Warren now in charge).

The sick just lay in the sun awaiting vehicles and only a very few Q and R Bns left. In the evening the rest were bedded down in a hut and given some food. Now leaving in dribs and drabs. Also I am told that Tarsau, whilst absolutely full, was given no warning of the descent of some hundreds more bodies. Lt-Col. Harvey can, in consequence, spare us no drugs and he reports that he cannot send any ether since they have only about enough for one case themselves! We still get at least five or six injuries daily from flying fragments of drills. Men have been hurrying like hell to put down their two drill holes of 60 cm and some finish shortly after lunch. In consequence of this foolishness, all drillers now have to do two holes of 65 cm each day and at this rate it will go up.

28 March 1943

All officers still working like navvies and the men are having a most trying time on the railway course. The Ns having made an effort at the 'evacuation' of the sick now assume that all men can work. They have left the hospital alone up to date, but they are drafted the night before and if people go sick overnight (dysentery etc.) they are forced out to work notwithstanding.

There are many very curious movements going on: Ns in lorries going through both ways, N engineers hurriedly withdrawn from English mountain camp one morning recently but work resumed today. Fresh Australians who are said to have arrived and to be at Kanburi have received letter cards from home. Also rumoured that there is considerable mail for POWs at Bampong??

Alan Woods and I working like blacks today on the water scheme, stark naked, as one becomes covered in mud hacking roots and shovelling in the creek bed. N tools are terrible: axes with slipping heads continually breaking and shovels with shoddy handles folding like tin. Kanamoto talking this evening and said two Tommies going back to Rin Tin for execution. Also two who escaped from Kanburi walked into Tarsau by mistake.

29 March 1943

135 from Konyu marched in today, mostly without boots. Arthur Moon reports that he managed to keep back sick and LDs. Dick Allan has malaria and infected sore of skin. Lt Smedley remains at Konyu and is doing good work getting canteen stores to the top of hill. Padre Bourke came up in the rain to see Grant: he has being having a rough time, being forced by Lt-Col. More to work as a labourer. No facilities for his job.

Although there is as yet no great falling off in the Regimental fund (apart from the $500 given to Capt. Hands) there are very serious danger signals through our inability to obtain pay for light duties men who must go to hospital or do full work; and the increase in sickness which is very marked. It will be extremely hard on the private, who will be left only 17 cents a day (1 egg now costs 8 cents). It is regarded as absolutely essential to the group that sick be well cared for. If we do not strike now it will be perhaps necessary later when there are many sick to take even more than the one-third contemplated. (The policy of making profits out of canteen sales was discussed and condemned as furtive and irritating.)

I had a most annoying experience today while working with Allan Woods. I climbed a tree to free another one we had felled from a vine and gave out with weakness in the legs and arms before cutting through the vine. I dropped the axe and was only just able to get down without falling. Definitely we are not the men we were. As a result my legs are badly skinned. New No. 1 at guard house: Cpl Sakata has taken over from Ikimoto.

30 March 1943

Maj. Corlette very sick with dysentery – blood and mucus++ and continuous, with severe pain. Looks rather wretched and I must say I am worried. Fortunately he still has a little sulphaguanidine and is taking it. Otherwise just fluids. I called on the new No. 1 and found him tearing strips off all N soldiers, fitting them out as orderly dogs with armbands and fixing up the usual record boards, name bands and other paraphenalia of N guard rooms. The little devils have been very slack lately. He also demands much more *keré* from us (expected). Does not seem very useful about the tent shortage or lack of boots. He is introducing PT and Shinto.

I am appalled at how wretchedly sick some of the troops look, yet it is difficult to hospitalise them with both Ns playing a game of grab for all men possible and now a great shortage of tents to cover them. (I feel wretched myself with legs now covered with scabbed, septic sores and a large, raw, septic mess on one thigh from my damn fool tree climbing. Horrible sleepless night last night and got eaten badly with bugs of all sizes.)

It is a frightful business at present to get men out to work each day to meet the N numbers. Poor wretches without boots and horribly blistered feet, which of course develop septic sores, are one problem; now there is a wholesale epidemic of gastroenteritis, probably infective. This begins suddenly with severe colicky abdominal pain and frequently paroxysms of vomiting and retching, then diarrohea with anything up to twenty or thirty motions a day, mostly watery but some turning later to dysentery (blood). A few develop joint pains and I have seen several troops of late with swelling of large joints, knees etc. Some have what they call 'rheumatism' affecting the feet, legs etc. A number of these men quickly show mouths and scrotum lesions if they did not have them at onset. So we may be dealing with the four Ds of pellagra.

The wretched conditions of living also apply: rain night and day at present so it is always a bit wet; wretched meals are just gulped down in the morning and not much time for other meals. We asked for more tents and instead they are being taken away so that 20 per tent is a common figure. Many men get dreadfully wet at night. Things can't go on long like this.

Some Australian troops went through here in lorries today – 8th Division Changi men among them. They seemed fit and cherful. More Australian troops rumored coming here but we do not know when. This evening some rat told Maj. De Cresp to go and indulge in unnatural fornication. I went very cold at the parade. I understand that sort of bitterness; we are the only people that a disgruntled and desperate soldier can curse from the back rank. Nevertheless, they are putting up a really heroic battle to keep going.

I explained the necessity of raising the levy to one-third of pay to troops, everyone contributing 2 cents per day to Regimental (Hospital) Fund.

Lt Smedley's idea of distribution of Australian troops coming in is as follows: 100 to our present camp, 200 to English camp at the top of the hill and 250 to a new camp on the river. This may be nonsense. He reports new Australian Bn will be called No. 2 Bn.

Arthur Moon reports less than twenty in hospital at Konyu (O & P) and he still has approximately 20 light duty men getting pay. Dick Allen is down with malaria and septic sore.

31 March 1943

Nip Sgt Major called today for particulars of our sick, was very polite, asking many questions about myself. He was 'very very sorry' all men must at present work terribly hard without rest; later we would have a rest. We must be very careful to look after men so they don't get sick! Useless to talk to these people.

Maj. Corlette had a wretched night or two but is better today. God knows where he would be without sulphaguanidine. That or M & B 693 is life saving for dysentery. The treatment of large numbers of men suffering from severe diarrhoea at present is difficult. At present we give charcoal, 2 tsp., and light diet or some Nip Creosote pills, and morphia to those with much pain, but we are running light on the last. Large number of cases of men injured with rock fragments from the N drills. With absence of both sufficient anaesthetic and light at night, apart from fires, very few of these can be got out and of course some go septic. No ATS to give them either.

I worked all this morning and on into the afternoon, finishing with over 90 hospital cases. The mornings are dreadful, seeing that many men are in too late at night or get sick overnight and are consequently included in the day's 'fit' for work category. They fall out on parade (some in a dead faint and out to it after struggling to parade), then a dreadful re-shuffle occurs to fit them into the over-strained camp duties so they can rest a bit. The day's figures have to be met, otherwise duty section men are marched out.

Evening sickness parade is the principal one at 1800 hours. In the wet it is difficult for men to do the one metre a head on the embankment and they are being kept on until they finish, straggling in after evening *tenko* (1900); thus they have their meal in darkness and all this mucks up the sick parade and hospital figures for the following day. The shortage of hospital accommodation and the financial pinch makes it necessary to drive out many very unfit men to work.

Ron Lum gave some particulars about his stay at prison in Konyu. Five weeks solitary, just in his clothes with no bed or bedding and a stone floor. He was tied up in chains at night, his hands behind his back. One meal at night, chiefly rice. Inquisition each night, thorough beating up for first week or two each day. After that just slapping and kicking in the shins with questioning. Specific torture methods: room with peculiar waddies and sticks for beating, knotted ropes and on one occasion he was tied with hands up, feet just on floor for half a day. Other trick is to pin one down on floor, head back over a block, and water is poured from a kettle down the nose (idea is to first make the victim drink about 6–7 glasses of water and the feeling of drowning is rather

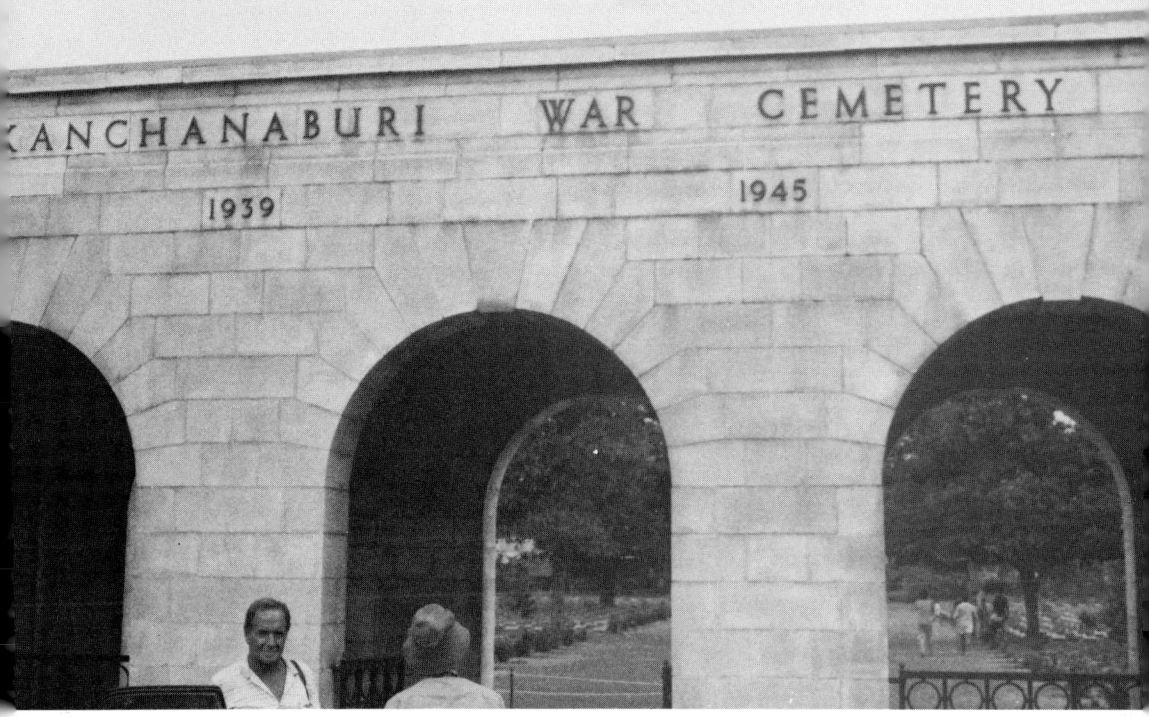

.chanaburi War Cemetery

.e of the headstones of the POW dead, in a peaceful corner of Kanchanaburi War Cemetery

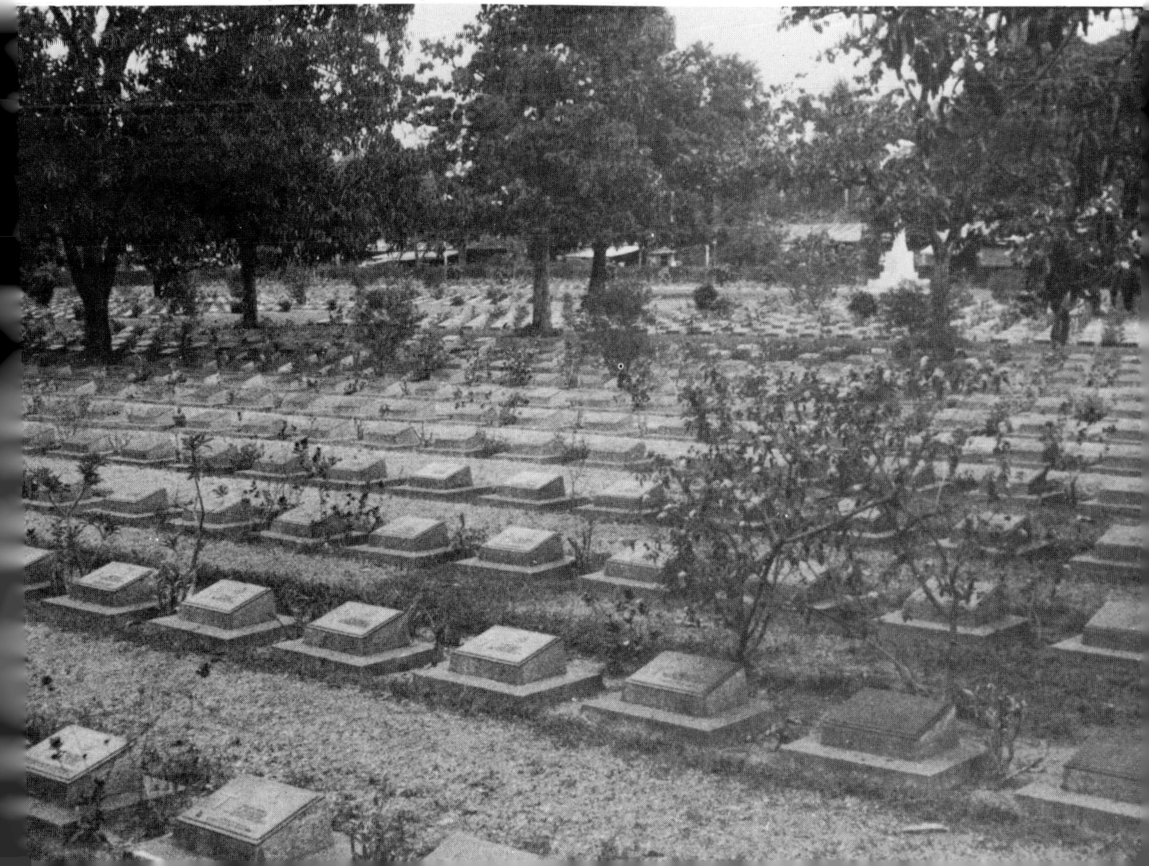

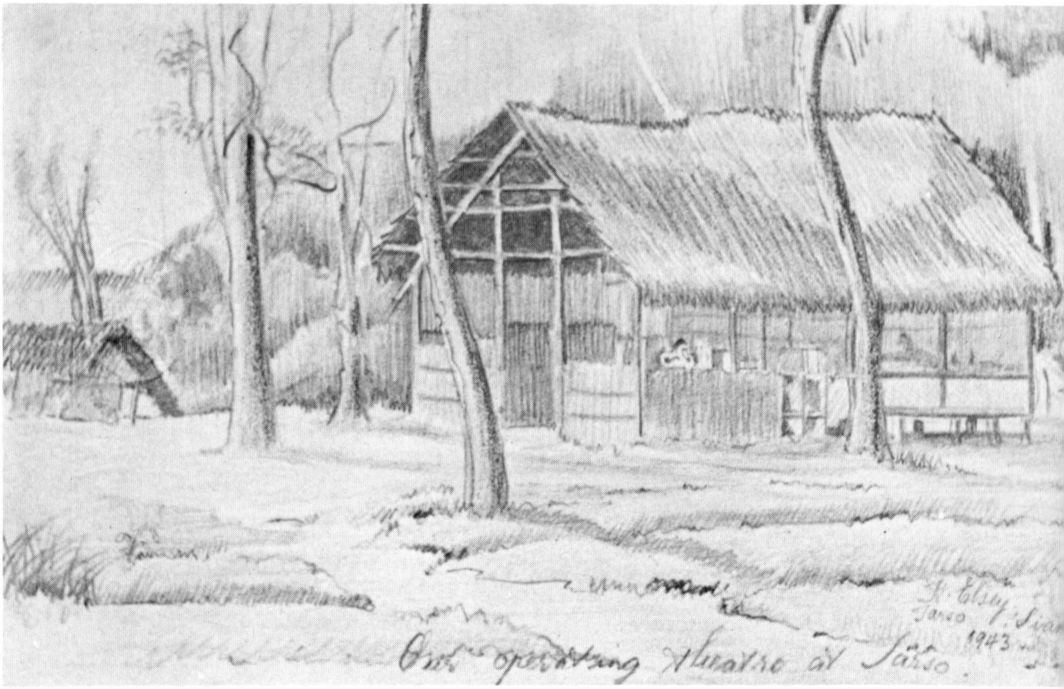

59 Operating theatre, Tarsau, 1943 (*T. Elsey*)

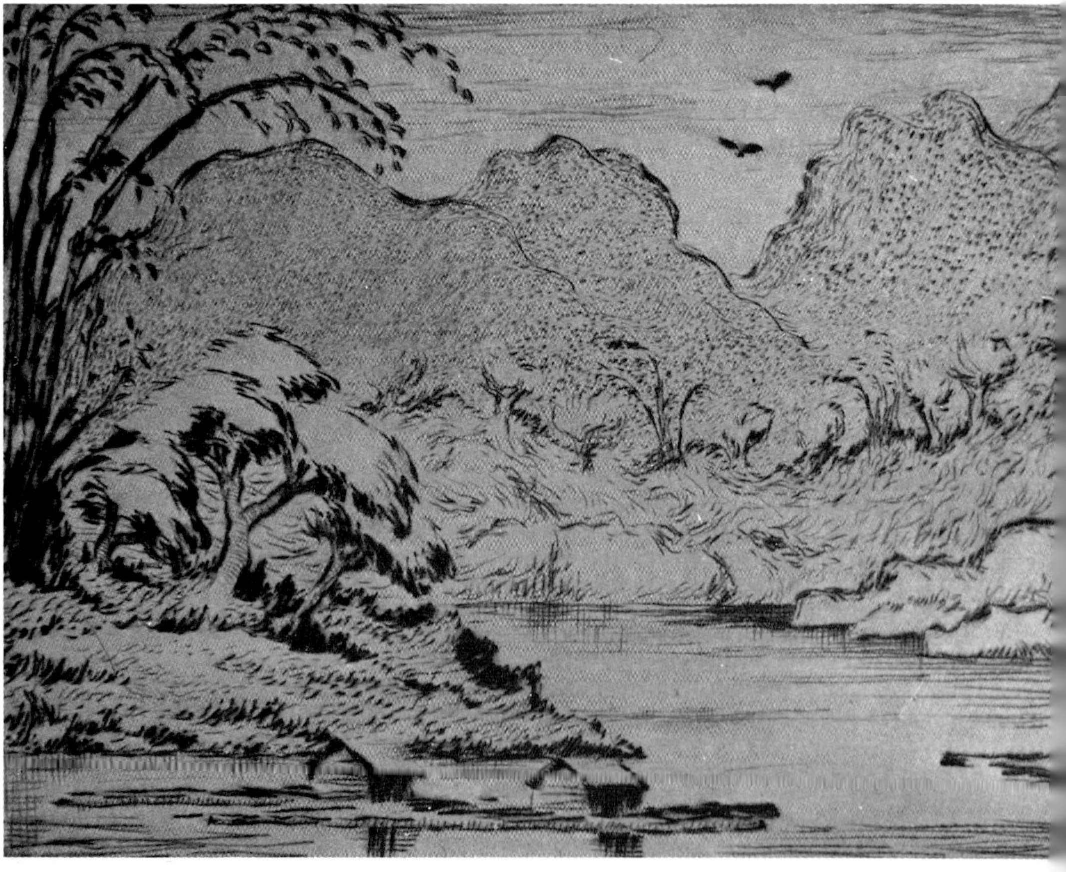

60 Kwai Noi River and Elephant Mountain, Tarsau (*Ray Parkin*)

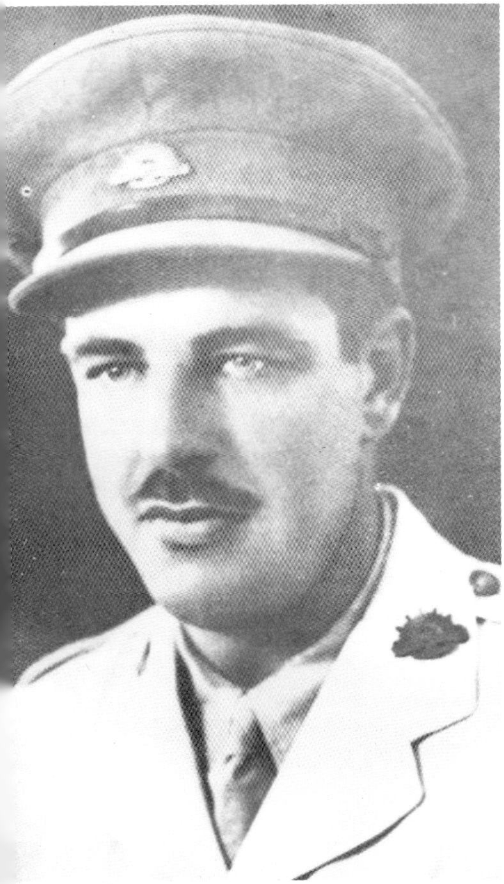

. E.L. Corlette OBE, RAAMC, dedicated and beloved
sician, affectionately called 'The Gangster'

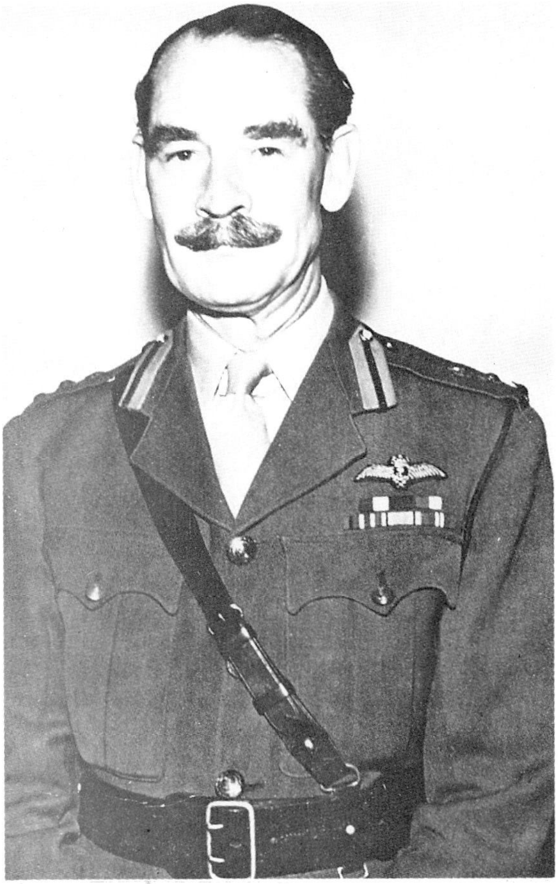

62 Col. Alan Ferguson Warren CBE, DSC, Royal Marines. An admired gallant officer and close friend

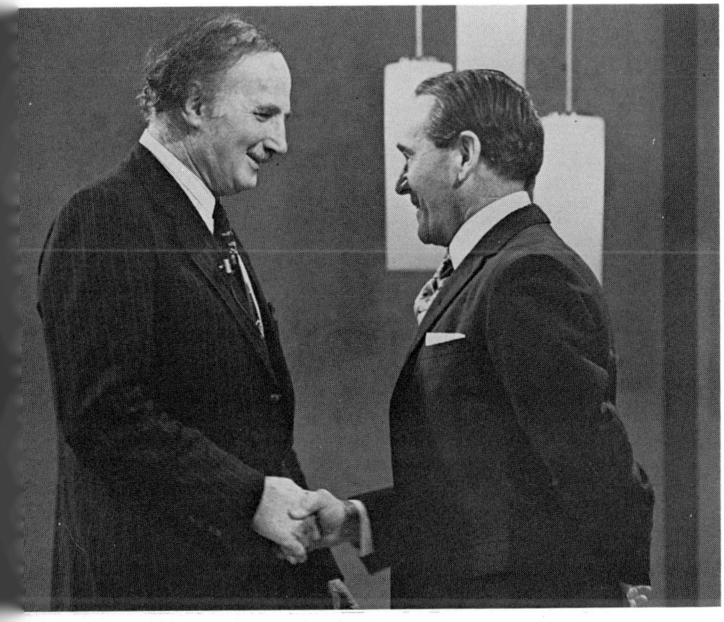

h Brig. W.W. Wearne OBE, *This is your Life*, 1979

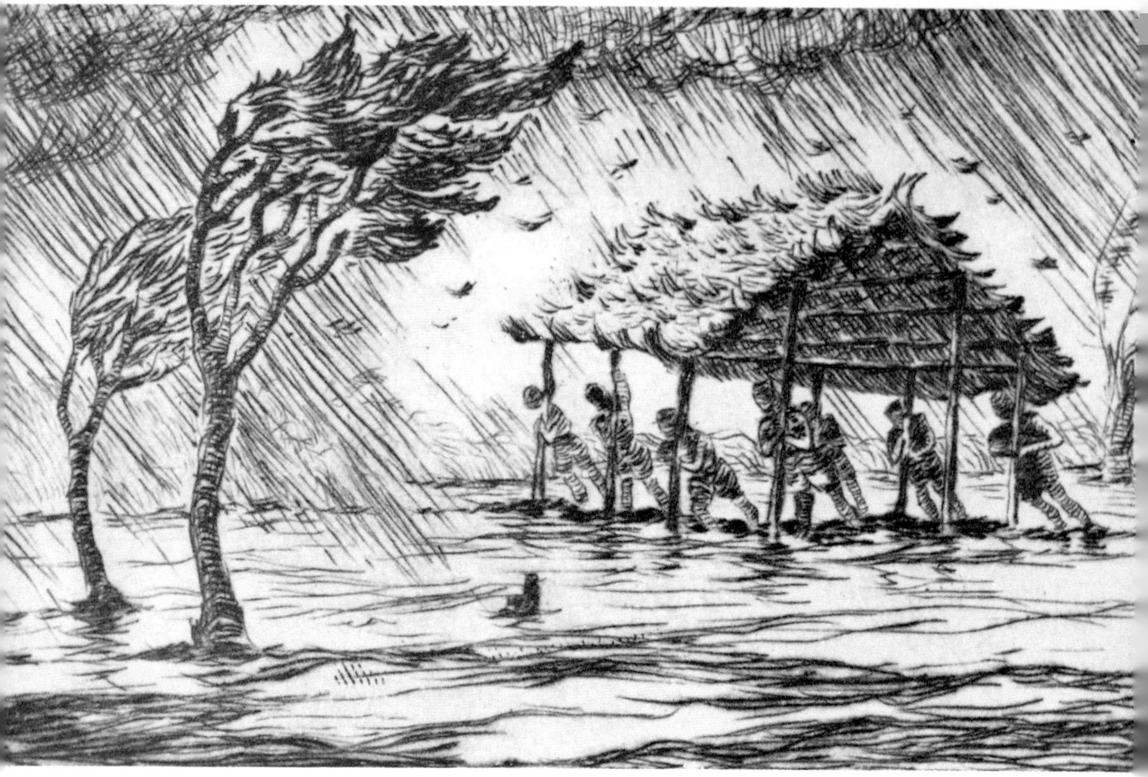

64 Saving the latrine shelter, 'The Caryatides'! – Tamuan (*Ray Parkin*)

terrible). One officer of 2/2 Pioneers was tortured in this way and by having papers burnt under the nose to burn sensitive tissues. In the end Ron gave in on his story of being a Chinese cook on a rubber plantation and said he was an Australian. God knows how he held out for so long.

1 April 1943

Maj. Corlette is getting better; I am still plagued with multiple septic sores and continually bitten by flies, sandflies, bees and every wretched thing that flies. Sick are rapidly increasing, the major problems being gastroenteritis and diarrhoea syndrome and septic sores and drill fragment wounds. This is aggravated by the no boot problem.

English camp probably on move up the hill and hospital said to go with it as a clearing station for Tarsau. Quinine is again growing short, therefore we decided to wipe out the ineffective prophylactic 3 g a day for all troops at present.

The latest news is that N policy is now to evacuate all those who are going to be sick for more than ten days. Name, rank, illness, estimated duration of illness. I am sending in a list of 29–old, debilitated and finished. (There is not a man in this camp who looks less than his age and most of us look ten years older; I am horrified at how old many men of 40–45 look). Claims against Ns for men injured at work in March equals 46 names.

2 April 1943

Maj. Wearne to Konyu to see Osuki but O away today. Billy reports that when the English camp shifts, Smokey Joe may take over the arrangments to deliver our canteen stores. Heaven preserve us then! English camp is sending 280 men away to Kanburi – Arthur has picked out 70 down at Konyu camp including Pte Ambrose, Pte Harrison W., Pte Crawley J.D., Pte Powell K.A. Pte Camerson is marked for evacuation.

A wretched row this evening: a sailor sold his gramaphone and 47 records to a Thai in the canteen for $35, than in the evening Ns said 'Please bring gramaphone' (they borrow it frequently). The storm began. Our man and the canteen Thai were thoroughly beaten up and Ns confiscated gramaphone *pro tem*. Crep and I were called to N office No. 1 and much trouble. i) Troops must not speak to Thai people ii) Must be no changy, changy – at this point produced the ace up the sleeve: a pair of N boots which they collected from Thais and claimed one of our soldiers had sold or exchanged. Eventually we got the chap away with threat of 'choppy choppy' tomorrow on *yasumé* day – of course the whole wretched business arises from their damn cupidity. Tension subsided with tea.

3 April 1943

Yasumé day but work from 0730–0900 for all and 120 men required to go to Konyu for supplies which makes a gruelling day for them. Ewan Corlette still off duty so another big day with an extra big sick parade in morning, avitaminosis parade at 1430 and sick parade in evening. An enthusiastic evening singsong; I don't quite know how they do it.

4 April 1943

Maj. Corlette returns to duty; Maj. Wearne from Konyu with Maj. Moon, Lt Smedley and party: P Bn, 21 includes the two officers, O Bn 8; total 29 (leaves Dick Allen and two ORs at Konyu).

Weather is fine again and the jungle is assuming a new coat of multitudinous shades of tender green. The atmosphere appears to have been washed ineffably clean and pure by the rains so that the sky is a serene, fathomless blue and everything assumes a marvellously clear outline. The light of great cumulus clouds appearing over the clear rim of our mountain world is most startling – I cannot recall ever seeing anything so radiantly white. It is as though everything had been washed utterly clean. The morning and evening sometimes positively hurt with their beauty, especially the lovely quarter hour before dawn when the whole sky is aglow with brilliant crimson bands showing through the clearly etched foliage in a brilliant atmosphere and the softest of pale blue.

Vividness and colours everywhere. Butterflies of every size and shade– predominantly white and yellow – fly in their scores in long chains or come to rest in little pools of mixed colours, the faint sway of their wings recalling a mass of yachts swayed by a slight breeze on a still lake. Staghorn ferns are extravagantly luxurious everywhere. Monkeys in a great troop swing carelessly across the face of our Western cliff on the great trees whose foliage is agitated as though by a storm.

There are some beautiful flowering trees, such as the 'Japanese ranunculas', a lilac-flowering acacia with a beautiful scent, light blue convolvulus and a tree with no foliage at present, only deep dark red blooms. Yesterday I saw a bird ruthlessly tossing these brilliant flowers about so that they fell in vivid little fragments. I have noticed a flowering tuber, white and yellowish white like freesia, peeping through the hard earth in the jungle.

Insects of every queer variety abound. Today, I saw a most curious one like a cross between a butterfly and a locust with a great horn in front (length 3 inches or so in all), and *wings* flecked brilliantly with red, green and blue to harmonise with mosses on the tree. Inner brilliant wings of black and yellow. Its progress from tree to tree is half jump, half flight.

5 April 1943

The Lizard was enraged at the increase in hospital figures last night and says that he will inspect today with a view to reducing numbers. This is due to the Konyu party (nearly all old and infirm) and the men selected for evacuation to Tarsau (39), who were put into hospital so that they will not miss evacuation. Consequently I ordered all men to stay in bed and told him it was not possible to 'parade' sick. At 1000 hours he inspected first the duty section then the hospital 133 patients – all in bed lying very quiet and still except for a few using the benjo. He stupidly argued about the figures until eventually worn down by the inexorable, relentless weight of arithmetic.

The food facts: ration is practically 500 g rice per day and very poor quality at that. This was augmented by canteen purchases including eggs, onions, fat, *katchang idjoe*, dried meat etc. Total expenditure: $236.

Capt. Hands called in. His men coming soon to the 150 kilometre mark (next door to us). He has 16 sick in hospital. Tanaka recently gave his Australian party 5000 eggs and they now have some canteen facilities. Hands got beaten up yesterday and has a very bruised face. Some Changi Australians are in his camp (500). Recently some 2100 Australians and about same number of English (2800) have come up the river. They are in good health and are a bit rattled with local conditions. Private soldier's pay in Australian now equals American, 14s 6d per day.

6 April 1943

Dick Allen staying down at Konyu with two ORs at present. Maj. Moon and Lt Smedley marched in with all rest of Konyu personnel less Capt. Allen, Sgt Reid and Don Blakeney. Maj. Moon will take over P Bn sick parades tomorrow.

7 April 1943

The Lizard continues to be a terrible thorn in the side. He insists that not so many men are to be allowed to become ill. There is, of course, ample reason for this unfortunate tendency: starvation rations, miserable, wet quarters, overwork, absence of drugs, poor sanitation – but, in addition, Maj. De Cresp. complained about the impure water, pumped by Nip filter pump from the creek and taken out in bamboo 'chatties' by elephant. The Lizard hotly defended the N pump and brought in a most amazing charge that our casks add unfiltered creek water to the tea! This is 'face saving' tripe.

I spent the morning benjo digging and in the afternoon went round the railway course with Reg Piper. With the rains there is a transformation in the horseshoe area around which the men work. The dry stricken trees and bamboo are putting forth a marvellous crop of new green leaves. It is however hot as Hades and on the rocks the men's feet nearly fry. It is also terribly close and humid.

All embankment works are now concentrated on a very large embankment at the southern end (approx. 30 feet). It is terribly hard work getting earth from between the rocks and soil must be carried 200 yards in places on rice sacks slung between bamboo poles. Continual 'speedo speedo'. And men have often been kept very late recently as they are again marked down to a definite task per day, Hiroda having conveniently forgotten his promise about 5 pm knock off. I saw him today and he edged off warily, avoiding me, giving a cautious gleam of teeth.

Drillers are still doing 120 cm and finish too early at 1300–1400 hours: they will soon get more work at this rate.

Rock clearing appears rather dangerous, with the possibility of taking a wrong step and falling down the precipitous slope.

One Nip enquired about Maj. Greiner whom he said was a good '1-hour man, work very good 1 hour'. The troops are fairly cheerful in spite of the dreadful gruelling time they are having.

8 April 1943

To Nip HQ. Osuki in bed with malaria (cold pack on brow and behaving childishly, alternating a weak at-death's-door aspect with getting out of bed and throwing himself down conversationally). My visit to Tarsau-Kanburi with next lot of evacuations was reluctantly approved.

A special Nippon present from supreme Nip HQ handed over to me – said to be for the troops' good work but that if they did not work well perhaps no more presents. Only stipulation was that presents were for men working on the railway course and people such as cooks who did camp work.

Milk (condensed)	tins	120	(10 bad)
Sugar	kilos	90	
Flour	bags	4	
Coffee Beans	kilos	68	
Cigarettes		5,500	'Horrors' in 3-castles packets
Towgay	kilos	90	

Also a box of 'flimsy toilet paper'. In view of my desire to get to Tarsau and because of the 'presents' I did not leave a letter I wrote to the I.J.A. criticising miserable deficiencies and economies.

Tadano, who has also had malaria and does not look well, asked if we had received rice polishings and peanuts. I say did not know about peanuts. He was interested: 'If not receive tell me – soldier take get (motions of slap, slap).' Frankest admission of any Nip yet! (Actually the peanuts were received.)

Discussed affairs with Lt-Col. Warren, who is having a bad time with men also continually driven to work when sick and sick figures mounting most astronomically though all unfit men sent to Tarsau before the shift. He is particularly worried about his officers being treated as privates and kept out working until extremely late hours at times, some of them having been struck and knocked about including one major (one man lost two teeth recently from a blow). He is having some trouble with discipline (one incident bordering on mutiny with men refusing to shift at night).

Maj. Marsh ex Changi is in charge of the newly arrived 18 Div. party (new battalion) and he gave me much Changi news.

In Darwin recently N lost 22/27 attacking planes. Supplies by air to China now greater than Burma Road. Churchill in his 25 March speech warned the nation of heavy fighting and sacrifices to come. Tojo: speech re naval losses – cannot and will not lose – fight on rafts if necessary!

Seven men evacuated to Tarsau today.

9 April 1943

Capt. Allen reported yesterday that his great problem was that soon he would be forced to leave the river camp, thus losing contact with that vital lifeline and the barges. Eggs are about the only thing which have kept the troops going and they are now very short. The position is grimly serious as is also the difficulty in transporting stores with no Konyu parties allowed. Arthur Moon was sent to Konyu early this morning to present medical stores requirements and arrange sick evacuation to Tarsau etc. He returned very shivery and in the throes of dysentery, a real pukka attack. He has a bottle of sulphaguanidine thank heavens. Jock Clarke has also been unwell of late. I remain a mess of septic sores (legs), oedema of feet and absent knee jerks.

Row today, with Sakata confiscating all 'present' stores and he is very annoyed that some issues have already been made (7 cigarettes each man). The beautiful idea is to get a list of men who have worked well each day and call them out for 'presento' at *Tenko* in evening. (You recall the weary flagging donkey and the bunch of carrots held before the nose.) This is enraging, as even these few stores might have alleviated some of our distress for a few days and improved the range of food.

10 April 1943

Much movement on the road – N soldiers going up, some with full equipment, many Dutch and other soldiers (sick) going back. This has been going on for several days now.

Only medicines in hospital are quinine tablets and charcoal which the sick grind up each day. Okada today said that I might have five more medical orderlies. Only medicine available he brought – 10,000 quinine tablets – and as usual, he said more stores would come in a few days! Also he decreed that light duty men must do work in camp e.g. dysentery 30 motions no good, 20 motions perhaps work, 10 motions *work*. This would not be too bad were it not for the fact there is practically no room for such workers in our depleted duty section and when men go out of hospital they have to go to railway work.

Following Okada's visit, Hiramura made a lightning raid on the hospital and when he found beds empty, he stated that that number per tent would do light duty. Maj. Corlette said 'benjo' but unfortunately very few troops actually at that site. After much compromise, 15 men were discharged, which equals 22 today. This is infuriating, since under the circumstances nearly all these will be on railway work tomorrow. Bret. Moore's twenty-third birthday tomorrow – special dinner tonight.

11 April 1943

No *yasumé* and as expected, a dreadful struggle this morning to select out of the sick and ailing those best fitted to go out and meet the engineer's numbers. A filthy wet day. Arthur Moon still very unwell but improving rapidly. After much negotiating, Lizard discharged only 15 men to light duty today following arguments with Maj. Corlette.

I visited the English camp where I saw Dick Allan; definite orders to go tomorrow, also the English are leaving the river site. At present he has only stores for 20 men and few eggs but he is hoping for a barge with some good stuff today which he is anxious to secure before leaving. I then saw Ns, O still in bed with cold packs on his head and behaving like a pettish,peevish kid.

After a time in conversation, Okado beckoned me with a weak imperious wave of one finger! and asked 'What?' I raised canteen store question: if Capt. Allen goes, there will be nobody on the river, no eggs etc. purchased. Men will then go sick and not work. He insisted that Capt. Allen go notwithstanding. Said N soldiers would go to that camp; they will stop the barge and buy the stores. (Thai traders need very special handling and gratuities, and if they have to deal with N ruthlessness, taking their goods and giving them damn-all, naturally they will go to more favourable customers. In any case the N control means we get robbed as well. This is disastrous for us. I hoped for nothing from the interview except to get them thinking over the importance of the canteen. I tried further argument about the fact that we were not allowed parties to go down and Capt. Allen had much stores: 'What was to happen?' O pulled blanket over head and groaned and interpreter said, 'Mr O now has bad head, very bad, please go way and come back!'

I was also informed that of ten bullocks driven up from Tarsau by our officers 8 had 'escaped', thus no meat. Very, very sorry!

At this stage I was asked to see Dalziel, a young man with scalp lesions, said to have a fractured skull from a falling tree. I found a fractured neck (C6) and quadriplegia. Marsden did not show any particular concern for the fact that the chap was still lying on hard bamboo slats just covered by a blanket and that the diagnosis was alarming. In fact he felt he couldn't cope. I made the halter extension and when by six hours, the lilo or mattress had not arrived, stretcher (very ill-made) had just arrived, Col. Warren gave me authority to confiscate one from an elderly officer who had otherwise no bedding, poor chap. He looked very thin and ill and it appeared a mortal blow! Dalziel was placed on the stretcher with the mattress and I had to leave, requesting Marsden to apply the weights.

On the way home I met several Thai cart parties. These apparently had nothing to sell but showed a great desire to buy me right out of clothes from head to heel, including my watch. Good watches bring enormous prices in Bangkok. The road today was almost impassable and difficult even for walking. Work on the railway was so difficult that men just could not go on climbing the embankment with earth. Finally, No 1 established an unusual precedent by stopping work at 1430 hours.

12 April 1943

Several officers not very well: Jock Clarke has been greatly troubled by repeated attacks of diarrhoea, and Arthur Moon is recovering from dysentery. (Houston is never very well and suffers from sleeplessness owing to the post-dysenteric arthritis of his shoulders and is pale and miserably under-weight.) Billy Wearne is the only one who looks anything like himself of former days. Hec Greiner looks large and burly but cracks up and goes to bed after any special exertion. The Lizard compelled Maj. Corlette, against all medical judgement, to discharge 15 men for inside work today, thus more and more sick men are forced out to work and a stand will have to be made, but with what? You can only argue with such people over a gun.

13 April 1943

Two clerks, Williams and Tanner, to Konyu HQ today to work on prisoners' cards. Can this work possibly mean mail?

	Total Strength	In Hospital	At Tarsau	Total Unfit
O Bn	446	71	26	97
P Bn	427	58	66	124
	873	129	92	221

These are official figures. Actually, many sick men are working.

Attempts to get a Konyu party today produced only six – 3 officers and 3 ORs. Maj. Wearne and I also went with a view to combining business with canteen store carrying.

Billy and I walked briskly to Konyu English working camp. A big conference was going on: Osuki, interpreter, Okada, Lt-Col. Warren, Bn Commanders E.J.W. MacNeilly etc. Subject: the number of sick men forced to work and the rising sick figure.

Numbers for 'all man' to wear given me; boots and shirts will come in a few days, meantime 'changy changy' sick men. *Letters* in a few days, from Australia! Everybody seemingly in childish good humour (laughter all the time). In the middle of this discussion O was playing round with a bottle of Scott's emulsion for 'Debility', pouring this cautiously down his throat then yelling for boiled sweets and tea. (He gave me a dose and a sweet.) Arrived home to gathering storm in more than one respect. Lizard demands 25 men from hospital for 'light work'; Maj. Corlette has only 7 ready for discharge. I directed him to discharge only this number and the fight is now on. I was summoned to the evening *kebetei* discussion and protested that already both battalions were sending light sick out to the railway course. The engineers frequently sent sick men home and said they were no good to them. The Lizard wiped me off and said tomorrow you will parade the whole hospital on the parade ground less those who cannot walk (fevers included, since only for five minutes). He would then select the men he wanted for light work. Meantime, he fixed the figures with engineers as follows: 0247; P 285 = 532 for railway work! An impossible figure with the men in their present condition.

The conversation went on for two and a half hours, with the Liz. being exquisitely polite. I offered to parade all the light sick for him tomorrow to show him. He agreed to entirely scrap the hospital patients' parade – regretted he must argue with such honourable gentlemen, but he really was terribly worried by the requirements engineers put upon him etc. Meantime he produced many cigarettes and some coffee and Nippon food. He refused, however, to face up to the situation and persisted in returning like a compass needle to the idea of subtracting 25 more men from hospital figures, not from working tally! Finally we all went to bed in a state of unsettled but polite evasiveness.

14 April 1943

Rose early expecting trouble. Paraded men for work less those light sick (27 by now) who were fallen in separately. I then said they were not fit. N orderly soldier Takata just roared and said 'Speedo Speedo'. I advised the men to take no notice, sit down and look sick. Eventually he ran off to bring the Lizard (obviously upset). I then said these are the men about whom I spoke last night – not fit to go to work Lizard had a face-saving scene and a long conference with engineer who earlier had apparently made it clear 'sick men no good'. Eventually all were given light duty in camp and those discharged from hospital yesterday were taken to N guard house to chop wood. They were then sat down and given some food and cigarettes. Incomprehensible people. Lizard said he was going to Konyu to see No. 1. I went completely through the hospital in the morning and with Ewan selected 15 men for discharge to light duty tomorrow (this a concession which the harsh circumstances make propitious). Liz. was very pleased.

The new numbers were issued to all troops. Mine is No. 1 O.

15 April 1943

No trouble over working figures this morning. Calico numbers go O Bn:1 (me) – 420. P:1–361, all ranks inclusive but excluding men at Tarsau.

Sanitation is still very defective, The hospital latrines are excellent – fly-proof box seats with automatically closing lids. One fly-proof latrine, deep trench type with 8 timber lids fitting very closely, is now complete. Another is being dug. There are not yet enough seats to close the big 'open' type deep trench horror which is breeding flies. This is urgent, as the camp swarms with flies. Other serious matters are the lethargy of troops, who frequently offend by defecating in the bushes about the camp. Lines are not kept clean and food scraps are left about. The lack of personal cleanliness of hands and mess tins is perhaps comprehensible considering their exhausted state. A foul open trench latrine is only 100 yards away from the kitchen and is to be closed at once. Rice placed in baskets for serving becomes covered with flies, so we are making big 'jackets' to protect the rice. Occasionally convalescent dysentery patients creep in as kitchen helpers. More than half the officers have had dysentery or enteritis. Accordingly a conference of Battalion commanders, 2 I/Cs, adjutant and QM was held. Officers are to be told frankly that it is absolutely necessary that *all* do manual work, since otherwise not enough fit men. Maj. Wearne to supervise allotment of duties etc. Some doing too much, others too little. Sgt C working on my X [wireless] with an astonishing modicum of apparatus including only [one valve]. Tonight was in contact with BBC Astonishingly good results – will summarise later.

16 April 1943

Liz. now allowing about 30 light duties in camp daily including the discharges of previous day (15 again today). A daily 'presento' is still being made to good workmen of the day. Drillers by stupid celerity in getting home have now had their work increased to 140 cm daily. Embankment men are now split into parties of 20 and used in a competitive way: the stupid fellows still fall for competition to some extent! (Selfishness I am afraid.) One would think there were plenty of trade union men about, too.

Today, a Konyu party of 23 was allowed: we dug up 9 officers and 14 ORs fit to go, including Major Wearne and I. Our stores were still down below despite the valiant efforts of the British to lorry all stores up after their day's work (they worked until 0200 hours last night). I called on Lt-Col. Warren and discussed news etc. Okada was rather preoccupied with a visiting N. Lt-Col. and uncommunicative: boots and shirts in a day or two. Letters come later perhaps.

Warren warned me re recent search of a nearby camp. Saw letter from 'Mackie': news of himself and 'Hookey'. They are at Chungkai, where there will, I gather, be a base hospital. The people evacuated there are largely of 'convalescent' type. There will soon be 3 base hospitals: 1 Kanburi, 2 Tarsau, 3 Chungkai. (Four Australian MOs are at Tarsau now, having arrived with the 2000 Australians who are at present there. One, Millard, wrote a letter to Ewen Corlette.) Ration conditions are, I gather, excellent in that part of the world as compared with us.

	Working	Non-working
Meat	150 g	50
Rice	750 g	650
Veg	500 g	–
Flour	100 g	50 grms

Canteen stores are plentiful and much cheaper. Many little canteens flourish in camp: coffee 5 cents, 2 eggs fried 15 cents etc (*à la* Java). Cattle can be cheaply bought and officers messes usually have a cow on hand. At Chungkai No. 2 Group and No. 4 Group are being re-organised – may be 5,000 strong soon. At present 1,120 including 850 Dutch. Four British ORs were recently shot for escaping (the ones we saw going down there in a lorry). Apparently Australian letters reveal that newspapers at home headlined the 'Epic last Days of Singapore' and the Selarang episode.

Information on Tarsau at present: Australians 2,000, British 1,600, some Dutch. Goods obtained from Konyu – most notable was 4,485 eggs, 23 rolls of tobacco. Maj. Wearne and I brought through 485 eggs, 4 rolls of tobacco and the medical stores. This was pretty heavy going up the hill; and those damn bamboo poles through the basket give the shoulder hell. It must be rather amusing for a Japanese to see the 'white lords' trudging the road with basket and pole while they roll by on lorries!

Medical Stores Collected

1 Bot. Kruschen salts		½ oz Salicylic acid
1 oz Pot. Permang.		1 oz Meth. spirit
Aspirins	Few Tabs	3 oz Mercurochrome 2% sol.
Sodium Bicarb.	Few Tabs	4 oz cotton wool
Acriflavine	Few Tabs	1 sq. yd. cloth suitable for bandaging
Rimaoni	Few Tabs	(Kruschen salts in lieu of Mag. sulph etc.)
Plasmoquine	Few Tabs	
Atebrine	Few Tabs	

The Nipponese came into the tent today when sergeant working on X using my bed.*

17 April 1943

From tomorrow reveille and breakfast will be at 0700,† parade at 0730, move off to work 0800. The idea is to finish work by 1700 hours. This move is termed 'changey changey'. The troops are already getting a terrible belting and are looking thin; also septic sores are a grave problem, there being very little to treat them with. Men in large numbers are working, although covered with these sores which cause much pain. Men move stiffly and miserably in irritable temper and become gradually more comfortable at work but upon stopping, the throbbing irritation and torment of flies makes rest impossible. Practically all officers are out working today except Dick Allen who has septic sores, Fred Smedley with diarrhoea, Houston arthritis and general debility. Nippon 'presento' nonsense goes on every day, upsetting the evening parade. Sometimes the same troops are picked out several times. Some silly asses have apparently fallen for the competition and on the embankment carried 130 loads of earth a day. As a result, this has become the standard which all are expected to do. Watching Nips when they see a stretcher load regarded as too lightly loaded reject it in the count, saying it is a 'presento' load. Sometimes they stamp the load down and pile rocks on it for extra measure.

The Lizard is polite to Maj. Corlette now; but expects him to discharge 15 sick men each day. Also as the sick have now risen to a total that makes the supply of 500 working men not practicable, he decided that tomorrow some light sick must go out to work (10 in one evening).

18 April 1943

Reveille in the first grey light of dawn. Men have to perform what toilet is practicable and have breakfast by 0730. As it takes a long time for 800 men to draw a meal some have no time to eat breakfast before they are on parade. It is anticipated that very soon they will be working as late in the evening as ever.

I was engaged with officers in digging latrines all the morning. Hec Greiner is sick again with dysentry, also Piper, Allen and Primrose. I went around the railway course with Brian Harrison-Lucas in the afternoon. Brian has had rather severe beriberi and it is necessary to go very slowly. I had a narrow escape from falling from the top of a cliff on the way. Rubber shoes slipped on the wet earth and I fell about 6 feet; fortunately I was checked by Brian's legs and catching a vine with my left hand. Things are a little cooler on the railway course and today work finished earlier than usual at approximately 1600 hours. I saw Hiroda and told him the men were getting worn out with no rest and poor food. If no transport is available some must go to Konyu to carry sugar etc. tomorrow. Some have already had no rest for one month. Would he lend his lorry? This was agreed and he would let me know the time tomorrow. Tomorrow is definitely *yasumé* day.

* X was the wireless set and the sergeant was Sgt Cawthron. It was a close shave.
† Tokyo time 0700 = 0500.

One man was struck in the thigh today with a flying stone from blasting – a nasty wound. Some clothing and Nippon boots of rubber and canvas have arrived for outside workmen. The Nipponese broke up the evening parade to issue these which they did in a most inefficient and time-consuming way, every Nip soldier rushing around and putting a finger in the pie. The issue: O Battalion 238; P Battalion 190: Total 428. Rubber and canvas footwear is useful but neither durable nor watertight; there was great difficulty with big sizes. Only boots were issued tonight – we have obtained permission to issue the rest of the clothing ourselves. This will be O 81; P 70: Total 151.

19 April 1943

Yasumé day with reservations. Eighty men from each battalion were required to work on the road as a change from the railway. Approximately half were back soon after lunch.

The engineer's lorry, though it did take our reps down to collect stores, refused to descend the hill and only brought a little bit of stuff from the engineering top camp after keeping the party waiting there for hours. Sixty pairs of shorts were issued to each battalion and 75 hats. Both of these of NEI Army pattern of green drill and green straw respectively. Practically no shorts were of any use, since they were made for the smaller pelvis and legs of NEI native troops.

A moonlight *yasumé* concert was well attended.

20 April 1943

Hitler's birthday! All at work again. There is a slight easing on pressure on the sick. The Lizard enforces 15 discharges from hospital each day but is tolerating a rising rate of admissions. A new feature being introduced is a special lighter duty tab worn by men doing outside work, i.e. going out to the railway but receiving consideration out there. It is, however, a killing walk there and back.

We are now seeing for the first time some really first class examples of pellagra rash. Five well-marked cases presented. Some are present on the feet, others fairly general wherever the sun beats on them, all over the trunk on skirtless men working on the rail. At first, a well marked erythema and even blistering, looking like sunburn, changing gradually to a brown scaling rash as a 'toadskin', typical of pellagra.

There are several much more severe cases of beriberi now. These show marked swelling of the face and legs and shortness of breath, liver enlargement, etc. Most of these have active ankle jerks. Owing to the shortage of eggs of late, there is a marked deterioration in the state of those troops receiving treatment for avitaminosis. Some have very bad mouths and scrotums. It is noticeable that the strong workers who throw themselves into work are now coming in looking very broken and will obviously not be fit for weeks, even with hospital rest and treatment. Treatment amounts to 'wood and water', in other words, charcoal and foment. Each man is now responsible for his own water supply, as the elephants have gone elsewhere, so we are cutting bamboos for the purpose.

21 April 1943

Shortly after 0400 this morning a 'plane or 'planes were heard overhead heading down the river and some thought they heard bombs or ack ack. This is the first 'sign' we have met with. Subsequently explained by HQ Clerk Kanamoto as an 'eccentric plane come, Chinese, Engine English perhaps, eccentric aeroplane drop bombs between Tarsau and Tonchin. Very, very eccentric.' Local chatter has placed the crumbs of planes as anything up to a squadron and a huge diversity of opinion as to the number of bombs and where! Billy and I acted as pole and basket pair on a trip to the ferry to collect canteen stores and as our first trip unhill carried two tins of guala, about 130 lb. (This is reckoned a bit of a record in these parts.) The trip up the hill is a killer, what with rain and slush underfoot, the intense heat and the nasty way a pole hurts the shoulder. A miserable wet day.

I discussed with Osuki the following:

1 Claims for men injured working. It seems that we will have no claims met out of all those submitted up to date as they have to be submitted as a swindle amongst workmen claiming – not as a separate claim. The Lizard will not let us do this, but he has now been given a written instruction by Osuki. Bang goes $274.70.

2 Canteen stores. The only concession against our trouble is that we can have the use of lorries going from working camp to working camp, but not for ferrying up from the river. I am given a written chit for a party of twenty to come down and do the ferrying tomorrow.

3 Permission for the two chaplains to visit our camp on evening of 24th and stay overnight, holding special Anzac and Easter services.

It is unusual to get a written chit from any Nippon commander or authority and I am sure this is due to a native dislike of irrevocably committing themselves. Much easier to deny subsequently the spoken word. Nip intercommunication seems to suffer a good deal from this dislike of paper.

X [Wireless] Attempt to reinforce Tunisia by troop-carrying 'planes was intercepted. Losses known to be at least 74 and sixteen fighters. J.U. troop carriers carry 70 to 80 troops in each. Said to be the greatest air victory of the African campaign. The RAF active in the North Sea. Two destroyers sunk.

The party returned with stores in rain and slush carrying eggs and tomatoes. Crep. and Bret. in last, very exhausted. Jock and Clive also very knocked out and several members of the ORs party useless for tomorrow. I was lucky in getting off on lorries six tins of oil, eight tins of guala, one bag of sugar and a few eggs. So on the whole, a successful day. The elephants were being used at several points to pull lorries out of the mud today.

22 April 1943

A party of 20 ORs with Billy and I set off to Konyu again for a solid day of ferrying stores. We left at 0830 and after arriving made three trips with stores which was as much as the chaps could stand. Even Billy was just about sunk on the last trip. All stores must be shifted up today and after that there will be no more purchasing at the river for at least ten days, as N troops are moving in.

This is alarming as we have very few eggs and will get no more for ten or twelve days.

Yesterday as our rail party was going out they passed a stray bullock, the usual thin, miserable creature. N soldier jokingly said '*Makan*' and one of the lads promptly hit it on the head with an axe before he could intervene. It was then skinned and cut up in the twinkling of an eye. The result was that it was carted first to the N engineers' lines, about 100 men, where all the meat was cut off the bones and the latter were then generously sent to us.

Today, after a similar episode, a Thai animal was again done in but this time we were given the lion's share with only the tongue and undercut being taken. The skin was buried to conceal the crime. Today we got up all our stores from down below and a good deal of British stores. They have bother in finding men strong enough to carry up guala or oil in tins. Today, tommies were carrying up dried fish and meat threaded on bamboo poles, about 14 lb to two of them (they were light sick). Osuki and the interpreter were extremely amused to learn that I, too, was carrying stores. Much laughter. How many trips? Three! Peals of laughter.

The Tamil coolies have walked from Bampong and they report conditions in Malaya are very bad. Work is scarce, rice very scarce. They have been receiving only about eight pounds of rice a month (normally they eat one and a half pounds a day). They accepted the offer of work at Padang Besar near the border, their rate of pay to be $1 a day plus food, and were just a bit disconcerted when the train did not stop until Bampong. Now they are told they are marching to Burma to work. They are most wretched as they cannot stand rain and of course $1 a day here does not buy much at all. They are clad in damn all and have no bedding some merely carry a glass bottle for water, some a small bundle. There were two women in a party of 400. Malayan people report that they require a lot of care and die like flies of pneumonia if exposed to wet. One offered Billy and I cigarettes.

It was a sad sight to see these poor wretches trudging their way up the deep slushy mud of our road guarded by armed N troops – a wonderful tribute to the new order in South-east Asia. A few spoke English and pathetically asked when the British were coming back to Malaya. It is reported that they spent the night in the English area next door in the open and wet. Just another of those dreary, homeless mass migrations of war along a road of sickness and death.

Blackout at 2200 as from tonight; fire out. Instructions were given if a whistle blew we must disperse to the bush.

23 April 1943 Good Friday

The troops are out working as usual. Our two clerks returned from Tarsau; they have merely been re-numbering cards. They report food conditions good there. Australians there now include 2/10 and 2/12 Australian Field Regiments, 4th Anti-Tank and 18th, 19th & 20th Australian Infantry Battalions. The rail is approximately four miles from Tarsau. Recently they have been working 22 hours a day altogether, with unequal shifts of approximately 13 and 9 hours.

Conditions at Tarsau have improved since the advent of a new N Lt-Col. Men do not have very far to go out to work and the rice and water are taken out to them.

The road is very bad indeed. Both sergeants had their faces dusted over for not being prompt enough in getting out to push. Once again a narrow escape for Horry Williams' spectacles. He reports some talk of mail arriving on the day of the Emperor's birthday, the 29th. I am as usual sceptical of this possibility. The Nipponese issue of soap to troops today was seven per bar, this giving a piece 2 in. × 1½ in. × 1 in. of watery soap. (Soap as provided in these parts, whatever the size of the piece, usually melts in washing a single garment.)

New claim for sick, injured working submitted, back-dated from 21st, included O Battalion 7 NCOs and 15 ORs; P Battalion 15 NCOs and 26 ORs. Williams reports that units are claiming pay for the trip from Changi so we too will submit a claim. These of course are the days taken in transit. Obvious preparations are being made to use this area for transit camping and many N notice boards are going up, also tent covers (not waterproof) are being flung over our skeleton huts. Two cwalis dug in for cooking and two floored tents have been erected for the Japanese. It is reported that a great number of POWs and also N are moving up this way. Many of these are now walking and some Australians are at present marching from Tarsau.

24 April 1943

Lt Smedley went to Konyu today with a few ORs to try and arrange a collection of canteen stores by lorry. He had much delay and finally in the middle of the night was forced to get 100 troops out of bed to pull the lorry out of mud. However, we now have all the stores we ferried to the top. The padres were reported to be in trouble at approximately 1915 hours as they had arrived without a pass and were threatened with being sent straight back. Typical of N intercommunication. Local Nipponese after gaining much face by this show let them remain at my intervention. They were then released from the guard house. Parr meantime looking thoroughly militant, Bourke as usual the church militant. As it was then impossible to find out if there was indeed to be a *yasumé* tomorrow, combined Anzac Easter services were arranged for 2030 hours just after evening *tenko*. The Roman Catholics in the chapel area (relic of Father Kennedy) and the C. of E. in the concert area between the tents. Rain had just fallen so the ground, of course, was sodden. It was in some ways as lovely an evening as you could wish to see. The huge dark menacing mass of 'Jack's mountain' was partly obscured by great trails of mist, the upper part extremely distinct and suddenly appearing almost terrifyingly close as mountains do just after rain. Glorious great grey-barked trees simply laden with lilac blossoms blazed brilliantly here and there amongst the lovely green. The sky was positively aflame with crimson banners and mass cloud formation broke the fading light into all colours of the spectrum.

Some hundreds of men attended the C. of E. service. A few round about preferred to busy themselves with a little cleaning up and the inevitable frying. As the light faded, the padres' candles and a few fires lit the scene fitfully. The theme of the address was suffering, the cross and the empty tomb. The suffering of which we had experienced something, only a little of that endured by millions of others, was not in vain; that if all suffering ended only in muddled stupidity the sacrifice of the Cross would not have been made. This service was followed by the Last Post and Reveille, beautifully played by Page. Then 'God Save the King'.

Then followed Holy Communion, for which the padre donned his robes of office. More than sixty communicants. It was a strange sight, the robed and beared figure fantastically lit by candlelight with book and vessels performing a solemn rite, the communicants moving forward out of almost complete darkness from the little surrounding islands of men around the fire.

Both padres were very pleased with the roll-up and voted it a successful evening. One of the features of the night was the difficulty in threading one's way back through the jungle maze to the officers' lines. In this valley with an overcast sky, it is black as velvet at night and I suppose that most of us have vitamin A defficiency. Some of the troops have to be led out at night.

25 April 1943

A *yasumé* day.

A thorough day of rest, washing and overhaul for all. Reveille was delayed about one hour so *tenko* was in daylight. The padres held hospital services before departing. Padre Parr reported about 30 more communicants which pleased him mightily. I have trouble with my X [wireless] which is technically very difficult.

Feature of the day was the arrival of 201 Australians at 1900 hours: officers 2, W/Os 2, NCOs 33, men 164. The officers were Capt. Gill and Lt Wyllie. These had been on the march for two days since Tarsau and were completely all in, just stumbling along in a strung-out line. Two had just collapsed – Capt. Gill and one OR, from exhaustion. The party was originally approximately 500, some 200 being left at Konyu South, the English camp. Lt-Col. McEachern and nine ORs, the latter sick I believe. Lt-Col. is at Konyu HQ, discussing allotment of duty with Osuki. Approximately 90 back at Tarsau, too sick to come on, so their wastage is already nearly up to ours. Those coming in were bathed in sweat, dirt and thoroughly all in, but otherwise looked in fair condition. I arranged an evening meal at 2000 and ablutions etc., also care of the sick. Maj. De Crespigney and Wyllie to the Guard hut to discuss duties tomorrow. These, I gather, to be of a light nature.

At approximately 0100 hours, I was using X and became aware of a new party having marched in – some 500 NEI army soldiers who left Java in February. These, following on the five-day trip from Singapore, had been marching with all gear for six days and still had two days to go, probably to Rin Tin. They reported extreme brutality on the way, so far only one soldier having actually died on the road. One of the three medical officers fell down and was kicked. The CO endeavoured to help and was struck. (This MO and a few sick were left somewhere en route.) The exhausted troops were just lying in a sodden heap on the wet ground, sick, miserable and sorry. I tried to cheer up the commander a little, gave him some local information and told him where our latrines were situated.

A letter was received from Capt. Wells for Okada, 23/4/43, notifying the fact that Tarsau had been instructed not to send any drugs at present as they have 3,000 men in the area and a devil of a lot of sick. For the same reason direction of IJA is 'No further evacuations of sick until a new base hospital at Tarsau under construction is completed'. This is an awfully nice arrangement for forward camps! Also instructions re classification of sick. Influenza to be shown under tonsilitis and 'other conditions'. Colitis, only minor alimentary disturbances to be included.

26 April 1943

Ten tents are being erected and bamboo cut for flooring for the new arrivals. This means 20 per small tent. Two sick NEI soldiers were given breakfast and later picked up by lorry. Our new S Bn personnel are engaged on inside work, chiefly their own accommodation and bamboo fencing along the roadway. As CO S Bn has not yet arrived the duty section has been fixed on a temporary basis: 22 men – 10 cooks, wood and water 5, clerks 3, blacksmiths 4.

Approximately 9,000 British soldiers will march through our camp, each party stopping for one day and night; the first party of 500 is due tomorrow. Twenty extra men of O and P battalions (10 each) to assist in the cookhouse to provide meals for troops in transit. Shortly after *tenko* some 200 NEI troops passed through, halting until 2200 hours. They also had been on the march for seven days and complained of unnecessarily harsh treatment from the escort. This seemed to be officially inspired these days.

27 April 1943

S on parade with our troops. Things are going smoothly. 0930 the first party of British transit troops marched in after a short morning march from Konyu. They are No. 7 Bn, composed of Manchesters, Gordons and Loyals commanded by Lt-Col. Stitt, 2 I/C, Maj. Buchan, Adjutant, Captain Peres, 280 ORs. Also a road party of various units under Maj. Woods RASC, 92 ORs and No. 2 Bn under Maj. Hill with Maj. Mollineux 2 I/C, 16th Division recce 128. They bedded down in four huts covered with tent covers. We cooked their evening and morning meal and arranged watering, bathing etc. Lt-Col. Stitt, 2 I/C and Adjutant lunched and dined with us. His crowd came to Thailand in October, the last camp was at Pookai 113 kilometres and there moving to 205 kilometres. A N general, Sassa, previously at Bampong, is now coming to Tarsau as GOC Prisoners-of-War Thailand.

Lt Osuki called in today and I gave him the claims for our movements from Changi to Tarsau, 20–25 January: Total 593.00 ticals, the rates being 25 c, 15 c and 10 c.

This evening Lt-Col. McEachern arrived about rice time bringing with him 3 ORs, the total thus now 206. He is about 37 and appears very pleasant.

28 April 1943

Shortly after *tenko* about 250 Dutch troops went through. The British party moved out at approximately 0815 hours and at about 0930 another party arrived, No. 1 and No. 13 battalions. 13 Bn a mixture of RASC, Ordnance,

Sherwood Foresters, Beds. & Herts. and a few Roy. Artillery. Commander Maj. Housecroft, 2 I/C Capt. Bates, Adjutant Lt Kidner. No. 1 Bn Beds. & Herts. Command Signals, Fortress Signals commanded by Maj. Dobbs, Middlesex Regiment, 2 I/C Maj. Flynn, Adjutant Capt. Garrod. Strength No. 13: 106; No. 1: 311: Total 417. Maj. Dobbs was interested in birds [wireless sets].

The theft of blankets, food and such articles as haversacks, packs, trinkets etc. has increased alarmingly with these transit parties. We have piquets night and day with only partial effect. Worst bag was Col. Stitt's party. He said 'These Manchesters'.

Okada came to the camp with Tadano and we were told that one MO must go to Kanchanaburi Base Hospital, so after a brief discussion Maj. Moon fixed to pack immediately. This is a serious loss as Arthur has done magnificent work with the sick and is one of the most thorough, loyal and capable souls living. Also the work here is quite heavy for two men and I have a great deal to do.

29 April 1943

It is ordered that officers move to a new site: I discussed this with the Lizard and a few concessions were obtained. The transit party moved at 0800 hours and a new one arrived. Three battalions, No. 5 – Lt-Col. Mapey, 20 RAOD (18th Div.) under Maj. Longdon and the remainder 2nd. Cambridgeshires totalling 328 (of these 21 were officers from the Malay Regiment, Malayan Volunteers and 2 Cambridgeshires). They were on an eight-day march and have done three days. No. 9 Bn Maj. J. Wyllie (125th Anti-Tank Regiment RA), 85 AT Reg. RA, 135 Field Reg. RA and 53 I.B. (5th & 6th Norfolks) Lt-Col. Dean previously commanding went back to Chungkai. This party left Changi on 27 October 1942 and moved to Wonlong where they stayed until the end of February. They then moved to Tarkilin, thence to Wampo and to Konyu. They think they are going to Suiji-Dogo about 220 kilometres. 'Z' Battalion Captain W.D. Harris 18th Div. Recce made up of Beds. & Herts. 75, 1st and 2nd Battalions, Cambridge 75, 18th Div. Recce 50, 18th Div. R.B. 70, Northumberland Fusiliers 70, Sherwood Foresters 30: Total 390. They left Changi on 31st March and had come up with 2,000 Australians under Maj. Quick. They were left at Tarsau by their CO, Lt-Col. Swinton, East Surrey Regiment and his brigade major, Tom Broughton, Royal Scots Guards. Swinton was previously commander at Wampo. We now know that Osuki is coming here with staff – possibly the Lizard is to go.

Today being the anniversary of the accession of the Emperor to the throne was deemed a half *yasumé* and men were back from work early. We were also informed that 40 men were to work at night tomorrow.

Lt Smedley, who has been to Konyu to buy fish etc, reported that Arthur Moon had gone on down south and Smedley was able to give him $60 as that wretch Arthur left without telling me he had no money. This is two months' pay in advance.

Yesterday I had a conference with Lt-Col. McEachern re the command etc. He agrees to co-operate with us on the present administrative arrangements, particularly finance and canteen etc., and until the question of his permanent abode with S Bn will not take over command of this camp. He is, I gather, a Lt-Col. of more than seven years standing. I find the sick a hell of a big job and to get through well over 100 hospital patients in the morning is almost impossible – thus I am working all day and fitting in administration at odd moments.

30 April 1943

Transit arrivals No. 6 Bn, Lt-Col. C.E. Morrison, said to be going to the 210 kilometre mark while Stitt goes to 206 with Mapey and Mollineux. There is to be a double camp formed at 210–213 kilo of No. 8, Lt-Col. Johnson, No. 1, Maj. Dobbs and No. 3, Housecroft. No. 6 Bn consists of Leicestershires, East Surreys, some RAOD. With the party is Maj. Black's hospital party, at present commanded by Capt. Hardy, going to establish a hospital at the double camp mentioned above. The 'Officers' Battalion' which includes several lieutenant-colonels is commanded by Lt-Col. J. Larkin and is going to 217 kilometres. Also going will be No. 10, Bn, Milner; No. 11, Pinecoffin; and two battalions of NEI troops. This group will be under Lt-Col. Swinton. No. 8 Bn Lt-Col. A.A. Johnson, largely Suffolks. He is a butterfly and orchid hunter!

Tonight Osuki and staff arrived; much 'changey changey'. This camp is now Hintok camp No. 5 and strength with that at Tarsau is 1,084 all ranks. Lt-Col. McEachern and I were summoned to O. who gave us the new duty section, drastically reduced from 124 to 70 all ranks. It was indicated that those officers not employed in duty section would have to go on railway work. We managed to shift a slight increase in clerks from nine to eleven on his original figures. (All wood and water carrying personnel are now axed). We impressed upon O. the severity of the canteen and food problem, stressing the number of sick, the necessity for eggs, meat, vegetables. Sick figures and types of illness were discussed. It was agreed that lights out be changed to 2300 and as an earnest of good intention O. gave me some cigarettes for distribution, approximately 2,000. I told him of Lt-Col. McEachern's seniority. At my request for five more tents he gave me three.

A hurried conference of battalion commanders, myself and Billy came to fix the new duty section and retain in camp all officers and essential duty personnel, regimental sergeant majors, canteen reps, etc. Some of these are carried as medical orderlies (3), Haddon, Williams and Turner. (Medical orderlies were not allowed to include officers.) Some on pump, the rest as HQ clerks, anti-malaria, etc. Although terribly reduced, I think everyone fairly happy as to fairness. Bugler to act as batman and cook to officers.

The new Mess Duty Section is as follows:

CAMP	OF	WO	NCO	MEN	TOT.	OF	WO	NCO	MEN	TOT.	OF	WO	NCO	MEN	TOT.	Total
Duties Cooks	1			11	12			1	10	11		1	1	4	6	29
Clerks			1		1	4	1			5	2	1			3	9
Medical Orderlies			1		1			8	5	13				1	1	15

Camp	OF	WO	NCO	MEN	TOT.	OF	WO	NCO	MEN	TOT.	OF	WO	NCO	MEN	TOT.	Total
Duties																
Anti-Malaria	3				3	1		1		2	1				1	6
Bugler			1		1											1
Pump		1	1		2			2		2				1	1	5
I.J.A. Orderlies								2	1	3						3
TOTAL:	4	2	3	11	20	5	1	14	16	36	3	2	1	6	12	68

Allotment of Duties

Cooks	Medical Orderlies	Clerks	Anti-Malarial	Pump	I.J.A.	Bugler
Lt Airey	Sgt Wiseman	Lt-Col. Dunlop	Maj. Wearne	W/O Exton	Sgt. Oliver	Pte
Sgt Cory	Sgt Turner	Maj. Greiner	Maj. Clarke	Sgt Griff	Cpl	Hesten
+				Gunner	Lawrence	
27 ORs	S/Sgt	Maj. Woods		Siganto	Cpl	
	Harrison-	Maj. Corlette	Capt. Brettingham-		Donellan	
	Lucas	Maj. de Cresp.	Moore			
		Lt Smedley		Sgt		
	S/Sgt	W/O Fyfe	Lt Houston	Thomson		
	Williams	W/O Phillips	Lt Wylie			
	S/Sgt	W/O Cock	+	Cpl Warren		
	Gibson	Lt-Col.	1			
	Sgt Haddon	McEachern				
	+	Capt. Gill				
	12 medical					
	orderlies					

In Hospital at present: Capt. Allen, Lt Primrose, Capt. Piper, Exton. Griff, Siganto, Thomson are Canteen reps essential for canteen work and accounts. It will be seen that two officers are unallotted and will have to be on the sick list.

Numerous working injuries recently – blasting injuries with rock and hit with a hammer on the head, etc. Ray Cameron was hit on the neck and the back of the shoulder – a large flying rock said to be about 25 lb – severe injury.

1 May 1943

O 107; P 95; S 13: Total 215. I discussed the sick position with Okada, showing him many severe ulcers and avitaminosis cases. His attitude: 'Now kill pig tomorrow. Fifty men better, etc.' Quite hopeless but good tempered. He is pleased with our anti-malarial work and our system of dams and pipes. A further transit party marched in consisting of Nos. 10 and 11 battalions and some 196 Gordons and Manchesters belonging to No. 7.

A N soldier, Kanamoto, replaces Hiramura as a 'writoman' at evening conferences to Maj. De Crespigny's delight. Workers' conferences at least go more smoothly even if no change of policy. Three pigs arrived today. Osuki insisted on a sty near the cookhouse and ration store. Maj. Wearne and I firm for over the creek. Honour was eventually saved with O. getting near boiling point by the RQM building a sty at another nearby site. A thin cow also arrived in a very bad state of health, was eagerly seized by Doctor Weary but the Nipponese soldiers took it away from him and insisted that it be tied up near their lines. No kill today.

Okada attempted to donate a forequarter of beef from the N kitchen for the sick. There was a great row and the meat had to be returned. Kanamoto was particularly enraged and swiped at Fred Airey, also saying we could keep it for ten ticals.

The first flight of Australian troops came through tonight, pausing for a breathing space at about 2030 hours. Maj. Parry in command. Destination not known but probably up towards the Three Pagodas Pass 230–300 kilometres northward on the Burma/Thailand border. 7,000 British POWs in Changi 18 April: 3,500 Australians, 3,500 English under the command of Lt-Col. Harris. Lt-Col. Kappé is in charge of the Australian contingent accompanied by Lt-Col. Pond. They were told to bring all heavy baggage with them and this (naturally) is at Bampong, including three pianos with band instruments, medical stores and officers' baggage!

Lt-Col. Harris is waiting at Tarsau; going forward to set up a group staff. During movement the force had the use of an ambulance van and a lorry. Six parties of Australian troops will go through, one each evening. Lt Airey will endeavour to supply coffee or tea. This party included Maj. Stephens, AAMC, and Capt. Mills, AAMC. They have been marching seven days, about eighteen hours sleep. About 20 per cent of the personnel are said to be unfit. This leaves about 7,000 Australians at Changi and soon, probably, only hospital cases and sick. 'E' Force went to Borneo under the command of Maj. Fairley.

Unit Canteen: a change in policy. No section accounts. Dick Allen, Turner, Hadden do all the accounts for O and P battalions. Canteen reps. take orders and distribute stores. Only three issues are made per week.

2 May 1943

The transit party today is Captain Cossa with 574 Dutch including nine officers. I spent much time talking Dutch and made my classic 'howler': '*Houvel menshen heeft u gedood*? Actually I should have said, '*Gesterf*', i.e., 'How many men have you dead?' *Gedood*: killed. He said he was only a ladykiller!

Sent for today by Osuki Chui who told us with a 'What a good boy am I' expression that there were now many stores for collection at Konyu, including 45,000 eggs at 7.2c, fish, sugar, oil, peanuts, onions, tobacco, soap and many oddments for which he gave prices. We subsequently found the basis of all this good work was a faithful Thai trader* who established contact with the English. We discussed the collection of stores; he was most vague, saying 'come tomorrow', and would not promise a lorry but said I could speak at the other end.

A little confusion on the part of the new 'writoman' Kanamoto and the

* Boon Pong.

working party allotment so that the routine is now as follows: Reveille 0645 hours; breakfast 0650 hours; fall-in for checking into working parties by RSM 0750.* Engineer overseers arrive and the party moves off at 0800 hours. Evening bugle call is 1945 hours. All men fall in and must be formed up by 1955 hours for second bugle. RSMs check and hand over to the adjutant who hands over to CO by 2000 hours when Nippon orderly checks the parade. Then retreat is blown. More Changi Australians came through this evening and were given 'rice coffee', Lt-Col. Kappé wearing still his blue brigade armband; Col. Kappé was cheerful but very tired. 'The Nipponese have a complete brigade to contend with now, ordnance, AASC, and everything complete!' I said, 'Well sir, I hope that you will remain together, because things are pretty rough up here.'

3 May 1943

I went to Konyu with Maj. Wearne and observed a new Australian camp at the old Thai clearing 3 kilometres down the road. This is Maj. Quick's camp and is Australian. It is in a favourable area for tent erection but looks very malarious. They are working on the stream, dams, ablution areas etc.

At Konyu had a quick conversation with Lt-Col. Warren, other officer a very tall ginger-coloured chap and a good type. The position with Warren is that his men simply cannot carry up all the stores for surrounding camps. They do this work after their daily work, consequently some arrangement must be made, either for collection by lorry or for other camps to send collecting parties to carry stores uphill from the river.

New Tarsau interpreter arrived today and detailed Maj. Wearne to carry in his bag! This looked like a British 'presento' leather affair. Warren tackled him as spokesman re the above problem. He said 'Will bring up at this evening's conference.' A good English-speaking Nipponese but not nice to know. 'Smokey Joe' is completely out of hand with his prices and a complete nuisance to deal with. Maj. Wearne and I returned with three S Bn men in a truck with the Konyu interpreter who is now joining Osuki and so he gave us a life. We brought 1,700 eggs and a few pumpkins. The interpreter promptly collared fifty eggs and a few pumpkins.

Changi letters: the following notes were particularly sweet:

Wife: 'You will be surprised to hear no doubt, my dear, that I have adopted a dear little two-month-old baby – I know you will love it.'

Sister: 'I am writing this letter for X [his wife] to give you the news as she is busy getting ready to go out to a ball.'

From fiancée: 'When you come home, you will have to call me mother, as I just couldn't wait and have married your father.'

It makes one shiver when there has been no letter from home at all! The AIF transit party arrived today, Maj. Tracey. No MO, Capt. Cahill having fallen out exhausted at previous stage. I talked to Osuki who promised to arrange a lorry to collect stores at Konyu river site. 'Send an officer tomorrow, etc.'

* We worked on Tokyo time, two hours ahead.

4 May 1943

Maj. Wearne after a lot of luck secured a lorry and brought it back. 2,400 eggs. Osuki made no arrangement at all. Okada has been making a blitz for discharge of sick men to 'light duty' each day. Some of these being given a special red tab to ensure very light work. The result is just the same. The local Nipponese work them like hell all day with very little rest and just completely knock them out, so they even request to be changed to the railway where the overseers at least have some sense. Okada's idea is that on the basis of some eggs, one cow plus three pigs arriving, all men should rapidly be better and discharged from hospital. Today, he insisted on thirty discharges. I stuck on fifteen and after Maj. Corlette had worked him down to twenty, went to see him in a furious fighting mood. He immediately capitulated and Brian Harrison-Lucas 'poured a soothing syrup'. He said that No. 1 had personally gone into the question and it was really and truthfully impossible. 'OK,' said Okada, 'Fifteen.' (Nippon unpredictability.) Transit party AIF Capt. Schwartz, 600 approximately. Also arrived were Maj. Bruce Hunt and Capt. Frank Cahill, Bruce Hunt had been beaten up savagely with a lot of sick at Tarsau. They are behaving with an unreasoning brutality to the sick.

5 May 1943

Maj. Wearne went to Konyu. In view of the fact that we now have about 500 avitaminosis cases in 1,000 it is hopeless to especially select them out for eggs and I have decided that only those in hospital plus a few very bad cases will receive them, especially the three egg a day ration. The remainder are allotted on a *per capita* basis. There are at present about 140 avitaminosis cases in hospital, many suffering from other conditions as well, particularly septic sores, malaria and diarrhoea. Payment of eggs: each case is to be considered on its merits on discharge, according to credit, etc.

Malaria is now most prevalent and there are large numbers of primary malaria cases included. Troops are warned about nets but unfortunately 20 men per tent makes net rigging most difficult and the tent horribly airless. Septic sores are a terrible problem. Practically no resistance to them in many cases and the men become covered with horrible sores, all over the legs, the arms, and a pustular rash in the armpits, groins and crutch, etc. Some leg sores are 2½ inches in diameter. Practically all we have for these is foments at present, a little chlorosol solution or coconut oil! I still have many sores on legs and now a sore mouth. Dick Allen, Primrose and Piper all ulcer patients. Officers for the first time showing signs of B_2 deficiency cropping up.

In the evening, Hiroda Chui in conference with Osuki and interpreter, and we are told that there are two propositions, both of which depend on the fact that work is to be increased: drillers must now do 200 cm daily instead of 140 (this work is very heavy and dangerous already; also the rock clearing parties would be kept very late indeed); or rock-clearing parties are to be reduced from 35 to 25. Drillers, of course, giving them some help. This latter alternative was chosen by W/O Shea, W/O2 Allinson and W/O2 Gascoigne and was fixed by Maj. Wearne and I with the Japanese in conference after *tenko*. Okada tried to seize ten men for work on the N HQ after work on the railway today, but when we protested he instead took twenty English from the transit party. Okada is becoming No. 1 menace around the place, continually insisting on more men being discharged from hospital who are unfit. He is very moody and unpleasant. There are some rumours of movement of troops soon, ? to form a new camp near the river.

TRANSIT PARTIES

Date of Arrival	Commander	Time of Arrival	Composition of Party	Strength	Date Departure
May 1	Maj. Parry	2030	Mixed Party ASC, Sigs, Engineers & 8 Div. Infantry units and 2nd 10 Field Regiments	450	1/5/43 2200
May 2	Lt-Col. Kappé	2040	2/29 Bn. AASC, Sigs, Engineers	600	2/5/43 2300
May 3	Maj. Tracy	2050	2/26 Bn. & 2 mixed Companies, 2/19 Bn. Engs., Sigs, AAMC	600	3/5/43 2230
May 4	Capt. Schwartz (Maj. Hunt)	2040	2/26 Bn. Remainder 2/15 Fd. Bty. 2/40 Fd. Bty. Engs, Sigs & sick from previous parties	600	4/5/43 2130
May 5	Maj. Johnson	2110	2/30 Bn. Some 2/4 Anti-tank & sick from previous parties	600	5/5/43 2300

6 May 1943

Men working on the drills in the railway cutting pin their faith to a sort of limestone powder from the rocks they are blasting as a panacea for healing sores. Bandaged on and left untouched it seems to have some value. These are terribly prevalent in the camp; probably 75 per cent have sores of some sort. Yesterday Maj. Wearne and Exton went to Konyu, returning with 2,250 eggs and a varying assortment of cotton, thread, toothbrushes, powders, pastes, pencils, notebooks, pipe cleaners and tobacco. Very little of each article. Today they managed 1,250 eggs. The lorry refused to go down the mountain road to the river saying it was too wet. Further transit party of Australians this evening, O/C Maj. Anderson. 2nd 4th Engineers, 8th Div. Signals, AASC AAOC and 250 AAMC were told at Changi that they would be establishing one of those wonder hospitals at destination. Some men were horribly tired but the spirit was good.

7 May 1943

A party of N soldiers (termed 'bridge builders' because of no very definite knowledge of their identity) have set up a new set of lines alongside the engineers, opening a new spring, and dismantling our 'P Phone' which was close to their area. Two foully dressed N officers, one a major, one a lieutenant, were in the area today seeing Osuki and later walking into my sick parade. Both were in flowing, ill-fitting drill and pith helmets, the more junior one with a pith helmet of Thai type and a star in front – a truly villanous style. He was quite polite however and merely wished to see some of our exhibits of sick, poor devils plastered with septic sores and dermatitis. These were viewed with polite grunts. Later they were seen on the railway course. The details of the Duty Section and engineer duties called for. No repercussions up to date. A party in transit from Chungkai and Wun Run, containing remnants of all battalions 1–15 which have gone forward today; in command Lt-Col. Young Malay Regiment with Captain Benson and Captain Gotla, both RAMC. The former Brigade Major of Chungkai, Maj. Christopher, was handling the messing. He and the colonel dined with us despite the rain. They are the first of three parties coming. Lt-Col. Williamson, the Camp Commander at Chungkai, is expected through any day. Chungkai will then be a camp for sick and convalescent men from other camps. Fred Airey was visited by a N captain today who expressed sympathy re the rations and promised more food: possibly a sort of army service corps inspector.

8 May 1943

O 122; P 115; S 27: Total 264:

I have been terribly busy with the sick as indicated by the figures, and consequently usually working almost from dawn to dark. In between time, I am incessantly interrupted and harrassed by the Nipponese who insist on there being less sick. The second party of British remnants went through commanded by Maj. Bowman of the Coldstream Guards who played rugger for Cambridge and the Army. These 1st Cambs. Norfolks, 4th Suffolks, 135 Field Battery, 125 Anti Tank, RAOC, RIASC, 1 AOC and East Surreys. Osuki was in a pathetic 'twit' this morning, sending for me and running around in circles: General Sassa is coming. After giving me instructions re compliments, etc., he then started running around himself to the kitchen and even the tent of the night cook shift. After all this, only Lt-Col. Ishi, Commandant of Konyu arrived. A large fat, elderly, bespectacled and untidy man. An inspection was made of the hospital and the commander asked what the sickness tents contained. Re dysentry: 'How long do you starve the men? No food.' Me: 'Usually two to three days. Sometimes longer, depending on progress.' Commander: 'Must always give no food for one week'! A great contribution to the medical problem!

Conveniently, the old boy failed to see the large number of men lying on the ground with no tents. Following departure, I heard there had been a big row about the sick figure and Laurie reported that Okada was personally blown up by the general to such an extent that as his car left he threw a tin of water against the bamboo fence lining the road. I was sent for and told to find 700 men for outside work tomorrow to which I yelled 'How?' so loudly that both O. and the interpreter jumped in their chairs. Conversation became angry and Lt-Col. McEachern arrived, causing a cooling down on my part.

After endless discussion, a final figure of 679 was allowed so that in addition to numerous half-sick men pushed out, I was forced to discharge 17 men regarded as unfit.

O. and interpreter promise ration improvements as a basis for negotiation about sick. Six pigs arrived today. Therefore, fifty men better tomorrow!

9 May 1943

I arranged a battalion commanders' conference and for the transfer of four tents to the hospital giving a total of fourteen. Canteen and financial matters were discussed, then I handed over the camp command to Lt-Col. McEachern, thanking administrative officers for their loyal co-operation and hard work which had made my work very easy. Lt-Col. McEachern was in no way anxious to take over, but I made it clear that I was now too busy with medical work to carry on efficiently with administrative work.

A combined English and Australian party of 'remnants' passed through again in the late evening. Okada gave an order that 40 men were to be discharged from hospital tomorrow morning to go out of camp for a few metres while the general visited the camp. He gave a solemn assurance they would not be worked and would come back to hospital later in the day. Meantime, the hospital statistics would be improved by 40. We do not trust any Nipponese word in the least but there is nothing to do but to comply. The men were advised to collapse if worked.

10 May 1943

A day of terrific 'twit' and window dressing, Osuki fussing round like a nervous schoolboy, after demanding a plan of the hospitals so that he could explain just what sick there were in each tent.

Feverish work had to be done in setting up all the paraphernalia of a new N HQ building and guardhouse and building suitable fences. These were all brought into apple pie order. Now O. began assembling the troops. Several practice assemblies in compliment paying etc. on the road before the guardhouse with McEachern Crep. me, Woods and Greiner on the left of the line. During one of these practices George Page, who was posted, blew his general salute or whatnot and we fell in only to find it was Lt-Col. Ishi arriving with a large lorryload of vegetables, rushed through just in time and prominently displayed. Finally, Major General Sassa arrived, bugles blowing etc. and did a fairly comprehensive tour of inspection, including kitchens, hospitals, water supplies and men's lines. Of course, O. made the most of Allan Wood's 'waterworks' and his newly acquired hospital knowledge. It even happened that the only soldier whose lunch was inspected was eating an egg. After lunch we were called out again to salute as the general departed to the railway site.

Late in the day 29 of the sick returned, terribly exhausted after a hell of a day. They were lorried about two kilometres out and then had to roll 500 lb oil drums, three to four per drum, some kilometres to the compressor party. They were warned that if they rolled off the mountain track they would have to get them up again. Finally, they walked home four kilometres over the hills. These were sick men, most of them covered with huge sores and many weakened by fever and various illnesses. This is the most horrible thing I have seen done as yet, apart from their executions. The most primitive of races would scarcely treat sick and starving dogs in this fashion.

Additional pay of 5 c a day 'Danger Pay' is to be given to men engaged on hammer drills, pneumatic drills, compressor units and M.T. drivers. Each day a numerical role for each battalion is to be stamped as follows indicating where and what each man is doing.

In hospital	Injured in Hospital	At work on Railway
Duty Section	Drawn pay	
Pneumatic Drillers	Light Duty in Camp	Men at Tarsau
		Men at Kanchanaburi

I departed for Tarsau with Okada but Osuki stopped us and sent us back, saying I was to go later. Wells asked me to see Maj. Marsden, who was sick. I found that he had had an attack of some five days of gastroenteritis, settling down to a severe pain in the right lower abdomen. There was a tender mass high in the right lower abdomen and to the right of the umbilicus. Most probably a retro-caecal appendicitis. I advised an Oschner Sherren regime where he was, rather than bumping down to Tarsau for immediate operation. Captain McNeilly, rather alarmed, said he would 'not be liking the responsibility', but I said I would see him if possible. Meantime, Osuki and Co. had left me to walk and I began the seven kilometre walk in a curious feeling of extreme heat and exhaustion. Two days ago, I also felt rather off colour; I suspect malaria, damn it.

Thirty men meantime had been rushed off to Tarsau. Fitter sick men were sent as it is a lousy journey, and as a result bitter complaints were made by Osuki and Okada that they were working men who should not leave the area. Shylock had nothing on these fellows in extracting the last ounce of meat from bodies.

Twenty-four men have been discharged with a struggle from the hospital today. After a bitter fight with the Nips when they were told that I would discharge no more sick men and that if they wished it, they must accept the responsibility for ordering the discharge themselves. Accordingly, they ordered the release of fifteen more, two with their arms in a sling. Yesterday's remarkable performance, which reduced the sick figure to the level of 214 (254 – 40), has fired them with ambition. They wish the same number of men to go out today. Needless to say, I told Okada what I thought of his lies and bad faith. Yesterday, of 214 sick, malaria 85, beriberi 19, others with debility, etc. 13, tonsillitis 3, circulatory system 3, acute colitis 6, other conditions, diarrhoea, etc. 50, urogenital 1, furuncles 1, other skin diseases 19, bruising 2, wounds 9, fractures 2, sprain 1.

10 May 1943

X [wireless] records on the ninth that North Africa is cleaned up: Bizerta to the Americans, Tunisia to the British.

Lt-Col. Harper and transit party went through today and also the Group HQ of Changi troops who have moved through since 1 May. This was 'diagnosed' by an ambulance car and a marmon with Lt-Col. Harris on one vehicle. These vehicles did not stop. Lt Houston 2/2 Pioneers, general factotum and secretary of the officers' mess, celebrated his forty-first birthday today. Fifty-four bullocks stopped on the road outside the camp and after an endless conference with Thais and Osuki, we were allowed to drive them to the camp. Osuki took all the spare money, 800 ticals, and did not deign to inform us if we were further indebted or not. I loaned 60 ticals to this cause. The engineers took two cows to leave 52 for our 'ranch'. The Nipponese of course will say when they are to be killed, etc. Hiroda Chui today approached some drillers and said that if they drilled 160 cm they could have a two day *yasumé*. He said 'Me no lie. Speak truth. 160 cm, get 2 day *yasumé*.' Of course, these goats then drilled the extra 20 cm in about the same time. A few fit and experienced drillers can do this but it will soon become the standard 'presento' practice.

This evening Okada, inflamed with the drink, slammed a knife in the table under the nose of Capt. Brettingham-Moore and gave an ultimatum to produce more men than were as yet discharged from the hospital by the doctors. Today we were told that a party of seventeen men, including 3 pneumatic drillers, 3 cooks and 1 batman, would accompany the Nips to a camp at the compressor site by the river. Henry Boyes was sent for medical reasons.

12 May 1943

Today I have definite malaria with a temperature of 103° F., a feeling of malaise and weakness of the back, my spleen feeling full and obviously palpable. I commenced quinine grains 10 t.d.s. but unable to go to bed and don't feel enamoured of my bamboo horror anyway. By error, the great cow scoop was entered as yesterday. It really occurred today. Maj. Wearne and Co. also had had a good scoop, bribing Nip lorry drivers to carry practically all our eggs and canteen stores from the river site to the HQ camp. They brought many stores back with them. It is a complete mystery what Osuki has done with the 800 ticals that he demanded and to what extent the cows are our property.

Maj. Greiner, Capt. Piper and Maj. Woods have supervised the building of the bamboo stockyard with annoying interference by the Nips who have absolutely no knowledge of how to handle these scraggy beasts.* We now have quite a ranch with 52 cattle skeletons and six small pigs delivered by the Nipponese after the general's visit. Okada now screaming for the figure to be reduced for sick again. Seven hundred men to go to work.

13 May 1943

More N POW cards issued, with very stringent orders re filling in: no date; address to be No. 4, POW Camp, Thailand, officers to delete all reference to

* Okada said: 'Men go out to jungle – cut and bring back breakfast, dinner and tea for cows!'

working or pay, the card to be addressed to someone of the same name as the sender, except in special circumstances.

The N guards are all in severe trouble today. They stole a portion of their issue meat from their store and were cooking it in our kitchen last night when discovered by the Schu Bon when they ran for the bush. Result today; a terrific blitz, very pleasing to us. Nips are working very hard all day on half rations and an absolute spate of drill tonight under Osuki, with a great deal of standing to attention and running, etc. and angry voices raised all day, presumably telling them that they are scum!

A further row with Okada re providing 700 men, finishing with the acceptance of 679. Lt-Col. McEachern visited Maj. Quick's camp and also Maj. Sneider's camp and Phil Millard, a doctor who has been playing up very well, sent me one pound of chloroform and 0.5 g of Pentathol.

Towards the evening about 500 Malay, Chinese and Thai coolies came into this area; they are quartered on the outskirts of our camp close to the N engineering lines. We are all forbidden to speak to them but they use our showers, etc. at times. They say their pay is $1 a day, although they have not received it yet, and they are railway workers (probably timber cutters). Contrast with our pay of 25 c a day, the price of one coconut.

A party of English and Australian troops halted on the road outside tonight. Contacts were difficult.

14 May 1943

Malaria giving me a pretty poor time. I went to Konyu nevertheless to see Maj. Marsden in response to an appeal from Maj. O'Driscoll. He had leaned heavily on Marsden (fortunately on the left side), and said 'Oh, come on Marsden. You must go to Tarsau. I always believe in taking a chance.' Marsden was not so keen. I found him considerably improved and I think around the corner. I walked some four miles to call on Capt. Millard and to straighten out one or two worries. He has been under the impression that most of his fevers were dengue, an excusable mistake, although of course they are malaria. His sick rate is about 25 per cent and he too is having trouble with the Nips.

Transit people today actually walked in to the skirl of the pipes! This was most memory stirring. They consist really of three separate parties moving north together.

Butterworth has had a severe malaria followed by severe and persistent diarrhoea and looks a shadow. I finished my march today with a temperature of 103° F. again and feeling pretty wretched but spent some time in the late evening putting up a severe scald with surgical toilet and Tannafax.

Some of the hospital unit went through today, well equipped, having bought a lot of stuff down at Bampong. They have plenty of anaesthetic. No amount of talk of my wretched state induced them to give me anything. One particularly maddening and stupid thing is that having difficulty in carrying all their stuff, of all things, the damn fool colonel gave the Manchesters 2,000 M & B 693 to carry up. Of course, they promptly 'flogged' the lot. Maj. Hodgkinson and transit party through at 2040 hours, the last of Lt Harris's party.

15 May 1943

My malaria now complicated by some dysentry with obvious blood and mucus. I have to keep going somehow. Maj. Wearne and party to Konyu and secured 6,800 eggs. All officers and those available for camp duties at Konyu are engaged in building a new hospital hut.

Letter cards were handed in to the Nips. In view of the censoring regulations, I have no hope that my last card was forwarded.

In the small hours of the night Sakata and Kanamoto roused several officers to round up escaped cattle who were browsing quietly.

16 May 1943

During last night, a party of some 25 English, Australian, Dutch troops arrived by M.T. from Tarsau under Maj. Morrison. They were established in two tent flies in the N house area. Morrison, a Medical Officer, Hygiene, said that he was the advance guard of some 3,000 troops under Lt-Col. Humphries from Changi and including 600 Australians from Makasura, Java, who were shortly to arrive in the area. He has orders to clear a camp for 600 in the vicinity of our stockyard.

Today, I left early for Tarsau with Okada on one of the most terrible vehicles I have ever travelled on. Even my water bottle was broken by the jolting and my malarial back and head were almost likewise. Quite a lot of the rail is unfinished between Konyu and Tarsau, even as regards the provisional levelling, but there is some evidence of sleeper cutting. Tonchin, I was told, is a real camp of death, men dying freely from M.T. malaria and also the amount of amoebic dysentry coming down from up there is most alarming. The death roll for Tonchin is very high.

At Tarsau. I managed to dig in with a pass to return the following day and I am in the charge of Haruyama, one of the few polite N soldiers in these parts. He proved a trump and ran around notifying me of times and saluting smartly.

Col. Harvey has 400 patients, almost half the sickness for the month of April, coming from Tonchin: 2,550 patient days. Their system of finance of patients in hospital is now breaking down, as forward camps are no longer sending them their proportion of officers' pay subscription. Unless Tarsau area allows the use of officers' savings accounts, they will not be able to go on as before. Conditions re food are better in the base camps than those up here, but it is awkward for convalescent men who are earning no money. The only stores Harvey had available were 28 bottles of quinine, absolutely nothing else. I felt there was a lack of enterprise shown in local purchase. They have for example, no gloves and their wounds always seem to go wrong. Short of drugs and dressings and everything that goes for treatment of sick. Several men usually dying each day. I like McConachie, the surgeon, a keen and pleasant Scot who says he only operates in life-saving matters in this country, which seems wise. Harvey reported that Maj. Moon was at Tamarkand near Kanchanaburi, SMO of a large new hospital said to be about 1,200. Jolly good show for Arthur!

I had a long talk to Maj. Hazleton and he gave me a rather liberal supply of stores as things are these days and promised to send more as soon as his dispenser was ready to pack them. Dispenser sick at present. Lt-Col. McEachern had promised some $55 for sodium sulphate purchased, so I gave him that out of my money held for such contingencies.

Cpl Hood had been returned from Chungkai and reported that the first death of our 1,000 men known was VX 23560, Private Oldham, G.F., brother of Slappy. He died of dysentery. He had a big funeral with some 70 Australians present. One other Oldham boy was drowned in Java so it is very sad for 'Slappy'.

I had some welcome dental work done by Jim Finnimore, also contacted Capt. Newton about X [wireless], stores and other things. Tarsau actually a filthy hole – insanitary – open trench latrines and filth all over the place. A good place to escape from really.

17 May 1943

Up early to return with Haruyama at 0800 hours but no sign of the lorry. Tadano who is *socho* in charge of the HQ squad was out in the square with two big squads of Nips putting them through the morning shinto pep arrangement. He interrupted the procedure to loudly call out 'Dunropo' and I saluted and smiled.

I returned with the following medical stores:

Test tubes 3	Bandages 4 in. 12
Ac. Glacial acetic ½ fl. oz.	Bandages 3 in. 20
Argyrol Bottle with 16 Tabs.	Triangular Bandage 6
M. & B. 693 Tabs. 200	Cotton wool 1 lb
Tab. Sulphomilomide 100	Lint 4 lb
Plasmoquine Tabs. 100	Water proof sheeting
Tannic acid 1 lb	Hot water bag 1
Zinc oxide 1 lb	Kramer wire pieces 5
Chlorosol 1 lb	Flannel (for formentation)
	Mosquito Cream 7 lb
	Mag. Sulph. 10 lb

News X [wireless] Confirm the fall of all Tunisia. The Russians have made an advance on the Donets front, a break through on a seventeen-mile front Smolensk and Novorisock captured. Discussion in the *Bangkok Chronicle* as to whether an offensive will not be speeded up before 1944!

Maj. Wearne and W/O Shea today found a track from the railway works to the old barge point, the English river camp. Men can go down for stores after work, each man to receive two eggs for the trip. Wood-carrying is very difficult. Lt Airey's cooks cut what they can during the day and about 50–200 of the working party coming in are required to carry it in. More N economy of labour! Pay was received in bulk for O, P and S battalions. The rest of S Bn is at Maj. Schneider's camp. Maj. Morrison and the new men across our creek are under the engineers and now have nothing to do with us. Nevertheless, we have to surreptitiously feed them and they use our showers.

18 May 1943

Maj. Greiner to Konyu with a small party to unload and count eggs etc. at the barge. In the evening 4,710 eggs were collected by the party of 30 volunteers under W/O Shea from the railway. These men went by the new bush track. The unloading party handled about 15,000 eggs in all. In the afternoon, at the request of Capt. Parker, I went to Maj. Quick's camp at about 5 kilometre mark to see a sick surgical case: an English soldier 27 years of age, grossly undernourished, almost to a skeleton, with a history of recurrent attacks of diarrhoea (but never blood in the motions), usual colicky abdominal pain, but last night terribly severe pain in the right lower abdomen and the abdomen in general. His temperature was 99.5° F; pulse 140 with poor volume. His heart action not very vigorous. His tongue was brown and furred and dry. He was dehydrated and had the stamp of impending death on his face. His abdomen showed gross rigidity and tenderness, maximum in the right lower abdomen. Quite definitely general peritonitis. Although a terribly bad risk, it was considered necessary to at least put a drain into the abdomen. Accordingly, a rapid preparation was made for operation. Lawrence and Taylor, who accompanied me, were doing yeoman work.

The operation began at 1930 hours. The patient was very sick throughout and his condition was poor after the operation. To my regret he died one hour later, although it was really merciful that he did. His condition was quite hopeless, and the operation was really a forlorn hope. I stressed before the operation how slender the chance was; he was seen by a chaplain and made his will. The spirit of this lad was excellent and illustrated that all the heart in the world will not serve when the body has been starved and broken and become diseased, owing to the methods of our deplorable hosts. These days, in which I see men being progressively broken into emaciated, pitiful wrecks, bloated with beriberi, terribly reduced with pellagra, dysentry and malaria, and covered with disgusting sores, a searing hate arises in me whenever I see a Nip. Disgusting, deplorable, hateful troop of men – apes. It is a bitter lesson to all of us not to surrender to these beasts while there is still life in one's body. It is squalor and degradation of body and mind. I could never go through it again.

The hospital figures are being steadily ground down thanks to the inhuman qualities of Okada who seems positively to gloat over human suffering.

The nominal role of all O, P and S battalion personnel is required, allegedly in connection with the sorting of mail. As would be expected, the Nips are not even faintly interested in the delivery of mail, which in this country is entirely haphazard. A few people are receiving letters but this seems always to be due to someone pinching a bundle from the central dump for people they know are forward. Most stupid rumours persist that O and P battalions are going back to 'rest'. Even Maj. Wearne has this damn silly idea in his head. I feel I know Nip ruthlessness better than that.

19 May 1943

A letter was received from Maj. Moon. He has 4 RAMC and 4 Dutch medical officers, RAMC orderlies and approximately 500 patients which he expects to rise to 1,000 or 1,500 shortly. The food position is better but it is very much a prison hospital and he cannot get out to buy stores. The financial position is not good and he asks us at all costs to continue giving fellows going down a little money. A prince of fellows, our Arthur!

Maj. Greiner again to Konyu and with the help of another volunteer party of drillers secured 4,560 eggs. Eggs are simply vital to the health of the camp.

Osuki Chui today said that he would return our 800 ticals given to him for the cows and we could kill one cow per day. Five kilos of meat to go to the IJA. During the day, the expected party to take up quarters across the creek arrived under Maj. Gaskill. Many Java officers and men were amongst these, including Captain Rees, and F/O Park, all members of my staff at Bandoeng Hospital.

20 May 1943

Heavy rain yesterday afternoon and most of last night, and the morning work parade was held in complete obscurity of dark and low-lying clouds. Our quarters are miserable enough, but the newcomers have tents with only one thin fly and one is drenched to the bone night and day. Okada, as usual, demanded extra hospital discharges last night but was defeated by a firm front. Maj. Greiner and party to Konyu again: 5,310 eggs were brought in. Work figures at 690 – it does not seem likely that even Nipponese ruthlessness will produce 700. There were unconfirmed rumours of cholera to the north.

21 May 1943

Capt. Allen and Sgt Page to Konyu with a load of baskets for carrying parties. All eggs now collected so that remaining articles, sugar, white-bait, salt, peanuts collected by thirty men of No. 5 party. Sixty men from No. 1 and 60 men from No. 5 have been employed in this porterage work for the last three days. Maj. Gaskill called and reported they are told nothing, promised everything, given nothing and generally pushed around with typical unreasoning brutality.

Maj. Corlette is down with malaria; I still feel very weak but am able to carry on. Work at present is extremely heavy, what with the pouring rain all day forcing one to go from tent to tent under wet and miserable, overcrowded conditions. Smooth organisation of sick inspection is impossible. Most of the day is consumed in seeing over 200 hospital patients and fixing discharges. At 1700 hours a sick parade commences but as the parties are frequently now not in until 2000 hours, one sees sick in drips and drabs until as late as 2130 even, in dark and pouring rain by candlelight. The wretched state of the sick and the inability to admit many poor wretches to hospital is getting completely on my nerves. I am ashamed of my irritability. The avitaminosis position is improved by the arrival of eggs. Beriberi is now rampant and a great number of men have frank pellagra rashes. I am also worried about amoebic dysentry and the absence of drugs to treat it. We are no longer getting the prompt response of dysentery to M. & B. 693 and I suspect these are many cases of amoebic. Collecting of wood for cooking is now a battalion fatigue as cookhouse men cannot manage it. No men extracted from the camp this evening. Work figures: 690.

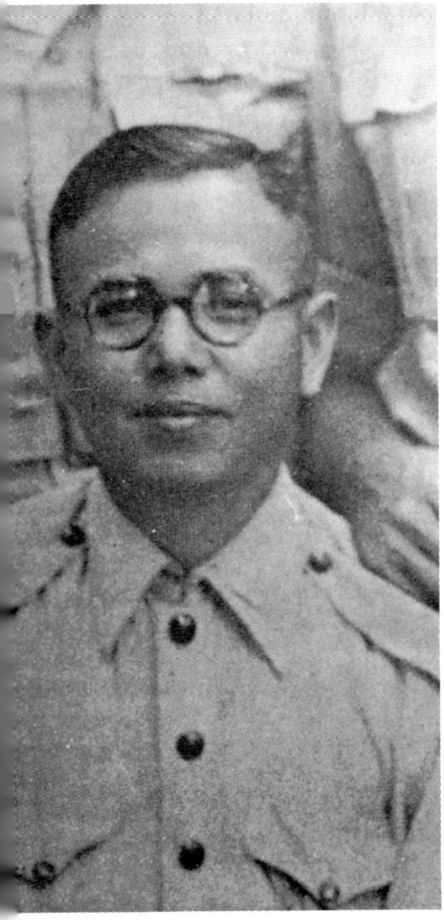

65 Boon Pong Sirivejjaphand as we viewed him trading on the Kwai Noi

66 Boon Pong with Ron Allanson after the war at Boon Pong Bus Co., Bangkok

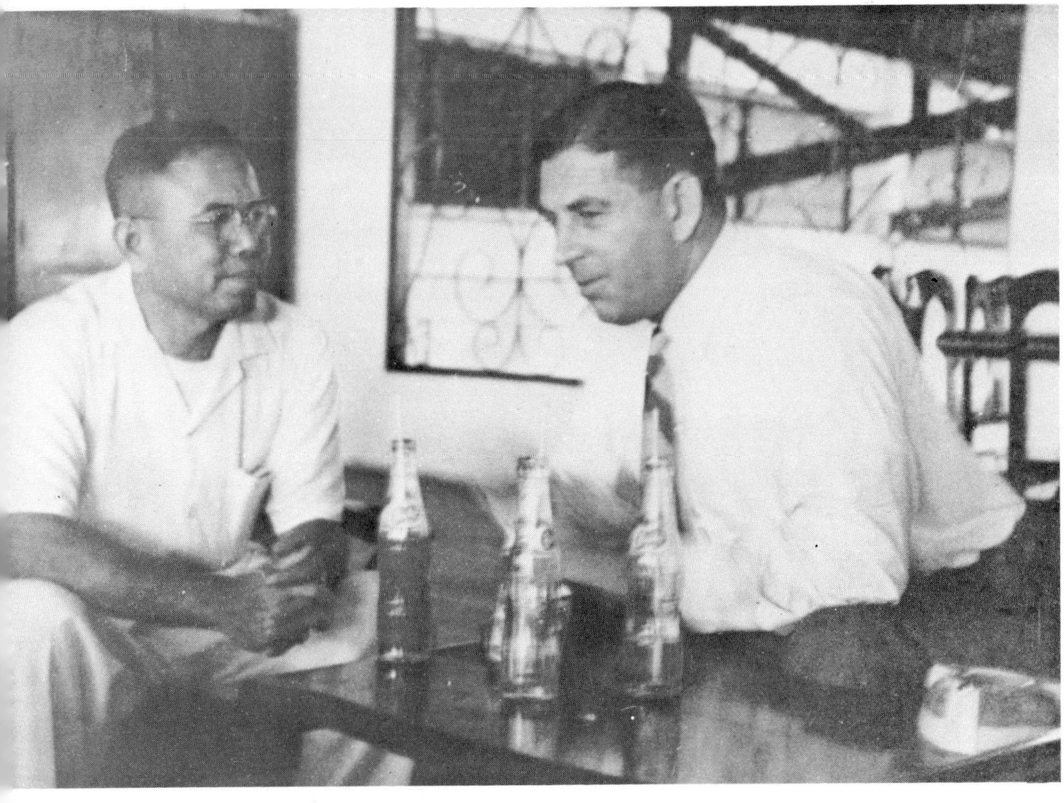

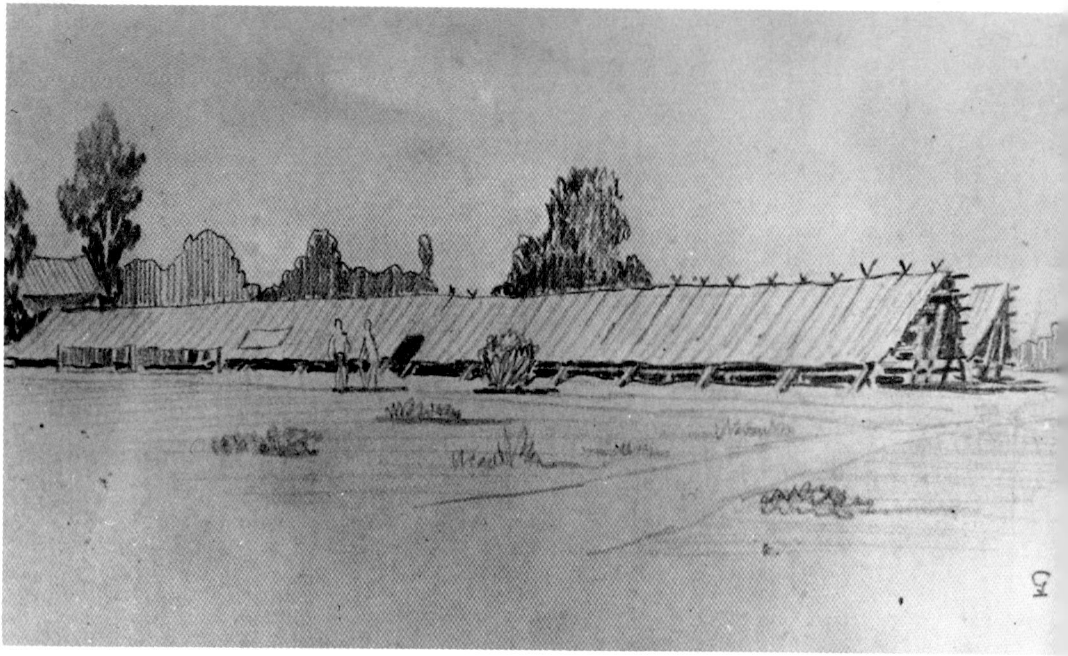

67 Original hospital huts, Chungkai (*S. Gimson*)

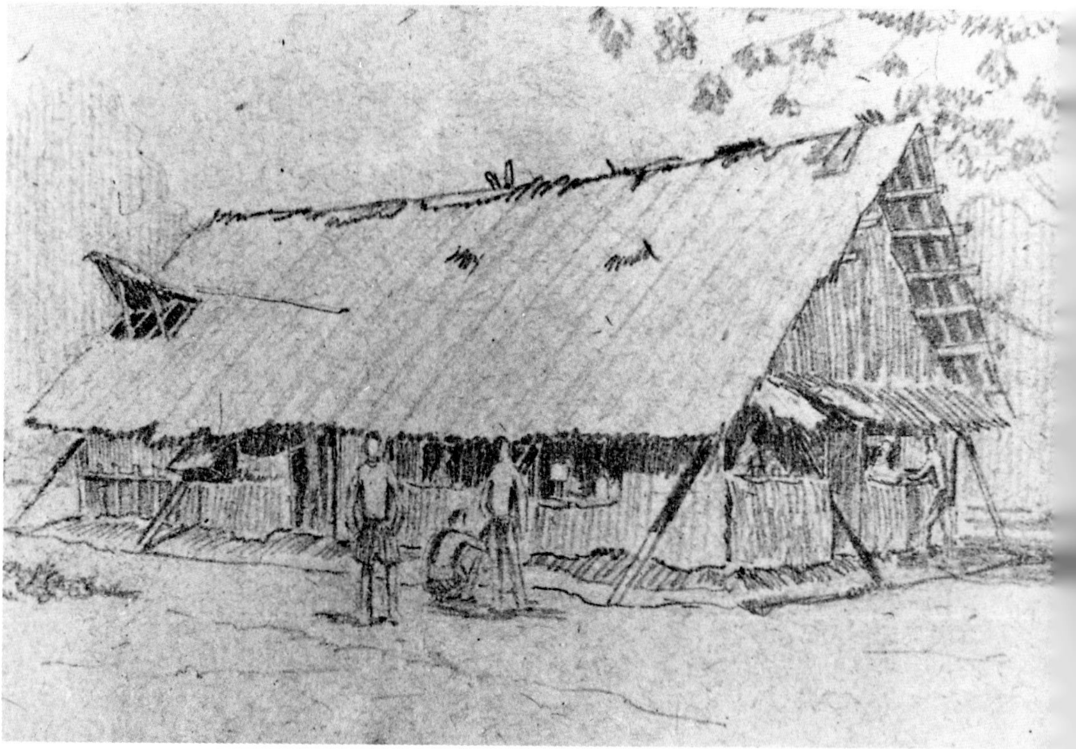

68 New hospital centre, Chungkai: from left, theatre, blood transfusion, dispensary, laboratory, dentist, office (*S. Gimson*

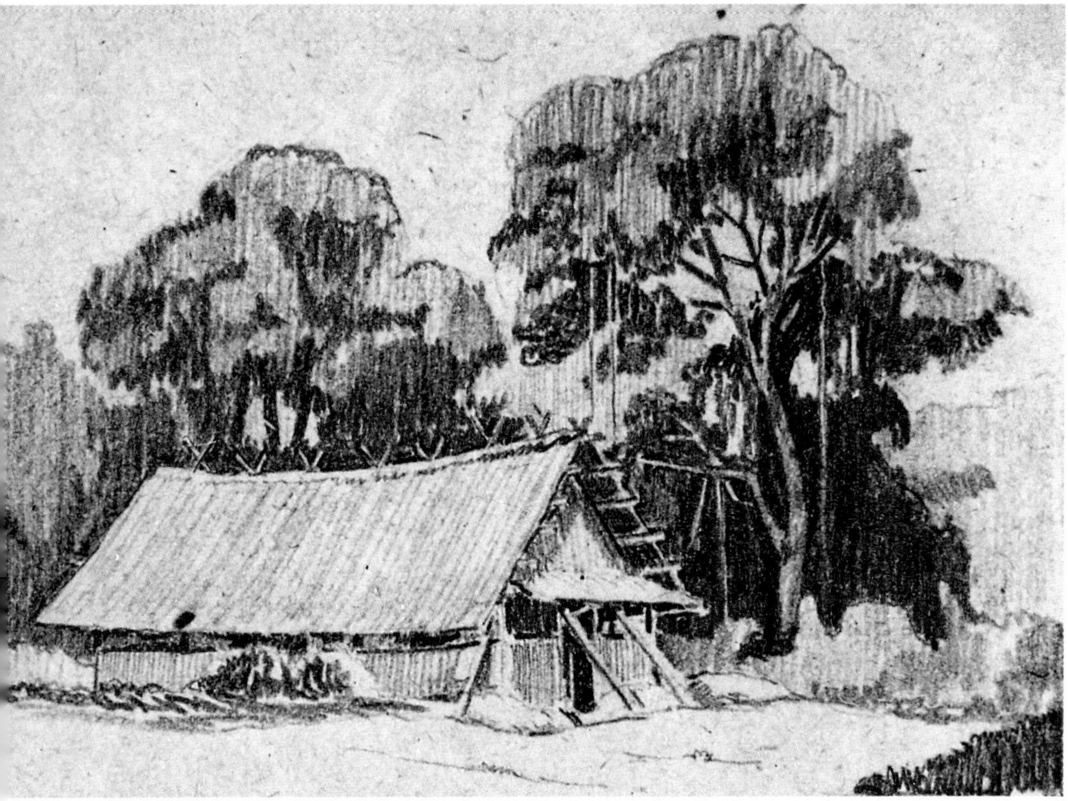

69 Medical officers' and padres' hut, Chungkai, 1944 (*S. Gimson*)

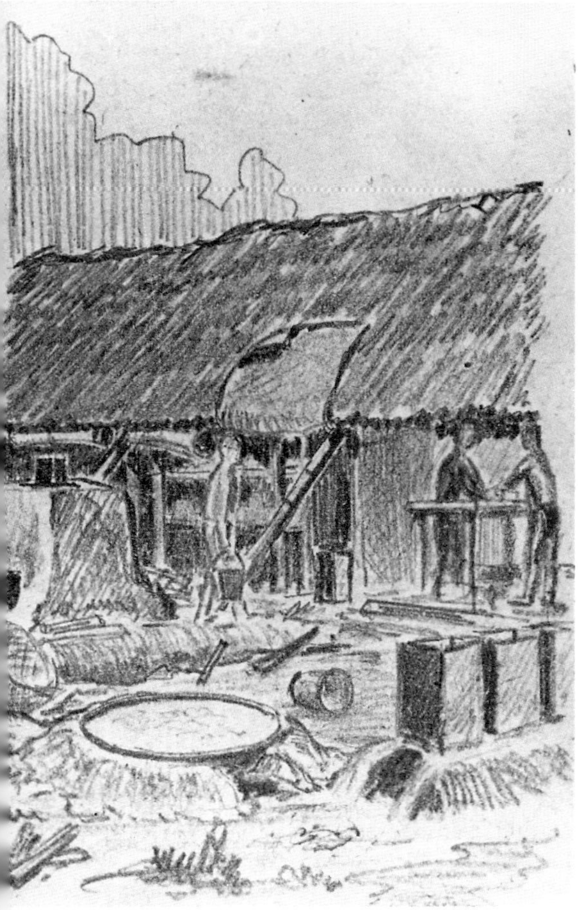

70 Cookhouse, Chungkai. Note *cwali* in foreground, left (*S. Gimson*)

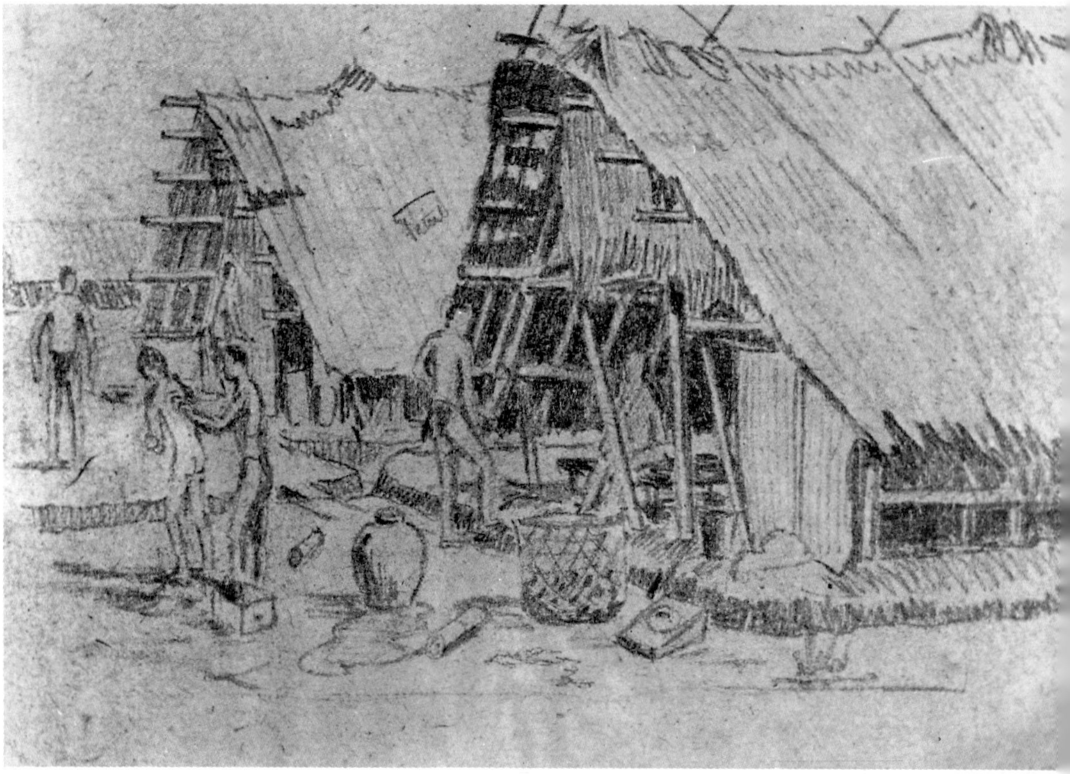

71 Skin wards, Chungkai hospital, 1944 (*S. Gimson*)

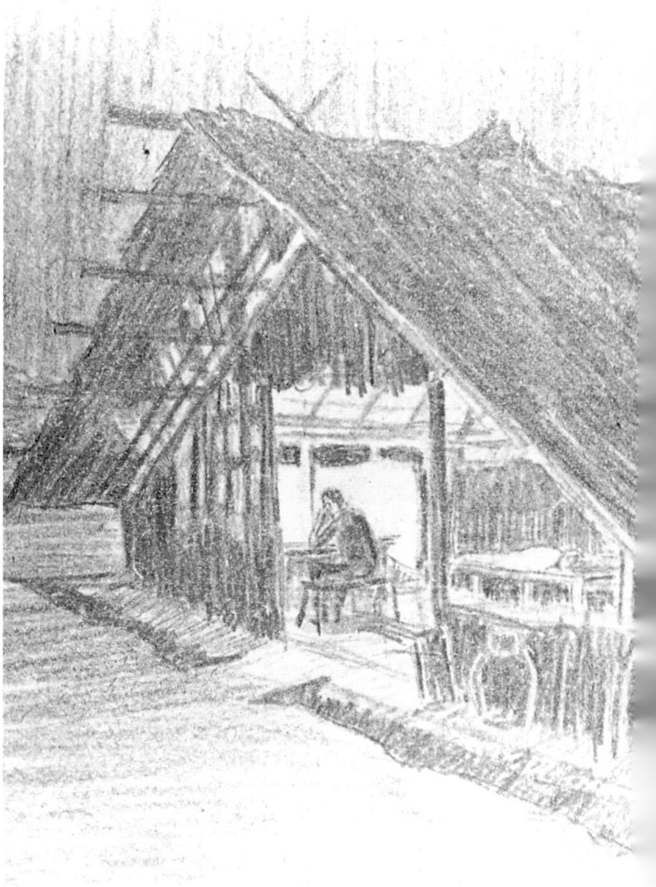

72 Night orderly, Chungkai hospital (*S. Gimson*)

22 May 1943

130 men were given a *yasumé* by the engineers today. No duties allotted except to collect two bamboos for the N cookhouse. Okada tried to use some of them for a Konyu party but was stalled off. Actually, the engineer officer subsequently complained about the men who had been given a *yasumé* by him having to do camp work for Osuki. The latter appears discomforted. The lads call him the 'Boy Choko'. Heavy rain all day and parties in very late. The roll call under the canvas-covered huts is a sea of mud, slush and dripping water.

The petty chicanery of time discrepancy has risen again. The engineers deliberately set their time half an hour behind this camp so we are handed over in the morning at this camp time and back again in the evening at engineering time, a gain of half an hour. Reference to this matter always provokes great mirth.

Further rumours of cholera by two fleeing coolies from up the line. Maj. Corlette is still stricken. Rain all night. My bed soaked as usual.

23 May 1943

Rain and mud everywhere. The troops must have hearts like lions to go out somehow. RSM of S Bn, W/O Cock, is down with malaria. No replacement allowed by the Nipponese; Lt Weilly doing his work. A party of 200 English and Dutch sick troops staging here behaved very badly today, breaking down bamboo fences for fires and taking bamboo bedding used by our men and there were numerous mean thefts of watches, food, personal articles, water bottles, etc.

24 May 1943

At last, *yasumé* day, when it seemed that flesh and blood could not go on any longer. As the troops put it, no matter how hard they are driven at the work, it just isn't possible to do the same amount in the driving rain. The Nipponese tried to counter this by working men longer and longer hours. Reveille 0900. Roll call 0915. Breakfast immediately after roll call. No wood-carrying parade (shades of a row between Osuki and Hiroda) but we are told we may collect wood for our own kitchen if we see fit – we do!

All transit troops on parade before Osuki and his rogues and they were told to disgorge Pte Middleton's watch and other articles, otherwise there would be a search. Of course, nothing was coughed up so they were all obliged to be searched by the Nipponese. This with no result but a great deal of inconvenience and rolling of their gear in the mud.

I obtained permission with difficulty for two NEI soldiers and an Englishman who were sick to be left in our hospital for the time being. Talk of appendicitis, etc. prevailed and the Nipponese were subsequently disappointed to hear there was to be no blood letting.

25 May 1943

Tuesday. The weather still much improved, thank the Lord. In the afternoon, 65 Work Party now abolished. These men *yasumé* in the mornings, leave camp at 1230 and return from 2000 to 2200 hours. Most men now finish work at approximately 1800 and, according to the difficulties of hill climbing in the slush, get home in time for late tea and roll call parade.

We are very short of funds owing to having still not received pay for the period 1–10 May. An appeal to other ranks for cash loan was very disappointing. The officers were cleaned out by raising the $800 to buy the cattle.

25 May 1943

One of our poor starving cows died at the wrong moment and the flesh was too far gone for the pot when detected. Another was just staved off from natural death by 'merciful intervention' of the butcher. Osuki Chui ordered a rendition of nominal roles of O, and P Battalion personnel with the new serial Tarsau number as obtained from Tarsau by S/Sgt Williams and Sgt Turner. An operation was carried out on Sgt J.E.C. Stephens, SX 8476 2/3 M.G. Bn for left inguinal hernia and hydrocoele of cord. Spinal percaine 12 cc. I was the surgeon. It has been difficult to do anything for these men who have developed hernia. The Nippon policy compels us to send them to work in great discomfort and we cannot arrange evacuations at present.

Stephens is at present in hospital with a lacerated leg getting compensation pay and as I may not again have good operating facilities as at present, including gloves, it seemed a good time to do this simple operation. A tent fly inner was used to exclude flies as much as possible and the boys built an operating table to carry a stretcher and capable of being raised or lowered one end. (Holes in bamboo upright to give the horizontal bar various levels.) Actually, all this took so long (as usual) that it was about 1800 hours before I made a start and then almost immediately it began to rain, spitting through the thin fly to my horror. This was checked by drawing some canvas over the top and from then on operating was reasonable and asepsis good by these standards. Bert Lawrence assisted and did very well indeed. Ken Walker and many other orderlies are ill at present.

No operation is simple under these conditions and as I said to Ewan, the strain is hardly worth the candle. Still, the team have to be kept on their toes for emergencies and a try-out of apparatus and facilities will cut the time down a lot. The spinal worked well and it was a chatty party with some spectators, including Budge Gill and Smedley, also Sakata who soon went out to relieve his stomach! Nursing conditions are difficult but he can be nursed on this stretcher.

Advice was received that there is mail ready for sorting for O, P and S battalions at Tarsau: each battalion is to send a representative for the work. I will believe this story when we see the mail.

Thirty more Other Ranks arrived at Maj. Gaskill's camp today. They are said to include Lewis Altmann from my Java camps. Considerable black market activity of late by men who stop river barges. They offer goods for sale at considerably higher prices but to their restricted customers in unrestricted quantity. Two windfalls today: 486.50 ticals, being the cost of eggs promised to us ages ago at Konyu which we purchased, and the 800 ticals spent on the cattle was refunded.

Osuki and Okada have both gone down below via Tarsau. Osuki's visit is causing the usual conjecture re movements, etc. Sakata is temporarily in charge and ordered us to remove the cow yard to another site after *tenko* to-night. He was at last dissuaded to allow this more difficult change to be done tomorrow.

A 'bootmaker' was discharged from hospital today to function as a light duty man for the present. Maj. Corlette back at work today and bang – down I go with dysentery, really quite severe. Trying to carry on and have not completely reduced my diet to fluids but have begun M. & B. 693 4 g in about 10 hours. The hospital figure is up to 213.

28 May 1943

I am properly ill today with fever and nausea and severe abdominal pain, aching back and weakness. Dysentery intermittently which means slushing outside in the pouring rain and mud. For good measure my bed got soaking wet last night. I never felt quite so poor in health and full of self-loathing. I am eating nothing, fluids just a bit, M. & B. 693 continued 2–3 times a day. I have a hunch that I have really got amoebic dysentery and have had it for some time. A mail party, Capt. Gill of S Bn, Captain Brettingham-Moore O Bn and Sgt Williams left for Tarsau by motor transport. Lt-Col. McEachern inspected the lines today and said that a party must be made available to clean up the lines each day from hospital personnel marked for evacuation. Maj. Clarke to supervise. A detailed inventory of our tentage has been made and signatures had to be given to Hiramura (the Lizard) despite deficiencies in odds and ends. We were notified today by the Nipponese by the death of VX 27889, Pte. C.E. Hay 2/2 Pioneer Bn at Tarsau, 20 May 1943 – dysentery. The pay book, medical cards and burial certificate were given to Blue Phillips of 2/2 Pioneer Bn. Pay was received by Capt. Allen and found to be 200 ticals short on our estimate. The Nipponese to investigate. Also officers' pay for April and May O and P battalion. Osuki Chui and Okada returned this evening bringing cholera vaccine and instructions for same to be injected tomorrow. Our request for flyproofing of a tent for the canteen stores was refused and we were given some fly-papers instead!

29 May 1943

Pouring rain and wet. I am feeling wretchedly ill. Dysentry i.s.q. and just able to take a little sugared drink. Continuing on M. & B. 693 one four-hourly with no effect. Maj. Corlette is carrying on with all work as I am flat out. Osuki, Okada, Kanamoto off to the 'high-lights' of Bampong. Maj. Woods is mending boots for his battalion and does a most excellent hand-sewn job. A second cattle yard was built today. Innoculation of cholera vaccine by the medical orderlies commenced at 1500 hours as work parties returned.

Fifty men were ordered to join the compressor gang. W/Ol B.H. MacKenzie to be in charge of the party. They have five buckets, three rice boilers and rations for three days. The N guard agreed to supply three tents.

Lt-Col. McEachern developed malaria.

30 May 1943

Still feeling very sick. Dysentery only slightly less. No lessening in blood and mucus. Today three doses of sulphaguanidine 3 g. Managed to keep down one plate of tapioca starch syrup, flavoured with lemon. I am increasingly convinced my affliction amoebic dysentery but Ewan advised me to hang on and give the M. & B. series a thorough trial. There is damn all in the way of emetine and drugs available anyway. Two men are very sick with dysentery, one having repeated haemorrhages (? amoebic ulcers). Kuwamura is acting as 'writoman'. Rain all day today and at 2345 hours the adjutant was called to get out a party of 100 men to salvage a bogged truck three miles along the road to Konyu. On return at 0500 hours, the men were given a drink of sugared tea and 20 N cigarettes each. A pitch black, wet and dirty night and the men came in bathed in mud. They were promised a half day *yasumé*.

31 May 1943

The fly problem is now terrific in the hot, moist conditions. The whole camp is just crawling with them, including a terrible concentration about all kitchens. Men with sores and such lesions are tormented with them. Kitchen hygiene in particular is unsatisfactory since there has not yet been a proper pit for kitchen refuse and the refuse is partly incinerated in ash heaps. These are now crawling masses of flies and require the strongest measures of attack. An inner tent fly has been borrowed from the hospital for cutting up meat, since otherwise this is a disgusting procedure. Some mosquito nets have been promised for the fly-infected canteen orderly room tent. Osuki refused a net. The camp is a sea of mud and God knows how the cooks go on keeping fires going in their open redoubts.

Three transit parties arrived today and they are compelled to stage tonight in the slush and mud under the so-called transit huts. The perished canvas of these offers no protection against the rain and the sea of mud under them never dries. These parties, comparising previously sick English, Dutch and Australian personnel from Kanchanaburi and Chungkai hospitals, are moving north to rejoin parties.

I am still a cot case, eating almost nothing, a bloody flux not much abated. Look a bit like a skeleton, I imagine.

1 June 1943

Nearly fifteen wearying interminable months as a POW. I wonder if twelve more will be all. Sakata has agreed to temporary alteration of evening roll call, 2000 to 2030 to adjust to later return of men from work. The evening meal 1900 to 1930 hours so that late parties may now get something hot. We are told that when roads are better we may send men to Konyu after work to collect attap for this camp, kitchens, etc. How noble! Majors Woods and Wearne went out to the compressor camp and found it a fair site with the personnel looking better for not having to struggle to and from work. They get canteen stores as usual. I took the plunge today and injected myself with emetine hydrochloric grains 1.* Jack Taylor is also ill with dysentery and sounds rather like an amoebic case. Lt-Col. McEachern is improving. Still heavy rain.

2 June 1943

Much better for the emetine, even today, and pains in the stomach much less marked. A blitz being carried out on flies and kitchen hygiene by Lt-Col. McEachern who addressed the troops about their manners. Capt. Brettingham-Moore, S/Sgt Wilson O'Brien and Harrison-Lucas returned today after a barge trip to Konyu and struggled through the mud. Captain Gill admitted to Tarsau hospital owing to developing a severe infection of the foot. The mail proved to be all 'big mistake': no mail at all for Australian troops at Tarsau. The road is almost impassable, knee deep in mud in parts and flooded in others. The following most welcome additions to stores were obtained:

Ethyl Chloride 1 oz Tubes 2		Chloroform	16 ozs. Bot. 1
Pentothal Sodium. 5 g No 5		Tab. atebrine	90
Chloroform 50 g No. 2		M. & B. 693	180
Amp. Camphor 20%	10	Tab. Creosoli	500
〃 Pituitary 0.5	6	〃 Stomach	150
〃 Digitaminum 1cc	10	〃 Sulphonilamide	20
〃 Novocanin 0.5% 5cc	5	〃 Hyd. Perchlorate	20
		〃 Aspirin	80
Zinc Plaster 1 in.	2	〃 Rivonol	20
Bandages 2 in.	6	〃 Sod. Bicarb.	50
Gauze (small pkts)	2	Iodine	1 fl. oz
Cotton wool		Zinc sulphate	1 oz
Sodium rolled	1 lb	Sod. Sal.	4 oz
Sodium Phos.	8 oz	Kenomine	4 oz
Meth. spirit	3	Mag. Sulph.	500g
Mercurochrome	16 oz	Pot. Permang.	2 oz
Hyd. Peroxide	10 oz	Stick eusox	1
Liq. arsenicalis	6 oz	Fe. Sulph. Exsiol	4 oz

VX 23359 Pte E.L. Edwards, 2/3 M.G. Bn died of dysentery in hospital at 1100 hours. This is the first death in our camp since coming to Siam. God knows the angel's wing must have been over us in view of the terrible mortality in all other camps up and down this line which seemed to be being built on bones. As Maj. Corlette recorded, this man was killed by the Nipponese just as surely as if he had been shot by them. In the absence of a chaplain I read the burial service,

* I collapsed under a tree going to the interminable *benjo*. The vultures gathered on the branches above, ignoring my feeble fist-shaking. There arrived from nowhere Capt. 'Legs' Lee RAMC, who felt my pulse and said he would give me some emetine. I said 'Rot – how much emetine have you got?' He said, 'I have six grains and you will have half.' I said, 'No way – you will need all that yourself.' He gallantly over-rode me and and prepared the injection, dissolving the tablets on a spoon. The following day I was sufficiently improved to throw stones at the vultures!

Lt-Col. McEachern and Maj. Greiner acting as chief mourners. Comrades of the 2/3 M.G. Bn and other units who were free in camp followed the cortège to the graveside. Military honours were paid and the Last Post and Reveille sounded at 1225. This sad affair, I am afraid, will be repeated many times unless succour comes before many more months pass. Suffering is written deeply in the faces and frames of almost everyone in this camp and there are many who cannot stand much more. Perhaps the only difference between myself and this poor lad is a few grains of emetine.

Konyu is a real camp of death these days – at least an average of one death a day and five in one day recently. They have started a new cemetery at the top camp as the other one is full and is too far away. Also, in Quick's camp there have been numerous deaths. The wet weather and exposure is an additional strain, making the work ever so much harder and the walk-out takes at least one and a quarter hours of slippery struggle, even for the strong men. Work is now finished at 1800 hours for most, 1830 engineer time. Thus the poor wretches rise in pitch dark and wet, leave with the first light after bolting their morning rice and return again in darkness after a gruelling day in the rain and mud. Many have no boots at all. The greatest difficulty is keeping clean, washing clothes which are wet all day, and the terrible over-crowding means disturbed rest.

Brian Harrison-Lucas reported Osuki suffering from malaria on the trip down. This required Brian to put cold packs on his brow and throat, etc. and to fan him constantly while he kept putting on childish turns. Arriving at Tarsau, he made a swaggering recovery and clattered in impressively, subsiding into the N hospital again next day.

3 June 1943

Still going quietly owing to the emetine therapy which is achieving the most satisfactory results and I can eat again with reservations. Oh, the depression of thinking about the things one has to conquer again. The jungle stew of odious dried radish, the stinking fish and whitebait, the coffee (so-called), and rice *ad nauseum*. At present I am cracking into a precious reserve tin of condensed milk, eggs and a little rice. This morning, Maj. Corlette's trouble began with an epidemic of food poisoning, severe gastroenteritis with agonising pains. Over thirty men were affected. Nineteen of these were so ill that not even the Japanese could get them to work. Various things are suspected: the most suspect – the tongue of a cow cured yesterday. More care is to be taken with containers, etc., which should at least be treated with hot water before use. Many of these men were S Bn and more drifted in later in the day, after a longer incubation period. S Battalion no doubt, after a long period of comparatively 'soft living' at Changi, do not seem to be able to take it like O and P. This is shown too by a tendency to lie in bed in the mornings, letting us and the Nipponese and figures go to hell. That is all very well but the Nipponese react by saying 'Produce more bodies from the hospital'.

4 June 1943

Further food poisoning today. Sixteen more men on parade unable to carry on and shifted to hospital, the figure thus leaping to 262 in consequence. Fortunately, Okada is still away. Sakata was furious but allowed the parties to proceed to work short in numbers. A N officer inspected the hospital and made searching and unpleasant enquiries as to the necessity of our Duty Section personnel. *Tenko* tonight was not held, as very few men were back by 2050 hours. Some light duty personnel not back by midnight. One man took five hours to struggle home.

5 June 1943

Three light duty men who arrived home very late last night were given a *yasumé* today. Of six men returned to work by Nipponese, five 'collapsed' on the work parade and were re-admitted. Permission received to kill two of our sick cattle today but one beat the butcher to it and was lost. All the cattle are weak, diseased and painfully thin. Rain of extreme violence after midday and the camp is a morass of mud and water. The cooks are making heroic efforts to keep going, cooking in the open and to avoid their dug-in ovens being completely flooded. I returned to duty today still under emetine treatment and very shaky.

6 June 1943 Sunday

Still violent rain. One man collapsed this morning and after much argument was taken to hospital. NX 35598 Pte F. Couzens of 2/19 Infantry Bn died last night of dysentery, bacillary. No laboratory confirmation of course. Aged 27. Next of kin, mother – Rose Couzens, Harley House Hotel, 11/12 Marine Parade, Brighton, Sussex, England. Buried 1315 hours with simple military honours, Lt-Col. McEachern reading the burial service, Lt Weilly 2/19 Bn as chief mourner. Paybook was extracted and entered in the official diary.

Thirty-one men are to go to Konyu to live at the River camp site and transport rations up the hill each day to be delivered by motor transport. Capt. Allen to Konyu and with the aid of 30 men from the drilling gangs got back 3,000 eggs and other stores. W/O Phillips went down also to help control personnel, some of whom are doing a lively trade with the Thais for their own profit.

7 June 1943

Notable for the return of those two prize bastards, Osuki a[illegible] 1 and Medical Corporal respectively. In general in disgust with life, shaved off my moustaches as a gesture. Feel rather strange without it.

Today notable for the beginning of severe, acute dermatitis of the feet. The feet become red raw with tinea, injury, and secondary infection; they swell grossly with redness, weeping and loss of skin. The poor wretches stand either in mud or water or on rocks all day and the feet never get dry. Those suffering the miseries of ever-present diarrhoea and dysentery, of course, are for ever getting up in the mud and slush at night and that makes things worse. The plight of these men is pitiful. They take hours to walk four to five kilometres in from work and just about cry with the pain of walking and standing on raw, bleeding feet. The Nipponese, of course, just bash them for being late to work or too slow. The wet season work immeasurably increased the misery of the men and doubles and trebles the labour of the day. Our neighbouring camp of five hundred odd men, who are living in squalor, short rations and misery, had already reached a hospital figure of 250 today when the Nipponese paraded all sick in engineers' lines and drove them out to work in the pouring rain and muck to the tune of 100 men, plus one medical orderly allowed. These Englishmen are frail stuff in most parts, skin and bone already and many will soon die. W/O Gascoigne and thirty men left today for Konyu for rice-carrying fatigues. They are to live in the old English Konyu camp on the river and will draw rations from the English main road camp. The hospital figure today is 261; the storm has not broken about this yet.

8 June 1943

Okada down to the hospital early on one of his mad, unreasonable blitzes. Must reduce the hospital to 200! He was savagely ignored. Levinson, a British nursing orderly *ex* No. 1 Allied General Hospital, Bandoeng and Makasura (one of the Clephan Bell, Altman, Levinson trio) and a Jew who was said to have done two years or so of medicine in London, was a rather anti-social chap who was suffering from dysentery and sent out to work yesterday in the purge. He could not struggle on fast enough and was struck and beaten with sticks by N guards. Today, he was found unconscious, obviously extremely ill, small pupils and coma. Maj. Corlette saw him and was rather puzzled. Thought of cerebral malaria, did a lumbar puncture, thinking also of cerebral haemorrhage, possibly sub-arachnoid from the injury of beating, but there was no blood. We looked in his gear for morphia. Death occurred and the diagnosis will never be certain, but an empty morphia phial was found with his effects. The N swine would not allow proper burial in our cemetery tomorrow but directed he be buried in the jungle like a stray dog tonight, thus avoiding the loss of any working time tomorrow. One thing is certain: that is the implication of murder by our hosts.

Our main medical problems at present are:

1 Malaria. Men are riddled with it and relapse frequently working under these ghastly conditions of exhaustion and constant exposure to wet; fourteen hours a day of strain is usual.

2 Septic sores and skin infections of the most florid type. These are quite evidently related to some extent to semi-starvation. The absence of adequate dressings and [illegible], in particular, increases the problem.

3 Pellagra and beriberi – the former affecting about two-thirds of the men obviously, and nearly all to some extent. The latter rapidly mounting to very severe cases now arising, for example, Ford and Sgt Little and Smith. I think that pellagra is definitely bound up with the ever present misery of diarrhoea. I suppose we will soon see dementia too. Painful feet are curiously rare in the pellagra of this year.

4 Dysentery and diarrhoea. The latter terribly prevalent and the former, ever menacing. A number of these are not responding now to the M. & B. 693. We have plenty of amoebic dysentery but amoebocide drugs are practically unknown in these parts.

5 The foot problem – related to the terrible weather and the absence of boots or unserviceable boots.

6 Diphtheria is amongst us without any anti-diphtheric serum and there are

now some cases of respiratory infection and odd cases of pneumonia.

Sick parades are now a wearying struggle going on until 2330 hours with poor devils practically crawling in along the jungle tracks in pitch dark and rain. Tonight Okada is howling like a wolf for ten more men to go out, yet already fifty men have gone out who are scarcely able to stand, let alone work. These not admitted at all.

The evening of the *kebetei* and the grand Osuki swindle. This gentleman, who raised money from his troops before leaving in various ways (kindly), brought us back 1600 ticals worth of cigarettes – 5,794 packets and approximately five months' supply at our rate of consumption. There are 116,000 Cat brand cigarettes, $2.90 per 200 carton. These are offered to us at 29 c a packet and when we demurred about the quantity and needing our money to buy eggs and the necessities of life, O. half blurted out that we had to take them because some of our pay had been spent on them! He then resorted to other devious lines of attack saying that if we were good boys and took the cigarettes, relieving the commander of embarrassment, perhaps he would induce Nippon to buy some eggs from the next barge for us. Vague threats about closing the canteen were included.

A long straf of diversion about the increase in the number of sick. Why? I told him a few reasons, feeling like a cat thrown out amongst thousands of mice. More lectures on co-operation and getting the sick figure down. I refrained from saying that a J.C. was the man required. Okada's demand for ten men was over-ruled after my sarcastic utterances that as Okada disagreed with my professional opinion he could give any orders he liked. He was in command – I was only the doctor and no doubt he knew better. After this lesson in 'co-operation', it seemed tactful to take the cigarettes and be diddled gracefully!

It was notified today that only pneumatic drillers, compressor drivers and blacksmiths would receive a specialist pay; not hammer drivers and drillers, etc. who are included in the present claim of 230 daily. The total will be 21 men and an increase of 5 c daily. 'Speedo' tactics on the railway have increased again and blows and sickening brutality are increasingly common. Hiroda Chui is responsible for their conduct which is accentuated in his presence. He frequently has been known to throw stones at the workers. So-called light duty is a travesty, the men being given exhausting labours at the end of the trek to the railway sector and are mercilessly driven and beaten. We are told that a certain amount of work will be done by the end of this month, whatever the cost, and that there will be no rest. A typical light duty day would be a track to Konyu, 7 kilometres and back, struggling with heavy stores. This would tax a strong man in present conditions of mud and slush yet it is regarded as an easy day. A very much worse fate can befall these men and as recorded above, some have been as late as midnight in getting back from work. Deaths are sickeningly common in the camps about us. Thirty-five died in five days at the Konyu camp.

9 June 1943

At conference last night, the reasons for the increase in sickness were discussed – long hours worked in incredibly difficult conditions; little or no footwear and no change of clothes; little or no medicines to treat most diseases; and inadequate rations for more than a year have left the men with little resistance.

As a result of this and a final side track concerning the men's feet, honour was saved by the Nipponese after consulting the dictionary profoundly, and producing a pinch of permanganate crystals. Thus, footbaths for 1,000 men and all to be better! I was then ordered to 'co-operate' to reduce the sickness and was called upon to accurately forecast admissions and discharges for the next ten days.

Twenty-six men on the work parade today were unable to stand on their grossly inflamed feet. An angry scene developed, with the N NCO in charge inspecting the feet and trying to make the men stand and walk. Eventually, he agreed that 13 might be carried to the hospital, the remainder he insisted must go to work but as a special concession they could go slowly and would not be bashed for being late. Okada later today came to the hospital and gave a 'pep' oration, saying that he now realised that we had terrific difficulties to keep the men well and at work. 'From the bottom of his heart' he thanked us for the work we were doing and the long hours we were on the job, often thirteen or fourteen hours in the hospital area a day. Also it hurt him, (again 'to the bottom of his heart') to see men suffering as these men were suffering, whether Japanese or other men. Nevertheless, we must keep going. If the figure rose any more there would be trouble from Tarsau and the men would be driven out to work. Please try even harder! This I imagine was sincere in the Nipponese fashion.

Maj. De Crespigny is ill with intestinal colic today, requiring morphia to quiet him. He seems to get this each time he takes Thai bananas.

10 June 1943

Maj. De Crespigny is improving. Hospital figure today advanced to 283. This morning was again a grim log-sitting struggle with men crawling or being carried to sit in front of the parade. After an angry exhibition of repeated efforts to make the men stand on their raw and bleeding feet, finally seven were allowed to be carried to hospital. The others crawled to work as best they could, some arriving back at 2300 hours and later. For example, Pte Kearney of O Bn who crawled much of the way back in black, dark and rain. Lord knows how they even find the way. Sick parade then goes on by candle light or crude oil light until all the men are in. Ewan and I take turn about.

I am much better after grains 6 of emetine hydrochloride, 1 grain daily by injection. This is not a complete course and I still have a little blood and mucus.

F/O Park kindly brought another 6 ampoules grain 1, but in view of the terrible shortage of this drug, I am arranging that this be given to another patient.

Our hospital admissions today were 56, discharges 29. Fifty-six is an all-time high. During the day, a grotesque little figure in appalling clothes with a Hitler moustache and a swinging stethoscope came to see me and Maj. Corlette. He said he was a N doctor from Tokyo University, wasted hours of our time in futile talk about my seven children and other topics. Declined eventually to see any patients because the paths to the hospital were so appallingly muddy and eventually settled down on the real business of trying to change watches with me. Wog! Ewan Corlette has found me 9 grains of E.B.I. and I am going to take it. One grain tonight then 2 grains nightly ambulatory.

11 June 1943

Okada did an early inspection and chased men from the showers, saying, 'Strong men, go work'. Simply won't tolerate men with fevers and sick men having a shower.

Lt-Col. McEachern to Maj. Quick's camp to discuss S Bn pay, etc. and on return he informed us that at Konyu, out of 600 men, 60 are now able to work. There were 25 deaths in May. Up to 11 June, 32. Six men are now spending their whole time digging graves. Six Australian deaths since arrival plus many tommies. Maj. Marsden RAAMC, AIF, of Lt-Col. Humphries' party, came down to our camp today to visit the British camp and spent the night with us. Those men in Maj. Gaskill's camp are in desperate plight. The Nipponese control their kitchen and all serving of food. They have been almost literally on just rice and they all look starved, wretched and exhausted. Another victim died today and was buried alongside Levinson in the jungle. Tonight thirty men were demanded to go and carry 50 kilo bags of rice from a bogged lorry 3 kilometres up the road. The terribly exhausted men almost reached mutiny and delay occurred in getting them.

Maj. Corlette did a fine job today. A message received about 1200 hours that a soldier had collapsed on the railway course of cerebral haemorrhage. He was brought in by Maj. Corlette and a party in torrential rain and Herculean difficulty, all soaking wet. Diagnosis: cerebral malaria and grains 10 of intravenous quinine given. Pte Lang Fraser of S Bn. He has had repeated fits today and is still comatose.

Received a letter from Arthur Moon and Lt-Col. Thomas, Tarsau re hospital finance.

12 June 1943

'O' 135; 'P' 104; 'S' 58: Total 297.

Special fatigue party not in until 0355 hours. Simply soaked in mud and could get in only seven bags out of twenty. The rest were left on the road.

A real ding dong row. Thirteen men unable to stand on their raw and festering feet. Screamed at and bullied by the engineer work parade NCO. He would not desist until three men were carried to the engineers' lines, allegedly to chop wood, the rest to hospital. Pte Murphy driven to work yesterday, today was found to be unconscious (again cerebral malaria). Given quinine grains 10 intravenously with good effect. Fraser is still in coma and fitting so given a further 10 grains of quinine hydrochloride intravenously. Interestingly, Okada has told us that log sitting is 'all right'. It gets his figures down for the day and of course he is not interested in the suffering of men involved. Nevertheless, he put on a bit of a show today, arriving with a big stick and threatening the log sitters and yelling, '*Kura*'. He then quickly settled down and backed me up a bit. The N doctor paraded all men who could walk today and without seeing a man, kicked 45 out by the simple expedient of having them walk past him and sending them to the left. (Okada to take the name.) Others to the right. Okada grabbed several men that he really had rejected. He was particularly 'death' to men covered in ulcers and dysentry and malaria patients. In a few cases, he reversed decisions when we argued, such as a man with acute dysentry being sent out. Being short of the figure he came for, he sent the malarias through again and turfed some more out to 45. I told him quite forthrightly through Brian Harrison-Lucas what I thought of this inhuman bestiality and eventually the concession was given that we would discharge some men we thought most fit but must produce 45. He left a silent, grim-faced hospital without any compliments being paid!

Drilling today was increased 2 metres. Men to work until 1930 hours. F/Sgt Fortescue and two other British soldiers died today. As a result of the N doctors' display, the hospital figures were improved by two! Figures: 598 working on the railway, including 69 light duties. The hospital, 295; 122 at Tarsau and Kanchanaburi; the Duty Section 70; Total: 1,085.

Two British soldiers, who were said to be unable to work because of their feet, were compelled to stand to attention until they collapsed, then forced to their feet again and again by blows and brutality for about an hour.

14 June 1943

Up betimes for the early morning sick struggle – staged three collapses of men who had gone sick during the night. Poor wretches, they were convincing enough – so much so that Okada suspected one of being cholera, yet advanced to feel his pulse. Gallant fellow! Things went more smoothly with Okada supporting me and six log sitters were sent to the Nippon engineering house, seven to the hospital either carried or assisted. Okada came up to our lines to tell us that there was a serious outbreak of cholera at Konyu in one of the coolie camps. 200 cases. The Nipponese are in a flat-tailed spin about cholera and some are actually walking about the camp in masks. No British are affected at Konyu as yet but some of them have died at Tonchin. This is bringing things near home, particularly as we have a few personnel at Konyu mixed up with the coolie force. All personnel not injected with cholera vaccine some days ago are to be done today, including Lt-Col. McEachern and me. The following measures were taken additionally.

1 All water to be boiled. All food to be cooked. No eating of fresh fruit or Thai cakes and other ready-made native foods.

2 All eating utensils to be cleansed with boiling water and containers were obtained by the Nipponese. 3 *cwalis* for this purpose.

3 All food to be covered by mosquito nets etc. Also, all refuse before disposal. Nipponese gave some large mosquito nets for this purpose.

4 Castellani's bottles for the kitchens. (These are to clean the hands.)

5 The Nipponese agreed to stop washing in our main water point.

6 General anti-fly and latrine campaigns. Nipponese are giving us some kerosene and oil for treating the latrines (which are of course a mass of maggots), and also for anti-malarial use (3 gallons obtained today and more to come).

Jock Clarke and Billie Wearne saw Kanomi at Konyu today and intimidated him with talk of 'chorrera', causing him to sweat freely each time the word was mentioned. Suggested that our Konyu men shift over to the old Australian camp away from the coolie labourers. Billie reports Lt-Col. Warren is ill with dysentery. With a terrible struggle and great pressure from Okada, who holds the Nippon doctor over us like the sword of Damocles, 41 men were wrung from the hospital and the sick figure reduced as above. The CO addressed the troops, telling them of the official notification of cholera – Bangkok, Kanchanaburi, Tonchin and Konyu, also a point to the north of Hintok, and stressing the orders given above.

15 June 1943

The log sitting game went on fairly smoothly at parade this morning, Maj. Corlette dividing the men into hospital and light duty at the N house. One man drifted in this morning of exhaustion and sickness, unable to get home last night so pulled a couple of sacks over himself and slept out on the transit road. He made his way back early this morning and was admitted to hospital. Maj. Corlette has done a splendid job on Lang Fraser; the lad seems to be coming round. Murphy of O battalion, the other cerebral malaria, is doing well too. Such splendid work atones for our three deaths recently.

Camp hygiene has improved greatly since the cholera drive and the co-operation of the Nips. Nipponese are letting up a little on the English camp after their six deaths recently. At present, only 150 are going out to work after the 500. This is an example of how inefficient brutality leads to very poor economy. F/O Bainbridge of Makasura camp is with them now. Nipponese camps in Thailand may truly be said to be camps of disease, misery and death.

Yesterday, pay was received for the transit from Changi to Konyu, also for the period 1–10 May. This pay was short and it was found that all inside Duty Section workers, except officers, were on old rates of pay: W/O 20c; NCOs 15c; Lance Corporals and privates 10c. We have decided to bring the pay for these men up to the standard of the others from our own resources.

All day, all available officers and men in the camp are employed on essential camp maintenance work, digging refuse pits, latrines, etc. Even hospital patients have had to do some of this work.

13 June 1943

WX 4131 Pte R.J. Watson of 2/3 M.G. Bn died at 1430 hours in the hospital today from dysentery. He was buried with military honours in No. 13 grave in our cemetry. Lt-Col. McEachern conducted the service with Maj. Greiner, Chief Mourner. Aged 24 years, he was borne to the graveside by his special chums, one of whom could not control his grief. Okada displayed great interest and represented the Nipponese. He went to the hospital area and said some sort of prayer over the body, then called for a leaf and water – dipped the leaf in water and sprinkled it over the body with further ostentation, prayer and bowing. Finally, he attended the burial service, walking with me behind the cortège and watching me closely as to the compliments paid, punctiliously saluting. He expressed his regrets that he was unable to pay his respects at the other two previous burial services. Naturally all this aroused resentment in other hospital patients under present circumstances. Poor devil, I suppose he has his problems too.

FOOTWEAR POSITION ADVISED – IJA

Bn	*No Boots*	*Unserviceable Boots*	*Require Urgent Repair*	*Require Mending*	*OK*	*TOTAL*
O	162	103	26	291	153	444
P	105	117	49	271	154	425
S	35	68	79	182	34	216
TOTALS:	302	288	154	744	341	1085

(To date repairs to 26 'O' Battalion, 22 'P' Battalion)

CLOTHING ETC. RECEIVED

Bn	Hats	Boots	Tunics	Shorts
O	90	16	60	175
P	70	15	50	125
S	30	4	20	100
TOTALS	190	35	130	400

Cholera near Tarsau reported today; 240 died in two days in the coolie camp next to the Australian officers' battalion. Tonchin: 3 British deaths day before yesterday.

16 June 1943

The log sitters again free from bullying this morning and seven were allowed to enter hospital. Osuki advised that 240 pairs of boots were to be sent immediately from Konyu, also 5,000 eggs as 'presento' from Nippon. Parties to collect them tomorrow were detailed.

17 June 1943

Weather conditions much improved, thank Allah. Log sitting now an established procedure. Crosses 4 in × 1 in of stout teak wood were erected over the graves of Ptes Edwards, Cousins and Watson, graves No. 11, 12, 13 respectively. Lt-Col. McEachern and I were obliged to lodge strong protest with Osuki Chui against half a dozen log sitters being unmercifully bashed over in the engineers' lines today. Two of these men I attended to myself: one Pte Bonzer, very bad feet and developed malaria today. Apparently aggravated by the lad's slowness and helplessness, a N soldier hit him on the back of the head, knocking him down. He developed a sort of hysterical fit which seemed to amuse the Nipponese and I was called in. Their laughter so enraged me that I lost nearly all control and advanced on them, calling them every 'cuss' word I ever heard. No doubt the meaning was caught, if not the actual words, and they backed away. I then highhandedly got a stretcher and we carried the lad away. Another soldier, De Wyer, who was tending the fire was beaten unmercifully over the head, first with a clog then a bamboo.

The Nippon NCO with typical 'speedo' incompetence hustled the men in a log hauling party in such a way that a log went yards out of position on the wrong side of a big rock. They were required to haul it over by brute strength and were straining at the job in a welter of sweat and exhaustion when suddenly the Nip began belabouring one poor chap over the head with a bamboo. In maddened exasperation he tore the bamboo from the Nip. This miscreant then seized an iron bar and began to thump him with this and to try and hit him in the crutch. He did his best to fend this off and was then stood at attention while one Japanese punched his face from the front and another from the side. Further beatings followed when the N sergeant was told he had attempted to hit the N soldier. P/O Parkin as an eye witness vouches for this story.

Capt. Allen reports that the Konyu central camp is now one vast hospital with no men working.

18 June 1943

Two British sergeants died in camp next door last night. The party who went to Konyu for boots yesterday were sent back with Nipponese stores instead. This evening, the Nipponese are celebrating and it is a wild and very alcoholic affair with noises recalling strongly the zoo!

19 June 1943

Still no canvas boots.

I was doing the evening sick parade at 2030 hours when Pte Harris of S Bn was carried in on an improvised stretcher. He had no lunch and in the early part of the afternoon was obviously too sick to work and was allowed to lie down. During the afternoon, profuse watery vomiting by the quart and pouring watery diarrhoea. Seemed to be extremely sick on arrival with the most terrible dehydration and no perceptible pulse. Cyanosed, shrunken, 'washerwoman's fingers'. He was speechless, but on questioning indicated severe pains in stomach and cramp in back of legs. Despite his pitiable condition he was quite conscious. Diagnosed cholera and at once isolation. He passed a typical rice water stool about one litre and began to sink rapidly.

S/Sgt Gibson though not well, assisted Pte Lacey who at once took on the unpleasant nursing job. Lt-Col. McEachern and I then went to the *kebetei* and interrupted a mahjong game. This was the one good thing in the whole affair. I felt like a small boy with a big cracker in the classroom or even an anarchist with a concealed smoking bomb at a W.C.T.U. meeting. What a twit! Osuki and interpreter visibly shaken and jittery, the former building houses with piles of mahjong pieces and nervously blowing and pushing them over again. 'What to do? What to do? Okada! Okada!' Finally, they did at least ask us what we wanted. I said the first thing disinfectant – Lysol, Potassium Permanganate, Hyd. Perchlor. etc. Then more in sorrow than expectation, drugs to treat cholera, also more innoculations of vaccine. Okada recovered his wits most quickly and said he would send to Tarsau tomorrow for these. They are completely unable to make up their minds what to do about the soldiers who carried Harris in, one Sgt Hall having drunk today from the same bottle. Finally said to come back early tomorrow for more orders. I would have loved to have yelled 'chorrera' into Korean house guards' sleeping quarters on my way back!

20 June 1943

NX 35973 Pte R.H. Harris S Bn died at 0120 hours today of cholera. The tent was rendered flyproof and the body sewn up in a blanket last night. All faecal and other excreta were treated with chlorinated lime and boiled before disposal. Immediately after morning 'pap' but before the egg, enter Okada, yelling for me and all other *shoko's* to hospital where I found a really amazing 'twit' going on. Osuki and Hiroda Chui, attended by several masked and nervous soldiers and Okada, all talking at once. Permanganate solution was thrown by our orderlies all over the tent and area inside and outside and were even required by the Nipponese to throw it over themselves to the point of drowning, clothes and all! They were demanding the body to be burned 'speedo' and almost succeeded in pushing in Hector Greiner and another officer as bearers until I got things in hand and arranged for the orderlies in charge of the case to do the carrying. All other *shokos* to make a funeral pyre for cremation.

The tent was removed to a remote site for erection as a cholera tent and all bedding, 'bali bali' materials and personal kit of the soldier burned on the spot. Meantime, the body was borne to the cremation pile of bamboo. Kerosene was liberally spilled out (this provided by Okada). Pte Harris was then cremated with expediency and simple military honours at about 1030 hours, Lt-Col. McEachern reading the service. Okada, Sakata and Hiroda were present at the ceremony. The engineer works' parade NCO speedily excused Sgt Hall from duty when told of the cholera association.

Conditions in the British camp are simply appalling. As a typical example, sixteen men from malaria tents were discharged from hospital today by the simple expedient of a 'surgeon' walking in with a stick and driving them forth without lunch or breakfast. The English camp were at last given one of our cows today but as usual the Nipponese supervised the distribution of the soup. The hospital patients got no food at all all day and only on protest given some 'pap' in the evening. The distribution of cow by the 'presento' method was an absurdity. They are allowed two medical orderlies only but these are at the beck and call of Nippon soldiers who use them in the morning for hygiene purposes, according to their own ideas. Accordingly, the latrines are so sited that the dysentery patients rarely reach them. The orderlies are allowed to tend the sick only after 1400 hours as a general rule. Twenty much more solid bullocks arrived for our camp this evening and the meal problem is very much improved.

The wrestling of Albert and Angus provides much cynical amusement in the officers' lines. Albert has been silent for quite a time. [This refers to difficulties with the wireless].

21 June 1943

Osuki Chui issued a certain number of boots to river camp personnel today and returned with an attack of malaria.

Okada today is convincing the N guards and others that Harris died of dysentery, not cholera but seems to have considerable doubts in his own mind and is all of a twit with anti-cholera precautions, even to the extent of coming out on the meal parades and chasing flies away and supervising the treatment of eating

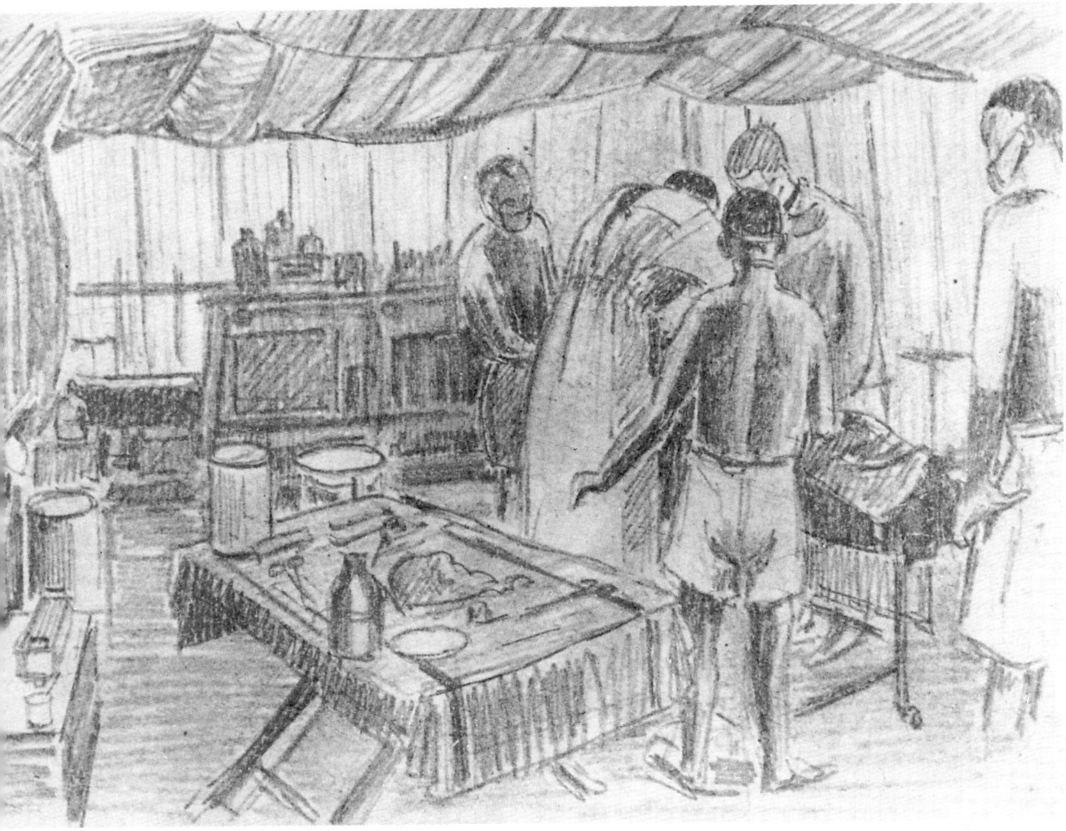

e author in the operating theatre, Chungkai (*S. Gimson*)

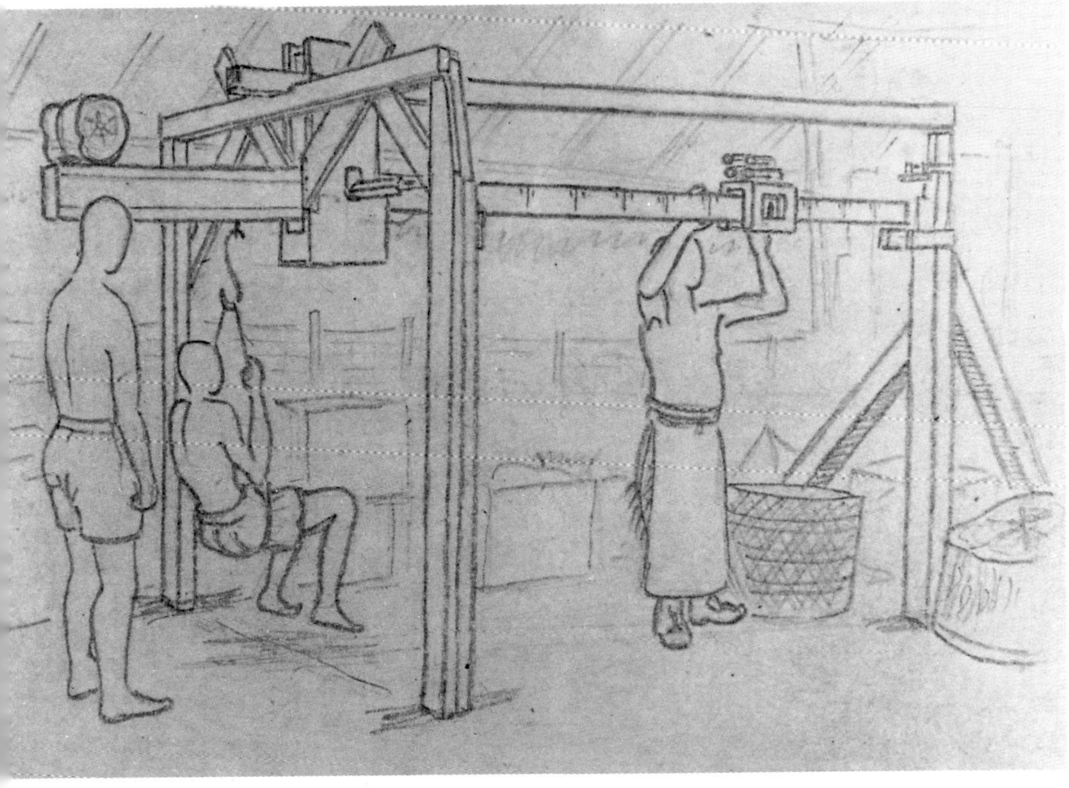

ighing patients, Chungkai (*S. Gimson*)

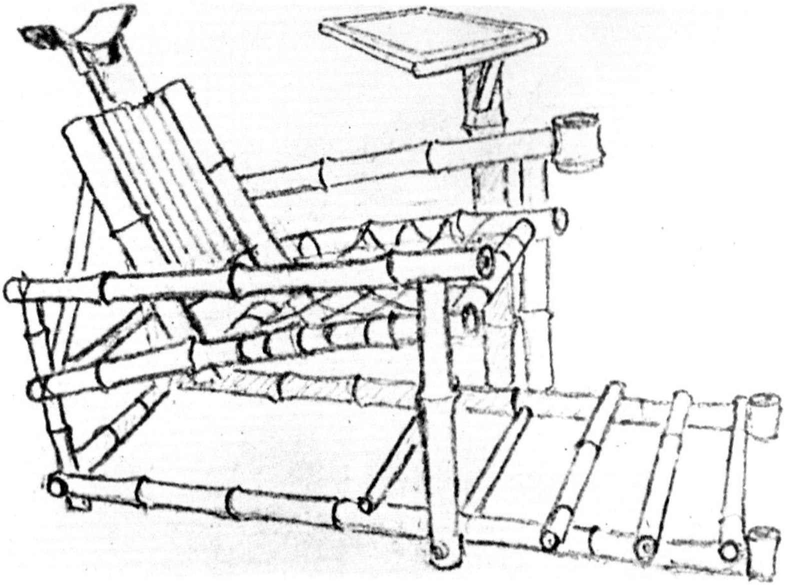

75 Dental chair, Chungkai (*S. Gimson*)

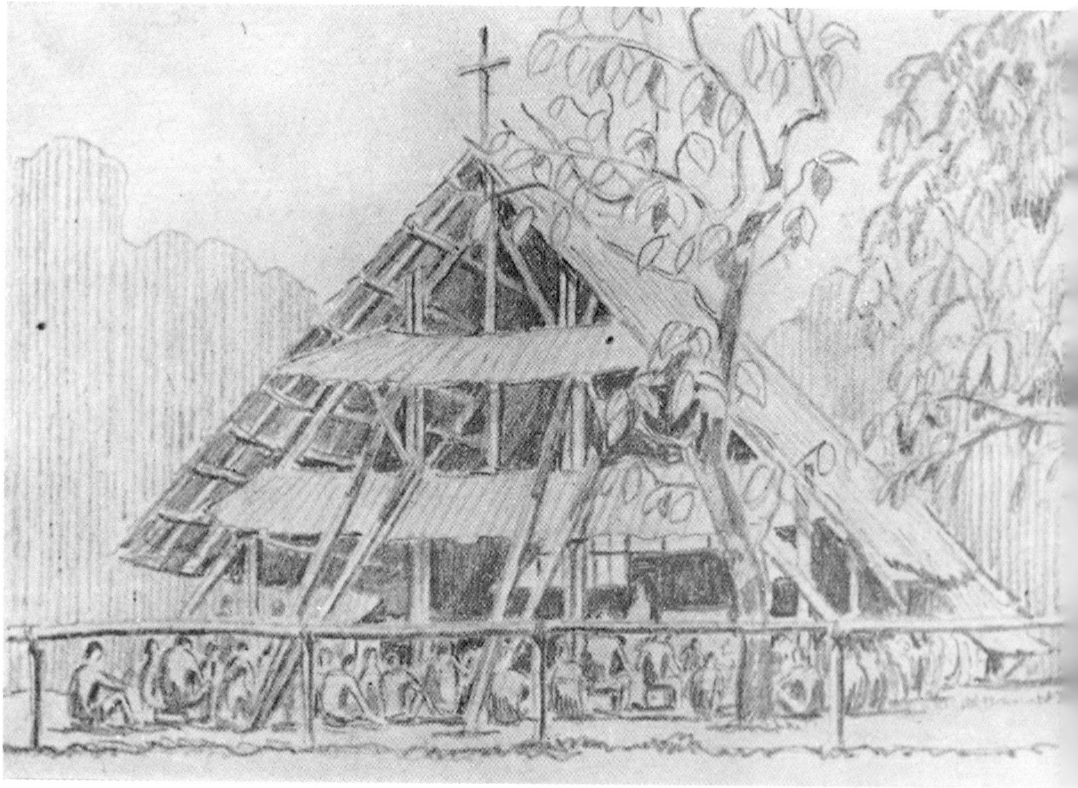

76 Chungkai church, 1944 (*S. Gimson*)

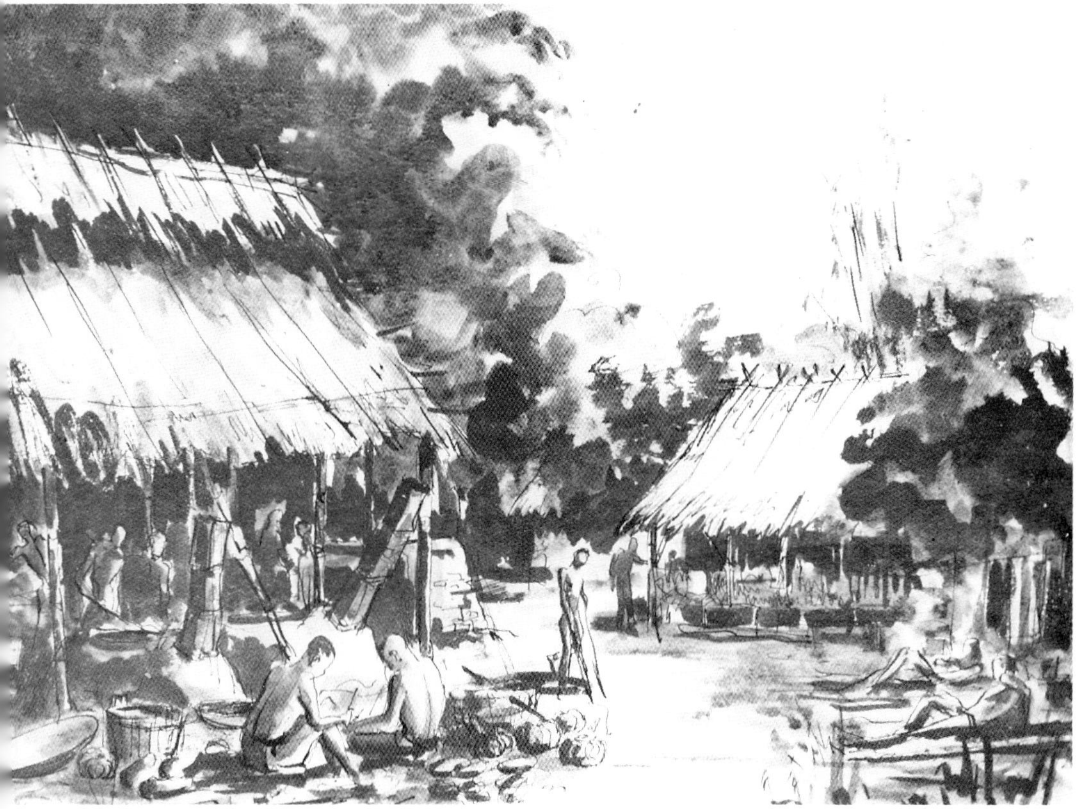

khouse and adjacent surgical wards, Chungkai (*Jack Chalker*)

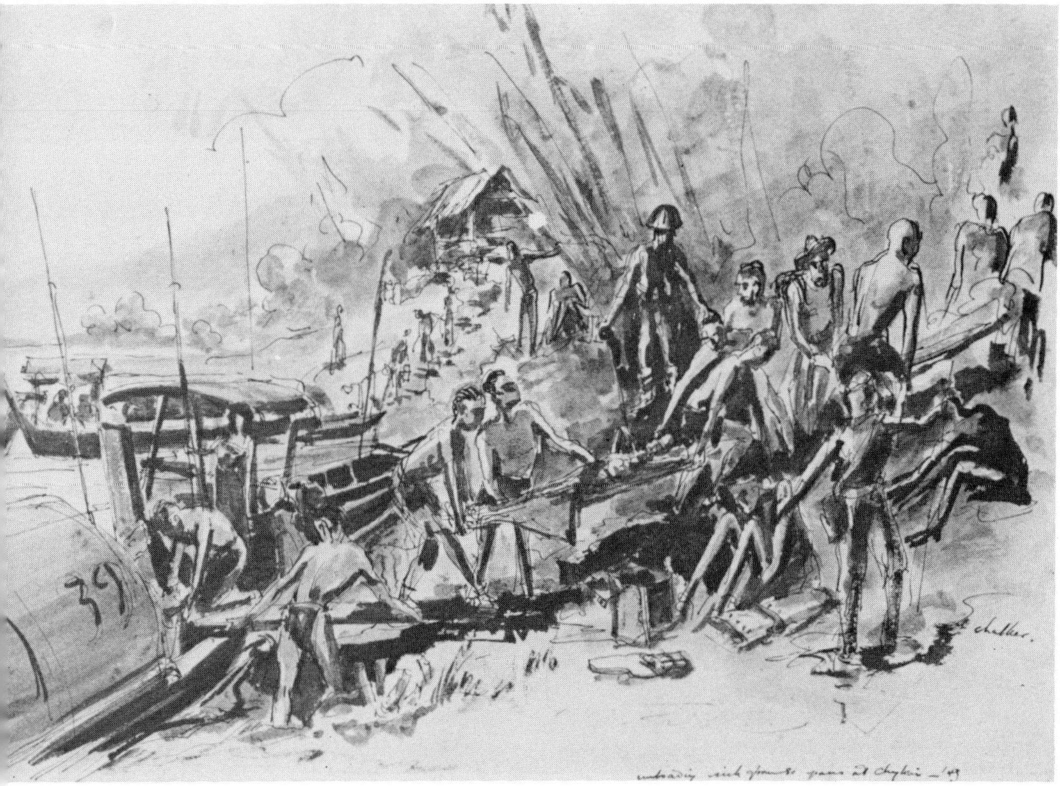

r barge transport unloading sick at Chungkai (*Jack Chalker*)

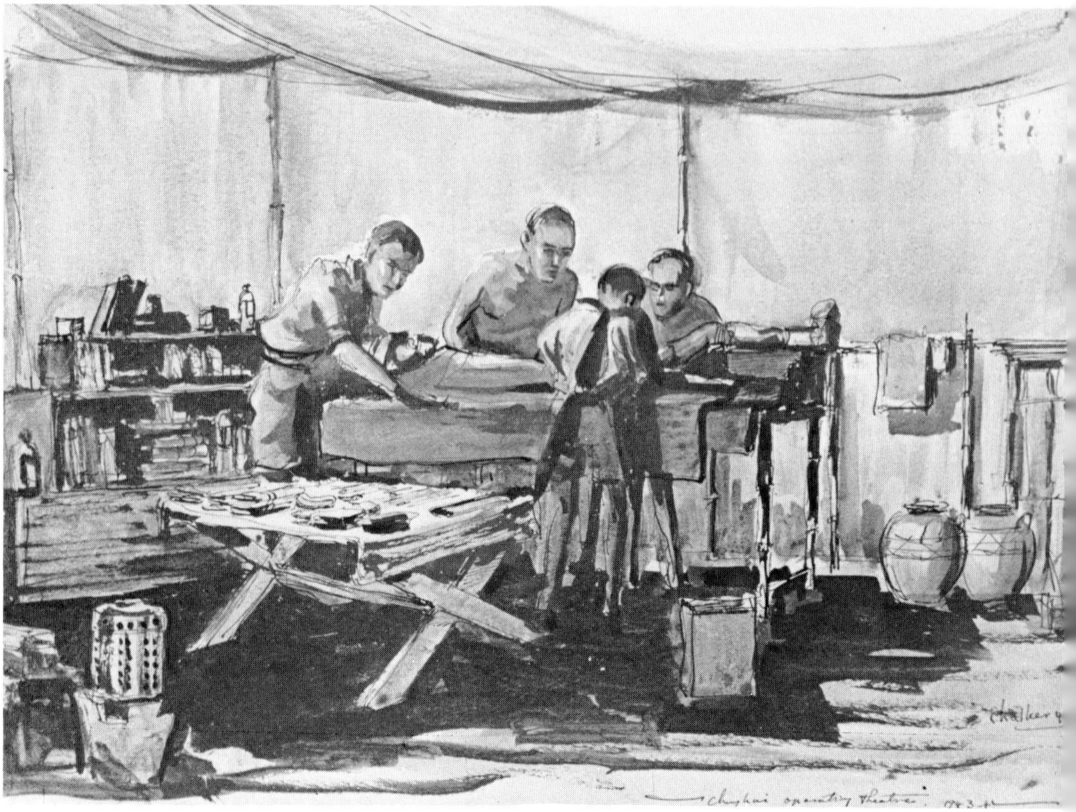

79 Improvised operating theatre at Chungkai. Surgeon: Lt-Col. Dunlop; anaesthetist: Capt. McIntosh (*Jack Chalker*)

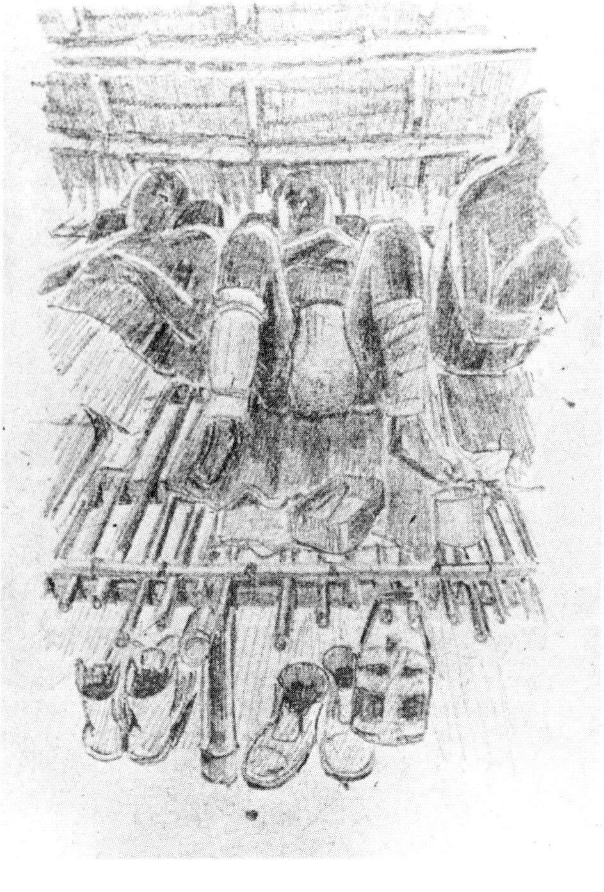

80 Chungkai patient with entire possessions (*S. G*

utensils with boiling water, etc. A gallant sight to see the brave Okada chasing cholera from the camp!

22 June 1943

The Duty Section received cholera vaccine 1 cc today and the rest of the camp will have it tomorrow. This is the thirteenth day without a break in the work. Maj. De Crespigny is arranging for collection in a suitable bottle of ashes of men cremated. They are then being interred in our cemetery and a cross placed over the site. Most of the camp are having cholera vaccine 1 cc a day and arrangements are in hand for the compressor camp and Konyu personnel.

22 June 1943 *Cont.*

Very serious troubles developed this evening. F/Sgt Oliver reported that 12 men were missing in the party arriving at the work site. There was a big blitz with mens' numbers being checked etc. This followed a minor disturbance this morning when each battalion was one short on works parade. No. 25 did not locate their man but 26 and 17 eventually did. Meantime, some were accounted for, e.g. Sgt Hallam (malaria), who was unable to get out, had checked in with the Nipponese in this camp and had been admitted to hospital, and one other man had come in with him and reported himself. No. 2 rock clearing party were detained at the engineers' lines after *tenko* time and a fruitless search went on for missing bodies. It seems that all gangs were checked and some others were also short, thus not improving the situation. The engineer sergeant came over, checking numbers against official records, and so far as possible Osuki Chui was helpful to us. A number of men, including the unfortunate Sgt Hallam who was dragged from hospital very ill with malaria (he had actually fainted on the way to work), were given an indescribable beating by the engineer sergeant and the other Nipponese. This included the following: blows with a fist, hammering over the face and head with wooden clogs, repeatedly throwing over the shoulder heavily on to the ground with a sort of fireman's lift action, then kicking in the stomach and scrotum and ribs etc., thrashing with bamboos frequently over the head, and other routine measures. When men fell to the ground, they were somehow got to their feet by such painful stimuli as the above and the dose was repeated. This disgusting and brutal affair continued for some hours altogether. After 2300 hours, five men were carried or assisted to hospital. The most serious cases were Pte F.C. Denton who was groaning with pain from kicks in the abdomen; Pte P.J. Moate whose face was unrecognisable with discolouration and swelling and lacerations; Sgt Hallam was quite collapsed with a temperature of 103.4, face grossly contused – contusions to the neck and chest, multiple abrasions and contusions of limbs and a sprained right ankle. The engineer sergeant instructed that all men were to work tomorrow. This is impossible, unless they are to be carried there.

1000 hours dramatic change to the condition of SX 6343 Pte J.V. Jarvis, aged 24, who was admitted to the hospital 18/6/43 with malaria, an upper respiratory tract infection and has been under routine treatment, typical cholera symptoms. Patient was isolated and given saline drinks, morphia 1/6th, rectal saline – a pint and a half at a time. By 2200 hours his condition was desperate and other means of giving fluids debated in my mind. We had only one ampoule Ringer's solution (½ litre). I decided on intraperitoneal administration and with the following apparatus administered it: record needle, rubber catheter, Thomson Walker syringe, then followed up with kitchen salt and ordinary boiled water at 'normal' solution strength 3 pints (equal one saki bottle) The patient's condition showed considerable improvement after this measure and a further 1/8th morphia. The boy is very run down and is one of two brothers in the same unit, another brother having been killed at Tobruk.

23 June 1943

New case of cholera today TX 1774 Pte W.R. Breen aged 33. He was recently suffering from enteritis and was forced to work on the railway, very weak and unwell. He was unable to leave camp today since prostrated with a fresh attack of diarrhoea and vomiting last night, and developed whispering voice, 'washerwoman's' hands and feet etc. He was transferred to the cholera tent.

Some boots were distributed today. Nippon pattern.

These days I spend 14–16 hours a day in the hospital area. This cholera is the last straw.

24 June 1943

Engineer brutality continues without check or abatement.

All hospital Castellani bottles to disinfect the hands have been placed at all benjos by Jock Clarke and all men are requested to use them. It is a matter for thought that the last two men almost definitely caught cholera in the hospital area.

Today on the railway course, Hiroda lined up his supervisors and read them a screed. Later we were told that the big drive would terminate about 30 June and we would then have a *yasumé* and do light jobs. Meantime, drillers must do 2.5 metres and all work output increases. Naturally the *yasumé* part of the story is probably another piece of deceit. Sgt Hallam collapsed today and apparently death was averted by Ewan carrying out artificial respiration.

25 June 1943

Cpl Ken Walker was today suddenly stricken with cholera, this following gruelling malaria and dysentery. By this evening, his condition was critical. This hit the CCS hard and I've got everyone straining every nerve. Kenny has a great fighting spirit but I feel gloomy about him.Another 2/2 Aust. CCS original, Pte Charley Mould, reported tonight with vomiting and the dread rice water motions: a definite cholera but not very sick as yet. Unfortunately, he has been working as a cook in our kitchen with *diarrhoea the last 3 days*.

Pte Fraser is also suspect and is isolated in the cholera area. Screams of bloodcurdling nature rend the air in the night hours: 'Help. Help!' Ewan's cerebral malaria case, Lang Fraser, absolutely off his head and abusing the Nips and demanding an axe to deal with them. I was sleepily conscious that public opinion demanded that I go down to the hospital to investigate and groaned with happy relief when Ewan said 'It's only Fraser'. I have made arrangements for Fraser to have hyoscine.

26 June 1943

A cholera death in the British camp today along with 3 others. Their state is pitiable but then, Oh Lord! hygiene is a menace to us who live alongside them. No. 2 rock clearing party left today at 0700 hours in darkness and no doubt will not be back until late tonight, poor devils. So the pace increases. Imagine those poor ill, exhausted wretches having to be got up, fed, issued with lunch rice and got away in black darkness after counts, etc. and to drag their way into camp again in the dark some fourteen hours hence. Some light duty men were included. Every morning, this process goes on of pulling out light duty men into railway parties. If they have boots, they are usually the first drafted. If they have no bandages, or only a few, and lack external evidence of malady, they are the next to follow. Eventually, the pathetic dregs of the light duties are allotted tree felling and hauling. (Most of them have no boots at all.) The task is the felling of 15–30 trees which have to be cut up, branches trimmed off and then hauled several hundreds of yards over rocks and jungle to the bridge builders (about 4–5 to a single log).

Death of Sgt S.R. (Mickey) Hallam TX 2361.

Facts: This soldier suffering from fever collapsed on the way to work 22/6/43; unable to carry on, he made his way back, reported his condition and was sent to hospital. He was diagnosed as having malaria and enteritis. On his own voluntary decision, he lined up with the other men who did not reach the railway that day and shared the sadistic punishment meted out as already described. He was mercilessly beaten up by the Nippon Engineer Sgt 'Billie the Pig' and his assistant, 'Mollie the Monk'. He was returned to hospital deadly pale, face swollen, neck and chest contused, abrasions to the knees and legs and a sprained right ankle. His temperature was 103.4 F., excited and sick. 24/6/43: He had two attacks of profound unconsciousness, am and pm. 25/6/43: A similar attack. Digitalis commenced. 26/6/43: Died in a similar attack in the early morning.

The Cause of Death given to the Nipponese: 'Contusion to the heart causing cardiac arrest – a result of beating by a Nippon engineer Sgt whilst suffering from malaria on the night of 22nd June, 1943.'

The cause of death is really a little vague, possibly the above injury, even malaria affecting the conducting mechanism of the heart. My theory is cardiac beriberi. In any case, he was slain by these Nipponese sadists more certainly than if they had shot him. Osuki accepted the 'Cause of Death' and said he would write to Tarsau about the incident. This sergeant was buried with the usual simple military honours at 1315, Grave No. 14 in our Camp 'Cemetery'.

Chaplain Marsden RC, who was in camp today, reported severe cholera at Lt-Col. Oakes' camp near Quick's (70 cases and many deaths). These men were also under Malayan administration and semi-starved. Pte Washington, a new case of cholera in our camp, today also acquired it in hospital whilst suffering from dysentery. Ken Walker is hanging on in a gratifying way and is, I think, a tiny bit better.

Private H. Bird (Royal Norfolks) was wired for a broken jaw by Jock. This occurred in the tommy camp yesterday as this lad was flogged about the head with a wooden clog and beaten down with a heavy bamboo until his face appeared cut to pieces. His jaw is badly mashed up and no one seems able to look after him over there so he will come to our hospital to be fed.

27 June 1943

Early rock clearing party again of 71 men. This work is dreaded by the men who naturally try to avoid being detailed. Of 10,000 eggs obtained from 'Charlie Chan', Nippon Sgt No. 2 here promises to buy 5,000 for us.

Another cholera death in the English camp today (9 cases suspected in all). Billy, Bret, Jock, Smedley are all suffering from dysentery at present. This is particularly trying as at the moment 'Happy' and 'Bish' are doing wonders with the evening ritual, providing roast steak and vegetables, sweet potatoes and pumpkin, onion gravy, 'bubble and squeak' etc. Also the evening stew has now become a thing to which we hasten home, quite thick and with obvious meat.

330 men were not home by 2030 *tenko* this evening and we heard how ten light duty men had collapsed at work this morning and had been shown some mercy because of the cholera scare. A Nip in Lt-Col. Oakes' camp apparently took the cholera to heart with such thoroughness that he endeavoured to bury a soldier alive the other day. He was first felled by blows with sticks and spades before being pushed into the hole. The Nip then insisted on the hole being filled in, thus burying the lad alive with this potential infection. The soldiers with the party refused to comply with the burial order and many were struck. Eventually the 'corpse' was rescued.

We were advised today that Hintok rations will come by road and to river party by barge. Osuki advised 30 men to go to the river camp 29 June.

A letter was sent to A.A. Moon, forwarding to him 210 ticals: 100 ticals O and P Regimental fund; 60 ticals – his pay; 50 ticals S Bn.

He was advised to use it at his complete discretion.

28 June 1943

The terrific drive on the railway continues and the 30th of this month will be the fortieth day without a break. By various Nip statements the 30th is fixed as about the end but I do not believe it.

WX 4144, Pte N.F. Dawe, 2/3 M.G. Bn died of amoebic dysentery at 0130 hours.

CO approached Osuki about a *yasumé* for the men. The latter said he would speak to the engineers but 'very difficult'. 'Charlie Chaplin' went with W/O Exton to the river camp and brought back for us 4,443 eggs. TX 1774, Pte W.R. Breen of 2/3 M.G. Bn died of cholera in hospital at 1345 hours. He and Pte Jarvis illustrate some of the difficulties of this dread disease. By working on them at all hours, we got them through the algid stage. They seemed a reasonable prospect, yet neither looked like establishing kidney function and became comatose after a stage of restlessness and delirium.

English today, 6 deaths – 3 cholera, a dysentery, a pneumonia, one inconclusive. Osuki regrets not much possibility of a *yasumé* but suggests possible course of events work finish about 6th–7th to middle of next month, then probably we move either to Konyu to build a station, or move to the river camp. CO requested to do reconaissance of the river and to find a suitable camp. In any case, when work finishes, *yasumé* for a few days then some men work, some rest.

29 June 1943

Early morning departure of No. 2 rock clearing party. The numbers this morning were reduced to 40. This gang suffers cruelly from the bashings of 'Billie the Pig'.

At 1800 hours today, SX 6343 Pte J.V. Jarvis 2/3 M.G. Bn died of cholera and uraemia. The eighth day of his illness, he was quite unconscious for the last two days and only began to secrete any urine just before his end. His brother was kept in today (specially admitted to hospital) and so was able to attend the cremation service. Cremation details were delayed until after the service and his departure. Jock Clarke took the service as he was a Roman Catholic. Because of the possibility of infection, I acted as one of the bearers and could not help thinking it was a terrible, sad and dreary little procession, dragging through the rough jungle tracks between the bamboos and dripping rain from a grey sky. The body, roughly sewn in a grey army blanket, sagged between bamboo poles on rice sacks and the dripping undergrowth brushed against the stretcher. The brother and a soldier friend, shabbily clad in Dutch oddments of clothing and without boots, picked their way painfully in the rear. I suddenly saw a bright crimson flower buried down among the green jungle undergrowth. I had an impulse to seize it and lay it on the body to add somehow a little touch of beauty and colour. However, being of stolid British upbringing, this impulse was never fulfilled. The whisper of the bugle playing the Last Post and Reveille reached the troops on evening *tenko* parade and Maj. Wearne called them to attention. This death hit me hard after all the intense work on the boy and his apparent great improvement before the uraemic manifestation.

Thank the Lord, Kenny Walker is making progress though rather like a pincushion about the belly.

30 June 1943

Seventy men required for early morning party today. Notified today of a large scale move of men to Compressor Camp: 80 now and 80 in a day or two. The CO detailed Maj. Woods as CO of this camp, Lt Weilly to accompany him, also 90 ORs from the Duty Section, cooks, etc. I am sending Frank Laycock to give three medical orderlies (Henry Boyes and Ray Denny are there already). Charley Mould became gravely ill with cholera today – relapse.

Jock Clarke has come to my rescue with a still [for use in intravenous treatment of cholera patients] and we have a design worked out. Billy Wearne is helping by persuading Okada to consent to the taking of a petrol feed pipe from a Nip lorry. This is on the engineers' lines. This was then passed through a large bamboo water jacket and the actual boiling vessel of 4 gallon petrol tin, leading to the petrol pipe by bamboo joints. Frantic work went on with this into the night and the glad news was received that the first saline made from distilled water would be ready soon after midnight. The still requires constant work in the changing of water in the jacket and stoking and changing bottles, etc. The output at present is about 1½ pints an hour. This may save many lives. Geoff Wiseman then makes the saline with kitchen salt, weighed out by means of Borroughs Wellcome's tablets. The whole is filtered and re-sterilised by boiling up the bottles in a water bath. Even with this filtration through cotton wool, some of the early samples were very murky.

1 July 1943

Out of bed between 0230 and 0530: transfusion for Charley Mould with the first saline obtained from the new still. This boy was profoundly collapsed and apparently unconscious, almost pulseless. After a saki bottle of saline i.v. (3 pints) he actually partly sat up, looked for a cigarette and began smoking. A most dramatic change in his general condition. Jock Clarke, Fred Smedley and Bill Wearne continued the work on the still all night and will keep it going today and so on indefinitely in hope of getting a reasonable reserve of saline. Charley Mould is still on his intravenous drip and is critically ill, despite every attention that we can give him.

Some 300 tommy troops moved through our camp and the English camp towards the river. They have come from Tonchin and a camp south and will build a large bridge in our area.

2 July 1943

Lt-Col. McEachern, Maj. Wearne and Osuki off to the river camp on a reconnaissance of the new camp site. O. smiting the jungle valiantly with his wooden sword. *Tenko* is becoming a joke these nights; 214 men still in the jungle at *tenko* tonight. The British camp had four deaths today, bringing their total up to 31. Some 200–300 Nips went through today. Small parties are frequently on their way through.

Bob Hadden was admitted to 'half way house' in the cholera area today, almost certainly a mild case. Sgt Reg Sheedy who had been in hospital suffering from exhaustion and general nervous prostration was admitted as a definite case and given intravenous saline.

QX 7586, Pte C.F. Mould of 2/2 Aust. CCS died today at about 1500 hours. Charley was one of the original 20 members of the CCS and was a fine little character – quiet, efficient and never giving anyone a moment's worry or bother. He was cremated at 1645 hours. Many members of the CCS, including Sgt Gibson, Dave Topping, Maj. Clarke and Ewan Corlette attended and I read the service. Another member of our small unit has passed on. The usual simple military honours were paid; an extract of Charley's paybook and bank book will be retained by me and put away with my paybook.

Sgt 'Horry' Williams went down with malaria today. Eighty more men will go to the river camp tomorrow. A N doctor called this evening to discuss the cholera situation.

I had a letter from Jack Hands and regard his performance as remarkable.

The original strength was 377 of which 307 still at Kinsayok, 69 at base hospital (evacuated), 1 death at Tarsau. Of the 307, 12 in hospital, 295 working on the railway. There is cholera at Kinsayok but not in his particular camp. Bowman, the guardsman who stayed here a day or two, is with him at present.

3 July 1943

A number of coolies moved through the camp to a site down near the river with news of a Nippon bridge on the railway collapsing last night and killing some English. This is not confirmed.

Three more English soldiers died today.

4 July 1943

Early morning party of 40 departed smoothly. Sgt McKerrow, 2/3 M.G. Bn runs this party well. Works parade was also smooth and the log sitters selected by us for hospital or light work as usual now. Dick Allen had his face slapped by No. 1 at the river camp, 'the Charcoal Burner', whom Dick had reported re the matter of a levy of 65 ticals on a Thai bargee. Osuki promptly made some enquiries into this matter but whether to try and seize the 65 ticals or on account of justice, I don't know!

Two definite cholera cases were admitted today including Pte Gray, an old ulcer patient of mine, also two suspects including Bert Lawrence and Cpl Whimpey. Bang goes my other theatre orderly who has been doing such stout work in the cholera wards. Walker and Lawrence now both out of action. The total is now 5 definite cholera, 4 suspects, 4 deceased. English deaths rose to 36 today. Forty men with two tents and a N store tent to go to the river tomorrow at 1030.

Osuki considers that we will all move soon to the river camp, site selected by Lt-Col. McEachern.

5 July 1943

Sgt McKerrow is now going to the river camp and S/Sgt Prosser takes his place. Forty men left for the river camp at 1030 hours, taking tents. Maj. Wearne and Maj. Greiner to the river camp to plan the new camp into detailed locations. Lt-Col. McEachern and I went visiting. I with great discomfort owing to the throbbing pain of a developing tropical ulcer on my right leg. Did not like to call the party off at the last moment. At Quick's camp found Capt. Parker AAMC, a very tired and run down man with cholera in his camp. He had two deaths today and said the total was about 40 and that over 200 men had been evacuated.

Konyu is a real camp of death. I found Lt-Col. Warren missing, having been evacuated with dysentery. The officers are living right up against an open latrine used by the hospital dysentery cases, so it is no wonder they are having trouble. Maj. Robertson was on deck, shaved and a little less wild looking! Hazleton was at Konyu, looking pale, yellow and very tired. He showed me a letter from Maj. Moon promising to send some Mag. Sulph. in a haversack soon; half for Jack Hands' camp and half for me.

Lt-Col. Oakes' camp is a shambles with cholera and the same starvation conditions of our tommys here. They have 96 deaths from cholera, etc. including 60 Australians. Lt-Col. Oakes himself is isolated at present as, with a blaze of science, the Nipponese arranged and took rectal swabs at the camp the other day, three on each slide. As Lt-Col. Oakes was one of the three positive slides, he was isolated while further investigation occurred. Concurrently with this scientific display, 150 exhausted tommys in poor shape were marched into camp into a cholera epidemic of considerable magnitude without innoculation. These are now dying like flies. Another similar hygiene effort was compelling all the dysentery and diarrhoea patients to pass faeces on the parade ground of the camp to detect 'malingerers'.

Returning to our own camp: 20 more cows were purchased for this camp today. We now enjoy a reputation for being very well fed around here! Osuki also reports more vegetables coming and is quite the 'white, little woolly lamb'. In spite of good feeding, very few officers are fit for normal labour. Even Billie Wearne has had a go of dysentery recently.

6 July 1943

Six English soldiers died in the camp next door today. The CO thanked Osuki for the cows and vegetables and after suitable flattery tried to get more definite information about the move, without results. One annoyance of the good meat stews these days is that many men now have enteritis so badly that any meat gives them an appalling attack of pain during the night so that they can only drink the fluid. Okada talked to me tonight, rather sympathetically, and when I told him about my problems with cholera isolation, etc., agreed that I might put the hospital figure up a little. This ended at 289.

The lettering of crosses for graves was finished today and Chaplain Marsden, R.C. blessed them and the ashes of four cholera dead. An R.C. mass was held in the Orderly Room at 2200 hours tonight, the padre spending the night with us. Jock Clarke still is working night and day under high pressure, meaning life and death to cholera patients. Officers work night shifts to see the twenty-four hours through. Sixty-two baskets of vegetables arrived today and I have to to dig up large parties of light sick hospital men for peeling them, now about 20 daily. My leg gave me just hell last night and will form a hell of an ulcer. At the present, it is all throbbing cellulitis and gangrene and pain from the ankle to the knee.

Sgt Raleigh, who has been in hospital with septic sores etc., today developed severe cholera. Cpl Bert Curry 2/2 Aust. CCS has severe pneumonia of which I have about twenty cases at present. Sgt Jimmy Little 2/3 M.G. Bn is in desperate straits and I am afraid sinking after a hard fight.

7 July 1943

The still was moved down to the creek and hitched up to the bamboo irrigation system, thus giving continuous irrigation through the bamboo. Fred Smedley and Jock arranged the site just above the old showers and built a fireplace and roofed the whole with attap. Very neat.

There are rumours that a crowd on the river arriving from Saigon have lots of emetine and so the CO and Billy are going out to contact them tomorrow. Conditions in Saigon were very good as the French helped with drugs, money, food etc. The French apparently are secretly pro-British.

There was heavy rain after lunch and the condition of the tents now deplorable – all splitting into strips and admitting water freely. This includes hospital tents. Cholera cases are now 18 with ten suspects. My ulcer is giving me hell and I have very little sleep.

8 July 1943

VX 38432 Pte C.J. Gray of O Bn died of cholera today in the reactive stage. He became delirious and wild last night. This is the lad who had a camera and films. These unfortunately had to be destroyed in a routine way.Maj. Greiner took the service. There was heavy rain this afternoon. The C.O. and Billy have been out to contact the Saigon party under Col. Hugenon. They had no drugs. They did not know they were coming here and so left them all behind. Chumps! Padre Headley who really belongs to the 'H' Force English camp across the creek is sleeping with us because the officers over there are 28 per tent. Fifty-six in two tents and these are decrepit. The deaths over there are 46 to date.

The still is working day and night, the officers doing four-hourly shifts.

9 July 1943

VX 45748 Sgt Raleigh, G.H., 2/3 M.G. Bn of cholera. A very gallant and truly fine NCO. He will be deeply mourned. Simple honours were paid and the last post.

Another 19 cows arrived today and 8 pigs. Excellent! 'Buck' Snow, who was with the ration party at Konyu, reports that some of their evacuees were seen going upstream by barge and there is mail at Tarsau for us. Don Buckley and Goldfinch said to be doing a roaring trade on the coffee stall at Tarsau.

Pay arrangements: the men in hospital injured at work will receive 10c per day irrespective of rank. 'Presento men' 5c per day instead of food. Nips also to pay 15c per day 'danger pay' to bridge builders and dynamiters. This leads to rather complicated readjustments.

The boys at H.Q. were very 'boozed' tonight and suddenly Tadano, my friend, called on me, absolutely lit up. He greeted me with boisterous manifestations of friendship and spent an hour or two of reminiscences and also gave us a lengthy lecture upon the state of the war and Nippon's legitimate aspirations to one quarter of the world. Mr Churchill was the villain. He said that he had noticed all Australians were very strong men and all Nips were very strong men. They had much in common amongst a world of weaklings! 'All OK and shake hands, if strong leader like Colonel Dunropo went home, became Prime Minister and explained these things to Australians!' He says he has greatly increased the POW ration at Tarsau. This probably correct.

Okada today says oil for anti-malarial benjo, etc. at Konyu. Eight men to collect it tomorrow. Also indicated much chloride of lime and perchloride to come for disinfection etc, and very welcome cholera vaccine for injection of personnel in the river camp.

Maj. Woods visited the camp today – he says that the Tarsau estimate of British deaths is now 2,300.

10 July 1943

There are 19 cholera cases. Men in hospital: 285. Death today of VX 56357, Pte L.E. Batten, 2/2 Pioneer Bn, of beriberi. He was buried in grave No. 16 of our cemetry. Investigation reveals that of our evacuated men, some are at Tarsau, some at Tamarkan and some at Chungkai. A few are working at 125 kilometre mark.

The output of the still at present is 40–60 pints a day if pushed. We are gratified in bringing about almost moribund men back to some degree of life. Conditions remains appalling in the British camp where there have been 56 deaths. The Nipponese have interfered in administration matters so much and there is so much starvation and apathy, that there is difficulty in even keeping up the water supply to 280 patients in hospital. Many men are lying in split bamboo right on the ground; there is much trouble with fouling of blankets. Also trouble in obtaining sufficient fit men for grave digging. They have given up cremating the cholera cases. Today I sent 50 ticals to Tarsau to Lt-Col. Harvey for purchase of drugs if possible. Mag. Sulph. in particular would be a great help.

It is interesting to contrast at present the mild behaviour of our inside guards with the screaming frenzy of the engineer personnel.

11 July 1943

Now there have been 27 cholera cases (10 mild) with 6 deaths. Those today included Fitzgerald, a debilitated pneumonia case, and Allsop RAAF, who was in a very low state of health. Lt-Col. Newey, Maj. McKay and Lt Forally of the nearby English camp called in for the evening meal. The notification was received of the death at Tarsau of TX 3464, Pte S.H. Burton, 2/3 M.G. Bn. Some white calico shorts were received today. We now require 420 pairs of boots of all sizes. Generally speaking, the men's clothing is shocking, some having sewn the most odd garments about their loins. Many have just a bit of tape around the waist and simply tuck some cloth round the crutch region. This we call a 'Jap Happy'. One or two have natty garments made out of sacking. Reg Sheedy looks decidedly picturesque in a sacking jerkin, no apparent trousers and a battered Wolsely helmet.

Work on the railway is said to be nearing completion and there are persistent rumours of movement. Maj. Wearne and 'Budge' Gill today went to Konyu.

12 July 1943

NX 68905, S/Sgt Booth, W.J. aged 52 was admitted to hospital. On 10 July, he was savagely set upon by N engineer, punched, kicked and struck on the head with a stick. Today he was required by the Nipponese to take charge of a party of 8 men to carry a heavy 'shoot' or 'skid' for logs etc. out to the railway. It was 1600 hours when they got back and for thanks, S/Sgt Booth was punched in the face and head, thrown repeatedly to the ground, struck on the head and body with a stick and kicked in the jaw by a soldier known to the AAF, as 'the Crow'.

Maj. Woods called in and took out a cholera vaccine for his men. Padre Headley set out for Tonchin. Bret. Moore went out to the river camp to help Maj. Woods. I am still hag-ridden with my ulcer of the leg and have miserable, sleepless nights. It is now a large indurated, sloughing, offensive crater but I do not think the tendons are yet involved. It is very painful.

13 July 1943

The cholera increased to 27 cases. Death occurred of TX 1739, Pte A.G. Brown, 2/3 M.G. Bn of cholera. Poor devil – he has been a patient of mine for a long time with ulcers. The following instruction received from a No. 1 to all POWs in Thailand is of interest.

'*Instruction to POW on my assuming the Command*

'I have pleasure to lead you to the charge of last stretch of railway construction wardom with the appointment of present post. In examination of various reports, as well as my partial camp inspection of the present conditions, I am pleased to find in general you are keeping discipline and working diligently. At the same time, regret to find seriousness in health matter . . . to my opinion [these] are due mainly to the fact of absence of firm belief as Japanese 'Health follows will' and 'Cease only when the enemy is completely anihilated'. Those who fail to reach objective in charge by lack of health or spirit is considered in Japanese army as most shameful deed. 'Devotion until death' is good . . .

'You are in the act of charge in colleague with Imperial Japanese army. You are expected to charge to the last stage of this work with good spirit by taking care of your own health. Besides you are to remember that your welfare is guaranteed only by obedience to the order of the Imperial Japanese army. Imperial Japanese army will not be unfair to those who are honest and obey them but protect such. You are to understand this fundamental Japanese spirit and carry out the task given to you with perfect ease of mind under the protection of the Imperial Japanese army.

'Given in Kanchanaburi, June 26th, 1943
Col. Sijuo Nakamura
Commander of POW Camp in Thailand

This surely requires no comment. We now know what we should substitute for food and drugs, sanitation, and the inadequacies of broken and bruised flesh. Unfortunately, the writer overlooks the fact that we really don't belong to the Imperial Japanese Army.

Cholera vaccine 1 cc was given out today.

14 July 1943

Osuki and co. went on a reconnaissance to the river area to select another camp site and was informed that in a few days all major construction work would cease. Except for the sick and a small remnant the inmates of this camp are very shortly to move to the present compressor camp site.

Today, I was called upon to excise an eye from a patient from the British camp. During this time, the poor wretch's boots were stolen. I suddenly felt something like a sickness of soul at the horrible aspect of everything: the lad's pitiful wasted frame, the distressing nature of the operation, the crudeness of operating arrangements and the surrounding vista of eternal rain and foul smelling black mud. Sixty-nine Englishmen have now died.

The following died today of cholera: SX 11385 Pte Williams, R.K. 2/3 M.G. Bn; TX 3526 Cpl Smith, E.J., 2/40 Bn; NX 49759 Pte Fitzgerald, W.J.W. 2/19 Bn. These were cremated, Padre Headly taking service. The cholera cases are 41 in all with 10 deaths, leaving 31 (7 new cases today – 3 deaths).

15 July 1943

Cholera cases now 36; 12 mild; 24 definite (5 new cases today).

Tarsau POW cards are being checked today;? in preparation for a move. *Tenko* was unofficially cancelled as all men were required to stay out on the job tonight and only 35 men came in to get the evening meal.

Cholera is a major thing in our lives these days. Ewan and I are completely extended, also all the medical personnel and those concerned in the flat-out, night and day production of the still. Also those concerned with wood and water supply, the digging of graves, and the collection of wood for funeral pyres.

Osuki today produced a special 'presento' of 720 packets of cheap Indo-China cigarettes called Black Horse; 48 tins of condensed milk and tins of Philippine margarine. These to go over 960 men, though Osuki said the sick were not to be included.

The men are to work all night tonight, though God knows why – probably a supreme gesture. The last bridge is almost complete and the rails are there waiting to be put across. Tonight is the sixty-second day of continuous extreme work without rest and the men are almost out on their feet. Eight men are at present receiving intravenous injections of saline and even then the sets have to be changed around. My stethoscope has gone into the crude administrative apparatus owing to shortness of rubber tubing. Beer bottles sawn off at the top, bamboo joints to rubber tubing and finally a sawn off needle as a canula. Of necessity, everything is terribly crude – kitchen salt, and our distilled water at times sediments fairly heavily. Asepsis is fairly crude. This cholera fight is the grimmest fight I have ever been in. Several CCS orderlies are now down with the disease.

16 July 1943

The weather is still absolutely foul and I think a good deal of the poor wretches out all night on the work. Deaths: VX 38410, Pte Topp, N.S.J. O Bn, dysentery ? amoebic; SX 6143, L/Sgt Sherwin, cholera (an early death after improving with saline).

Three stills are now working flat out with officers' shifts over the 24 hours and maintain an output of over 100 pints a day. The medical stores given to us by the Nips this week were the first reasonable contribution we have received; although not in any way adequate, they do at least contain some useful dressings and even drugs. Even a small quantity of morphia and local anaesthetic is included.

We were required by the Nipponese today to sort out men as follows:

1 'Very, very strong men fit to go for a long march.'
2 'Strong men.'
3 Sick men. Not better one week (i.e. to go to Tarsau).
4 Cholera sick and also 'die here' men (too sick to send to Tarsau).

As usual, we compromised and reluctantly included about 200 men as 'very, very strong', but at the same time told Osuki now that no men really were very strong.

The men out last night got in at 0445 hours and reported that the rail was now across with the first train, a diesel engine rail layer. The rail layers are a small gang of very well-fed tommies and numerous Tamils.

17 July 1943

Working parties are still being called for heavy work. Deaths: QX 12701, Pte Lofthouse, J.W., 2/3 M.T. of dysentery; VX 37693, Pte Freeman, R., 2/2 CCS of cholera; WX 5200, Cpl (A/Sgt) Robinson, W.J. of dysentery.

Robinson was a highly skilled little wrestler and a most gentlemanly fellow. Roy Freeman, 2/2 Aust. CCS horribly emaciated and run down with a big ulcer of the leg, most depressed and unable to put up any fight. Dear Nippon to have produced those conditions of semi-starvation, emaciation and filth which renders weakened frames suitable seed for cholera borne by our co-workers, the Tamils. Robinson was buried at night in the light of acetylene flares. We are still cremating all cholera deaths. Arrangements are under way for the move tomorrow. Ewan volunteers to stay here with the heavy job of looking after the sick. He considers my general run down state and ulcer of the leg would make it impossible for me to manage. Nevertheless, I have stubborn ideas of my own. I have never handed over the hard end of a job to another fellow yet.

18 July 1943

Arrangements under way for the move to the compressor camp site tomorrow. Osuki and Okada are very jubilant, obviously expecting pats on the back because we are all to stay here while other camps are combed out and go on up the railway to further construction work. Okada summed up our function as a 'shush pusher come' with actions – 'shush pusher' indicating an engine and presumably the train falling over. Australian men fix 'shush pusher' indicating the action of righting train. Then all men *yasumé*! This indicates rail maintenance perhaps, but I have no doubt the work will not be light! Today, in spite of requests for some men in camp to prepare for shifts – digging new latrines etc., the engineers have taken every weary soul – light duties and all – to do work in connection with their shift.

I have decided to stay on, despite my leg, as I simply cannot leave this awful mess to Ewan or anybody and the greater part of my unit remnant will be here. The hospital is to be shifted between 0930 and 1000 hours tomorrow. The tents to be struck at 0930 by company personnel before move, disinfected and all patients promptly moved up to the new buildings – two long barracks, one very incompletely roofed and *kebetei* and 'Texaco' Barracks (occupied by Nippon guard). All tents are wanted for the river except the actual cholera tents. (Cholera hospital to stay in its present dreadful location of course). I am to have a general duties squad of 11 men, including an RSM, W/O Topping, as Dave has dysentery at present. W/O Exton will stay on for the present to sort out the canteen arrangements and supervise recording; also, W/O Fyfe, who is in hospital with an ulcer of the leg and recovering from pneumonia, will give a hand. 9 cooks, Sgt King, Cpl Walsh, Cpl Bourne, Pte Hannagan, Pte Nelson, Pte Duncan, Pte Sidler, Pte Bailey and Pte Burns. Pte Nelson and Cpl Bourne are at present in hospital and are replaced by Pte Mitchell and Pte McScady. Nursing orderlies: S/Sgt Gibson, Sgt Harrison-Lucas, Sgt Wiseman, Pte Thomas, Pte Tarran, Pte Hanley, Pte Brown, Pte Lacy. (Nip approved Duty Section 8.) Sgt Cory, Pte Price, Pte Binns, Pte Cahill, Pte Butterworth, Pte Harris, Pte Taylor, Sapper Knighton. (Hospital patients but working and paid by regimental funds.)

Officers: Jock Clarke and Fred Smedley very decently volunteered to stay on with me and after a little discussion about Smedley this was approved by CO. Some senior admin. officers should stay on as I am very busy with medical work and the number of personnel staying on here will be about 370, a large chunk of the present camp. CO did not seem to be keen on losing senior officers but eventually he directed Maj. Wearne to stay for the present – this to my great delight. It was decided Maj. Corlette must have five nursing orderlies. Stores were shared amicably (and some regrets on my part about instruments necessarily given up from my set). Maj. Corlette will take one still and two intravenous apparatuses as he will probably soon have cholera cases. SX 8061, Sgt Little, A.J., died this afternoon at 1800 hours. Poor Jimmy – it was a relief to us all as he was just going to pieces. This is my second AIF patient to die since I arrived in Java with the exception of the cholera deaths recently. I have never seen anyone go through so much before dying. He was buried in the rain and wet tonight with the usual simple honours. Oh, the whispering of that bugle through the jungle is all too common lately. More and more fine, virile men of yesterday being quietly borne away, roughly stitched in a blanket to be buried in the jungle much after the fashion of a dog. This despite our natural efforts to give the ceremony a little dignity.

Also before I turned in after midnight, Corporal J.H. Smith died of cholera.

19 July 1943

Up early today for the move – all engaged unpacking and striking tents.

One hundred dysentery and diarrhoea patients (these separate) in the large barrack across the road; forty beriberi and other assorted diseases in the incompletely roofed barrack across the road; remainder crowded into *kebetei* (for the most part the patients with ulcers needing much treatment) and the malaria cases in 'Texaco' Barrack. The cholera cases remained in the present terrible site down in 'cholera gulch' amid the mud and slush.

This day developed into a rather terrible one as there were 17 new cases of cholera, some of these being sent back from the march out to the river camp. The cholera area is a dreadful quagmire. At night, the place deserves a circle in Dante's inferno. Extremely low, inferior N tents, all leaking. Patients lie on rough bamboo bedding a few inches off the muddy floor and one works bent almost double. The only light at night is the fitful flicker of crude oil lamps improvised by wicks of fibrous materials suspended in condensed milk tins of oil. Patients vomit in gushing fashion into bamboo containers and indeed often all over the place. The orderlies have made little bed pans out of cut-down tins placed in little wooden boxes but of course nothing can deal entirely with the gushing faecal contamination. With these intolerable cramps and abdominal pains and delirium there can be no silence and the air is full of groans, cries for relief and curses in weak, husky voices. Very little morphia is left and few have morphia now. They look so dreadfully emaciated and unrecognisable almost from the beginning and their discomfort is terrible. What can one do really with a blanket and ground sheet and some clothing for a pillow at best?

The saline drips, although they bring relief from cramps, cause their own special misery in that they necessitate lying quietly without much movement of one arm which remains extended. The symptoms and signs of this disease are unforgettable. The piteous shrinkage and dehydration, the earthy cyanosis, faint husky voice, agonising cramps and abdominal pains, rapid breathing and icy cold breath, the clammy almost pulseless cold limbs and terminal restlessness and delirium. One rather disconcerting aspect of the patient is cholera sleep – the habit of sleeping or lying with the eyelids open and the eyes turned up so that the pearly whites stare from between the lids. Almost all complain of roaring in the ears in the early stages. Four men died during the night and another one, Von Steiglitz, slipped into raving, confusional insanity.

Those brought in included Pte Ladyman, A.B. Costin and Gray. Gray collapsed on the way in and was finally collected by a party from this camp getting back after midnight.

Over in the English lines they have suffered 100 deaths in two months: nearly a quarter of their number.

20 July 1943

Three cholera deaths. Maj. Corlette has 12 cholera patients. He has not been able to get the still working efficiently. I have now arranged to send out a quarter of the still output as saline per runners who arrive frequently. This fresh outbreak makes things look pretty grim. The strain on the intravenous apparatus and equipment is now acute. Working well, the two stills can put out about 120 pints a day.

The big thrill of the day was the arrival of letters from home. The first were over eighteen months old – these June and July, 1942 include Mother, Father, Cynthia MacCausland, Mr Allen, and Helen who wrote the most lovable letter in June, thirteen long months ago. Poor darling, she would have been shocked to see me having these stuffed in my pocket in the cholera area so as not to touch them, me with two days growth of beard, shabby, haggard, growing very old and grey and limping about with my tropical ulcer burning like a coal. I have taken a thrashing the last few months with malaria, dysentery, beriberi, and tropical ulcers, not to mention almost complete lack of sound sleep of late. The letters I read later and Helen's was so adorable that I felt something suspiciously like tears in my eyes. Billy, Fred, and Jock are doing grand work. I am delighted to hear that Billy's letter revealed him as an OBE and an oak leaf [i.e. mentioned in dispatches]!

This was a really terrible day and night. Deaths: VX 13362 Pte Baker, R.C., death on 3rd day, severe case; RAAF 401054, Sgt South, E., late uraemic end; NX 41437, Pte Drabloes, S., late uraemic end; WX 12097, Pte Todd, A.C., acute algid stage; NX 35638, Cpl Carter, T.M., late uraemic stage; VX 20803, Pte Clements, E.G., never rallied from the algid stage.

All dead on the 21st, i.e. after midnight of 20th.

Bill Aldag and his party are doing excellent work cremating the dead in great pyres, four at a time. This is now heavy work.

I was terribly sorry to see Sgt South of the RAAF go, as despite his terrible emaciated and run down state, he made a most gallant fight and nearly made it. South had a charming whimsical way in his illness and enquired anxiously more than once if any Nips had caught the disease yet! In the latter stages, he got rather delirious and I overheard him gently requesting Ian Wynne to remove the pan from under him. Ian said, 'No, Eddie – you haven't got a pan there.' He said, 'Oh, all right, then don't bother to take it away! My God, I do feel uncomfortable though.'

21 July 1943

Endless streams of wretched coolies from Malaya are plodding their slippery way up the jungle road. Those who speak English frequently have sad words to say about the recruiting methods of Nipponese used to secure their services. A powerful factor seems to be starvation in Malaya since the rice ration is reduced from the normal 8 katis a week to 3. These poor wretches are dying up here in countless thousands. A number of Nipponese soldiers have also passed through recently, plodding resolutely through the mud in single file.

22 July 1943

Total in camp 367; hospital 337. Today was another severe reverse from the point of view of cholera deaths (6), including Jimmy Findlay, a quiet, semibald, sandy haired little Salvationist, a member of the 2/2 Aust. CCS. He had no strength to speak of and was old for this terrible grind out here, but quietly and heroically stuck it cheerfully for months, only to be done in by this cholera in the end, and finally so defeated as to beg to be 'finished off.' No more struggling out to work on lame and bleeding feet without boots. Sgt Cowan, who died today, was typical of the well-off Australian landowner who came away in the ranks. I was looking at a picture of his wife and children today and the incongruity of things struck me – that men with comparative peace, comfort and security at home should be obliged to go to war and to suffer hunger, hardships and privation along a grim road leading to such a miserable death in a little quagmire in the jungle.

23 July 1943

Thirty-seven men were discharged from hospital to camp duties. The cholera hospital – one new admission (Pte. Atkinson); deaths, 2.

I arrived back in the camp to find our kitchen surrounded by grazing cows from the English camp, accompanied by a party of tommy cowhands (very immature) and a tall patrician-faced, very 'noble' British major. His face was very lofty and haughty and he was in the act of having the cattle taken back to 'our corral' (the one we built for *our* cows), since 'we are obviously not wanted here.' It seemed Fred Smedley had naturally objected to the cows fouling and ploughing up our camp around the kitchen.His loftiness, remonstrating: 'But old boy, they're only grazing and won't do any harm.' He was overruled firmly by Smedley. He then said, 'Well, old chap, can you suggest where I can take them? I don't know the area.' Fred refrained from the obvious advice! He then did a recce and said, 'Well, I will take them up to this little glade.'

Freddy: 'Oh no, that is the officers' lines and kitchens!'

'Well old boy – surely they won't mind?'

Fred: 'Too bloody right, we mind!' Hence the scene which met my eyes on arrival.

The camp situation at the river is pretty grim as regards hygiene and Ewan is very busy with the sick and the cholera patients. Okada has the latter fenced into a compound and has things passed over the fence. Two hundred men are working for the engineers. There has been an increase in the Duty Section out there to approximately 70. It seems that practically no men are available or allowed to bring in rations or canteen stores to us. Men come in here to the old engineer lines to carry out stores etc. and we asked that they carry in stores to us. Stores have been very plentiful on the river but the difficulty is getting them in (1,800 eggs at the moment are practically going bad).

24 July 1943

I am having a campwide blitz on the beards and the long wild locks. Each barrack has an NCO in charge of such arrangements and there is much clipping of hair and shaving.Jock and I have both contributed our razors to the cause. We now have satisfactory latrines constructed in the vicinity of the wards and the usual arrangements for hot water used in scalding eating utensils, etc. Some hand-washing bowls are up in the dysentery ward area and the patients are co-operating well in keeping the place clean.

25 July 1943

Cholera cases remaining number 55. Six deaths were known to have occurred at the river camp, all from cholera: also it is rumoured that Ewan has the fever again. The English camp had 9 deaths today.

In view of our now very straitened circumstances with so many men in hospital, plus the recent evacuation of 60 men from the river camp and reduction in pay to the old rates, I am revising the whole policy of extra eggs and diet accessories for patients. Our present consumption of milk is 15 tins a day, mostly cholera and dysentery patients. My scheme for eggs is as follows. All patients in hospital receive one egg per day, the very sick two eggs or even three (maximum). If they have money or credit, they pay for them. Patients discharged from hospital have to buy all eggs against their money or credit. This rate of expenditure will far exceed our means and cause us to draw heavily on the regimental funds. Because of the talk of evacuation, I think this is justified. In any case, the men are at a critical stage in their health and require a special effort at present.

Tomorrow I am introducing bowel irrigations for chronic dysentery cases. I hope this measure may bring some new hope and morale amongst them.

26 July 1943

Maj. Wearne and Jock Clarke visited the river camp today. Ewan Corlette has had another session of malaria. The total cases in hospital there are 108, including 29 cholera and 50 malaria approximately.

It is reported that there is a further epidemic at Kinsayok and Rin Tin in which spots appear on the face and trunk, whether smallpox, typhus or plague or what. Lt-Col. McEachern now apparently in charge of the remnants of E, J and W battalion at Konyu and there is a general scheme that a hospital be formed at the Konyu river camp. All Hintok personnel to be either at the river or shifted to this hospital.

27 July 1943

A hard fight all day with Bombadier Tulley, a case of cerebral malaria.

I was asked to send a further 20 patients out tomorrow. Argument seemed useless as Osuki had ordered it, so I stressed that many of the men discharged were fit only for very little work, no good to walk to the river camp and that I could not bring canteen stores and rations if 20 men were sent away. Of course, they have to go.

I actually had time for a game of chess tonight. I usually work steadily from 0800 to at least midnight and sleep very poorly owing to the constant prickling irritation of my tropical ulcer and the necessity to stir up further painful reaction by about two-hourly trips out of bed (owing to the notorious Hintok bladder). The frequency and loss of control of most camp inmates is quite astounding.

28 July 1943

WX 4120, Pte Ladyman, J.M. 2/3 M.G. Bn died of cholera. I discharged 6 from hospital, admitted 4, transferred 90 to the river camp.

The ground is so miserable and slippery here when it rains, even without carrying a load on the back one gets a sensation like an inhabitant of a skidding car and much energy is used in standing up. I find the work here relatively easy to cope with at present and in contrast, poor Ewan Corlette is extremely busy. How very odd, when I thought I was doing the right thing by staying here.

Streams of Tamils continue to go north, also endless herds of cattle driven by Thais and Nips.

29 July 1943

No deaths. No fresh cholera admissions. Weather improved with the sun shining a bit; one or two downpours during the day. The bamboo shoots are growing about an inch a day in a simply miraculous way. The herds of cattle going north interest even our sick men and definite efforts are being made to grab the stragglers. One of these was nicely secured today but the wretched animal bellowed so sorrowfully after the herd that the Thais looked around and came running in with the inevitable axes and knives. Cpl Cully tried to bluff and said, 'See, this is Nippon cow.' But the Thais called our bluff by screaming even louder, 'Nippon, Nippon', and with little resistance offered took the beast away. I was a somewhat self-conscious witness.

Letter received from Lt-Col. McEachern states that Osuki now commands the Konyu group at Hintok. The combined camps are known as no. 3 camp. He controls the above camp as Camp Commander. All fit men from Hintok and Konyu to go to the river camp (some have already arrived). All sick at upper Konyu to go to Konyu River camp, the former to be occupied by Tamils, etc.

There are no directions about the sick in this camp. No new cases of cholera at the river for 54 hours.

30 July 1943

The death occurred of NX 38460, W/O 2 Jentsch, O. 2/1 Heavy Battery, of cholera. W/O Jentsch was one of those war tragedies who had been mentally unbalanced ever since Timor (he was relieved of responsibility there). He has for weeks been saying that he was going to die. His last day was his happiest, for in the morning he pressed me to promise him that I would not let him miss the hospital ship and this beautiful delusion went on until the end. He was full of bustle getting ready; his car at the other end to drive home! I called to the Nip guard room in the morning and Harry Haruyama told me to prepare for evacuation of all sick to Tarsau and make out nominal roles etc.

I was very surprised to hear today that amongst a large hospital party which had recently come up from Changi, were Bruce Anderson, Jock Frew, Drevermann and Tim Hogg. These are all acting as MOs to the Tamil camps without medical stores and presumably with little to do except to make hygiene rules and bury the dead. In companionship I suppose, nothing but the Nipponese – what a life!

W/O Charlston, who was bowled over by a great mass of rock with injuries to the legs and back, developed a suppurative arthritis of the right knee. I could devise no really effective means of immobilisation at the time in those dreadful, low, little N huts. Today we made a Thomas splint from wire, twisted double, in a padded ring and slung him with a Heath Robinsonian collection of stones for weights, cotton reels for pulleys, untwisted rope for cords, a Nipponese canvas boot and a canvas spat for a traction apparatus. Perhaps I will be able to correct a horrid and fairly well developed flexion deformity.

We officers have moved to a splendid little shack made by Jock and Smed. Last night I had my first really decent sleep for weeks without pain from my leg.

New surroundings and bed – delightful, after the constant squeaking and rustle of rats on the little canteen corner and a collapsing bamboo horror.

31 July 1943

Ewan's letter, which arrived yesterday, contained a complete list of deaths at the river camp to date – all cholera. Only one cholera in the last three days. The medical orderlies are coping at his end and he sent me three precious grains of emetine which I propose to give to Jack Taylor.

My own camp: 17 men were sent to the river camp today in response to Nipponese demands for 20. None of these are very well at all. Beriberi is rampant now! Most of these are wet beriberi but some of them have nervous signs as well. Another worry is that men are saturated with malaria and get fresh attacks with any exertion, particularly in the wet. Some seem to get attacks as frequently as every seven or eight days, even when they are taking quinine. We have no atebrine.

Personnel in camp today received 3/4 cc of Pestis vaccine all around. I don't like this as it is weeks old at least, but no harm done. Called over to the English camp to invite F/O Park to stay with us and to say goodbye to departing English officers who are moving out, when I heard that QX 6383, Lt Hutton, A., an Australian of 2/10 Field Regiment was very ill:? cerebral malaria. I asked to have a look at him. It was dark, he was in a tent but he was quite unconscious, incontinent and befouled, breathing quietly, temperature 101° F., his pupils equal and reacting to light, his plantar reflexes normal, knee jerks were not elicited. His spleen was easily felt. Captain Phillips thought he was very likely cerebral malaria and had given him intra-muscular quinine. I thought the diagnosis was likely to be correct but said I would see him, both in the morning and in the evening.

1 August 1943

I saw Lt Hutton. Earlier he seemed improved and recognised one or two people. Later when seen, he was incontinent – a sodden, stuporose bundle in a leaky tent, no-one left behind having any time to do anything for him. Accordingly, disregarding Col. Newey's order, I sent a stretcher party and just whisked him over here with F/O Park's consent. I said I would take responsibility. Later, the Nipponese consented to the *fait accompli*. I began to doubt the diagnosis and suspect toxaemia from some infective disease, enteric or typhus.

In the wretched English camp, some 70 souls are left with damn all but rice and after talking it over with Billy, I felt we must help them with rations, sharing some of ours with them. F/O Park has been left no money, and no canteen stores have been arranged.

Fred Smedley will dispose of their dead as they cannot cope. He is a grand chap to have about. At present we have quite a big undertaking in the cemetery arrangements. Bob Fox and Steve Wade are doing an excellent job with crosses, the particulars being burnt into the wood split from jungle trees. However, the cemetery area is rather small and it would be terribly hard work for our few sick men to clear more jungle. As most of the dead are now cremated, the area given to each cross is therefore only one-third of the burial area. The ashes are placed in bottles which contain the particulars written on a slip of paper. Seeing all the rows of crosses and piles of crosses awaiting erection today, I agreed with Ivor Jones when he said the last two months have been a bad dream.

2 August 1943

Billy, Maj. Wearne, received a note from Lt-Col. McEachern advising him to move to the river camp today as re-organisation was taking place. This nettled me not a bit, as of course the correct procedure was to make the arrangements through me. Accordingly, I wrote a note to go with Billy pointing this out. Billy will see if anything can be done through Col. Newey, as no money has been left for F/O Park to buy canteen stores for the English sick, who have been left here with inadequate rice and staff. I have been told that the whole of H Force receives full pay from Singapore; accordingly, my informant says, he does not quite know how to spend his money! I commented, 'Ever think of buying a few lives? I was reliably informed that one officer is saving his for an instalment on a car! It seems that Lt-Col. Oakes and his AIF officers are putting in all money over 20 ticals, however. (This reverses the Bandoeng form).

3 August 1943

No deaths. It is still terribly wet and I fear more cholera cases will crop up. The Nipponese have taken the copper tubing of one still, leaving us with two stills now. Fred Smedley did a fine job draining the cholera area today.

Jock Clarke has severe diarrhoea again and spent a miserable night in the wet last night. Today I have him in bed with morphia grains ½ by mouth.

4 August 1943

No discharges and no deaths; cholera: 52.

Maj. Wearne reports a great gathering of clans at the river camp where O P S T E J W Y Battalion remnants are being assembled and a bridging company and a composite party from all battalions. There are about 750 men at present and they will soon be 11–1200. It seems very probable that the fit men will soon move up to Kinsayok. Evacuations are going on at Konyu very slowly.

5 August 1943

Lt Hutton, who has been distressing everybody with his continuous moaning cries and delirium, has become quiet today. A ration party of 20 went to the river and brought back some canteen stores with approval at the river end. Our Nipponese were objecting but were told that no other stores, vegetables, etc. were available for collection – hence the canteen stores. F/O Park contracted malaria and enteritis.

6 August 1943

Ken Walker emerged from cholera isolation after 42 days as the first of our 'violets in December'! W/O 2 Frank Charlston, suppurative arthritis of the right knee, had his right knee joint drained. The operating is becoming rather difficult with no gloves, no dressings or swabs, etc. The anaesthesia in this case was Pentothal 0.5 g after morphia ¼ and atropine 120th grain. This was perfect and the patient's condition very good throughout. He was finally put back on Thomas splint and extension. It is perfectly surprising the anaesthesia which can be got with Pentothal, even 0.5 of a gram and morph. ¼ in these debilitated patients.

7 August 1943

Maj. Corlette is holding 38 cases of cholera today, some new; mild cases include Ernie Blakeney. Great trouble with feet in the wet – dermatitis starting as pustules, some proceed to ulcers and grossly swollen feet.

Butterworth went to Konyu today (without anybody's permission) and reported no canteen stores there but almost 1,000 sick men awaiting evacuation at lower Konyu.

Malaria is absolutely rampant here – for example, eight of the 52 cholera patients have fresh attacks. Re-infection must occur over and over again. Malaria has a deplorable effect on ulcers, which begin to spread even before the temperature rises.

8 August 1943

Off to the compressor camp with Jock Clarke. In spite of finer weather yesterday, the track was horribly wet and slippery in places. Much amusement watching large monkeys swing about in the jungle trees with marvellous agility. My leg is now healing famously and I have only one ulcer of any size. This is shallow and about the size of a shilling piece.

We thought of the jungle trail with its bamboo thorns and sharp stones as a sort of *Via Dolorosa*. Few trails have been trodden with more suffering. For months spent and exhausted men picked their painful and slippery way along it, often in pitch darkness and in rain with raw and bleeding feet. Some 80 of them died at one of its two ends.

We trod for a time along the Nipponese railway, the cause of it all, and smile with bitter humour at its crude and snake-like course. Every possible fault exists except that for the most part the rails are parallel. At times the rails are up in the air above the sleepers; sometimes the sleepers are up in the air attached to the rails! The sleepers are not even faintly regularly laid – just like so many matches tossed down by a giant hand. The rails are spiked down approximately 1 in 5 sleepers. There is a curious switchback railway effect in places supposed to be level. Often one rail is higher than the other and to look along the rails is to see a most disconcerting zigzag – a 'Snakes and Ladders railway'.

At one place, the rail is carried over a ravine by a most crazy wooden bridge which has repeatedly fallen down and is now held up by stays. At this new point, a new embankment and cutting are being built by Tamils to skirt and avoid the bridge. However, the rail has passed on and trucks drawn by diesel engines are carrying fresh rails and sleepers up to Kinsayok. In the wake of the railway is left a wreckage of humanity, stupidly broken by inefficiency and design.

The river camp is horribly wet. I first saw Lt-Col. Newey who was as usual bursting with good war news, none very likely to be correct. I found Corlette doing sick inspection in bare feet with an unpleasant dermatitis of the said feet and a rather fagged and wild look in the eye. He has had one hell of a time of late. Our officers are installed in a most roomy attap hut, all with tables between beds, etc. and very comfortable. Lt-Col. McEachern was having a malarial attack so I gave him some atebrin – also sat on his bed and broke it. I had a most excellent meal of *katchang idjoe* which was quite thick, recalling Makasura and mashed potato and liver. Meat is now quite plentiful at the camp. The smart conversation of the day:
Jock: 'What sort of a chap is Major Quick?'
Allan Woods: 'Oh, all right, but the troops have a saying: "There a back up if you're Quick"!'

Most of the officers appeared fairly well and in good spirits. Jock did a little dental work for Ewan. I gossiped and called on Lt-Col. James who was in his tent, trying to avoid the many leaks.

I saw Osuki who looked very fat but not especially cheerful. He apparently is learning English and asked awkward questions, such as, 'Shall, will, could, would, what use? or 'perhaps maybe' or 'What is difference?' I told him about perhaps and maybe with an illustration: 'Perhaps you Japanese win the war, but only maybe!' He asked, 'English lieutenant pronounced "leftenant" but American "lootenant" – why?' The boy shoko really is an *enfant terrible*!

Osuki had today donated 800 pomelos and a number of eggs and some sugar to the camp. It seemed that the hospital at Hintok is not on the distribution list for these. Jock and I finally got a dozen eggs and much tobacco and slithered our way home, slipping back nearly as much as forward.

9 August 1943

Seven of the 11 admissions today were 'cover ups' as the Nipponese were again on the war path for men to go to the river camp. They insist I send out fifteen to the river tomorrow, despite my protests re canteen and ration party difficulties. A sergeant in 3 M.T. ('Honest John'!) today admitted having gone to Konyu on a secret excursion to purchase stores to sell to his comrades at a profit. This despite the fact that as an enteritis patient, I had been excusing him from all major duties. Meantime, other men carried stores up from the river to him free or at cost. Cpl. H. went on a similar excursion to the river while a malaria convalescent and excused duty. There are a few troubles here concerning discipline. I have just to mention an 'up the river' threat and that finishes trouble.

10 August 1943

Cattle duffing is causing much amusement here. At present about six bullocks are tethered up in the camp and in the jungle and no doubt N credulity must be a little taxed as to the co-incidence of how we find one wandering loose each day. We have explained that many cows are loose in the jungle. Can we send out men to look for them? Len King, one of the world's unconscious humorists looks after them nicely and leads them around for grazing and watering. I am pleasantly surprised to see that by severe economy measures the last two months I have a little credit left out of my Nipponese pay, less contribution to the troops' fund, etc.

Mess 1.6.43–19.7.43		11.70
		20.55
		32.25
	Pay Net	38.24
	Credit	$ 5.99

On the strength of this, I have distributed my last $10 reserve over the CCS lads in cash gifts. It worries me that I have been able to do damn all for my own lads owing to having to put all my spare money into the general fund. Jock Clarke and Ewan, who recently sold watches, have done a good deal of late in a very generous way. The financial axe falls very heavily now, owing to the huge preponderance of sick over workers; from now on the hospital expenditure must be cut to 10c per head per day for each patient. We have been spending more than this on milk alone. 12 tins a day at $2 = $24. I have to cut expenses for 200 patients down to 200 ticals.

11 August 1943

I was annoyed today to find that our carrying parties have been buying goods for cash from the canteen at the river camp and retailing to patients back here, some at a profit.

The boy wizard 'X' [wireless] actually produced the goods late tonight. The fall of Sicily seems imminent and the Russians are nearing Krakow. The Nipponese are in trouble in their last stronghold in New Guinea. Also pressure in New Guinea about the Solomons which is getting strong. The RAF are doing big stuff over Germany: 13,500 tons of bombs on Hamburg in six days.

W/O Charlton's knee seems to be doing fairly well. The following camp chit chat:

'Where are you off to Ivor?' – to Ivor Jones, who has been working hard on the cemetery.

Ivor: 'I am going down to the cemetery to have a really good cry – would you like to come along?'

12 August 1943

Cleaned up the day's work early, shortly after 1200, and left with Fred Smedley for the river camp where I was in time for lunch and found Lt-Col. McEachern about to come and see me about matters of camp and hospital finance. The following grim position outlined: from 21–31 July a grand total of earnings of AIF personnel was $1431.75. This of course is now incredibly lowered by much additional sickness (the sick are not paid). Thus the new rate of hosptial expenditure to be 5c per man per day, less than a quarter of the present expenditure. O and P Battalions' – the last balance sheet shows

$4,075.17; during July, only $380.00 was received, and $2,300.30 was spent on hospital and kitchen, so that the actual capital in cash is about $2,000. The Nipponese are always about two periods behind in pay, so that the regimental fund meantime finances the group and keeps things ticking over. The new policy regarding pay is that all ranks' earnings are deducted one-third of pay to the fund. Rest of the pay is pooled plus danger pay, 'presento' pay, specialist pay, and paid evenly by rank to all earners, whether inside or outside and 'cover ups'. I discussed this with the CO telling him that with the proposed rate of hospital expenditure some sick men will die, but that this must be faced if the strain on the earner was becoming too great. I stressed the fact that 'luxuries' should be avoided in canteen trade.

I saw many sick with Ewan, amongst these, the Aboriginal, 'Pinkie Brockman', terribly emaciated with dysentery following cholera and a large mass in the lower abdomen, obviously dying.

The river camp is nearly 100 cattle short and some of the smart lads are apparently killing them in the scrub and selling meat. Home in good time over the railway cuttings and the big trestle bridge – a horror on which I get my old stupid height giddiness reaction.

13 August 1943

S/Sgt Gibson is having his leg badly pulled by all and sundry owing to his being told that a Tamil had died in the engineer lines. Gibbie then arranged for a cremation and the party went along and were about to carry the corpse away when he suddenly moaned and showed distinct signs of life. The party was cancelled. Also so were Fred Smedley's arrangements for a Christian burial! As Ewan has about 400 hospital patients out at the river, I strongly advised that another doctor, AIF, be got from Konyu where there are several. The CO promised to try and arrange this. Ewan has no thermometer and almost no drugs. Bob Haddon and two others came out of cholera isolation today.

14 August 1943

Weather is fairly pleasant with some brisk showers. Jock Clarke and Fred had a very amusing and fruitful session of bee hive robbing, acquiring some honey and beeswax for cobbling boots.

15 August 1943

Death: VX 30258 Pte Souter, F.R., 2/3 M.G. Bn, aged 23. Tropical ulcers, malaria, enteritis, beriberi. Finally cardiac failure. There was no sign of impending disaster with this patient. He was a tall, pale freckled boy, very thin; rather large but healing tropical ulcer and recent malaria, still under quinine treatment, no recent enteritis or obvious signs of beriberi. I am rather worried lest quinine may be a factor in these sudden deaths where there is malaria and beriberi.

Some of the men working have now been at work without rest for over 80 days. Work is not of the 'speedo' type now, but the hours are still very long.

16 August 1943

The Nipponese have asked for discharge of 10 men tomorrow.

A huge black and yellow 'death's head' spider has his residence near us and we watch with great interest his trussing up and insatiable gobbling. Bob Fox and Steve Wade feed grasshoppers to him. Sgt Keith Neighbor came up today from the river camp to sketch the cemetery and a little hut for the stills, etc. Jock, Fred and I live very cheaply in the mess these days but 'Bish' Hera Singh makes very tasty meals considering the ingredients. A recent innovation was a rich pudding. I am doing very well owing to Jock, Fred and F/O Park being troubled very frequently with enteritis. That of Jock's is rather worrying and of course amoebic infection should be excluded if one could. We play a good deal of chess in the evenings.

17 August 1943

We are replacing the decrepit Dutch crosses over their ten graves in the cemetery and have an excellent sign board on a large tree. 'Hintok, Australian and NEI POWs' Cemetery', surmounted by a rising sun. Lt Hutton is sinking fast today.

18 August 1943

Death occurred of Lt A.A. Hutton, 2/10 Field Rgt at 0210 hrs. He has been in a practically unconscious condition for a month.

The shock of the day was the return of Osuki with the announcement that we start moving sick tomorrow – 240 men to be transferred each day on 20, 22 and 24 August by barge. It was decided to send our sick to the river camp to stage: an alternative to Konyu. The Nipponese are not allowing any outside workmen for the carriage of the sick and it will have to be done almost entirely by the evacuees themselves. The rack up the cliff and the ladder was discussed and it was decided that we must get them up somehow. I am thinking that some of the stretcher feats have been incredible. (Witness Bill Aldag and party getting in 'Curly' Gray at midnight after hours on the jungle track in black darkness and rain. Finally having to lower poor 'Curly' down the cliff, tied onto the stretcher, by the light of fires top and bottom). It was arranged to send 10 stretcher cases and 20 walking sick tomorrow. Discussion occurred as to the officers' going down for sick administrative reasons and Capt. Brettingham-Moore and Capt. Piper and Lt Houston, Maj. Clarke, and Lt Smedley to go. Major Clarke was my decision and a very hard one – there were never two better fellows than Jock or Fred Smedley and they have given the most magnificent service up here. Jock is ingenious with tools and full of ideas. I am sending all the men I possibly can who are not required for some essential duty. The nursing orderlies present a severe problem as they are almost all sick and worn out and when the sick go, they may be hammered out to work and more 'speedo' duties. For the sake of the troops up here, I feel I must keep the main hospital group together. 'Budge' Gill returned with me from the river camp out of his own kindness of heart to act as an early courier tomorrow. We arrived just on darkness and preparations for the move kept me busy until after 0200 hrs.

19 August 1943

The departure of the first batch of evacuees – 10 stretcher cases, 20 walking. These were the less sick men as I have some hopes of going down with the last barge-load to try and arrange smooth transport for the very sick. After correspondence with Mac, I found this policy will have to be reversed, the Nips having made arrangements for very sick men first. I feel extremely sad today that nearly all the old O and P men will be going down terribly broken, some of them like W/O Charlston and Abbott and many others, and I don't think a number of them will see the day of liberation. This is one of those big break-ups that occur from time to time when tried and trusted old friends depart. Altogether, during the last few weeks, with the cessation of the fiendish 'speedo' attentions of the Nipponese, we have been happy here – really quite happy. This happiness is a strange thing. I find now that my policy of keeping our group of Java party men together was in the end a failure, excellent though the results were for six months, I just didn't quite reckon on the inhumanity of the last three months or the cholera. On the whole, the lower spirited NEI men will perhaps do as well as any others. They decided early they could not cope and would prefer to give up and die, with the result they would be taken out when the going was good and in large numbers. Whatever a man has in his body and spirit it is certain that the last will be extracted here and he will leave bankrupt.

The local Nipponese have not had word of the move this morning and acting only on my information were very much in a flap and very jumpy. It was with difficulty that we stopped them sending off all our fit men as bearers on a carrying excursion of their own.

Alf Denton was detected with some stolen N sardines in his pack. After a few preliminary wallops and threats with a bayonet, Haruyama took over the situation and brought him along to the *kebeitai* to stand at attention with a large placard on his chest including the label of the sardine tin and the words 'Stolen – one tin of sardines, 19.8.43 – Pte Denton, A.W.' This sight caused much mirth but the irrepressible Denton was not particularly abashed.

The river carrying party arrived at about 1200 and departure was delayed until after lunch. All evacuations to be completed by 22 August 1943 except choleras, so far as I know at present. A wet miserable day so that the bearers of six per stretcher had a heavy struggle. All patients got up the ladder OK. The cemetery was complete today with even the Dutch crosses.

20 August 1943

Forty were evacuated, including 10 stretcher cases. At the last minute, only 30 men were found to have arrived from the river camp for carrying due to the Nipponese not supplying fit men for carrying and only evacuation cases were available. Two more bearer parties were scratched together, some rather sick.

I witnessed the job of moving these up the cliff in the rain and the mud – a very sad sight. Charlton, Abbott and Tully were tied onto the stretchers and bullocked up the ladder rung by rung, the rear bearers supporting the stretcher poles on their shoulders. Other men managed to get up with assistance, some having to have men behind them to lift their feet up each rung in a combined pull from above and a push from behind to hoist them up that distance. Beriberi knees are particularly bad on steps; thus the strong men leave in the shadow of that cursed mountain. Many of the bearers are in bare feet, typical ragged tattered figures, emaciated and hag-ridden with sores.

I am approaching the Nipponese through Mac to request that I be allowed to go down to the base hospital at Tarsau to throw my energies into the huge sick problem. The only catch is that I would feel a worm evacuating myself while there are even a few of my original command left in the area.

21 August 1943

In view of the heavy work of the bearers themselves, mostly sick men, I severely pruned the stretcher list today, believing that the cases omitted will get out somehow if their gear is carried. Osuki says 'No', to my Tarsau request; I may go down later with a N medical clerk. I am allowed to shift the cholera cases tomorrow.

22 August 1943

Tarsau evacuations 48; 3 cholera stretcher cases transferred. Fred Smedley and Jock Clarke have gone. After an hour or two, I felt rather lonely and restless and decided to carry some medical gear out to the river. On the way, I found Sam Compton collapsed half-way up the cliff and took him back as a ? cholera for observation, then set off again. I found all patients eventually – I got out Dave Topping, rather shaky, and also Jock Clarke, very wan on arrival. Don Thomas, was shivering with malaria after work, so I admitted him to hospital and arranged to bring his gear out tomorrow. I arranged to transfer myself to the river tomorrow with the rest of the cholera patients and most of the other personnel, leaving W/O Exton in charge for the shift, which surprisingly enough will necessitate 500 man loads – that being the only way to shift gear here. Some of the lads like Jack Brown, 2/2 Aust. CCS, have become nearly as good as the natives at shifting loads with a pole. They almost have the same jog trot.

I called to have a last powwow with the local Korean No. 1, Yamamoto, and told him of arrangements tomorrow, to which he agreed. I then thanked him for having been a very kind No. 1 and that I hoped he would soon be made a general – to which bait he responded, by producing a pommelo, bananas and cigarettes, etc. and made all sorts of kind enquiries re my wife and seven children. [fictitious for prestige]. He asked if I had only one wife, as seven children seemed rather a lot to ask of one woman. He has, on his own part, a wife and three children whom he has not seen for three years. People in Japan are very tired of war, he said, and never thought it would be so long – 'Now, perhaps – another three years? What did I think of Nipponese men?' Answer: 'Sama sama all men – some good some bad' He said: 'Yes some very bad men in Nippon – but some good.' Brian Harrison-Lucas did the translating. Gus delivered the goods on both our last two nights with excitement, snapping of fingers and calls for me. [Refers to wireless news! Gus-Sgt Cawthron.]

23 August 1943

S/Sgt Gibson, Sgt Harrison-Lucas, Sgt Wiseman, Pte Lawrence and Lacey went with me and arrangements were made for Bunny Brown to get malaria at the river (spurious of course) so he took all gear. The personnel left – Corrie and Hanley and 9 cooks; 10 hygiene people; 3 convalescents. When Bunny went sick at the river, that left a total of 23 at the mountain camp, leaving two convalescents of which W/O Exton is one (W/O in charge of the camp). As we left, they were just killing the last of our duffed bullocks to go around the 23 men.

I arranged with W/O Exton to close down the canteen, transfer stores and obtain stores directly out here. I was grieved to hear of the death of another CCS man, Sapper C.L. Watson, who died of bacillary dysentery on 8 August after being evacuated with chronic malaria.

Blue Butterworth insisted on going off with my heavy valise roll so that I had no more than an average heavy load and was thus able to give a cholera patient a hand. Much mirth when I arrived looking like Father Christmas and also rather hot from making a false turn down the mountain near the river, thus getting nearly stuck on a soft slope with masses of fallen bamboos and loose stones rolling down from the cutting above. Some 200 yards of sweat to get back on to the track again. All the officers are looking fairly fit for POWs. This surprised me less when I found out how well they are feeding. The following medical officers are now in the camp besides Maj. Corlette: Capt. Parker, Capt. Wright, Capt. McNeilly, Capt. Matheson, so there were MOs to burn.

I saw Lt-Col. James today and discussed the camp medical arrangements. He agreed to a common camp hospital quite cordially and said that the only difference that might arise would be in [comforts] and diet supplied to patients. The present hospital site appears to be too small to take both our infectious cases, dysentery and the other cases. A new site was looked over with Maj. Wearne.

I was dismayed about the local sick fund arrangements. The CO has already written to Tarsau telling them that as now nearly all men are sick, they cannot support sick that have gone or are going down via Tarsau. (This is correct but it does not mean that we can do nothing.) As all sick men will be gone and some money will be collected from danger pay, 'presento' pay etc., there is no need to have a subscription from working pay (at present one-third of all pay). I opposed this point of view, stressing that we had really reached a point, 5c per man per day, when it was doubtful whether, in many cases, a patient could be kept alive. Soon, whatever force was left behind, the proportion of sick to fit would be about the same and no funds would have been accumulated to meet the contingency. Also, money collected into funds was much more wisely spent on the whole than by individuals; further, it would scarcely be right to disclaim responsibility entirely for evacuated men. Billy Wearne suggested as a compromise that the levy on all pay should be one-fifth the earning rate.

Further departure of 130 evacuees today.

24 August 1943

Evacuations to date, 20–24 August inclusive, total 469. All CCS men and Java Ambulance Car men are still here including Fred Smedley and Jock Clarke.

There are signs that the Nipponese are getting jumpy about the number of men going down. Seventeen CCS men are down for evacuation tomorrow which will leave only 24, Ewan and I included.

25 August 1943

A bombshell was dropped on us by the Nipponese that no further evacuations were to take place today. The incredible statement was made that some of our cholera convalescents sent down still had cholera. N doctor must come and examine all men before any more go down. (Probably Okada was at fault sending men down without a glass rod test being done, for I am sure the cholera story is nonsense.) This holds up the evacuation of 299 men.

This is our 231st day in the jungle from 25 January to 25 August. 24 May was the last official *yasumé* day for all men. Therefore, work has been in progress without halt for 93 days. Even on previous rest days some men were forced to work. It has rained on 110 days of which 43 were full wet days. We have had eight storms and one hurricane with an extreme destruction of our belt of jungle which missed the camp by less than a mile. It was reported today that 220 men have died in 13 weeks in the Hintok English camp.

26 August 1943

It was a big day for Hintok, since what Okada calls the big 'shush-pusher' arrived in these parts, welcomed by all Nipponese and awaking the jungle with shrill echoes from a loud whistle. An intense celebration by the Nipponese, who had a special dinner and smoke social, at which Hirota presided at a table with cigarettes and beer for all and also much saki. Nipponese rank and file squatted around in a square. There was much singing and clapping of hands and other simple amusements. Molly the Monk was the only one who could find nothing to sing – this one would expect. Proceedings were enlivened by a fight between 'Bill the Bastard' and 'Happy' with Pop looking on disapprovingly. 'Bill the Bastard' was rescued from suffocation by a most efficient stranglehold.

Other celebrations about the place included the Tamils who were celebrating the coming of age of two young boys. After much beating of drums etc, they appeared to go into a hypnotic trance and had to be revived by buckets of water. Then one of them forced a piece of iron through his tongue, seemingly without pain or blood, and led a wild procession around the camp, running, yelling and beating tomtoms. Muhammadans were also said to be celebrating Ramadan. We alone seemed to have nothing to celebrate.

27 August 1943

The Nipponese celebrations went on today and what do you think! a *yasumé* for all in camp – the first for three months and three days! I am having a certain amount of difficulty regarding hospital workers as De Crespigney, under pressure of Kanamoto, wishes to cut the inside workers and supply more outside workers. This is supported by the CO since Kanamoto seems to be able to arrange pay swindles. Crep's economy figures left the hospital with but ten men which raised a storm from me. Finally, we have 18 as a result of no benjo workers. I object strenuously to all this. We go out of our way to send men out to work just to please Kanamoto whose largesse, I am certain, will not depend just on his good humour. Again, I am willing to send Red Cross personnel out to work to spare sick men, but I do not like the assumption that of necessity they go out just as other men. There are few enough of them left and they are very important to the health of the troops, quite apart from the breach of international law.

28 August 1943

The N doctor arrived for 'glass rodding' at about 0900.

A timely hint is given of the likelihood of a search tomorrow morning. I presume Osuki is not keen to have any contraband found in his camp!

29 August 1943

Total hospital patients 488; Australian patients in general hospital 331, of which 303 are to be evacuated. All men and all officers were on parade at 0930, including all hospital patients, except bed patients and all medical orderlies. Osuki and other guards searched the camp, going through all gear (cholera area omitted and very little attention to the hospital). Hiroda's search of the nearby camp was very strict, including the cholera area and inspection of the surrounding jungle. 'X' [my wireless] survived the search.

George Stilley has been having progressively worse cardiac attacks and this evening, despite all efforts, a second collapse and death.

Okada agreed that all men should now receive quinine grains 6 three times a day as a prophylactic dose. He was startled when I referred to a case of typhoid named Bliss. Brian corrected me and I then said, 'Major Corlette at first think perhaps typhoid. Now get better so think malaria. Case very, very eccentric!' It seems Okada does not regard typhoid as an acceptable diagnosis since it brings repercussions from Tarsau, so the merry game of deception goes on. Lord knows what N statistics really mean. It is not permitted to return men as having dysentery – all dysenteries were changed at a stroke of the pen to colitis. Later this also fell into disfavour and a stroke of the pen made this 'other conditions of the alimentary tract'; yet when the men die, we return the death as dysentery without comment.

30 August 1943

Total hospital 511. Called to Okada who is grave and stern: number of hospital admissions always greater than discharges – why? This, of course, is easy to answer, because all sick men were now admitted for evacuation with same effect as moving to a new camp. After a little discussion, I arranged the evacuation of a further ten men with Okada, explaining that I was 'very eccentric' so had now better change the number.

31 August 1943

I am now very desirous to evacuate all O and P Battalion that I possibly can and in particular, get as many CCS men as possible out of the area. I fear a move up the river will occur very soon.

1 September 1943

Results of swabbing were all negative so that cholera men will now be speedily evacuated. All remaining personnel were put through the 'glass rod' test today. In the event there was a sudden barge flutter and we commenced a mass evacuation. I decided to go down with the party.

2 September 1943

Breakfast in Lt-Col. Knight's mess run in 4 Royal Norfolk style; he was not especially cordial. There is to be a meeting re finance today but Lt-Col. Harvey said I am not invited because it is really a camp matter. 'Like hell,' I said, 'I see – you have the meeting then we'll have another one to see if we agree with you.' This little sarcasm was ignored or not noted.

There have been some pleasing signs of late as regards medical stores and emetine in particular. Certain gentlemen have supplied some 72 grains and offer a most hopeful avenue for either free supply of drugs or supplying a cheque for medical purposes.* I reported to Harvey the position as regards the camp remnant and the six medical officers – also mentioned my CCS personnel and their possible usefulness. The following arose during the morning: Maj. O'Driscoll approached me re the transfer of Captain Colin Christy and his 'appointment' to the hospital to assist him. I said coldly in the presence of Hazleton: 'I do not understand how appointments are made here.' He said, 'Well you have to be evacuated to get here' – this information, frankly given, was of interest.

Chungkai is said to be the base hospital for No. 4 group but it cannot be established that evacuations do not occur to Kanchanaburi and other hospitals. Those evacuated are termed 'walking' or 'lying incurables'. Walking drafts go by railway, lying by barge. Chungkai is said to be an excellent camp from the health point of view, the rations being good (meat issues about 5 oz per day). There is a most excellent canteen run by the camp at a big profit and this way the diet is reinforced up to about 8 oz a day. Drugs are said however not to be so plentiful as here and to summarise, pure debility cases do well there but cases requiring much treatment not so well. The N regime is apparently helpful.

The present number in hospital and convalescent section here is approximately 2,300. I have no exact knowledge of the medical organisation as yet but Col. Harvey is CO, Finnemore AIF Dental, as registrar, Maj. O'Driscoll RAMC Convalescent Depot, Maj. Hazleton, AAMC doing pathology and apparently has some control over AIF interests (not very much I fear). Capt. Street, Dysentery Section, has control over emetine and I believe is impartial and fair. He appears to me in addition to be an excellent doctor. McConachie (Surgical) has done good work with poor instruments and now Millard has surgical interests. I regard the surgical wards of the hospital as sound. Convalescents, however, produces the most alarming rumours, the main complaint being the absence of any treatment to speak of.

At 1100 hours drafted the new sick from Hintok with Hazleton into Medical,

* Boon Pong and the underground.

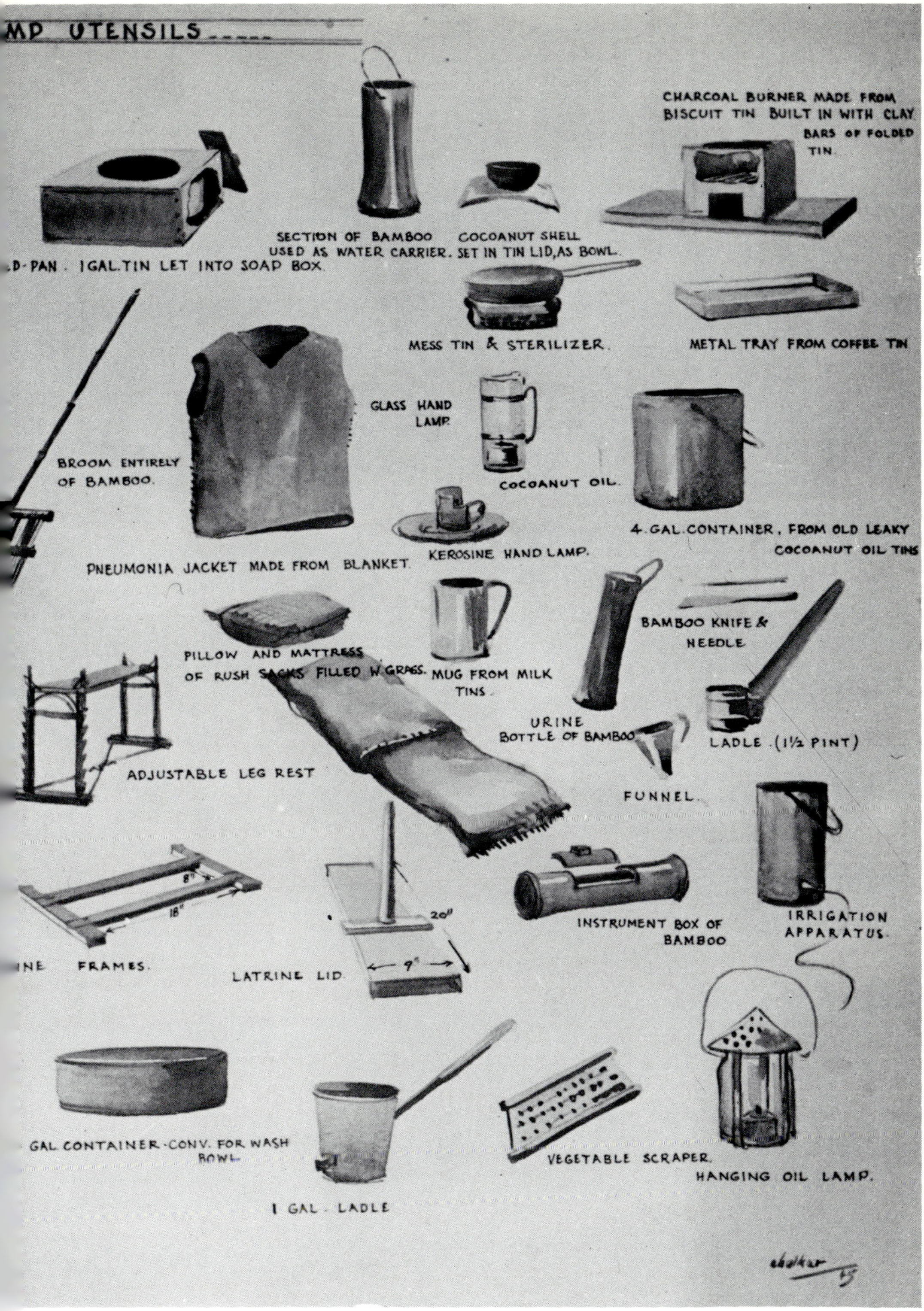

p and hospital utensils (*Jack Chalker*)

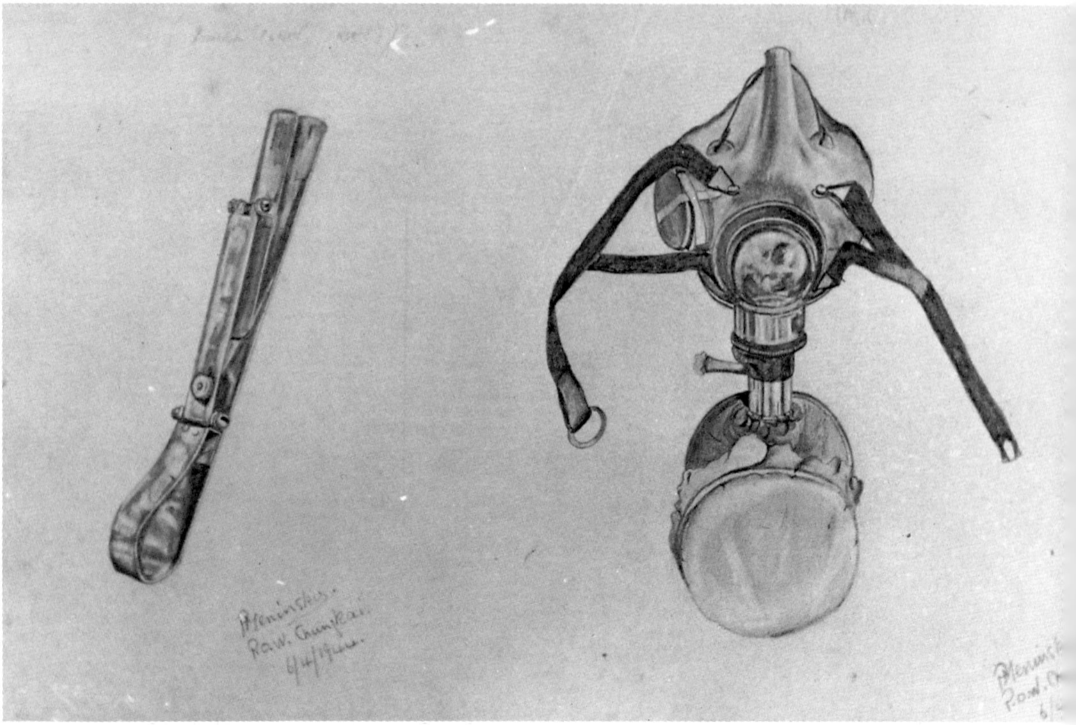

82 Improvised anaesthetic mask and bowel clamp (*P. Meninsky*)

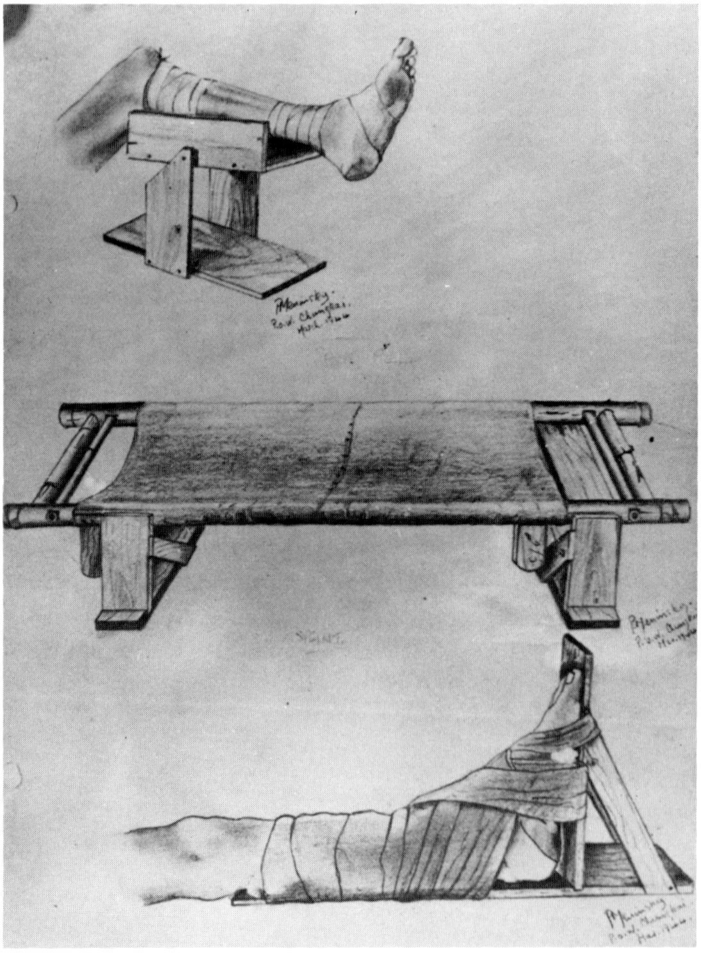

83 Leg rest, rice sack bed, splint foot ankle (*P. Meninsky*)

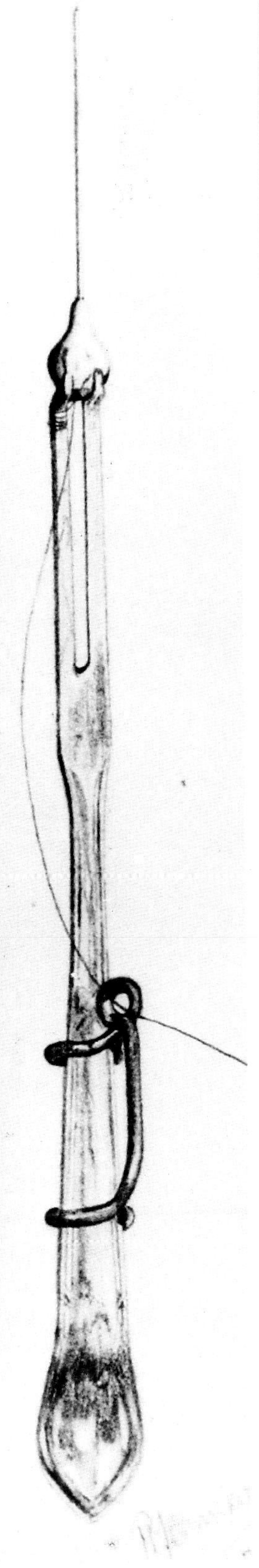

gical snare made from portion of
rk, hypodermic needle and wire
Meninsky)

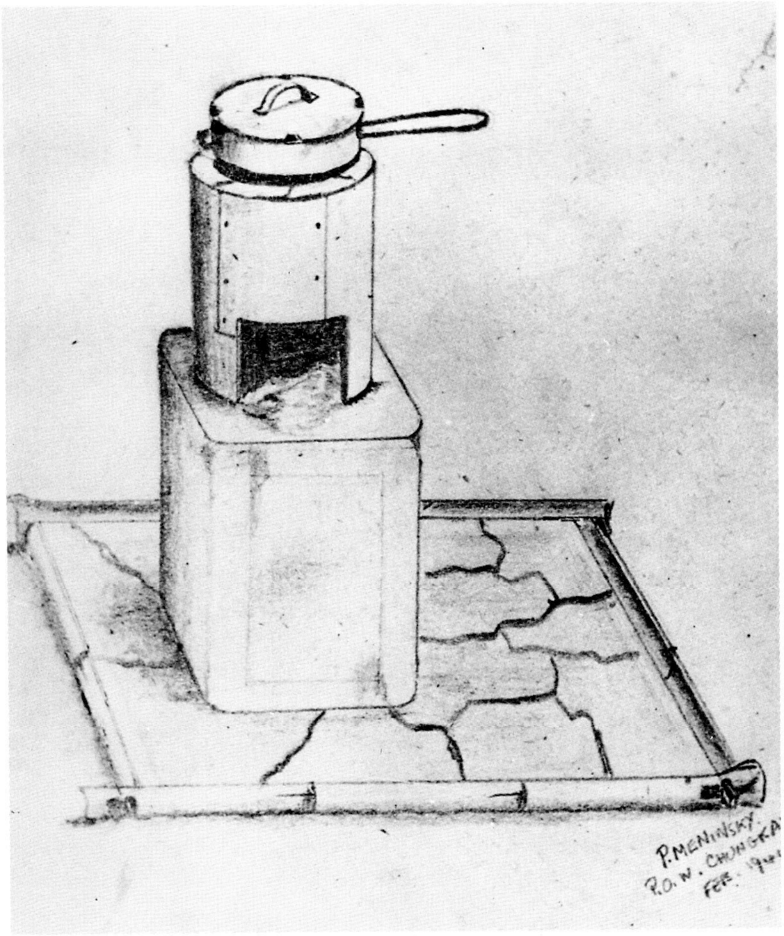

85 Portable steriliser – charcoal stove, tin and baked mud (*P. Meninsky*)

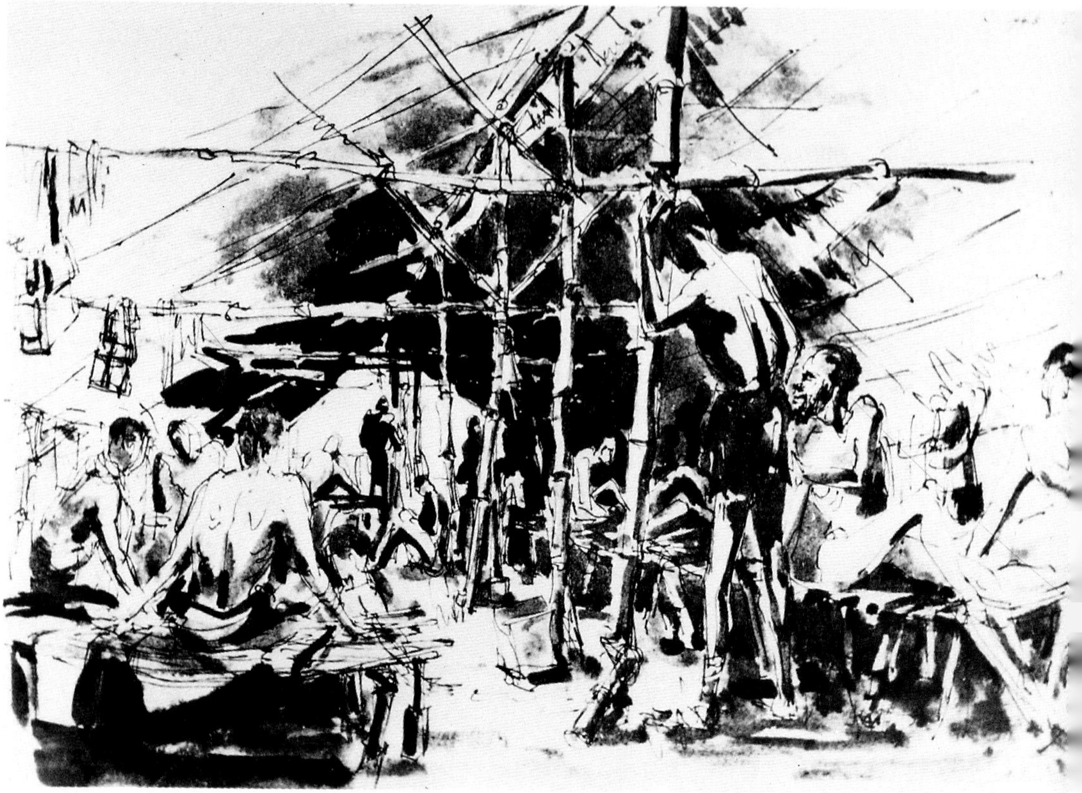

86 Chungkai, decrepit hospital ward (*Jack Chalker*)

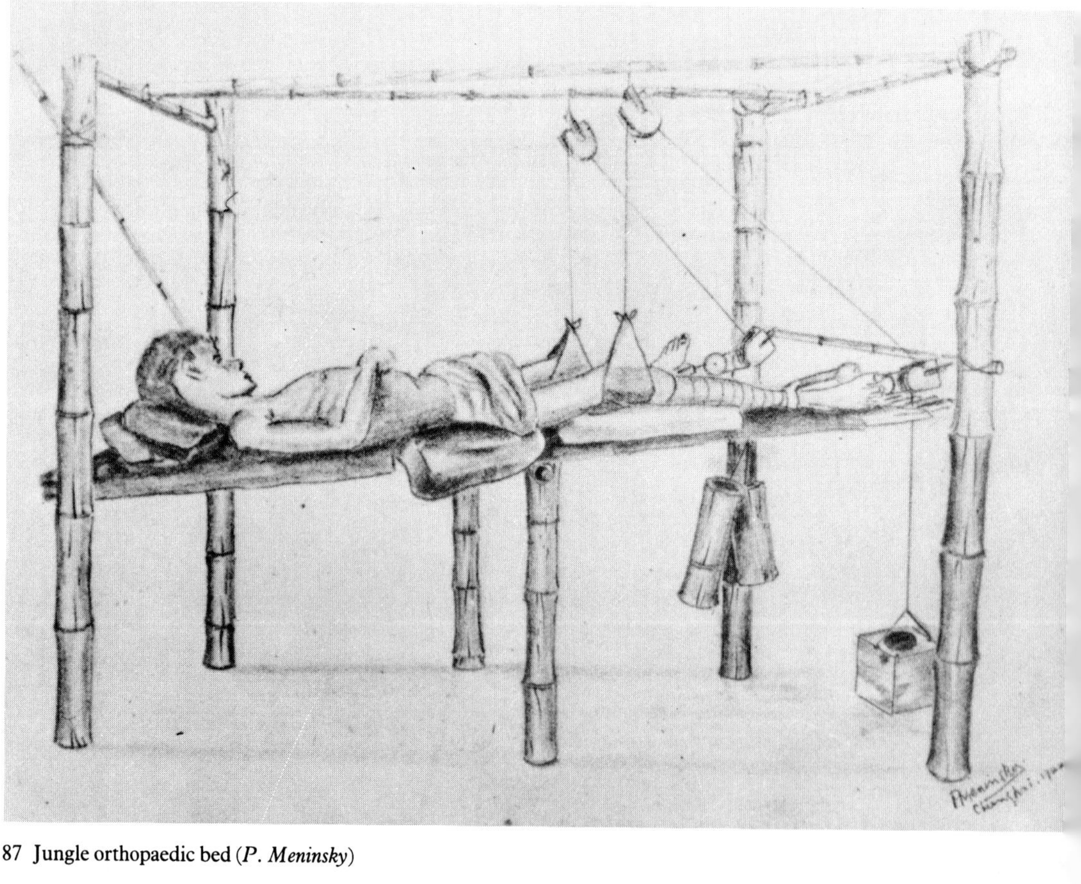

87 Jungle orthopaedic bed (*P. Meninsky*)

Surgical, Dysentery, Convalescent. In my ignorance of the above rumours at the time, I sent too many men to Convalescent I fear. Hazleton and Finnemore promised to endeavour to keep the CCS personnel in the area and to employ them – a relief to me.

I gather that the 'A & D' book records [medical records] are well kept here by Lt-Col. Thomas. I visited Lt-Col. Warren who has shaved his beard and looked remarkably like Anthony Eden in moustache and profile. I discussed finance with Lt-Col. Thomas in the presence of Warren and Lt-Col. McOstritch. Increased rates of pay will operate from August. The Tarsau arrangement is that all ranks pay 10 per cent of pay to a messing fund and all officers above 1st Lt also 15 ticals to hospital fund. It is requested that we subscribe 5 ticals to a special contingency fund for No. 4 group, mainly to avoid the possibility of being left without further income.

I found Padre Bourke in the officers' ward with beriberi (very cheerful); Padre Thorpe has been in the guard house for a few days for 'jumping a barge' on the way to Kanchanaburi after his wild tour up to Kinsayok. I saw many patients today and did a general reconnaissance. Last night chilled to the bone after the trip, and now have fever today. A blood slide tonight.

3 September 1943

I inspected many wards superficially by calling on patients. Newly arrived sick patients today and did a general reconnaissance. Last night chilled to the bone quite definite that the N quinine supply is causing some most nasty complications, including sudden death or Stokes Adam's attacks, wild maniacal states, etc. This may be due to quinidine and other alkaloids being present. The Dutch theory is that they are using green bark and much quinidine. The cholera evacuation cases have arrived from Hintok, including Jim Murray and Dick Leftwich.

4 September 1943

A day of incessant, annoying preparations for departure. Continually told 'Leave after rice'. Finally saw Osuki who was in Tarsau on the 'aboriginal jag'. I asked him if I could go to Chungkai and he said 'No. Go back Hintok.' In the evening I saw Tadano who said tomorrow 0830.

Still many distressing reports re the convalescent section and the absence of treatment. Poor Ted Abbott died last night and Fred Smedley attended his burial service. Bob McGuire is terribly sick and weak and I am afraid not very long for this world.

It seems that 'No. 1 all POWs' is visiting Tarsau soon and the Nips are showering benefactions on the place, granting all reasonable requests re sanitation, buildings. Also the local doctor, Moroko, is preparing a report for the Red Cross.

5 September 1943

I went to the river and was told 'No barge for Hintok' and was turfed out. Tadano took me back, gave a few rapid orders and a pass was given. 'Great mistake!' A very smooth trip and the weather was beautifully fine, with white fleecy clouds in the blue sky and brilliant green jungle reflecting in the placid river. The Thai barge crew, besides myself, two Nipponese, a Chinaman and a Thai, were very hospitable and soon ceased trying to buy my watch. They gave me an excellent lunch cooked on the barge, also pomelo and cakes. Arrived Hintok approximately 1500 hours. All this camp are under warning to move, presumably upstream. Some discussion occurred as to whether I should go down to Tarsau. I feel this is a matter for CO to decide, as I do not care to evacuate myself along the usual lines!

6 September 1943

C.C.S. Remaining in Jungle Lt-Col. Dunlop, E.E., Maj. Corlette, E.L., S/Sgt Gibson S.A., Sgt Harrison-Lucas B.P., Sgt Wiseman G.K., L/Cpl Bourne J.D., Pte Brown A.A., Pte Leacock T.G.A., Pte Duncan D.E., Pte Geraghty T.J., Pte Cardier A., Pte Mansfield T.J., Pte Tarren D., Pte Hanley R.M., Pte Denny R.R., Pte House, Pte Boys H., Pte Browne J.A.L., Pte Butterworth M., Pte Badham E., Nursing Orderlies: 10.

The following CCS Personnel Acquired Cholera in the Recent Epidemic: S/Sgt Ross J., Sgt Haddon R., Cpl Lawrence A.G., Cpl Walker K.H., Cpl Leftwich R.W., Pte Murray J.B. and Driver Hayes K.N. All except Hayes and Haddon caught the disease in nursing duties. Nat Hanley is at last down with malaria and as far as is known only Maj. Moon and Jack Taylor have not yet had malaria out of the 58 CCS coming to Thailand.

2/2 Australian CCS as at 6.9.43
118 left for Middle East; 77 remained in Java after evacuations. Of 58 who reached Thailand there are 5 known deaths. Seven men 'wagged' it from work on the railway and were caught after much delay and checking of working parties. Punishment was dealt out by the Nips, one with a slipper the other with a fist. All these men were felled to the ground but nothing done to them while they were down. Hiroda came in at the end and said 'Next time – sword'. The second threat of this sort. His presence produced another round of punishment dealt out with the usual ferocious yells.

7 September 1943

CO reports an amusing conversation re cattle which are all penned in the yard after recent heavy losses. 'Claude', the interpreter, first suggested 'Men go bring food and water to each cow (and these over 400!).' This 'very difficult'. So next suggestion as regards cows: 'OK, men take cows out but only for short time. Morning meal? Midday meal? Evening meal?'

The CO naturally suggested that the eating habits of cows did not exactly correspond with those of *homo sapiens*!

I spent a day overhauling my surgical equipment, some of which has gone rather rusty. Many Nips to see me about their health. Very neurotic! One tried to get me to remove his appendix today. Yesterday I treated one to a dose of mixture of mag. sulph, quinine sulphate, and other unpleasant ingredients plus permanganate of potash. Today merely sago flour and iodine – a very good colour. One heaped coals of fire on me with a tin of jam which I gave to the hospital. Drugs are short, hence these harmless nostrums.

8 September 1943

Corlette and I much *yasumé*. I am taking atebrine at this stage for my malaria, my spleen having enlarged again. An English soldier named Lyons in the next camp committed suicide by diving off the rocks into the river. Things are very quiet. A move expected very soon.

9 September 1943

Disastrous encounter today, trying to extract a lower molar in an English officer. The tooth fractured and broke up leaving the roots in the gum – forced to desist.

10 September 1943

An amusing morning inducing the Nips to give me some disinfectant to treat latrines. I screwed them up from one bottle to two after threatening them with 'all men cholera and dysentery'. I did not mention that we already had ten bottles. Of course complete stock is inadequate. What is needed is a gallon of crude disinfectant. In the evening 20 men were warned to go to Kinsayok tomorrow; all sick P Bn to go by barge. We are all to follow them up in the next few days.

11 September 1943

Billy Wearne went off on the barge with draft of 20 sick to Kinsayok.

12 September 1943

Major Wearne arrived back; he regards Kinsayok as a 'fattening paddock' Huts are to be erected for all; a football ground has been prepared and recreation has been encouraged. The commander of the camp is Lt-Col. Lilly; also in the camp is Lt-Col. Hugenon of the Saigon Battalion. Decided to go up with him tomorrow and look into the medical situation.

13 September 1943

Things at Kinsayok are very much at sixes and sevens. Each group that arrives here is having a separate duty section of its own, separate kitchens and medical arrangements. The duty sections are large and include 'batmen', both as such and 'covered up'. The SMO is Maj. Bennett, RAMC. Each group looks after its own sick, the hospital being run by a 'Soviet of captains' but no common policy, no common stores, no arrangements for diets or special segregation of disease. The SMO appears merely to consolidate the returns to the Nips.

The Australians transferred are now attached to Capt. Trevena, Q Battalion, for messing and hospital arrangements with Capt. Godlee (Tim). The local Nipponese are not particularly nice, much attention to the *keré* and slapping. No. 1 Korean private, Yamoka, administers the camp apparently as Hatori Chui does not take any interest this days. Okada is medical sergeant, which is not so bad.

Jack Hands was reported to be a great favourite with Tanaka and has gone up river – promoted to local major and camp commander over two British majors (a doubtful compliment) – and he has now done well for the AIF. I met Lt-Col. Lilly; our conversation was limited to 'How do you do?' and his then walking away! He co-operates with the Nipponese. Hugenon refused to absolutely, and has at least on one occasion been before a firing squad, when he told them to go ahead.

Sanitation poor, with only one big latrine for all, sixteen seats, right at the back of the camp, for 1,100, including 74 officers. More latrines are being put down, of the open type unfortunately, though otherwise well made. Flies as usual and an offensive smell. For ablution a little stream pouring down to the river with a walk of 440 yards. This is also, alas, used by numerous Tamils [They were a sanitation risk.] The ground here is moderately sandy – much more pleasant than at Hintok (the black hell of Hintok).

14 September 1943

Central direction here is negligible and irritating with difficulties in the simple problems of accommodation and feeding of troops. For example, there are over 30 *cwalis* here and therefore enough to cook for 2,000 men by Hintok standards, yet MacDonald, the adjutant, is emphatic that each group can cook for no more. Billy is more than holding his own in these arrangements.

15 September 1943

Called to the hospital by Okada and given a lesson in dressing ulcers with saline, then discussed plans for the new hospital and OKd. my ideas re longitudinal beds and operating theatre, medical store and office. He said I must be No. 1 and that all medical stores must be placed in the medical store, not issued out all over the camp. I imparted this policy to some medical officers who expressed grave concern. It seems to be the only logical one anyway. I do not wish to supplant Major Bennett as SMO unless this course is desired by the camp authorities.

16 September 1943

Lt-Col. James arrived with a party from Hintok in the early afternoon; no preparation for their reception had been made and the troops were kept standing in the pouring rain while talks with the Nippon No. 1, Yamoka, went on. Eventually very leaky tents were handed out and the men had to erect and floor them in the rain and wet – a pretty bloody show! Some sick arrived again, also some medical stores which I took over. Okada today called for a list of men for evacuation and I eventually presented a list of 96 men, of which 36 Australians were from Hintok party. Called to office and told, 'Here, conditions good, food good, pay good, very many doctors, man get better. Why evacuate?' I was told to reduce the figure to 50 so the AIF list from Hintok were peeled to 18.

17 September 1943

Lt-Col. McEachern and party arrived by barge; the party includes Maj. Corlette and Capt. Parker. It was decided that the party was to go into a new hut, just being erected. We will open our own kitchen area for the Hintok group for the midday meal tomorrow.

18 September 1943

Maj. Woods party arrived from Hintok; these also were able to go into huts. The weather is still foul. This party includes CCS men and most medical orderlies, 'Gibbie', Harrison-Lucas, Wiseman, etc. They have all been working on 'speedo' work, shifting large quantities of wood down to the river barges for use by the 'shush pusher'. The Kinsayok party will be allowed ten nursing orderlies, some wood and water carriers. The AIF allotment is 6 nursing orderlies and 6 wood and water carriers and this is not too bad. MacNeilly is quite satisfied with his allotment. At present, most of the Hintok British are being looked after by Captain Allen, RAMC.

19 September 1943

Major Woods party, three officers and 50 O.R.S., including two hospital. 0 – 26; P – 22; S – 33; T – 18 = Total 99
Sunday. Today down to the river barge to see 'table tennis man' who had some medical stores for sale. These included Vitamin B_1 tablets, 6,000 said to be each 300 i.u.; three bottles of iodine 20 fluid oz; acriflavine solution 1%; cotton wool; 12 precious grains of emetine hydrochloride. A discussion with Capt. Pavillard, who has placed an order and I am to send an additional request to the agent [Boon Pong].

My men are working on an M.I. room with a shelter for fire and patients' foments, etc.

At my suggestion, we had a meeting and decided to suggest the following to the camp authorities:

1 That the hospital be placed under central administration with a definite staff. M.I. rooms to continue to be run on the present group basis.
2 Non-expendable stores to be pooled for hospital and general camp use.
3 It is recommended that the hospital have its own kitchen or, failing that, its own special diet kitchen arrangements. Supplementary rations: a fixed rate of expenditure per patient per day be arranged (at least 10c).

Harvest Thanksgiving Service today. Very well run by Maj. Walters, Lt-Col. Lilly and Mac taking part in the service. All attending asked to make gifts for hospital patients, eggs, etc. I crept in late with a wretched two eggs in my pocket – all I could find!

20 September 1943

Before men move off to work here and after they return, they are required to sing under control of the Sgt Major in charge – thus even if every soldier does not have a baton in his haversack, certainly every Sgt Major must! Favourite songs highly approved by the Nipponese are 'He'll be coming round the Mountain', 'Daisy' and 'Sons of the Sea all British Born'. 'Rule Britannia' has been employed but 'Britons never, never will be slaves!' rang rather hollowly.

I was busy arranging distribution of Harvest Thanksgiving products, when there was a hurried call of 'Speedo, evacuation men go barge today'. Misunderstanding that we're to go and finally only 35 men out of 50 left on the barge, including five Hintok group, AIF people. These all had their boots taken from them before leaving, presumably to walk in bare feet now until some other area issues them, if ever. Asked by Okada to arrange evacuation of a further 35 men tomorrow so total 50. Am arranging evacuation of CCS men, Bourne, A.A. Brown, T. Mansfield, Geraghty. By Lt-Col's suggestion, Caption McNeilly is to go.

We discussed today a Nippon court martial arising out of the shooting of a British soldier with cholera who was the first case in the camp. To spare the lad being shot at repeatedly through the tent, the British Adjutant of his battalion, Lt Primrose, shot him personally. This did not spare the camp much subsequent cholera. Asked to Lt-Col. Hugenon's mess to talk about Greece and Crete and the middle east generally. This was rather delayed by a surge of *keré* practice by all officers and W/Os. On the way back, I got bogged right over the top of my shoes in foul mud and the sole came off one shoe – a serious matter. I finally found my way to bed in the dark, muddy and miserable. As usual, rats course over the bed and mosquito net all night, keeping up a continuous war of nerves – just occasionally scurrying over one's body where it projects against the night and of course upsetting one with a shaking of the net – so much so that I gave a yell and lashed out when Paddy woke me with a hand on the knee the other day.

21 September 1943

Warned by O. that Lt-Col. Ishi is coming and we must improve our working percentage! He is obviously in his blackest mood and will not speak English. I saw Lt-Col. Lilly today with Maj. Bennett and our proposals re medical arrangements for the camp were approved in principle. The finance question is to be settled by the group and battalion commanders. The groups have now been re-named as follows: O, P, S and T are *yama* = river; E, J, Y and W are *kawa* = mountain. Some of the other groups and battalions are named *sakura* = cherry blossom; *yuki* = snow and *mishi* = road. Okada (now the *gunsho*) states that the correct spelling for the camp is Kinsayok.

22 September 1943

In the afternoon word that a railway accident has occurred – it seems that the steam train had been derailed three times between Tonchin and Kinsayok. Several N soldiers on board said to have been badly injured also 20 U Bn men were brought to this camp for attention: of these 10 were injuries and 10 were sick. The injuries, almost all sustained from jumping from the train, were not very severe. Okada says that all livers of bullocks are to go to the sick and arranged collection and distribution in the hospital. Letter from Maj. Clarke who was doing work at Tonchin of dental nature. He reports that things are going well at Tarsau with the exception of death of Driver George Washington and poor old Bob McGuire. Jacky Taylor and Dave Topping are much improved. Many of the boys of 2/2 CCS are employed at Tarsau. Jock also reports on an unsuccessful attempt by Maj. O'Driscoll to slap 'Slappy' Oldham – the latter eluded him and asked him to try again, promising a speedy K.O!

More *keré* practice this evening in aid of Lt-Col. Ishi's visit.

23 September 1943

Whole camp being stirred into unusual activity and considerable ferocity by Okada, who insisted on all heavy sick (excused duty in lines) being paraded and 100 out of 162 on parade were put to work carrying attap from barges as a show in the colonel's presence.

Later I pointed out to Okada that boots were taken from sick men yesterday, yet today they were being sent out to work without boots. Okada promised that they would be given some boots. The results – nine pairs of uppers with a few rags as soles – utterly useless. The men were worked all day until 1900 hours. The evening picture was rather amusing – boots, it would seem, were for issue to railway employees and outside workers without boots. Many hundreds of bootless men lined up. Nip, Yamoka, in charge of parade, then stated that boots would be issued only to sunburnt feet men (of course many men have recently been wearing all sorts of ragged remnants on their feet). Those with no boots were to show hands. Some, discouraged by his previous remarks, did not put their hands up and were sent away. They were then told that any men remaining who did not have sunburnt feet were obviously deceivers and would be punished. An inspection of feet was carried out and all those with pale feet were severely slapped and sent off. Owing to a mistake some were sent to the wrong group and were still more severely dealt with by mass slapping. The Dutch Eurasion troops were the most fortunate – all being passed as having sunburnt feet! Finally, it was announced that 60 boots only were available out of the 90 left so some would have their names taken as approved for boots. Thus, no doubt, Lt-Col. Ishi was informed that all men now had boots, except 30 for later issue.

Medical arrangements: all doctors to 'tap tap' (in other words to percuss) chests: Lt-Col. Ishi would see. At first, we were all to perform outside in the big barrack near the river on dry land, but later O. consented to some of us doing our normal duties in the M.I. room areas.

Received a letter from A.A. Moon who relates that now 3,000 patients are at Tamarkan with total deaths of 127. The equipment is very scanty, the food is fair and the canteen good; there are 250 officers. John Disse is a patient, also Visse.

24 September 1943

Plans for hospital, now much improved on a separate site on Japanese HQ, discussed with Okada. The kitchens are to be handed over for use and all medical officers to live together in a 'medical house'.

Some clothing was issued. The first people requested to step forward were those with loin cloths only! There were indeed some men with loin cloths only.

25 September 1943

Futher modification of plans for the new hospital. Three huts are to be 35 m long.

26 September 1943

Work on the new hospital begun. Despite approval of plans, the Nipponese commenced to build standard barrack huts. I interceded and Okada, who was in a good temper, allowed some alteration in beds etc. in the hut being constructed and said other huts were to be according to plan. He said I (Dunropo) must attend and watch the work. This resulted in my being kicked out by an infuriated N soldier in the afternoon who intimated I had no business to be there talking to the sergeant-in-charge of the works. Maj. Bennett and I are having a keen competition as to who will be 'number one' and live with 'O' in 'special house'.

O. says all work will finish here very soon about 10 October. There are two possibilities: to go to Saigon and build a big bridge over the Mekong (very good house and very much rice!); to go to Penang where there is good house and ? not much rice.

Malaria is the most prevalent illness – about 60 per cent of admissions. The number of O and P Bn men who have not had an attack of malaria is now almost certainly less than 10.

27 September 1943

Pressure less intense following the departure of Lt-Col. Ishi; Okada requires about 40 sick each day from the heavy sick group. The great clothes drive and repercussions continued. Several men got into severe trouble for having more than one pair of N issue shorts (the most recent are light, pale blue, thin cotton affairs tied with a string round the waist and looking remarkably like female under garments). The penalty for having more of these articles than permitted is in general a confiscation of almost all clothing in one's pack.

I am doing a good deal of dental work of a crude nature at present, pulling very decayed teeth. My technique of extraction and mandibular block is improving a good deal.

28 September 1943

Today Lt-Col. Hugenon turned a soldier over to the Nipponese for striking a sergeant major. He was given a trying time, including much kneeling in the sun, sitting back on the heels, sphinx like, whilst buckets of water were poured over the face followed by blows, kicks and a few bouts of just usual beating up. No gross bodily damage was inflicted. 'The Cat', a sergeant major, was finally called to see the latter part of the punishment. Finally, both parties were lectured by Yamoko. The soldier; not to be so impetuous and headstrong. Next time punishment would not be so light (and indications of terrible things indeed). Then to Lt-Col. and RSMs: must remember that young soldiers require careful handling and tact! Discipline must be enforced; but must make allowances for youth, etc. and must exert tact! In this case the soldier had been punished and you must now be careful not to victimise him and make it clear that his crime was now forgotten. Admirable!

A party from Kanchanaburi staged here on the way through to Rin Tin – arrived in darkness tonight.

29 September 1943

Cholera vaccine 1 cc injected. The total hospital and bed down figure for the camp ranges from approximately 250 to 300, depending on the energies of Okada! The latter is most frank at times and does a preliminary inspection of Pte Rees' figures and at the times of Lt-Col. Ishi's visits, he may ask the figures be 'adjusted' to an acceptable level. This co-operation has certain dangers, as O. might well then 'rat' on us and hold us to our figures; it also requires considerable mathematical ability in leaping from true to false figures.

30 September 1943

Fifty more men to go to Tarsau, the provision for O P S T being 12 men (*per capita* allotment). There is no great pressure of work here now and the weather is slowly becoming more pleasant. Oh, the relief of having this wet season nearly behind! It has done more to break men's spirits than almost any other factor. My tropical ulcer is still unhealed after some 3 months but I am lucky in having got through a recurrence of malaria without worse retrogression. Not to mention the improvement as regards dysentery.

1 October 1943

Re-grouping into 3 battalions. Camp is now under Lt-Col. Hugenon, Lt-Col. Lilly having gone up river with some 200 + to a nearby camp. Evening parades are now introduced and sick parades accordingly altered to 1900 hours. *Kawa* and *yama* remain one group in the new organisation. I am doing a good number of dental extractions and find they are not exactly a 'soft snip', some requiring so much rocking that all the bystanders have their mouths open in sympathy. Also do some conservative work with zinc oxide and oil of cloves.

2 October 1943

Last night some men went through this camp being evacuated from Takanoon. They were in a very poor condition, large ulcers and gross septic skin lesions, ulcers etc. They report that local conditions are good; the Nip Lt-Col. in charge is considerate and gives them good food. There is a big hospital there – Max Pemberton doing much surgery on ulcers, etc. All speak highly of him. Deaths in the area apparently about 10 per cent. They know nothing particularly of F Force, who are up past Nikke, but think they have done very badly. There are apparently now over 1,500 men in hospital at Takanoon.

3 October 1943

I was involved in a curious fracas today. Okada called a meeting of all medical officers at 1700 and gave us a little pep talk through 'Pop', the interpreter. He asked to see the sick and the kitchens, behaving throughout in a rather humorous way. When coming back from the AIF kitchen, I passed the N 'bath-house', where I did not notice the presence of two N soldiers bending over buckets, naked and covered with soap. They 'kurra'd' me and called upon me to explain why no *keré*. After saluting, I stood to attention whilst they washed off the soap, preparatory to dealing with me. Okada came up, took in the situation and rescued me, saying with much laughter, 'Colonel Dunroppo must remember salute Nippon soldier.'

About two hours later, I was entering my barrack when hailed by a soldier outside the office about 50 metres away. The officers never salute the office when entering this barrack as it is well away. I did not notice the 'kurra' so was called out and as usual stood to attention and saluted. It was the same soldier who had made trouble in the bath-house. He at once advanced with his rifle and took a swing at my face which I countered by raising my left forearm and deflecting the blow smartly, he nearly falling over with shock. I was then summoned to the guardroom and went with some qualms, hoping that I might be able to protest to some other Nipponese. On entering, my assailant who was equipped with a heavy length of bamboo about 3 ft long and 4 in across stood me to attention and then struck at my face with all his strength. I deflected two blows with my left forearm, suffering some damage to the same. He then struck three heavy blows to my left leg, one hitting over the peroneal nerve with a horrid numbing effect of the leg suddenly going to sleep and inflicting two lacerations. Desperately fed up, I disarmed him and threw his stick away. Mad with fury, he seized another lump of wood and was again deprived of it. He then kicked viciously twice, aiming at the groin, kicking my thigh. Then a sequence of still more heavy, murderous lumps of wood which piled up behind me. I was resolved to give him a K.O. and pay the penalty when Hannamurasan, the small clerk of the office, rushed in and stood both parties to attention and wanted explanations. On my demand to see Hatorisan, Camp Commander, he finally agreed and dismissed me.

I then went to Lt-Col. Hugenon and we went to report. As the interpreter was not there, I saw Okada, showing him my abrasions to hand and forearm and bruises, cuts and abrasions to the leg. I told him of the subsequent developments and asked him if he would take me to the commander. This he did and introduced me, apparently referring to the incident. I then further explained in English, making a strong protest. Hatorisan pondered this for a long time and finally said 'you must avoid such incidents with Nipponese soldiers!' He made a half promise of investigation, after first saying that it would not be possible to find the soldier as I did not know him. I suggested that Hannamura could help there and he was quite considerate.

4 October 1943

I discussed evacuation of sick mentioned above with Okada who said I could go down to Tarsau with him and the sick today and stay a few days.* There was a

* I discovered afterwards this was a strategem to get me away from the vengeance of the two Japanese soldiers.

rush departure in the morning. We arrived at Tarsau shortly after lunch and Okada went off. The patients were hanging about for hours but were finally drafted away when he had still not returned. I found it necessary to carry some 19 of the lying patients up the bank from the barge on my back.

I later saw most of the hospital staff including Harvey, Hazleton and Jim Finnemore. Fred Smedley and Budge Gill are not happy about the progress of many men and particularly criticised the Con Depot and the M.I. Room arrangements in the lines. The Con Depot food is very unsatisfactory, despite an extra 3c a day allowance for each patient. Medical arrangements in the Depot were not adequate to treat sick men; many have become worse and have lost their legs or died. For example, Bliss of S Battalion has lost a leg. Many have huge ulcers, attributed to a lack of attention until they become major problems.

5 October 1943

I discussed finance provisionally with Lt Ross of Lt-Col. Warren's group, who is now doing hospital finance. Lt Barrett is the camp pay officer. He considers the Tarsau hospital position as very sound at present: in August the excess of income over expenditure was 1,248 ticals. The September excess will be greater because the hospital canteen has shown a very good profit (has now been put on sound lines) and despite the provision of 3,000 ticals for ordinary and special diets, only 2,300 was expended. Eggs etc. ordered did not arrive. As hospital funds stand now at nearly 11,000 ticals, they could carry on for some three months at the present expenditure without any further income at all.

The latest information is that there are still 40 kilometres of rail to be done from the rail heads, now approximately 120 kilometres and 170 kilometres from the north. An escape party of 8, including C.R.E., were told that five 'died in the jungle'; the three survivors were sentenced to imprisonment for a term of years. There were severe repercussions to the camp naturally.

The hospital ulcer wards: four large ones can only be described as horrendous – 'a butcher's shop'. The stench of gangrene is horrible, sickly sweet, and nauseating. Except for Pte Abbott, I have never seen ulcers like these and they are not limited to the lower legs but include the thighs, buttocks and upper limbs. Evidence of cross infection is quite irrefutable. Huge numbers of men with naked, necrosed bone exposed and sloughing great masses of tendon. I was most particularly shocked at changes in the condition of men who were all doing well when I saw them last and are now in great danger of loss of limb or life. This infection writes its grisly tale on the face and frame very quickly, the pale, lined, harrassed face and haunted eyes telling of toxaemia, pain and loss of sleep – I well remember the pain and sleeplessness myself. The worst of these ulcers are exposing about two-thirds of the tibia in the lower leg and most of the tendons of the leg.

On enquiry, I found that standard ward equipment consisted of a couple of old forceps and a blunt pair of scissors; containers and dressings are terribly short. Orderlies are not very well trained to say the least of it (witness one wiping pus and slough from forceps on the back of his hand!); dressings are not kept in sterile containers and handled. Obviously, no sterile set-up between cases and it is submitted that there are neither sufficient containers or time to arrange this (towels, blankets and all sorts of fabrics have been called in for foments, etc. but are quite inadequate). The general policy of treatment, heat and eusol in the early stages, then sulphanilamide. I think they use this sulphanilamide too early; they employ practically no ointment bases – they have not used beef suet – and there is the most inadequate use of splints and elevation. The complaint there is that there is not sufficient fabric or other padding available to pad splints. There is an obvious shortage of hot water. I do not think the orderlies are capable of thorough toilets of ulcers, removing sloughing tissue, even if they had the instruments.

6 October 1943

Conversation with Lt-Col. Harvey: I told him frankly that the hospital medical arrangements were under some criticism, particularly the convalescent section, and that some of the men sent down had deteriorated badly. Present officer-in-charge of the Con Depot is unsuitable; the medical arrangements are inadequate; and the food and cooking is poor. I also criticised the failure to sterilise eating utensils and the urgent problem of the ulcers. They need more instruments, more containers, and to pay more attention to the problem, which he confessed had escaped his attention up to date. I offered my help, since there is an excess of doctors in Kinsayok, but he suggested only that I paid similar visits to the present one.

The financial meeting was attended by Lt-Col. Knight, Harvey, Warren, McOstritch, Cdr Lusker, Maj. Humphries, Capt. Bryant, Capt. Pusey and Lt Barrett and Ross (was ever such a mass of authority given over to deciding so little in dollars and cents?). The balance sheet for September and the estimates for October were discussed and the agenda included: officers' subscription (agreed to be $10: $7 hospital; $3 messing); the hospital special diets (increased to $2,000 – the only dissenting voice was Cdr Lusker who thought more should be spent on drugs. I thought food before drugs, excepting emetine); the Reserve Fund (reported $5,207, almost all collected.); the Con Dept (criticism of kitchen and, according to Lt-Col. McOstritch, also of medical arrangements. Harvey dealt with this, recommending a change of kitchen staff. He had confidence in his QM, Ross. He did not refer to the medical arrangements.); and the central canteen arrangements.

A side light on the Con Depot is that Dick Allen developed fever this afternoon, but as the sick parade was held this morning, there was no provision for treatment and even when taken to Hazleton with O'Driscoll absent, he was told it was too late to arrange a slide or for quinine. In disgust, he asked if he could take his own!

7 October 1943

There is a strong desire on the part of evacuated Hintok men that I stay down and look after their interests. My CCS orderlies frankly expressed their disgust with the local ward equipment and nature of toilet to ulcers, etc. Capt. Street in charge of dysentery, and Vardy (Medical) seem to have great respect from all; few have a good word for the convalescent personnel.

8 October 1943

The AIF admin. officers were very pleased at the result of the meeting and are going ahead buying extras for their men. In the evening a hospital birthday night with McConachie, Vardy and a Dutch doctor having a combined birthday party. The band played merrily outside, including George Page and his trumpet.

9 October 1943

W/O Mepstead's ulcer is now of gross proportions, exposing about 8 in of bone and deep tissues of the leg, threatening to ringbark the leg. Amputation was decided on and McConachie suggested that I do it. Mepstead agreed that it was better to lose the leg and to have some hope of getting back to his wife and family. His position was in the Tramways Board and he was sure that they would find him employment.

As a general anaesthetic was considered to be available, I was told chloroform would be used. The patient was not properly shaved and was waiting for the barber to fix this when he had a nasty collapse. After a lengthy pause, Lee replaced the mask and apparently considered him fit to proceed. I had no more than cut the flaps when he was seen to be in white asphyxia and completely out to it. Lee then gave strychnine and other stimulants and began artifial respiration without effect. In about ten minutes he was pronounced dead. I then rapidly made a midline incision to admit four fingers of the right hand and did a vigorous cardiac massage. Slowly the grey/white of the face changed and became suffused with some blood, at first cyanotic, and later the dead eyes looked a little more alive. At last, to my excitement, the heart began to beat, stopping after a few beats. I continued to establish regular beating and introduce 1 cc of adrenaline solution to the heart producing vigorous beating. The eyes changed, the pupils slowly coming down. Artifical respiration was now continued vigorously and after a seeming age, he began to breathe in a shallow way with a sort of Cheyne Stokes rhythm.

Hurriedly and in great nervous tension, I closed the abdomen and then finished the leg amputation, lower third of thigh. The patient was packed with hot bottles, head down, left in the theatre. Maj. Hazleton arranged a blood transfusion. The sad fact is that his heart must have stopped for at least five minutes, probably nearer ten, thus I consider that extreme damage would have been done to his higher centres and he would not recover consciousness. The lad has been really a friend of mine and has depended on me a great deal. The nervous strain of the whole business has been extreme and I feel depressed and shaken. Damn chloroform as an anaesthetic – I am certain this would not have happened with ether. The Scottish school are crazy about the damn stuff and of course ether is very scarce and uneconomical in the tropics.

In the evening I was told that I could go back tomorrow and to report at 0815 with the two dental patients. I am extremely worried about many things at Tarsau but felt it best to leave with a sad heart at this juncture.

10 October 1943

Away after a great rush and much waiting about at Nippon HQ. Mepstead is still alive but has not recovered consciousness, as I expected. I saw Padre Thorpe at Tonchin and took on some more soldiers going to Rin tin – a very hungry day, I had four eggs but shared them with soldiers. Fortunately in the evening, a friendly Thai gave us a bowl of rice and a little egg and vegetable dish. The river barge Thais are in no way intimidated by the Nipponese. The passage took about twelve hours and I slept most of the time when not reading the *Diary of Samuel Pepys*, provided thoughtfully by Lt-Col. James. I feel very tired and have not slept well at Tarsau.

The first hut of the hospital is almost completed and is reasonably satisfactory (my design, with the beds running longitudinally) but in spite of all promises, are being built on the same cramped lines. The new M.I. room and quarters for MOs and nursing personnel have been got ready in the Nippon Q store and it seems likely that we will not get the present Nippon HQ building. I believe the promise of the kitchen still holds.

11 October 1943

Recommended to Lt-Col. McEachern and Lt-Col. James that one or both go down to Tarsau to discuss problems with admin. oficers and recommend appropriate action. They, however, consider it better for me to go back, armed with a diplomatic letter from them, expressing my own criticisms.

I find little or nothing done about reorganisation of the hospital since I left so as a first step, I arranged medical staff ORs to be clearly defined and those marked cookhouse, wood and water, etc. to be available for hut-building duties.

It seems likely that some admin. officers were beaten up in Kanchanaburi over a matter of wireless sets and map found; they suffered severe injuries such as a broken jaw, broken arm and ribs and two have subsequently died. This type of beating to death can scarcely be termed punishment officially and no trial was carried out. These are only rumours.My assailant of last week has apparently given more trouble and one of the Nips in gossip said he had been sent to Tarsau for 'attempting' to hit 'Col. Dunroppo' (my God, I like that!). Lt-Col. I. has much reduced the hitting since I left apparently. It is now apparent that I had been spirited out to escape being done to death by this character.

12 October 1943

Discussion today with Lt-Col. Hugenon, McEachern and James so that I can run a hospital kitchen for all, look after stray troops who arrive in camp without officers or resources and purchase drugs, etc. without having to collect money from each group. I advised the utmost importance of settling a common scheme of officers' contributions, preferably the same as at Tarsau. We set the provisional allowances for patients at 13c per man per day, and all officers are to subscribe $10 per month to cover this. Surplus money not spent is to be sent to Tarsau.

13 October 1943

I am to approach Okada for permission to leave for Tarsau in a few days. A curious thing happened last night when six of Capt. Pavillard's men sent down with me to Tarsau a week ago arrived back in a working party – one of these labelled 'T.B.', one a case of amoebic dysentery and none fit for work. On arrival in Tarsau they were given one day's work before seeing a doctor at all, then seen and marked attend 'C', which they described as hard work. After one week, they were only too glad to leave Tarsau in a working draft. Pavillard is furious! All admin. officers are worried about the number of deaths and lost legs down below.

14 October 1943

The new hospital hut is going on well. Much talk of an inspection by a visiting general soon.

The numbers in hospital on 15, 16 and 17 October were 255, 265 and 267, plus 21 from outside camps. I frequently get rebuked by the Nipponese about the sick figure rising. Today, I had words with Okada after refusing to supply more than 20 heavy sick for working. He finally called for the interpreter, who after repeating the request said, why more sick everyday? I said, 'Am I almighty God to answer this question. Did I make this fever – this unhealthy jungle? Am I responsible that the Nipponese made these men prisoners and then worked them so hard and gave them too little food? Look at them with their skin stretched over their bones! The Nipponese are responsible. Why do you not ask: "Why do men die?" Look at that cemetery – does it surprise you that men get sick before going there?' This outburst shocked poor old Pop – he looked very uncomfortable and said, 'Then I take it you do not think more men are fit to work,' and hurried away with O. who looked as sulphurous as the Prince of Darkness.* I then worked out a whole organisation scheme for the entire Kinsayok POW Hospital under my command.

18 October 1943

The new hospital seems to be working quite efficiently. The kitchen capacity has been increased to take 6 *cwalis* which is quite adequate for all purposes. The weather is greatly improved with clear, hot, fine days and cool starry nights (not cold). Okada is ubiquitous and appears to work very hard in the interests of the sick. He is mortally afraid of Lt-Col. Ishi whom he detests.

19 October 1943

Uneventful days on the whole.

X [wireless] reports that in Italy after the fall of Naples the 5th and 8th Army

* My outburst to Okada was in part motivated by a plan to insult him to a degree that I would be sent off to Tarsau.

are not making much progress where German resistance is strong. Very hard fighting on the Dneiper Line; it looks as if Germany will see the winter through.

20 October 1943

Today I had a stinging malarial attack, feeling unwell for two or three days with malaise and restlessness at night and this morning a bone shaking rigor lasting about two hours, working up to an extremely high temperature (last recorded 106). I felt I rather lost count and was too muddle headed to convert Centigrade to Fahrenheit at that stage. I passed completely out with a curious delusion of being incarcerated in a block of glass, completely unable to move but with a curious detachment so that I floated above watching my pulse from the throbbing motion transmitted to the mosquito curtain. Became delirious and said stupid things. Maj. Corlette came and inspected the corpse and called for intravenous quinine. Surprisingly I answered him, 'Ewan, you may think that I don't know what's going on fixed in this block of glass, but I've been watching my pulse which is quite irregular and if you give me that quinine, I will be dead.' Ewan looked perplexed and confused and said to Gibby, 'Well sponge him for an hour and if he's not better he must have the quinine.' My temperature slowly came down with sponging and quinine by mouth.

21 October 1943

I was still prostrated and rose only for a short time in the afternoon to discuss hospital policy matters and finance. Provisional examination of finance reveals that we are exceeding our income estimates.

22 October 1943

It seems probable that along with 50 men for Tarsau evacuation, two or three medical officers are to go, in accordance with previous decisions made by the camp commanders. I will have to go. I have decided to take Wright. If an English medical officer is to go, it will be Capt. Allen, as he has the least troops remaining here. The men for evacuation are being picked out, I wish S/Sgt. Gibson and Butterworth to go with me too.

23 October 1943

I returned to normal duties feeling rather feeble and ineffective. I finished the evening in reprobate fashion, Bill Wearne and I being thoroughly ticked off for playing chess after lights out. Lt-Col. McEachern was also in the line up for *kiotské* etc. A party passing through from up river, evacuated in charge of a Dutch MO, Capt. Stahle.

24 October 1943

Departure of Captain Stahle and party. I gave Captain Stahle 200 ticals as a temporary loan from Maj. Wearne from O and P funds. He will buy drugs for us. I told him that if he could not get back to Kinsayok, I would be at Tarsau and he could deliver the drugs to me there. We discussed ulcer treatment and he

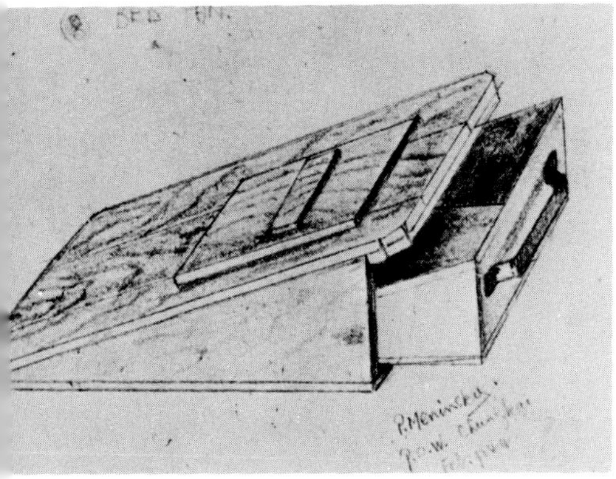

pan made of wood with tin container (*P. Meninsky*)

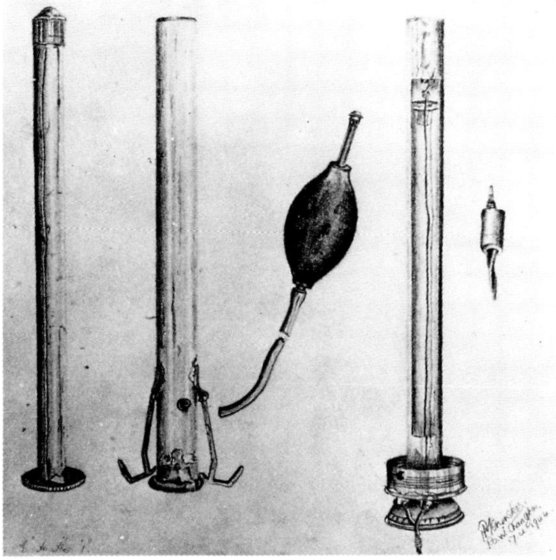

89 Jungle sigmoidoscope. Improvised tin tube electrically lit and with air inflation for viewing the bowel (*P. Meninsky*)

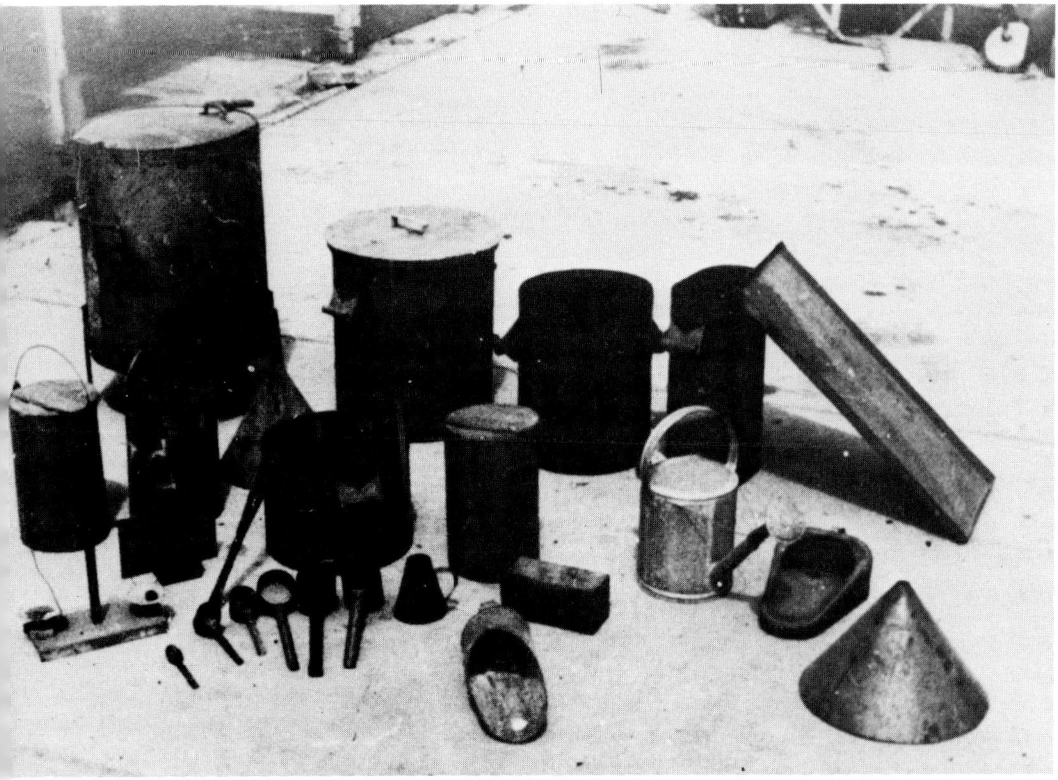

.ing untensils

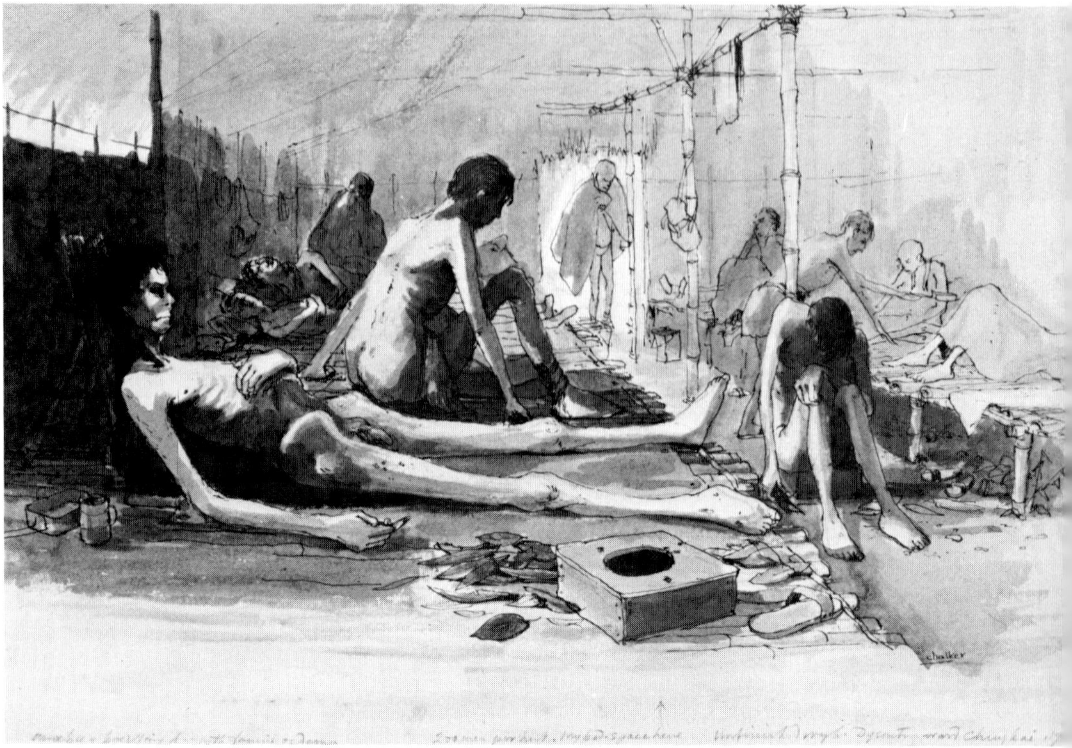

91 Dysentery ward, Chungkai from Jack Chalker's own bed space, 1943 (*Jack Chalker*)

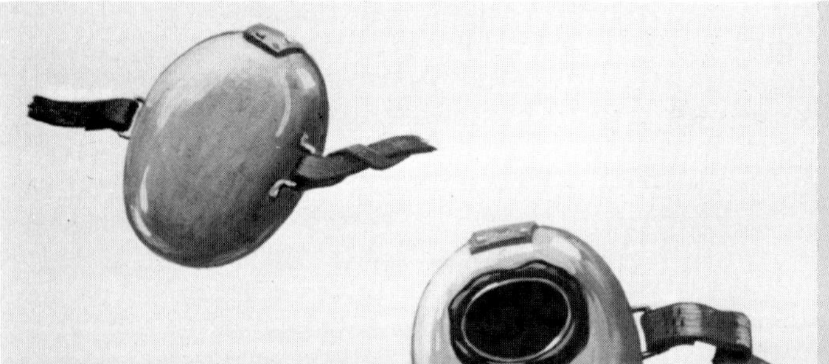

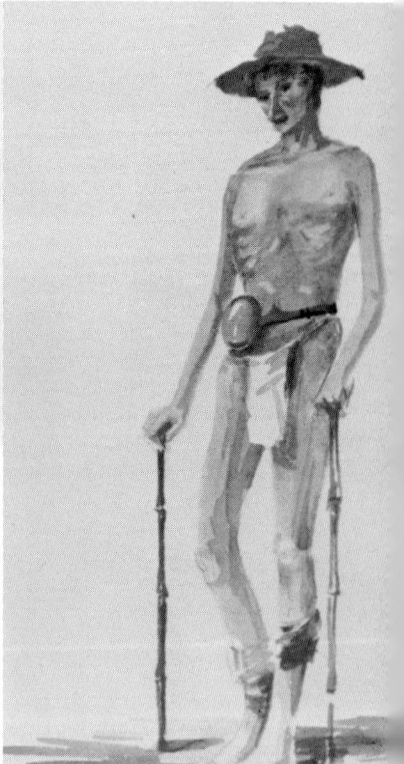

92 Ileostomy bottle (above) made from Dutch aluminium water bottle with pack straps attached, Chungkai 1943. Drawing (right) shows how it was worn (*Jack Chalker*)

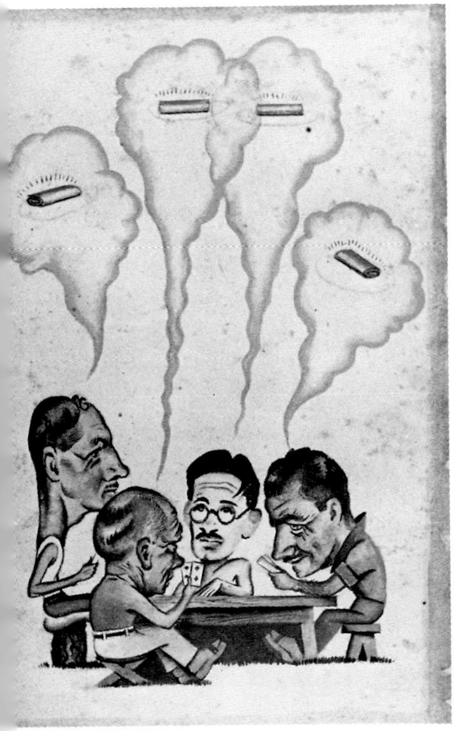

ıtract bridge: playing for omelettes. Pairs: A.A.
on and D. Hirst, E.E. Dunlop and 'Bill' Taylor (Hirst
Taylor were champions)

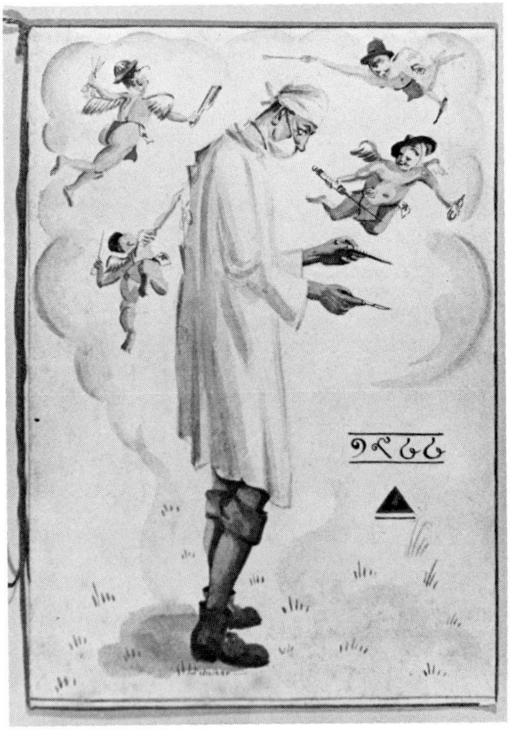

94 E.E. Dunlop operating, attended by seraphic theatre staff (*Jack Chalker*)

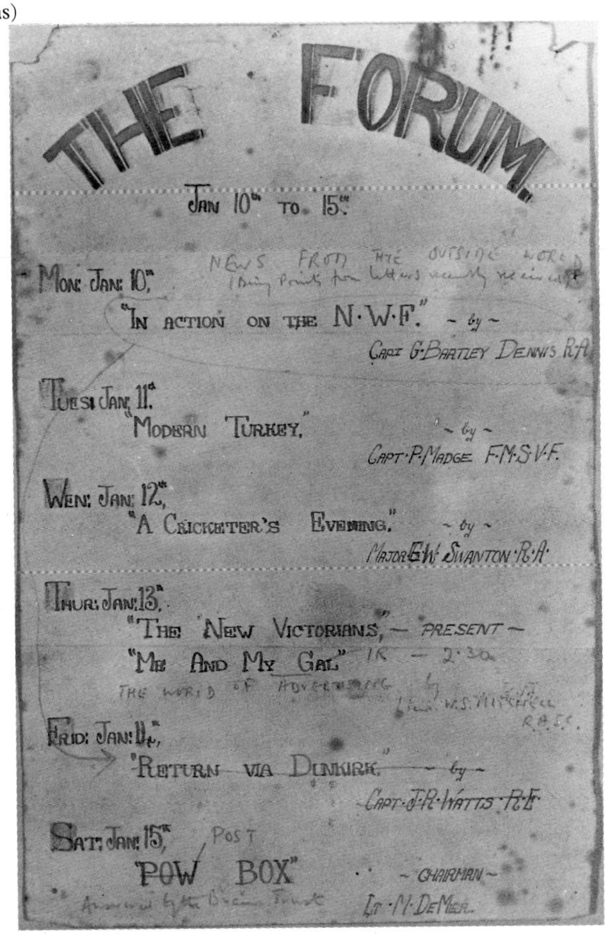

95 Poster for lectures and entertainment, 1944

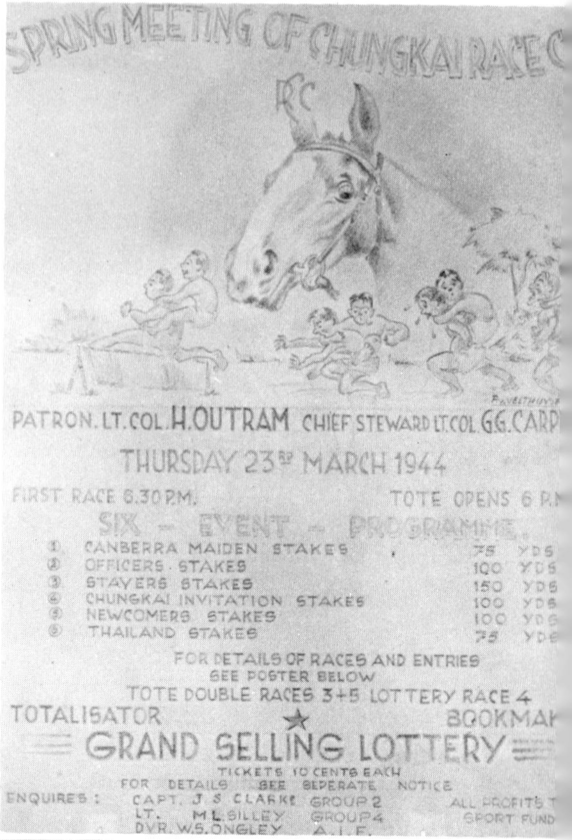

96 Poster for the Spring Meeting of the Chungkai Race Club, 23 March 1944

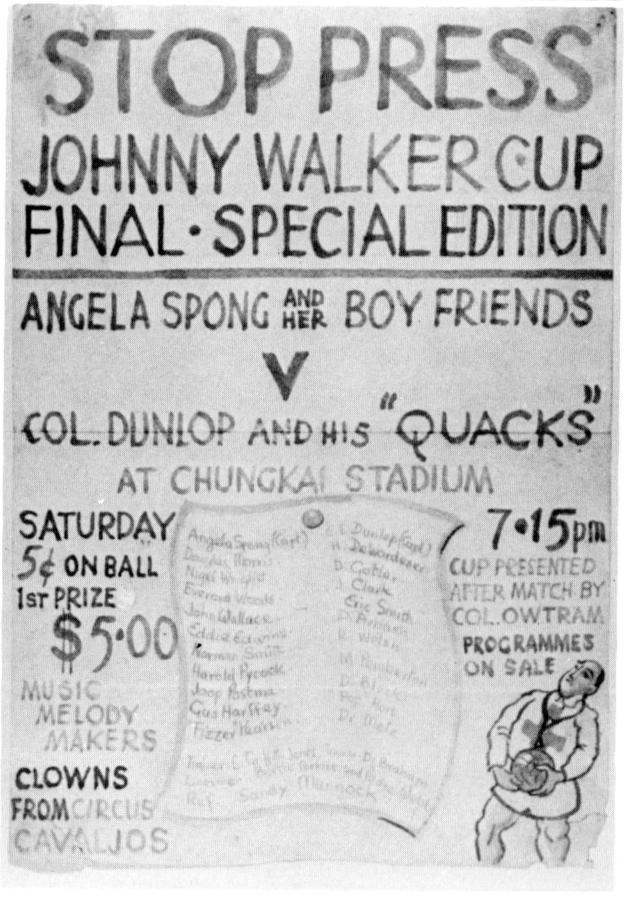

97 Poster for the soccer match, hospital *vs* camp, Chungkai 1944

said that at a large hospital in Java the routine was to curette the ulcers clean and treat with carbolic acid applied on cotton wool pledgets, just enough to whiten the tissues, then dust in iodoform and close with dressings for a few days until offensive (iodoform 1 in 10 with sugar is economical and quite effective). This routine may have to be repeated in some cases. He commented on the quick relief of pain with this treatment.

8 Tarsau

October 1943

25 October 1943

Departed for Tarsau at 1100 hrs with 50 sick plus Capt. McEwan, one dental patient, Reg Wright and I for transfer. We were met by Lt-Col. Harvey and other medical officers on arrival. Jock Clarke is looking fitter. Tarsau camp now has a formidable system of parades: a great deal of time is consumed in numbering and checking all the troops (all ordering and numbering is in Japanese). I am at present in the lines, sharing a bay with Lt-Col. Thomas. The hospital today obtained some most useful drugs and money – 3000.*

Things are much the same, with difficulty in purchasing foodstuffs for the hospital in sufficient quantity and in accordance with estimates.

26 October 1943

Total in hospital is 2461. Admitted 12; discharged 7; 4 deaths.

Discussed my function in the area with Col Harvey. I am to take over the hospital and convalescent depot from tomorrow and to be responsible to Harvey as SMO. I would assume responsibility for discipline in the area. Devoted the day largely to general reconnaissance and saw a number of old patients. The lads flatter me by showing extraordinary pleasure that I am now going to stay here.

27 October 1943

I inspected the ulcer cases with 'Monty' – a great improvement in many since the hospital acquired some iodoform which gives rather speedy relief of pain and good granulation of wounds. Don Thomas is doing good work in the ulcer ward. 18 amputations have been carried out.

The present organisation of the place is as follows: Lt-Col. Harvey SMO; Registrar: Capt. Finnemore; *Coy. Officer*: Maj. Mason.

Hospital, *Wards 1–15:* Maj. Hazleton AIF

Surgical	*path.*	*Medical*
Capt. McConachie	Capt. Cohen N.E.I.	Capt. Vardy
Capt. Millard		Capt. Smith
		Capt. McNeilly

* By grace of that magnificent man, Boon Pong.

Capt. Street
Capt. Lodge
Capt. Westcamp NEI
Capt. Wright AIF

Con Depot (Wards 16–24)
Maj. O'Driscoll
Capt. Pitt
Capt. Lees
Capt. Boston (NEI)

QM: Capt. Ross; Adj.: Lt Henshall; Clerk: S/Sgt Williams
Sgt Ogilvie – Senior Nursing Orderly

Hospital Staff: there is no definitely fixed duty section and convalescing patients do a good deal of the work. The hospital maintenance section, war repairs etc., is under Lt Higgins.

Lt Atkins is at present in charge of Hygiene and Sanitation. A provisional inspection reveals most problems here. The open-type latrines are very close to barracks, flyblown and offensive; these are also frequently used as swill tips and there is also the problem of disposal of offensive discharge and dressings from the surgical section. The main swill tip goes into the river but the water is rendered very still by numerous barges and some refuse floats back into the ablution area. There is cholera in the hospital (2 cases) and the area is too congested so that the cholera tents (which are not flyproof) are about 20 yards from the nearest wards. There is no disinfestor though some disinfection of clothing and blankets is carried out by boiling. The following are urgently needed:

1 Men to make a hygiene section of 40, including 4 carpenters.

2 Tools for hygiene work: shovels, 10; picks, 4; chunkels, 4; ropes, 1; axes, 1; parangs, 1; crosscut saws, 1. The tools are at present drawn in defective quantity at 1000 hours. As they are required earlier, it is requested that they be issued as a hospital responsibility and locked up in a special carpenters' shop here so that we can achieve earlier issue.

3 Materials: sawn timber, cases, etc. from the canteen and from the Nipponese. Wire, 8 gauge; oil, 10 gallons per week; kerosene or other fuel oil for lamps and latrine lights, 2 gallons per week; disinfectants, crude; bamboo ties and attap for Lt Higgins. Boilers: *cwalis* for sterilising eating gear, 7.
Containers: assorted tins (at least 70).
Drum: 40 gallon for disinfestor.

4 Cart: For carrying ash, swill and wood to boilers.

5 Hospital fence: more area required for suitable siting of latrines, etc.

Measures to be taken:

1 'Thunder boxes' required for use of transit sick in particular, as these foul the area

2 Ward masters must be made responsible for the hygiene of their ward areas and to ensure removal of contamination by 0900 hours.
3 Most urgent need is for fresh deep, covered latrines (one under construction) It should be provided with flyproof seats, etc. Special traps should be constructed for refuse and garbage. The containers for these are most unsatisfactory. Soakage pits are also required for the surgical wards
4 Lighting of latrines: oil lamps are required.

The following works are urgent: rebuilding of defective and leaning barracks; a new hut to contain the medical officers; clothes' lines between wards; some new wards if space and materials are available; splints, especially for legs; stretchers of bamboo type; artificial limbs; back rests for beds; Crutches.

Lt-Col. Harvey will do all official liaison with the camp authorities and the Nipponese HQ. Transfers occur at 1430 hours daily from hospital to the camp area.

28 October 1943

I carried out a general inspection; the convalescent kitchen now seems to be on a more satisfactory basis. O'Driscoll appears polite and co-operative.

A Nipponese medical major called in today with a captain and another officer. They were especially interested in the ulcers and wished to know requirements for treating these. These were, of course, given in plenty, with special reference to anaesthetic materials, catgut and operating material, iodoform, sulphanilamide, antiseptics and dressings of all sorts. They were shown the only skin grafting case that has been done here by Monty. We explained that there was insufficient local anaesthetic; perhaps they may give some help, as they noted some particulars.

I had just gone to bed tonight when I was called to see Pte McCann, 2/3 M.G. Bn: very acute abdominal pain and vomiting with abdomen grossly distended, visible peristalsis ++. Only slight relief with an enema. Confidently diagnosed intestinal obstruction. He has had previous operations for hernia on both sides and an undescended testis removed on the left side. I borrowed a petrol pressure lamp from the Nipponese. Laparotomy through the right lower abdomen. We finished at 0200 hours, had a cup of tea and reported to the guard without event, but nearly got into trouble with the sentry for standing inside the gate studying stars!

29 October 1943

Pte McCann's condition is satisfactory. A conference of administrative officers was held today at which I discussed the hygiene problem and steps requested, ward masters' responsibilities and the necessity to reduce the numbers in hospital. The Con Depot patients are to be sorted out weekly into sick, improving but not fit and fit for either working parties or unemployed.

More medical orderlies are needed and a training school is to be established. Twenty convalescent patients will be the first trained.

A scabies treatment centre is required for ambulant cases; the disinfestor is to be constructed.

As there are six troublesome mental patients, a mental hut with a fence is urgently required. Anti-malarial work: an officer should be obtained to carry out this task – some Malayan planters have a good knowledge of this.

I arranged for Capt. Wright, AAMC, to commence work in the medical wards of the hospital and in the lines with O, P, S and T personnel.

Sadly, a VD patient, an unusual thing, was called to the HQ to explain his infection (? acquired in a Thai village). He left the hospital area and decapitated himself by placing his neck on the railway line with an oncoming train.

30 October 1943

Perhaps the greatest problem with the hospital now is the nutritional diarrhoea cases. Diarrhoea is frequently much more nocturnal. Many of these are going downhill and finally find great difficulty in taking food. Probably the B_2 factor is the most important.

31 October 1943

Exploring the possibilities of carbolisation of ulcers in the acute, spreading stage. I brought down a little acid carbolic for this express purpose. Apparently the treatment is giving good results at Non Padok (Maj. Smith RAMC).

We require tulle gras (this is a vaseline impregnated mesh) for skin grafting, I am going to approach Westercamp for balsam of Peru, the Nipponese for some soft paraffin and mosquito netting, and a suitable knife for grafts. A skin grafting programme would greatly improve not only the rate of healing but the general morale.

1 November 1943

I inspected Phil Millard's ulcer ward. He is a most painstaking fellow and is getting good results. The ward staff and equipment are still primitive, but they are coping better.

2 November 1943

I investigated today the question of any waste of blood, bones or brains of beasts killed. I interviewed the camp QM who promised to lay on all the blood etc. possible. Socks are required for artificial limbs. I presume these could be knitted from donated woollen garments. I feel the hospital and Con Depot could be more closely linked, particularly on the A and Q side. Work on this area is slowly coming along but there are endless obstacles. I may create a healing ulcer ward under Maj. Hasleton and am investigating skin grafting possibilities first.

Lt-Col. M'Kellar has been detained for some sort of investigation.

3 November 1943

I commenced ward work today typical ulcer wards with nothing at all exciting about them. Ward equipment is very poor and the scabies problem is terrible. Some are just covered with impetiginous sores. Dressings are negligible and bedding mostly filthy. The scabies problem must be attacked immediately and there must be a crusade against dirt and uncleanliness.

Irrigating cans and sterilisers are urgently wanted in the surgical wards. Close supervision is required as to blankets.

Captain Brennan (dentist) at the hospital has been questioned by the Nipponese authorities but is reticent naturally. I gather that other officers are being questioned. Lt-Col. McEachern has been seen in the camp under escort.

5 November 1943

I discussed with Lt-Col. Thomas the increase in expenditure of the hospital, the special diets and messing of the sick. The monthly financial meeting was fixed for this morning at 1130 hours. I was to attend but to my surprise at 1030 hours was sent for by the *kempis* along with Maj. Williams of Konyu origin.

* * * * *

The actual circumstances of this near crisis were quite different from those recorded, because they were too sensitive to record at the time.

I arrived at Tarsau Camp under something like arrest by Okada, carrying my wireless set and much other contraband, diaries, maps, compass, etc. The *kempis* (Nipponese Military Police) were engaged in a wireless search and investigation and had already beaten some officers to death and badly injured others. A *kempi* search must have been fatal for me. However, Okada made it clear that I was his personal prisoner and pushed me through the *kempis*. I managed to hide most of my contraband and the set, but incriminating material was sewn into the sides of my pack, top of my cap, etc. I saw Lt-Col. McOstritch who was Camp Intelligence Officer and told him I had just brought in my set. He looked a trifle white and said, 'Well we need that like a hole in the head!' I said, 'Why worry about a hole in a detached head!' There was a council of war after Lt-Col. McKellar's arrest and when Lt-Col. McEachern also disappeared, I knew that I was at risk.

The only policy we could arrive at was never to admit having seen a wireless set under any circumstances and to lie glibly about camp rumours.

The evening of 4 November was enlivened by some grim accounts of *kempi* tortures, conduct of Nipponese trials and a sad account of the death of Page, my old rugby-playing friend, following capture in the second long range heroic raid on Singapore. Page's courage and bearing won him respect and a senior officer after his trial recommended that his life be spared. However, the Commander said, 'No', and – in effect – that such a heroic exploit in the great tradition of the Samurai could only have one appropriate end: beheading. The sentence was carried out respectfully.

Following my arrest, I was first thrown into a small cell where, to my disgust, I found in a concealed pocket of my shirt some wireless news whose cryptic nature no longer seemed clever. This I chewed up and swallowed. Curiously my prolonged interrogation was not accompanied by a search of my gear in the lines. I hoped that it would be dispersed by friends. Some hours of patient interrogation as to my doings ensued, with whom did I exchange news, what did I knew about the war, what were my movements from camp to camp, with whom had I had conversation, etc. Suddenly after some four hours, there was a dramatic violent change. The interrogating officer, 'Stone Face' jumped to his feet and pulled down a screen with Japanese characters and a tracery of connecting arrows. Pointing to a rather central character, he said, 'You are this person – we know all about you and your set – you will be executed but first you will talk'. I was clapped in manacles and he deputed two soldiers to flog me with lumps of firewood each time my answers to questions, though verbose, finished up in the negative. I thought of the dead British officers beaten to death in this way at adjacent camp where all this started. I maintained my 'innocence' under steady beating, but pined for a cyanide pill.

At last I was told patience was now exhausted and I must die. I was pushed and flogged along to a tree and my manacles changed to encircle my wrists behind the tree with my body and arms taut about the tree, my bare belly exposed to four bayonets wielded by an execution squad of four, making the characteristic belly grunting, blood-curdling yells, working themselves up to 'the moment'. I was told by the interpreter – the one in the party with long hair – that I was to have the grace of 30 seconds, which were grimly counted in Japanese. My eyes were locked on the flinty, impassive face of the 'interrogating' officer. Strange thoughts flitted through my mind, 'This can't be me. I don't feel frightened enough. It's just unreal!' I thought with ironic amusement of a time at school when for an escapade I anticipated expulsion and disgrace. My reaction then seemed far worse, more horrendous. I speculated whether anyone would even know how I died.

The egregious voice of the interpreter – 'Now ten seconds to go. Have you last message for relatives. I shall try to convey.' I shifted my gaze to his distasteful face and said contemptuously: 'Last message conveyed by thugs like you – no thanks!' The bayonets were withdrawn and poised for the last yelling thrust when I saw a flush on the face of my executioner who raised a hand and cried, 'Stop! He will suffer a lot more than this before he dies – untie him!' The manacles were transferred to the front and I suffered a bout of heavy beating without further interrogation.

At length I was pushed into a cell, squat-legged, facing a wall to await execution and presumably meantime to improve my attitude. A guarding sentry struck me with a rifle if my erect body slumped. As a ridiculous distraction I tried to recall Keats' 'Ode to a Nightingale' and watched a small lizard enviously.

Evening and, of all things, I was suddenly hauled forth to make up a team of 'lags' to play Japanese guards at 'circlos': a species of quoit was hurled back and forth and the point was lost if it was dropped. The game on our part was to be played in dead silence whilst the Japanese made raucous laughter and derisive yells at trembling hands and, in my case, bruised limbs and hands. My old friend, Dr John Diver of St Mary's Hospital London was particularly unsteady, and the Japanese concentrated on him calling 'Diver! Diver!' Well, the Japanese won 6–5. There were a few frustrating opportunities in turning to attempt communication in a stage whisper out of the corner of the mouth.

Back to the cell, manacles, and wall contemplation, some flashes of Keats' ode. A conundrum – 'If I had that pill would I take it now?' More 'encouragement' to sit at attention, legs crossed. It seemed too painful to think of home, my beloved Helen, or past life.

Again I was roughly taken out for execution, the same grizzly ritual, the same tree, but this time an air of grim finality: just the sound of steady counting and the horrible grunting yells with cold steel at times meeting my skin – but again, surprisingly to me, the last second reprieve.

This time I was taken in manacles to a small metal-framed pen which contained a Thai with, I thought, a good deal of Chinese blood. His manacles rested easily on his slim wrists, whilst mine sunk in even more deeply as my hands swelled. I rested on my back, hands raised most of the time. His conversation was to point at me pistol fashion and say, 'You – bang!', to which I wearily returned the compliment. Later, the ever present sentries pushed in rice and I envied him his monkeylike agility and mobile hands whilst I made such heavy going attempts to eat. Knowing the type of torture which went on in the place and having heard the screams of anguish, I frankly wondered whether I had the fibre to take it. For example, handcuffs behind, hitched with a rope over a beam, standing on a high chair, chair kicked away, dangling with a double dislocation of the shoulders – real torture then begins, eyes, testicles, etc. 'Yes,' you say, 'I have the set – you can have it'. But then the Judas pit opens: 'Who gave you the set? Who supplied the batteries? With whom did you communicate?' All unthinkable. I sweated it out until the following evening with a little more rice and intolerable pain in the hands.

My impassive companion was removed and tidily shot – my turn again, now almost hoping for a quick clean end. Shooting seemed promotion. My interrogator astounded me by resuming parley, inviting me to sit. He said, 'Colonel, you must understand that though you have not talked, that others have and we know that you are guilty.' Me: 'If they have talked, they are liars. Why don't you give me a fair trial to throw the lies in their faces!'

After a while, he looked at me in a sort of puzzlement and said: 'Is it that you really have not done these things or that you will not talk?' I laughed and said, 'Have I not spent all this time telling you that I know nothing?' Then to my utter astonishment; 'Colonel, if I were to release you this time, would you have hard feelings against the Japanese, hard feelings against me? We *kempis* do but do our duty.'

I said cautiously, 'From all I have heard of you *kempis*, I feel that I have been well treated.' I thought, have we some curious affinity? My manacles were removed and I was given beer and cigarettes. Suddenly I realised that prisoners' eyes would be on me being treated to the fatted calf, obviously as a reward for telling all, and this dimmed the surge of joy at my release. *Kempi* professionalism to the last.

I was subsequently called on once a month by *kempis* who looked me over. 'Colonel, how is your health? We *kempis* know that you are dangerous spy!'

At the fag end of the war, I faced 'Stone Face' in one of General Slim's 'identification' parades. There, without tunic or belt, holding up his trousers with one hand, face strangely gray and drawn. Our eyes locked again and I said,

'Interesting specimen that; but I have not seen him before.' However, what hope would a *kempi* officer have. 'We Kempis do but do our duty.'

★ ★ ★ ★ ★

6 November 1943
Total Hospital 2422. O – 166; P 145.

8 November 1943

I had a discussion with McEachern on the importance of a senior AIF officer coming down here to integrate Australian battalion activities and to look after AIF interests. He has approached Nippon HQ and they approve, subject to consent of Kinsayok.

9 November 1943

A weekly conference of hospital heads of departments with Lt-Col. Harvey attending. The following is to be adopted: Lt-Col. Harvey is SMO of the area and deals with me as CO of the hospital area. Under me in the hospital is Maj. Hasleton, divided into Medical (Capt. Vardy) and Surgical (Capt. McConachie), the A branch which is under Maj. Mason and Q branch. The other branch is the Con[valescent] Depot where Maj. O'Driscoll reports to me. The Q officer required is about the rank of major to correlate the work of kitchen arrangements in the hospital and Con Depot and in particular to be responsible for supply and maintenance of all equipment and for the activities of working groups, carpenters, tinsmiths, etc. As the needs of the hygiene group are at present supreme, Maj. Clarke is temporarily in charge of works and will fix priorities. Lt Higgins remains in charge of all camp building maintenance.
Indent for Drugs requesting purchase. This has been given to Lt-Col. Harvey.

Capt. Wright is in charge of the Scabies Unit. The disinfestor and boiling unit has been shifted to a new area and is nearly ready. A mobile team is to deal with the place ward by ward, ensuring thorough disinfestation of clothes at the same time as adequate sulphur treatment is carried out under their supervision. Sgt Ross will be the NCO in charge. A 'scabies' crusade is to be launched, emphasising cleanliness of the person and ward; every man must wash or be washed daily, and soap issues have been increased. Bedpans and utensils are to be washed between use and boiled daily.

There is an urgent need to increase special diets greatly to cope with the extreme prevalence of nutritional diarrhoea; these men simply can't cope with rice and stew and beans. This means increased expenditure. The expansion considered necessary is from 50–450! This will be a financial bombshell.
Hospital & Con Depot. An evening call of medical officers to attend any urgent sick must be carried out.

Food must be covered with mosquito netting at the kitchen-end serving point and sterilisation of eating gear must be arranged urgently.

All officers are to be accommodated in one ward. There will be no difference between the hospital and the Con Depot when the new hut is built.

Isolation is unsatisfactory at present. A new centre is needed.

10 November 1943

One case of cholera today. I addressed Ward Masters re defective hygiene and cleanliness of wards and the camp in general and warned that I will inspect the hospital and the Con Depot weekly.

I carried out the first Thiersch graft here today on a man called O'Sullivan with a large clean knee ulcer. A sharpened table knife cut the graft fairly well. We had some chloroform anaesthetic. I amputated the leg of Pte J.J. Gardiner, 2/3 M.G. Bn. He had a severe ulcer of the left leg and a nutritional diarrhoea.

11 November 1943

I am most worried about the steady small incidence of cholera which may become epidemic if they don't do something about it.

12 November 1943

Another case of cholera – most alarming. I put my views strongly to Lt-Col. Knight and Col. Harvey today, stressing the importance of containers and the sterilisation of gear, more care in handling food, etc. I don't know why all these trivial difficulties hold up important works when the things that you need are always available through unofficial channels. No help except the suggestion to buy. We supply 1000 eggs daily to patients; their needs are 1500. I have temporary authority from Col. Harvey to increase purchases to 1500. I am afraid I am bumping expenditure up sharply but it is necessary.

13 November 1943

Some success attends the work drive. One big latrine is practically completed and fitted with flyproof lids in two rows, an extremely deep latrine with a central tip for infective fluids, bedsores, etc. Two others are on the way, also an Otway pit. The tinsmiths and carpenters are doing excellent work producing all sorts of articles for the hygiene squad and wards; irrigators, splints, sterilisers, bedpans, containers of various sorts. There is an annoying shortage of wire, nails and containers, crude oil etc. Jock has plenty of solder now (acquired by devious ways) and we have enough containers, wood etc. to commence sterilising eating gear in every ward. This begins today.

Today I inspected all wards and the kitchen in the hospital area. Many grossly defective arrangements in handling of food, bedpans, soiled dressings, etc. Refuse disposal is shocking – a genuine attempt however has been made to clean up the wards and hospital area which has much improved.

Another Thiersch graft on a patient named Cameron. A further cholera case or two today making things look black.

14 November 1943

I had a further attack of malaria, feel cheesy, but am not going to bed this time. At long last, after many months, my right leg ulcer has healed.

The cholera is now serious affecting a number of the sickest cases in the hospital; a definite link with the hospital kitchen seems emphasised by the large number of people on special diets who are affected. The Nipponese were approached about a tented cholera area outside the congested hospital area (I asked for this before). Tents were obtained in the late evening, only one proving serviceable, so a complete transfer could not be done. Special measures regarding cooking and handling of food and sterilisation have been introduced. Mike Smith is to be a full-time cholera officer. Just at this time, of course, saline has been allowed to run out. Still to be worked at pressure day and night. Extra bowls and other articles were ordered today; I doubt if they will be forthcoming, though requested from the Nipponese. Damn this closing of stable doors after the horse has bolted! Everyone has had ample warning about cholera.

15 November 1943

The new cholera cases were transferred last night to a tented site in the jungle outside the hospital. Most lay on the hard ground and were well and truly tormented with ants and other insects. Today the cholera tents in the hospital area are being transferred. I am arranging for the stretchers to be got off the ground as soon as possible.

New cholera cases today, five from my ward, including Cameron (the skin graft). The whole of these were on Special Diet No. 2, I have now no doubt whatever that this is more than a coincidence. Lt Moroko, Mr Ozechi and other N officials did a partial inspection of the camp and discussed measures to combat cholera. When informed of the foul water drawn from about the Thai barges which we wished to be shifted, a filter pump was promised and later handed over. We asked for crude oil and kerosene in quantity and fly traps for the latrines of wood and wire netting. Maj. Clarke was given materials, including some much-needed nails, to construct some on a Nip model. Some good may come of this visit.

Lt-Col. Thomas is concerned about the hospital expenditure and asked me to see him and outline the policy. Accordingly, Captain Vardy and the hospital messing officer, John Day, worked out the new scheme and cost and I later explained it, stressing that now was the important time to increase expenditure because of the great prevalence of nutritional diarrhoea and dietetic disturbance for which we have no drugs. These patients cannot eat an ordinary camp diet and, although at present they are helped by the battalion welfare measures, these are spasmodic and depend upon precarious supplies. It would be better to put everything into a strictly directed medical effort.

If a major effort is made, the number of people being supported in hospital and the Con Depot would be rapidly reduced. For example, those with scabies and septic sores should readily respond to the present treatment, and once men are built up they can resume a normal diet and thrive on it.

All fit working men should be messed outside the hospital area. General messing will continue to be on the basis of 5c per man per day, hospital or Con Depot. Special diets are to be recommended [see Appendix I]. To my relief, Lt-Col. Thomas promised his support. He spoke of dysentery and cholera menace and asked if I would get Castellani bottles and other measures introduced into the lines.

16 November 1943

Received letters for many P battalion personnel per Fred Smedley. None for me. These brought cheer to many, including CCS men. Poor Jack Henshaw, 2/2 Aust. CCS died today after a long drawn out deterioration beginning at Hintok. He was changed immeasurably from his old self to a grey-haired skeleton. Nutritional diarrhoea, or I suppose really terminal pellagra. This is the fifth cholera death in the Australian CCS.

17 November 1943

Major Marsh reports that 442 men have no blankets in the hospital or Con Depot, 1300 have no jacket or pullover, it is sad to see some sick men with practically no other possession that a G-string and a rice sack. No doubt many blankets have been sold at one time or another, but then starving men will sell blankets. Perhaps some official N help may be forthcoming, or failing that, perhaps something could be done with a special appeal to the camp. Nothing is too old, nothing too torn, etc.

18 November 1943

Marsh today obtained quite a lot of new N issue matting for patients, including the operating theatre. This is badly needed. He has an idea of a weekly bulletin to be issued to the camp setting out the hospital position and its needs. This could launch the clothing appeal.

One new cholera case today. Of this outbreak of 39 cases, 29 patients have died to date. This very bad result must be expected in view of the appalling condition of these men before their infection.

19 November 1943

Major Marsh obtained today 300 mats to use in the wards covering this ghastly bamboo bedding. Some old mats can now become windbreaks around the ward.

The days are now beautifully fine, the nights cold and very keen. It is a lovely sight in the mornings to see the valley mists part and frame the mountains in a delicate pink, draped by golden wisps of cloud. Today I took the new orderly class and spoke to them about the common complaints of the camp, particularly scabies, dysentery, cholera and tropical ulcers. I illustrated problems of dressing clean and dirty cases by demonstration then showed them something of theatre asepsis.

Since iodoform ran out we are having greatly increased difficulties with tropical ulcers which are showing a backward trend in some cases. There seems little prospect of getting more. Captain Todd RAMC considers that a saturated solution of potassium permanganate gives excellent results. Just a pledget of wool saturated in the solution and wipe out the ulcer with a slight scraping motion until no healthy tissue comes away. He states this is the standard treatment in Malaya.

20 November 1943

Captain White, a Malayan planter, is looking into the anti-malaria work. He requires a squad of 20 men, including five officers, and permission to go outside the camp to do some of the work. This request has been passed on to N HQ. They would deal with both hospital and camp areas – this is the time after the rains when such measures are usually carried out. The salary of *chusas* is now increased vastly. I believe the situation now is that I receive 50 ticals per month, pay to the camp hospital and messing 20 ticals and collect 30 a month – princely! Thus today I was able to give Blue 5 ticals and Dave Topping 5 ticals (the latter is suffering still from amoebic dysentery and for a long time has had no income). There has been no further case of cholera. The camp hygiene is now much improved. I spoke to Captain Vardy about the formation of a diet committee, the object being to control the puchase of food, ensuring the very best use of the money spent on it, and to look into its preparation and distribution. At present the hospital messing officer, John Day has too much autonomy.

21 November 1943

On my advice, two Australian ulcer patients today had their legs amputated. Both had extremely serious extensive ulcers and were losing ground rapidly with nutritional diarrhoea. I regard both as bad risks, because few of these severe diarrhoea cases get better, even if uncomplicated.

22 November 1943

Discussed with Con Depot the requirements to open kitchen arrangements for an extra 250 men: some extra staff, four *cwalis*, 14 buckets, 2 crosscut saws and two axes.

I called a meeting to try and increase recreation and entertainment activities in the area. Lt-Col. Knight and Lt-Col. Harvey attended, also representatives from every group. Maj. Swanton had many ideas. The expanded activities should if possible embrace not only concerts and entertainments, quizzes, competitions, talks, etc. but also an arts and crafts programme (especially for limbless men) and education activities, lectures, talks, classes and readings, since there is a great scarcity of books. A committee of five members should be elected: three for general entertainment and concerts (Lt Jennings, Capt. O'Grady and Capt. Thoms), one for arts and crafts (Major Marsh) and one education and library activities (Major Swanton). Voting then was simple since there were only five nominations. I was interested to involve Major Swanton. Lt-Col. Knight did not show any particular enthusiasm.

23 November 1943

I roughed out a request to the Nipponese for a rather comprehensive entertainment, recreation etc. scheme. Two concert nights a week are required. Some difficulties may be met with obtaining lecturers on educational subjects and rehearsal facilities for musical items.

24 November 1943

I got the new diet scheme floated today with the necessary transfer of patients and staff to various kitchens, etc. This greatly increased expenditure on food has caused a comment, most favourable.

25 November 1943

I talked to Lt-Col. Knight about the new welfare recreation scheme and also pressed for blankets, I moved into a new *shoko*'s house right on the river and with a commanding view of the broad expanse of river, tangled jungle and the rugged mountains in the background. This hut includes Reg Wright, Padre Bourke, Padre Thorpe, Major Marsh, Lt Higgins, Capt. Smith (Mike) Capt. McNeilley and Capt. Westacott. I have a whole bay to myself so have asked for an extra bed to be inserted for the use of visitors, etc. My bed is composed of round small bamboos lashed together, hard and irregular like the hobs of hell.

A survey has been done of deaths in the hospital and causes. Number of admissions since the July census until 25.11.43 = 5946. Number of deaths = 364. Number of cholera cases in the recent epidemic = 40; the number of cholera deaths in the cholera epidemic = 29. (One of the cases included was only a suspect and died of amoebic dysentery. He was buried in the cholera area.) There is in this list an endless reduplication of diagnoses under different nomenclatures and a number of the diagnoses given are not primary causes of death. I consider it extremely important that the hospital records be improved and that uniformity is reached in diagnosis.

The 'captains of the men of death' were dysentery, cholera, malaria, deficiency diseases and tropical ulcers. Dysentery was much the most common cause.

26 November 1943

In consequence of Lt-Col. Knight's appeal to the Nipponese for blankets and bedding for the sick, Maj. Marsh received for the hospital 250 rice sacks (hemp), 300 mats and 200 rice mats of fibre type. These are most acceptable and I have asked him to go on with supply of these to those without blankets. Very sick men have priority of issue.

27 November 1943

I inspected the Con Depot today: some improvement. Many beds urgently need repair, but there is an extreme shortage of bamboo.

Supported by me, Tommy has built quite a fine fowl yard and this has been filled with fowls purchased by John Ray for patients, including just one massive duck called Donald who is well able to look after his interests. Today, the first fowl came into laying and the first egg was conveyed with due ceremony to Harvey (who has gastro-enteritis). Dick Allen came to dinner today.

28 November 1943

After much pressure on my part, representations were made to the Nipponese for a big purchase of drugs and eventually Fakudasan went down to Kanchanaburi to see what he could purchase for us. Emphasis was laid on such essentials as emetine, vitamin B1, iodoform, sulphur, carbolic acid and anaesthetics and surgical dressings. For the latter, bolts of cloth were regarded as an economical purchase. The net result is deplorable: only the most negative amounts being obtained.

We are informed that as from tomorrow the new No. 1 will be Captain Susuki (Lt-Col. Ishi is going to Burma). The F Force deaths are now probably 2,600. These men are all on the move down, leaving about 200 in the Burma hospital too sick for movement. There are 30 left out of some 400 Manchesters.

29 November 1943

I was dismayed to hear that the case sheets have not been preserved here (even with the shabby state in which they have been compiled) but were destroyed after the patient left hospital. It is incredible. Thus only the A and D book is a permanent record and even so, the diagnoses have not been satisfactorily completed by the clerks. I discussed all this with Henry Phillips; the requirements are to be not only the keeping of the hospital case records, but also each soldier on discharge is to be given a small card stating his period in hospital and the diagnosis with a brief précis.

30 November 1943

Education and talks scheme is moving along well: Swanton tells me he has the programme well in hand. Lt-Col. Warren reports that someone is selling four-gallon tins in his ward, so the 'house detective', Bonzo Mason, was called in to look into the problem. Removed an 8 in. sequestrum from the leg of a tropical ulcer patient.

1 December 1943

A monthly bulletin of hospital matters was for the first time presented to the camp today entitled *Hospital Bulletin*, 3 December 1943, commencing: 'Since July of this year Tarsau Hospital has grown from a camp hospital into a base hospital for the whole of No. 4 group. It is through no fault of our own that it is one of the most scantily equipped hospitals in the world.'

On 30 November, the total patients were 2407; of these 135 were in the critical medical ward and suffering from serious malaria or advanced avitaminosis, 200 were in the critical surgical wards with large tropical ulcers, 120 were suffering from amoebic dysentery, 220 were suffering from chronic diarrhoea and bacillary dysentery. There have been 341 deaths since 1 August. On the surgical side there were 27 amputations, and 10 men are now on crutches. There is marked progress in the ulcer patients. Special diets have been most beneficial. The main obstacle now is a shortage of drugs, especially iodoform and dressings. There were seven mental patients.

Diets: The new scheme of graded diets was introduced on 24 November. Some C Diet men in the dysentery ward showed a gain of 1 kg over five days.

2 December 1943

Performed an appendicectomy on a patient Sgt Snooks, AIF. His convalescence was uneventful.

Discharges from the Con Depot are urgently needed to take some 300 men reported to be coming in from Krian Krai.

3 December 1943

The nights are not particularly cold just at present; the days are hot. Cold weather in Thailand seems to come with the full moon. An amusing half hour listening to Marsh, Father Bourke, McNeilly and others after going to bed. Marsh explosively and violently took exception to the fact that Maj. Swanton, Turner and one other were taking advantage of their position on the hospital welfare committee to prosyletise their views as 'Christian fascists' (i.e. Anglo Catholics) and to that end depicted Franco as a knightly soldier of God! Padre Bourke took up the cudgels on behalf of Franco and swept in a mighty blow by saying, 'Seeing that you for months have taken advantage of similar welfare committees to prosyletise your own views to troops, I hardly see how you can take exception to others doing it!' How extraordinary that so many of our enthusiasts in politics and social economy etc. should devote so much time in evangelistic fervour, addressing these poor shipwrecked devils.

4 December 1943

A meeting about the unsatisfactory medical records and nomenclature. In view of the grave loss of health and the disabilities of so many troops, we should make every effort to preserve accurate records for subsequent pension and disability assessment.

The A. & D. book to be maintained as usual. We also discussed diets, complaints about food, the distillation of crude alcohol for medical purposes and Q matters.

Unfortunately John Day regards his department as a closed shop and co-operates neither with Marsh nor particularly with the diet committee, the hygiene officer, or even myself.

5 December 1943

The Dutch members of the camp had a visit from St Nicholas bringing gifts.

6 December 1943

Nippon HQ have warned us of a probable evacuation and in consequence we are preparing rolls for sick. There is likely to be a 10,000 bed hospital down Bampong way for all sick who need special treatment; others will probably go to Chungkai.

A new office is being erected close by our officers' hut on the river bank. Here were are to have a Nippon interpreter, 'Uncle Chunkle' of Kinsayok (a very nice old chap) and Matsudadasan and one other soldier who will directly administer our hospital affairs. I am to have a portion of the office, together with Col. Harvey.

7 December 1943

Monthly finance meeting held at HQ building, both Harvey and I in attendance, mainly about the great increase in hospital special diet expenditure for which we require 6,000 ticals for the month.

250 ticals from November and December canteen profits have been set aside for Christmas. My masterpiece at the tail end of the meeting was to request a therapeutic 'egg fund' to give the patients eggs directly in lieu of drugs. At least half of the expenditure of $1000 is to be met by a direct canteen allotment. A very satisfactory meeting.

8 December 1943

Cold and clear at nights. We had a balloon debate with me defending science.

9 December 1943

A party of approximately 300 arrived last night from Krian Krai, three dying on the way by train and one shortly afterwards. I developed malaria again yesterday so was not awakened for their arrival. All arrangements were made with O'Driscoll to have certain patients treated for scabies and discharged in readiness for the party, but when I tackled him about it this morning, he said that Lt-Col. Harvey had told him it did not matter. Thus neatly foiled, I passed the matter on to Harvey with some rather pointed comments on the whole affair. Another source of anger to me was that the poor devils did not get a breakfast meal until midday. Many of these have the very severe type of tropical ulcer and are extremely sick; if we do not get some iodoform soon, we are going to have a spate of amputations, I am afraid. Last night was intensely cold; God help all these poor sick wretches with only a bag to cover them.

I introduced the new system of medical records today. A real controversy blew up today between Vardy (Diet Committee) and John Day, Messing Officer. Vardy has written an irate letter re recommendations ignored, particularly referring to the unsuitable cooking of beans which affect bowel conditions very adversely. I discussed tactfully with John Day the many difficulties that he was causing me: unsatisfactory distribution of food, hygiene, failure to co-operate as part of Maj. Marsh's department, unsatisfactory feeding of Krian Krai sick and lastly the Diet Committee's letter.

10 December 1943

John Day, after sleeping on it requested relief of his duty. This is a source of relief to me.

I asked Lt-Col. Harvey to approach the Nipponese re the possibility of charcoal fires in the wards. The nights are terribly cold and men get up and wonder about in search of fires. Those confined to bed with painful conditions suffer terribly. The Nips again are requesting a return re men for evacuation.

11 December 1943

The Nipponese have asked us to join them on Christmas Day in mourning for our dead in Thailand. Religious and other feeling is that Christmas is hardly a suitable day for this purpose.

12 December 1943

As many of the ulcer patients cannot sleep with pain and cold it was arranged that that tea be served in the early morning, although the clatter wakes some other people up. In most of the wards, only about half the patients were sleeping. Some actually prefer to sleep in the open on the ground since they have very little bedding and on the ground less bedding is required underneath. Something must be done to give increased warmth or many men will die. I signed for pay today including pay for a number of incapacitated officers.

13 December 1943

The Nipponese supplied a number of rice sacks today to keep patients warm. Altogether, 3,900 received, and 1,000 rice mats.

The new messing officer, Captain Service, is a New Zealander, an Otago University and New Zealand University rugger forward. School of Mines man – full of energy and co-operative spirit. Lt-Col. Warren recommended him and I have had to do a little wangling to get him across. I think he will be the goods. The drug position is worse than ever.

14/15 December 1943

No entry.

16 December 1943

I gave a talk to patients on Ward 5 tonight, choosing 'Palestine' – a curious experience, because one talks in the dark completely unable to see one's audience and is conscious of other people lecturing away in the next ward. At times one has an impulse to yell, 'Are you fellows still there and are you awake?'

17 December 1943

A special 'order of the day' for the new Nipponese commandant, Captain Susuki, was read on parade.

Kanamotosan brought me greetings from Major Moon who is well and thinks he will be at Chungkai during the next month. The new hospital office is now complete. Planes, regarded by the Nipponese as allied, not infrequently fly over at night. Air raid precautions are strict: to extinguish all fires and lights and not even smoke in huts. All men are to go to hut and stay there on pain of shooting. It is suggested that the sick be made to get under the beds if we are attacked. This no doubt brings cheer to our fellows.

18 December 1943

I am arranging for a sigmoidoscope to be made out of tin and some auroscope parts. Unfortunately no spirits of salts for soldering and they are trying with resin. Maj. Swanton is to come on the staff officially.

19 December 1943

Planes were over for a long time last night. The Christmas spirit is in the air and considerable preparations are being made to give all the troops the best time possible under the circumstances. All battalions are doing something special for the troops in the way of gifts, cigarettes, money, etc. We have provided for an extra expenditure of 25c per head on Christmas meals.

20 December 1943

A long discussion with Major O'Driscoll today on the necessity to increase the turnover of patients and allow sick men in the lines to come in.

21 December 1943

The treatment of scabies patients in the Con Depot is now under way.

22 December 1943

'Balloon debate' before a huge crowd: Boadicea, Christopher Columbus, Nell Gwynne, Florence Nightingale, W.G. Grace and Will Rogers. We were in costume parts, I as Boadicea complete with trident and helmet etc. The troops seemed to enjoy this buffoonery greatly and it was certainly rather amusing. The spirit of the place is decidedly bucking up and the batteries of speakers and nightly entertainments is now most impressive.

23 December 1943

Called over to the lines today to try and interest the camp in Christmas lotteries for hospital patients. By enlisting the support of Lt-Col. Warren and Lt-Col. McOstritch, I raised 50 ticals in no time. I was discussing religion and philosophy with Warren when suddenly I shot a fierce malarial rigor. I returned back to the hospital to do a minor operation having to stand in the sun until I stopped shaking and began chattering of teeth and shaking of hands just as I finished. I feel wretched and my leg ulcers have broken out again. Bill Wearne arrived today from Kinsayok to attend a funeral service. Also Jack Hands, both tremendously well. Despite malaria, I had Billy and a few of the boys along for a nip of my Christmas bottle of Thai whiskey. Frightful stuff! Grand fellow, old Bill. He produced another 500 ticals for O and P funds. All is well at Kinsayok. Ewan is particularly fit and there is no news.

24 December 1943, Christmas Eve

Christmas pantomime cancelled this evening because of air raid worries. Combined Nippon, British, Australian and Dutch memorial service for the dead in Thailand at 1900 hours in lines where a suitable large cross and dais was raised. All Nippon officers were present and massed troops at the camp. Two wreaths were laid on the cross by bearers representing homage of Nippon army and our own. The service was largely conducted by Padre Alcock with Nipponese contributing addresses, particulary the new Nippon commander who lauded our achievement for a Great East Asia in building the railroad. Unfortunately, I was light headed and weak with malaria and all I recall of the whole service was a desperate effort to avoid fainting. I wish this malaria would improve with time. Every fortnight a bit thick. My blood film is simply choked with parasites B.T. and gametocytes. Bill Wearne practically brought me back to bed. He and Pavillard are leaving first thing in the morning.

25 December 1943, Christmas Day

Very good spirits prevailing. Visiting of patients in the wards commencing very early. I was shockingly embarrassed by my wards treating me to 'For he's a Jolly Good Fellow'! The height of optimism was reached by one lad who told me that he considered that now the pessimists said February and the optimists March!

I am completely sunk financially owing to repair of my shoes 6 ticals, Christmas presents to the 2/2 CCS of tobacco, cigarettes, tins of meat, 10 ticals, and similar small presents to batmen and ward staffs. But what the hell!

An excellent presentation of *Cinderella* in camp in the afternoon. The audience, which includes most of the Nipponese officers, was seated in the open before an excellent little stage built of bamboo. A gasp went up when the curtain swung back revealing the 'ladies' and elegantly costumed men. It is simply amazing what can be done in the way of dress and costume design by mosquito netting and other scraps of cloth, plus silver foil, tinsel and oddments. A most convincing presentation, the only amusement being caused by the well marked scabies and ulcer marks on the legs of the 'ladies'! I saw only the first hour, then came back to the hospital for the Christmas service at which I read a lesson.

In the evening 'Pop' Vardy as Father Christmas accompanied by a Crazy Gang of Brennan, 'Legs' Leigh, Sydney Pitt, Hazleton and others, did a grand tour of the wards making great revelry and investing the ward masters as sisters with a pair of tin 'pectoral projections', a cowl with a red cross, a shepherd's crook and a bottle with a teat. A lottery was drawn in each ward of 2 ticals first prize; three prizes of 1 tical and a few bars of soap. Sydney Pitt nearly broke his neck several times with acrobatics. Marsh did much of the organising and finally joined the procession as Nell Gwynne. Finally, the party assembled in the concert area and continued their buffoonery investing other officials: for example Harvey, with a large tin fish; Dunlop, an outsize in knives! Tommy Atkins was the most unceremonial, being treated with a final presentation of a thunderbox which was placed over his shoulders with his head through the hole and a jerry firmly jammed on his head. (Spectacles fortunately still intact!)

Bad feeling against the Con Depot staff (the Con Depot meal was a flop) was increased by them not attending or taking much interest in the men during the day.

26 December 1943

I am absolutely satisfied that the Con Depot staff makes smooth running of the area impossible through their complete autonomy, separate office and either conscious or unconscious obstruction. I have recommended to Harvey that the whole staff (officers) be relieved of duty. NCOs and suspected kitchen racketeers are to be checked over carefully. He concurred, I then had the painful task of breaking the news to O'Driscoll, who took it well enough.

27 December 1943

A Cinderella pantomime was shown today before a huge audience of hospital people; almost all patients were there, many fainting and weak from the sun. Tremendous enthusiasm and tumultuous applause.

28 December 1943

The whole area is now to be hospital, with a single office and admin. staff. Division into medical, surgical, dysentery and infectious wards is to be organised on heavy sick and light sick basis. Thus as far as possible the patients requiring diets will be concentrated in the acute or heavy sick wards.

Three instructors in Arts & Crafts are permitted by the Nipponese with a view to the production of 3,000 clogs (100 men are working with knives and wood); 300 stretchers (with bamboos and rice sacks); food containers (to replace mess tins); water bottles of bamboo etc., bed pans and ward equipment.

29 December 1943

Maj. O'Driscoll and party moved out today to the lines. Maj. Swanton by Lt-Col. Harvey's instruction also went to the lines but is now apparently the hospital amenities officer.

30 December 1943

A valuable supply of drugs arrived and 3,000 ticals [this was due to the wonderful services of Boon Pong, the river trader]. The barge liaison we made separate to this also producing some drugs at fabulous prices including 1 lb of iodoform (Evans) and 1 lb of phenol pure – an absolute Godsend. A handful of drugs, 900 ticals; iodoform 1 lb, 200 ticals. This changes the ulcer position immeasurably.

31 December 1943

An amusing ruction re the confiscation of a certain still worked in the Con Depot by a Gordon Highlander NCO There seemed to be an amazing number of shareholders preparing for Hogmanay. Unfortunately, some hospital vegetables were detected in the brew and the ethics of the whole thing was in doubt. Eventually, as we can use the spirit medically, I decided that the shareholders should be paid out from hospital funds. (A terrible thing to happen of course on Hogmanay Eve).

New Year's Eve: Spent some of the afternoon with Lt-Col. Warren, who is a man of parts, courageous, capable, many faceted with immense joy of living. I had a little New Year's supper with Tommy Atkins and Bishop (librarian) under a moon on the bank of the Kwa Noi. It was serenely beautiful and the sounds of camp revelry in the background were soothing. Later I returned to the mess, where we began singing sweet, nostalgic and melancholy airs. Somehow, we do not have the heart for more boisterous revelry. Never before have I felt such a dypsomaniac urge. I would have given anything to get so drunk that the pain of memory and twanging of taut nerves would quieten. Helen I think of always and sometimes the graveyard of these last bitter years is rather unbearable. Eventually, we packed up a little after midnight and the padres had a midnight service which was well attended.

Later in the chilly morning, Jock Clarke, Jim Finnemore, Phil Millard and I made a huge omelette on a charcoal brazier and discussed the war and the future. Happy New Year to you Helen, wherever you are! Dare we hope for too much in the coming year!

1 January 1944

Deaths for the last month only 50. A definite improvement on the previous months. I still feel profoundly miserable today and for the first time really in my POW existence, my nerves are strung to breaking point. I plunged today into work to try to forget: two operations, one a rather interesting case, Douglas 2/2 Pioneers, and Zitter, J.V.R. Dutch Army.

In the evening, Jock Clarke and I were sitting very miserably in my mess hut, no lights to speak of and I unburdening my troubled spirits, when who should arrive but Joe (Korean Joe), obviously gloriously tight, noisily and uproariously happy and wishing to felicitate 'Dunroppo *chusa*' on the New Year. I tried to rise to these heady heights of heartiness too. Joe is a quick and human fellow. He sat down on the bed and instantly sobered, saying, 'You not happy – no alcohol. Why?' I said, 'POWs very poor Joe and whisky is no good. Must set an example!' His spirits absolutely dashed, Joe sat shaking his head sadly and saying, 'Very very sorry!' Finally, he left quietly and even two days later again expressed his sorrow. A great-hearted old ruffian our Joe.

2 January 1944

A most astonishing diaplay of statistics required by 'Uncle Chunkle' today. As usual, he spent hours trying to tell me what was required but did not succeed very well. The following were finally prepared:

Total sick in camp	Hosp.	Lines	Total	% Grand total
English	1644	367	2011	65
Australians	691	276	967	80
Dutch	131	258	389	54
TOTAL	2466	901	3367	

Total 'fit' in camp	Lines	Total	% Grand total
English	1074	1074	35
Australian	209	209	20
Dutch	325	325	46
TOTAL	1608	1608	

Deaths 1/4/43 to 29/12/43: English 470 (69%); Australians 78 (11%); Dutch 128 (18%). TOTAL: 676

There is much stir about movement and it is known that most of the sick will soon be evacuated to Nakom Patom and Chungkai. The former is to be a new 10,000 bed hospital. 5,000 ticals has been sent to HQ Tarsau, I think through the Swiss Legation. It was decided to use this on food for the sick. No. 4 group sub-division leaves 2,750 ticals for this hospital area. I discussed this, amongst other questions of hospital expenditure today, with Lt-Col. Thomas, who says that I must be able to put up a case for continuing expenditure at the present rate as finances were going steadily down.

3 January 1944

Still more statistics for the Nipponese, even weights and heights and the effects of Thailand on the same requested.

4 January 1944

Death, 1 (cholera).

5 January 1944

Death, 1.

6 January 1944

Deaths 1. 909318 Gnr. Harper, H.W.J. 118th Field Rgt RA. A tropical ulcer of the left leg and amputation. Today with chloroform anaesthetic.

7 January 1944

Deaths 2. There were only four deaths for the first week in January, a bit of a record I should think. Nevertheless, the sick figure is not falling off and indeed there is actually a shortage of beds. I primed up Lt-Col. Warren and Lt-Col. McOstritch, saying that I thought it would be a serious mistake to reduce hospital expenditure at present and that probably the only solution was increased officers' subscriptions.

8 January 1944

There was a financial meeting at camp HQ at which I spoke. The expenditure on diets, was definitely reducing the death rate, and my impression was that the camps and units who had achieved the best results in Thailand were those who had made the most flat out expenditure on the sick; reducing expenditure would mean writing lives off. I felt that at all costs we should continue at the present rate and endeavour somehow to raise more money. Finally, Lt-Col. Warren proposed (seconded by me) that we raise officers' subscriptions and this was passed.

9 January 1944

Lt-Col. Knight asked me to write a letter setting out the need of continued hospital expenditure at present in order to put the position clearly to the camp. This was done.

10 January 1944

Lt-Col. Harvey walked in with a bombshell that I am to go down to Chungkai. This is a blow, as I understand that Chungkai is likely to be a light sick hospital and the big stuff will go to Nakom Patom. Also Chungkai is an 'ancient civilisation', with everyone well dug in so that I suppose I will be like some rude Goth descending on the Forum in Rome. All the old boys who avoided movement north and those who speedily tore back are of course down there. My only consolation is that Arthur Moon may be there. It seems that there are about 8,000 sick at Chungkai and the deaths over three months have been 500, so I suppose there will be plenty to do. How much nicer it would be to start afresh in a new area than to tackle the awful business of fixed views and lethargy of long established camps.

11 January 1944

'Uncle Chunkle' returned and confirmed most of the above about Chungkai. He thinks that Arthur Moon really is down there. I have picked out about eight 2/2 Aust. CCS men to go with me: S/Sgt Gibson, Sgt Haddon, Butterworth, Brown, A.A. Lawrence, Walker, Murray and Binns. Most of these are rather sick, particularly Gibson. The few remaining fit CCS men are mainly at Kinsayok. Jack Taylor is rather sick at present and weighs a little over 5 stone. I fear he will never leave Thailand, A party of 300 fit men are to go down to Nakom Patom to prepare the hospital.

12 January 1944

I saw Fred Smedley (OC AIF details) and gave him 200 ticals from O and P funds to take down, the remaining funds being held by him for P battalion to be handed over to Dick Allen. This will ensure a little money at Nakom Patom. I am arranging for Brettingham-Moore and Terry Croft to be included in the draft for Chungkai so that they can look after O and P Battalion men.

13 January 1944

An excellent show in the hospital area, 'Me and My Girl'.

220 sick arrived from Kinsayok under the care of Capt. Matheson, which is now cleaned out of sick. The hospital is to close. Consequently, bags of doctors and orderlies up there have no work. Okada has written standing orders for MOs! Parade 0815, 'tap tap' [percussing chests] until 1300, *yasumé* until 1500 then 'tap tap' until 1800. No bridge until after dinner.

14 January 1944

McNeilly and his party got away to Nakom Patom. There is much speculation as to the future of No. 4 Group and the sick disposal.

Jack Marsh is getting on magnificently on the Q side. He works in the arts and crafts section which is making a great variety of articles: artifical limbs, bed pans, charcoal sterilisers, bowls, buckets and pails, trays, brooms, pneumonia jackets, lamps of various shapes, urine bottles, ladles, mugs, pillows and mattresses of rice sacks and straw, funnels, irrigation cans, latrine covering lids, flytraps, leg rests, instrument boxes of bamboo, washbowls, vegetable scrapers, clogs, stretchers, even bamboo needles and scalpels. The 3000 clogs in production were roughly hewn from wood and then handed over to the Arts & Crafts patients to complete the work with pocket knives and webbing equipment for straps.

15 January 1944

Amusing conversation with 'Uncle Chunkle' who expressed slight exasperation and dissatisfaction that Germany had not won the war; particularly unfortunate in just failing to take Egypt. Spoke very highly of the British Navy but disparaged the American Navy, in which he said too much attention given to quarters and shore leave, dances, etc.! The Nipponese fighting army was like a 'desperate vagabond' fighting a rich old man with a top hat, a watch and many valuables. He is quite a pleasant and well informed old chap.

16 January 1944

I am to be off 'speedo, speedo' in the morning. Hence everything very hurried, but finance arrangements completed. I left a few surgical instruments with 'Monty', including abdominal retractors 2, tissue forceps large, Spencer Wells 6 in. forceps, six 8 in.

9 Chungkai

January 1944

17 January 1944

I seem fated to move in January! Party of 201 with 16 officers, including myself, Capt. Gaden, Bret.-Moore and Maj. Robinson. Also my eight CCS orderlies. Capt. Moroko said that I would be CO at Chungkai Hospital, which would be mixed No. 2 and No. 4 group, and introduced me to the Chungkai interpreter who accompanied the party. We finally entrained at about 1100 hours. There was a good deal of delay on the journey, it being very hot in open trucks, and the troops were not allowed to leave the train. The railway wound its way through almost untouched jungle.

We arrived at approximately 1700 hrs and marched to the camp. I was simply astonished to see so many well-remembered O and P men standing by the road without a leg. There were over 100 amputations about the place and some thirty odd had died. I was deluged with old friends wishing to see me and finally delighted to see old Arthur Moon who was doing surgical work.

A huge fellow was sorting out the sick and I walked up to him and told him my name was Dunlop. He replied, 'So's mine!' He is exactly my height and is surgical registrar here. A few of the party were then put into the hospital and the remainder bedded down in a large barrack to be sorted out. I speedily met Lt-Col. Moore, Lt-Col. Hill, Lt-Col. Outram, the Camp Commander. McLeod was commanding No. 2 group, Lt-Col. Riches, No. 4 Group. Lt-Col. Stitt of the Gordons also present. As I thought, Chungkai is a very 'ancient civilisation'. Everywhere men are selling cigarettes and amenities and rackets are not stamped down, but are made official and glorified. God knows how many brands of cigarettes are manufactured in the camp, including filter tips, sold at approximately ten for five cents. Very spacious camp site, huts not bad, the hygiene, as usual, is not good.

18 January 1944

Rations are much better than Tarsau: rice is plentiful, meat 4 ounces daily, I believe, and vegetables are considerably better. Many troops are quite plump. Fixtures of the area included tennis court and football ground. Gardens are also being cultivated, but unfortunately are up on the higher ground. The hospital area, being down on the lower ground, was flooded last wet season, most of the patients having to be shifted.

I called on the amputation ward today and had a talk to some of the lads. One Hargreaves of 2/3 M.G. Bn has lost both legs above the knee. On a casual inspection, the amount of skin infections, scabies, etc. is just about as bad as Tarsau. Excellent features of the hospital here are a transfusion centre where defibrinated blood is used. They have given over 300 transfusions with very little reaction since they started the technique. This is actually run by lay officers and is a show-piece. There is an excellent remedial exercise and massage team (this work is done in the open air); skin grafting is done in quite a big way. A good deal of improvisation has been carried out with theatre equipment and most of the operations are done with spinal anaesthetic technique, using solutions introduced here by Captain Markowitz, an energetic Canadian Jew.

The most amazing thing of the day was calling on Lt-Col. Barrett, RAMC, who is SMO. He received me quite cordially but obviously either did not know or would not admit to any change in administration. So after tea and a little polite conversation I retired to await some clarification of the position.

19 January 1944

There is a central camp finance fund administered by a committee. Hospital finance is administered by a hospital sub-committee.

In the afternoon, a sudden bombshell from Maj. Black (2 I/C of the hospital), who announced that Lt-Col. Barrett and Captain Marcowitz were suddenly removed by the Nipponese to another camp. Hence it is now assumed that I am SMO. I discussed the hospital organisation with Maj. Dunlop and Maj. Black.

A further 200 light sick patients arrived from Tarsau today. There was an air raid during the night, a number of planes being overhead, and some anti-aircraft activity. The objective seemed further off.

20 January 1944

I had a look at the work of the Transfusion Centre and was most impressed with the defibrinated blood technique and the general efficiency of the team. I had afternoon tea with Lt-Col. Outram and discussed major policy. As SMO it was most desirable that I be regarded as part of his camp staff. The hospital arrangements were to some extent a domestic matter but the utmost co-operation was desired, and I wished to give hygiene and Q matters first attention. The camp workshops are more or less under the direct supervision of the Nipponese who use the men and materials for designs of their own; the hospital workshop is a starveling with only one workman and practically no materials. I met the Hygiene Officer, Captain Lewis, and was not very impressed.

21 January 1944

Camp and hospital hygiene is extremely unsatisfactory: shallow, open latrines for the most part, very offensive and badly flyblown and used as both a deposit for excreta and refuse. The dysentery wards are particularly bad. Deep latrines require revetting with bamboo or timber and none is available; there are no materials for latrine covers, no oil or disinfectant. The scabies centre has no disinfestation and no large drums for boiling. As at Tarsau, almost everyone is covered with scabs and sores. Something must be done in this direction. NB: Necessity for a hospital hygiene officer.

I saw the N medical sergeant; he at once promised me the new operating theatre which was spoken of at Tarsau. I was informed that tomorrow a party would arrive from Kanchanaburi to take rectal swabs from all men.

22 January 1944

The Hospital Finance Sub-committee met and I suggested that expenditure on food would be best handled by a hospital dietician and we should combine forces into a suitable diet centre. This was agreed and I then suggested a diet committee with three medical representatives, plus Sqn Ldr Taylor (Messing Officer) and Captain Fisher (the Chief Welfare Officer).

The weather is excellent for swimming and at a swimming carnival recently the Dutch proved particularly strong swimmers, carrying off most contests.

The 2/2 Aust. CCS men now in Chungkai are Lt-Col. Dunlop, Maj. Moon A.A., S/Sgt Gibson S.A., Sgt Haddon, R., Cpl Walker K.H. Cpl Lawrence A.G., Cpl Roberts, L.G.J., Pte Binns, K. Pte Brown, A.A., Pte Butterworth M., Pte Murray J.B., Pte Gray T.J.E., Pte Harrison W. (a local sergeant), Pte Ambrose W., Pte Simpson, F.C. Pte Crowley J.D. Pte Powell, K.A., Pte Cameron J.A.

I attended a concert – an oldtime Music Hall style of show. An orchestra (very good) and a fair stage, but no lights were allowed owing to blackout requirements! Rectal swabbing by a Nipponese party was going on lustily, dealing with twenty at a time!

23 January 1944

I met the camp APM and Maj. Richardson and we discussed the prevalence of flogging blankets and clothing and discrepancies in dead men's kit and ways of stopping this. The Diet Committee met (with A. Dunlop and I also in attendance) and it was then left to prepare suitable diets over the next two days. The patients were then to be classified and the scheme costed.

I did my first operation in this camp – an amputation of the leg in the lower third of the thigh. No. 1872786, Spr. McNeill J. age 35. Ulcer of the left foot and leg involving the tarso-metatarsal bones.

24 January 1944

Rectal swabbing again going on today for the hospital and remainder of No. 4 Group. Also a preliminary inspection of the hospital in readiness for a further inspection by Kanchanaburi commander tomorrow. The turnout was fairly good. Some of the inspecting party wished to see an operation by Maj. Moon in the theatre – an amputation of the thigh. This spectacle proved rather too much for many of the party who began to perspire and depart, wiping their brows and rather pale! I was asked for a plan of the new operating theatre 'speedo'.

25 January 1944

I took the plan for a new operating theatre to the N medical sgt, I also a plan of a disinfestor for blankets etc. along for approval and was told that an attempt would be made to get timber in lieu of metal drums, providing we pay for it.

The inspecting officer, a lieutenant-colonel arrived shortly after 1200 hrs. The actual inspection was negligible, consisting of a walk as far as the camp gardens!

26 January 1944

Three NEI medical officers, de Hahan, de Jonge and van der Muellen, departed hurriedly this morning on a request from the Nipponese. This leaves in camp Shombury, Rennies and de Schnell. Col. Outram went with them to Tamarkand and saw Brigadier Varley and Lt-Col. Coates.

A meeting of all medical officers took place today. They were asked to select cases for the new diet scheme under the Diet Committee's guidance. Six diets have been prepared to meet all contingencies. The scheme could then be costed. A hospital hygiene officer is to be appointed to help in hygiene and supervision works; weekly inspections will be held by a commanding officer and a full turnout is required. A new officer is required for the skin clinic and scabies centre following the departure of Capt. van der Muellen. This will follow a sort out of ulcers and skin complaints; ulcers are to go into ulcer wards.

27 January 1944

A Group Commanders' Meeting. Lt-Col. Outram, his adjutant, Lt-Col. Riches, Lt-Col. McLeod and self in attendance: a very friendly meeting.

28 January 1944

At meetings of the Hospital Finance Sub-committee and the Camp Finance Committee, the diet scheme met with full approval. This will mean a slight increase in expenditure, bringing the hospital up to 11c per man per day on diets and welfare 1c per man per day. This will mean a finance of about 3,000 ticals a month debit, the reserves being at present approximately 5,000.

I received emetine 64 grains and morphia 100 ampoules grain 1/3.*

30 January 1944

Moves of ulcer, malaria and skin wards and their reorganisation were all supervised by Maj. Moon very ably. The allotment of medical officers was decided in the afternoon by a meeting of Maj. A.A.L. Dunlop, Maj. Moon, Maj. Black, Maj. Reed and myself.

It is very evident that acute medical ward provision is not adequate. I was called to see an AIF soldier, Capt. Dorrett, yesterday who was dying with double pneumonia (and probable septicaemia) in a general ward. He was lying on the common bamboo platform looked after largely by the patients on either side of him.

31 January 1944

I attended a meeting of welfare officers attached to the hospital. They seem a very keen and helpful lot. I outlined roughly the new diet scheme and we discussed welfare generally, particularly help with patients' ablutions and cleaning

* This was supplied through the underground (Boon Pong).

their clothes until we have an adequate hospital laundry and disinfesting facilities. Suitable instructors are to be obtained to get men working at arts and crafts in the hospital, thereby helping them acquire an interest in life and possibly some useful skill and knowledge for their post-war existence.

1 February 1944

The sort out and changeover of patients occurred yesterday so that the hospital is now at least grouped on a basis of disease. The diets are now in operation. The equipment of the ulcer wards at present is shocking. It is no surprise to me that the hospital has had 112 amputations. Just part and parcel of this is the fact that there is only one hot water point for a hospital of 2,000 odd men! No proper bowls or basins, no boiling water, no sterilisers. The main medicaments in use are Hyd. Perchlor. lotion, Eusol emulsion (= chlorinated lime solution shaken up with oil, 0.5% chlorine). No proper ointments; very little iodoform and apparently no sulphanilamide. No irrigators are being used. Maj. Reed, a keen chap, is doing everything he can to get some equipment into the wards and to get treatment going. On my specific request, the medical personnel from Tarsau have at last been absorbed onto the staff of the hospital.

2 February 1944

I spoke to the parade of hospital personnel expressing pleasure at the work being done(!) and requested that they set a good example to the area in behaviour, personal cleanliness and cleanliness of quarters. They must do everything in their power to help keep the hospital spotlessly clean and see that patients are kept clean and their morale maintained and built up (a general 'pep talk').

3 February 1944

My first day in the ulcer wards: the equipment is appalling. The patients are almost all scabies ridden and many have impetiginous sores all over them. No use has been made of beef or other fats for ointment. I am at once approaching the camp command for a supply of beef fat and am urging the construction of ward sterilisers and irrigating cans. There is no boraic acid for boric ointment so I am using carbolic ointment 1% as a sort of universal dressing. Something must be done at once to deal with scabies and infectious bedding and clothing.

Today was a sports day with the RAMC fielding a team against other battalions. All performances were pretty ghastly, but it is a good sign to see this sort of thing going on.

4 February 1944

Some local newspapers were allowed in camp and reveal that fighting is going on in Poland about Sarny. Things much the same as one would imagine elsewhere. It is good to have some news again. I am having a real crusade (without much luck up to date) to get a reasonable number of water points for the hospital.

Planes were overhead today and there was a good deal of ack-ack fire. Some soldiers laughed at Nipponese soldiers running to shelters and were taken to the guardroom and punished. This was their own fault.

Today about 12 'bed down' sick on a swimming parade for ablution were struck with bamboo for not going out to help with a rice barge that was stuck in the river sand, although not requested to do so. The Nipponese NCO in charge of discipline listened to the complaint and inspected their wounds.

There was some plague about and today we began pestis injections: all personnel to have 1 cc. An operation was carried out on a pilonidal sinus, 5775706. Cpl J. Wilson, Norfolk Regt.

5 February 1944

A concert today with a band in new open air amphitheatre and Lt-Col. Outram as the star performer in a selection from musical comedy: *The Student Prince* and *The Desert Song*. He is a fine singer. The large Hintok trees round here with their great scarlet blooms are a magnificent sight at present, the haunt of myriads of birds. Dust is the main *bête noir* of the camp.

6 February 1944

I have at last got the Camp Sanitation Officer sufficiently interested to have a try at making a steam disinfestor. His model was not very satisfactory but will do with some alterations.

The number of men on diets appears to be rising steeply which is rather annoying since everyone had an opportunity to select his cases a few days ago. Major Black (amoebic dysentery) has made an obvious under-estimate. We all have to do an essay for Nipponese HQ on certain aspects of the war. This is required of all officers not in hospital or 'bed down'. Also some 2,000 Other Ranks.

7 February 1944

Hospital inspection. It was a fairly creditable turn out with all the wards at least making a good try. The standard of cleanliness was good. The first ward steriliser was introduced into my own ulcer ward today and irrigators are coming into use. I will have to establish my own hospital workshop, despite the difficulties of tools etc. I have enlisted a tinsmith today to get things going. Fat and ointments are now available for the wards.

I carried out an operation of thoracotomy for a purulent collection in the right lung with local anaesthetic today. 6426763 Pte. Butler, T. 1Vth Suffolk Regiment, aged 26.

8 February 1944

Of some 2000 odd POWs who have filled in questionnaires, all seemed confident that the allies would win the war.

Today, an officer named Bill Bailey returned with some information about Nakom Patom. Huts of wood and bamboo and attap roofing are being built on a much more lavish scale than in other camps. The beds are platforms of wood – 7 ft wide with a 6 ft passage. The road is to be concreted and considerable attention has been given to the construction. The great difficulty is that the area is in low-lying paddy country in general but at the site two wells have been sunk

200 ft without having struck good water. The malaria problem is bad with many fresh infections apparently arising. The mosquitoes are extremely trying.

Nakom Patom village, said to be a sacred town, is characterised by a very large temple known as a wat. There is a aerodrome two miles away. Fruit is cheap and prices better than here at present.

I played rugger today for the RAMC. It seemed strange to be running again. We were licked 8–3 in the 'seven aside'. I scored a try. Touch rules re tackling with Maj. Dunlop as referee – all very strange!

9 February 1944

Absolutely desperate re seeing nobody on urgent hospital matters and can get nothing done. Reported with Lt-Col. Outram to Sgt Hirodasan and told him of my many troubles and no I.J.A. medical sergeant ever available. (He goes to the gardens each day!) I managed to secure some hearing and at once asked for tools for the hygiene work as at present there are only three shovels for the entire sanitation of the camp and all the latrines are in a shocking condition. I requested materials for the construction of deep latrines, hot water points for the hospital, containers and preferably attap shelters; I was told it was no good talking unless I had scales ready with amounts needed. I replied that I would be glad to produce scales. I asked for satisfactory M.I. room accommodation, a Q Store and an operating theatre. I was told that the men were really very well. Many were now 'fat' and I should get them to do more PT and more '*yasumés*'!

9 February 1944

There was a night air raid with apparently many planes. Anti-aircraft guns were in action. I operated on a man named L/Cpl. Nind, W. 5th Beds & Herts. No. 88531. He had encephalitis in Changi in May 1942, diphtheria in December 1942 at Tarsau, malaria at Tarsau in January 1943, then, on 9 March 1943, he was attacked by an elephant. He suffered large tusk-inflicted wounds in the left thigh and also in the coccyx and sacral region where there was a deep penetrating wound by the rectum. In November 1943, an incision was made over the sacrum for a pus pocket. When seen, he was found to have a long sinus with an opening just posterior and to the right of the anus, the other one opening to the right side of the mid sacrum. The operation was with spinal anaesthetic, a probe was passed along the track approximately 5 in long. I opened up the tract and excised and curretted the wound. It was packed with paraffin gauze. [Later, on 14 February, this very big wound cavity was slowly healing with continuous packing. On 1 May 1944, he was almost healed.]

I had a short conference with Lt-Col. Outram and the camp sanitation officer on the scales to be submitted to the Nipponese for requirements for hygiene purposes, etc. The camp sanitation officer clearly is the greatest 'waffler' I have met yet! I had to insist sharply on estimates for deep revetted latrines. The general idea seems to be because nothing can be expected, it is no use asking! Outram himself is a very good player. Finally, I submitted a formal letter on these points including requests on the scale of supply for tools for latrines and hot water points.

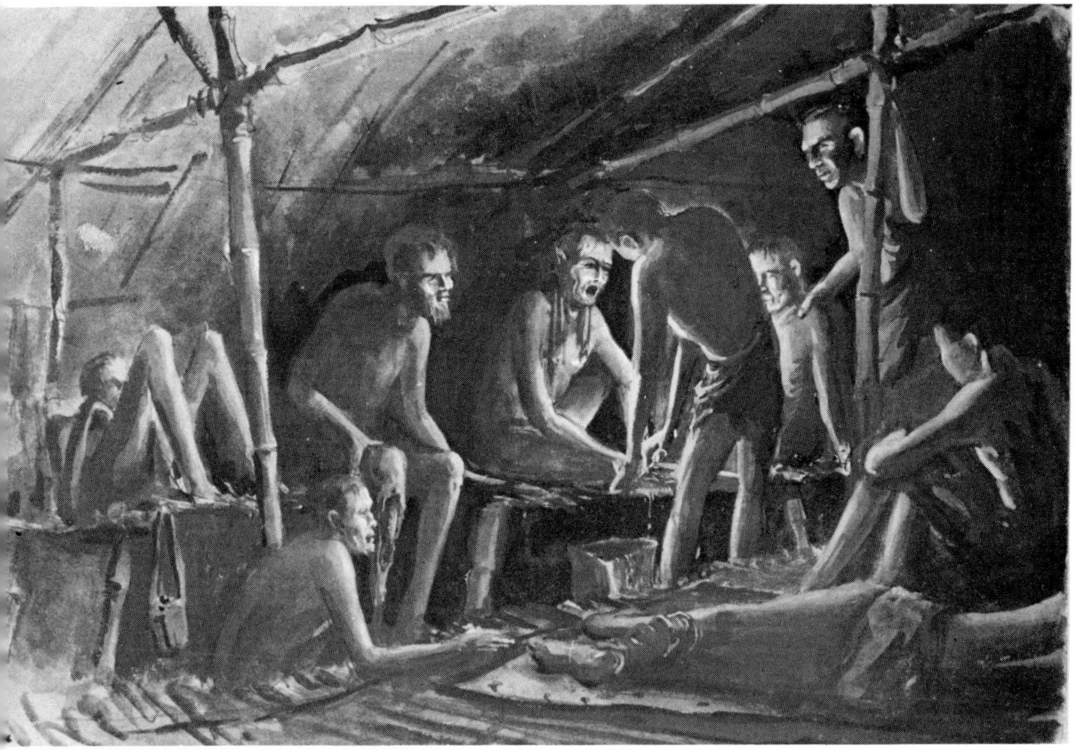

ɔpical ulcer ward, Chungkai hospital (*Jack Chalker*)

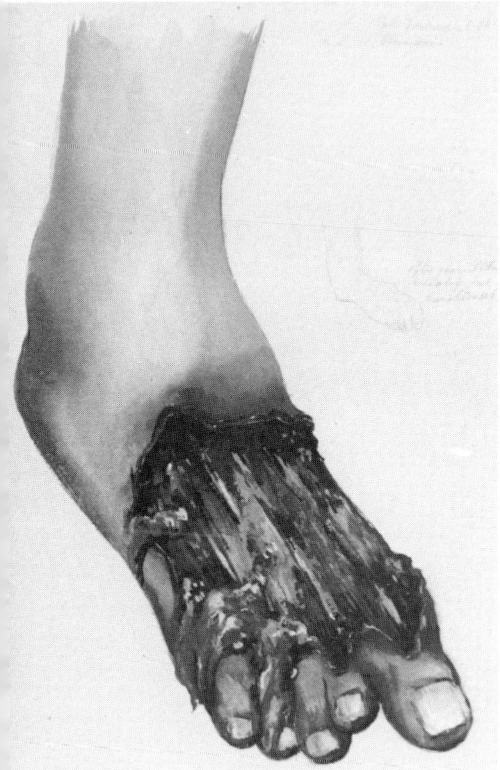

ive spreading tropical ulcer, (*Jack Chalker*)

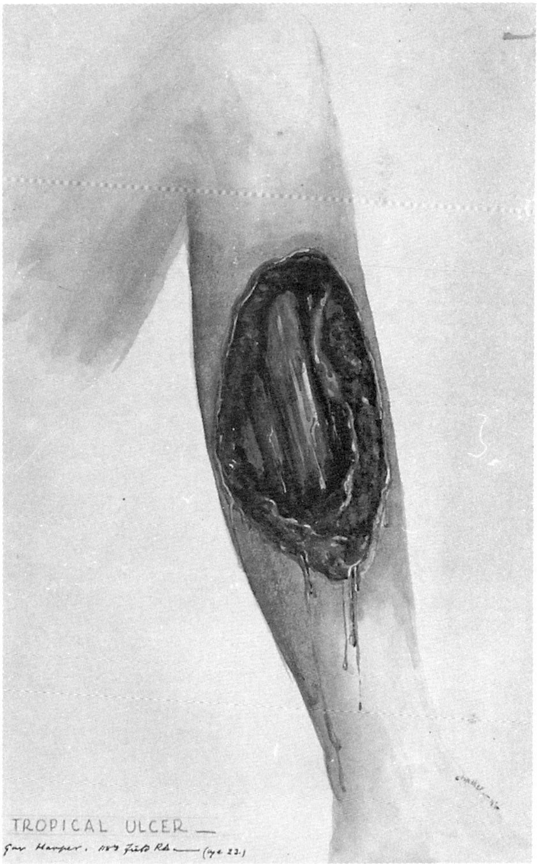

100 Spreading tropical ulcer in British gunner's leg (*Jack Chalker*)

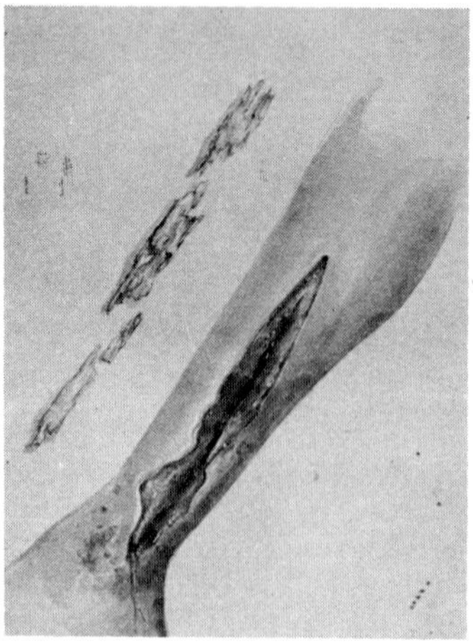

101 Sequestrectomy. Removal of dead bone following tropical ulcer (*Jack Chalker*)

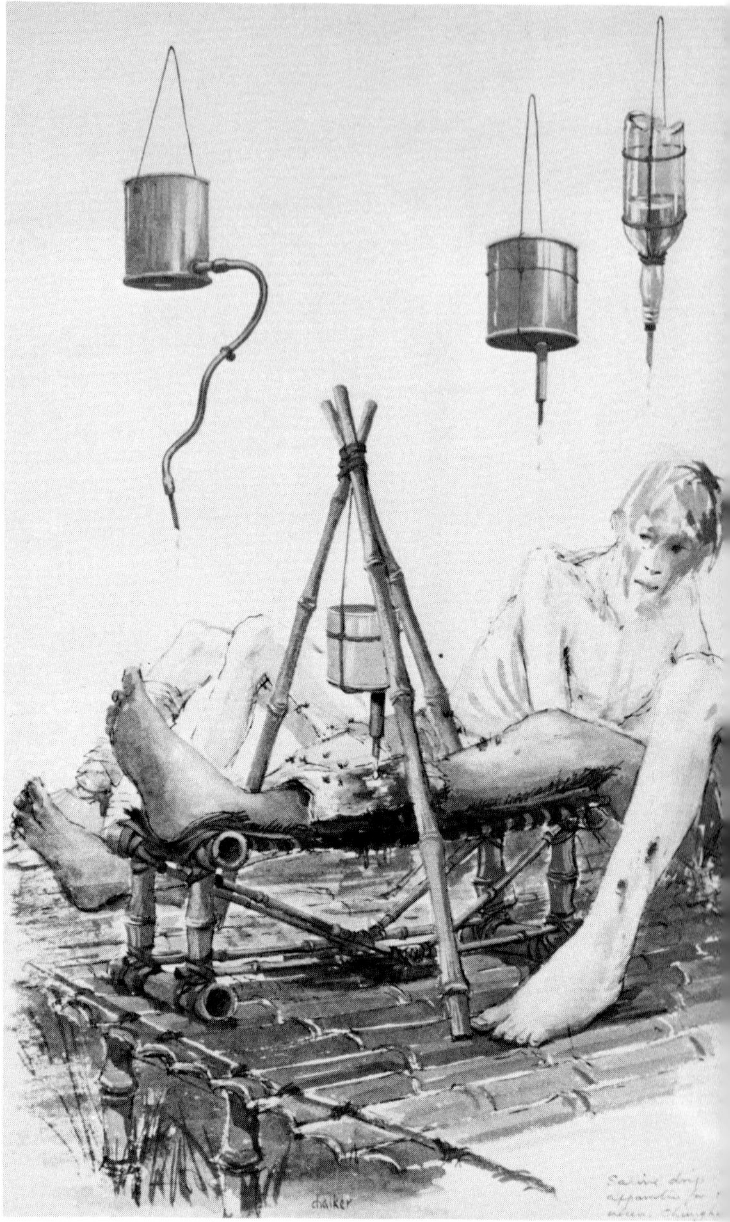

103 Saline drip aparatus for tropical ulcers, Chungkai 1943 (*Jack Chalker*)

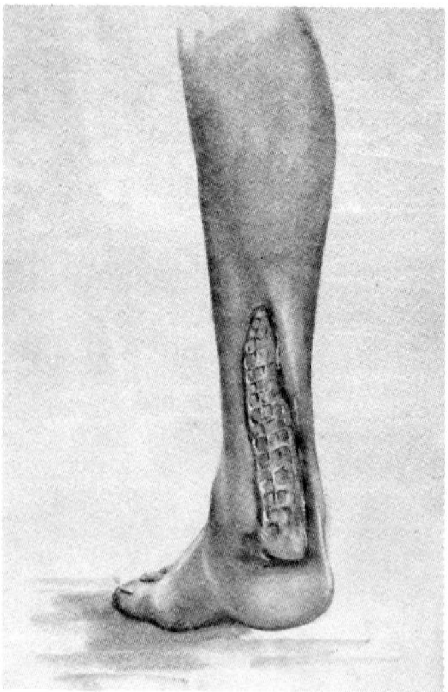

102 Tropical ulcer, loss of Achilles tendon (*Jack Chalker*)

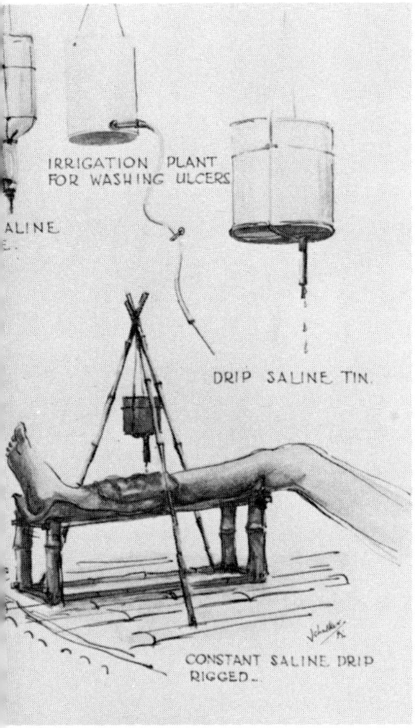

aline drip and irrigation cans and bottle
ack Chalker)

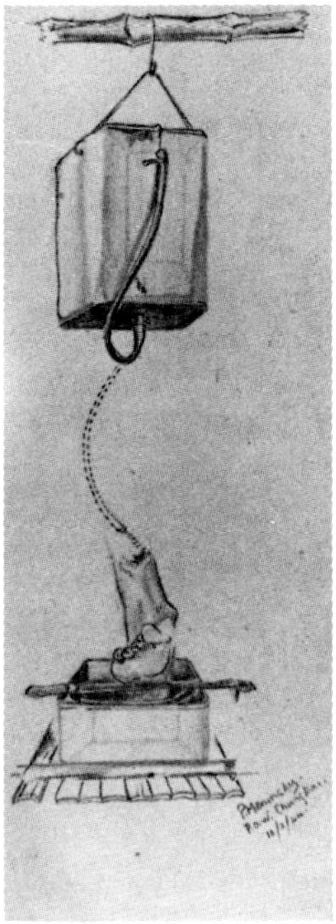

105 Irrigating can. Mass toilet for tropical ulcers (*P. Meninsky*)

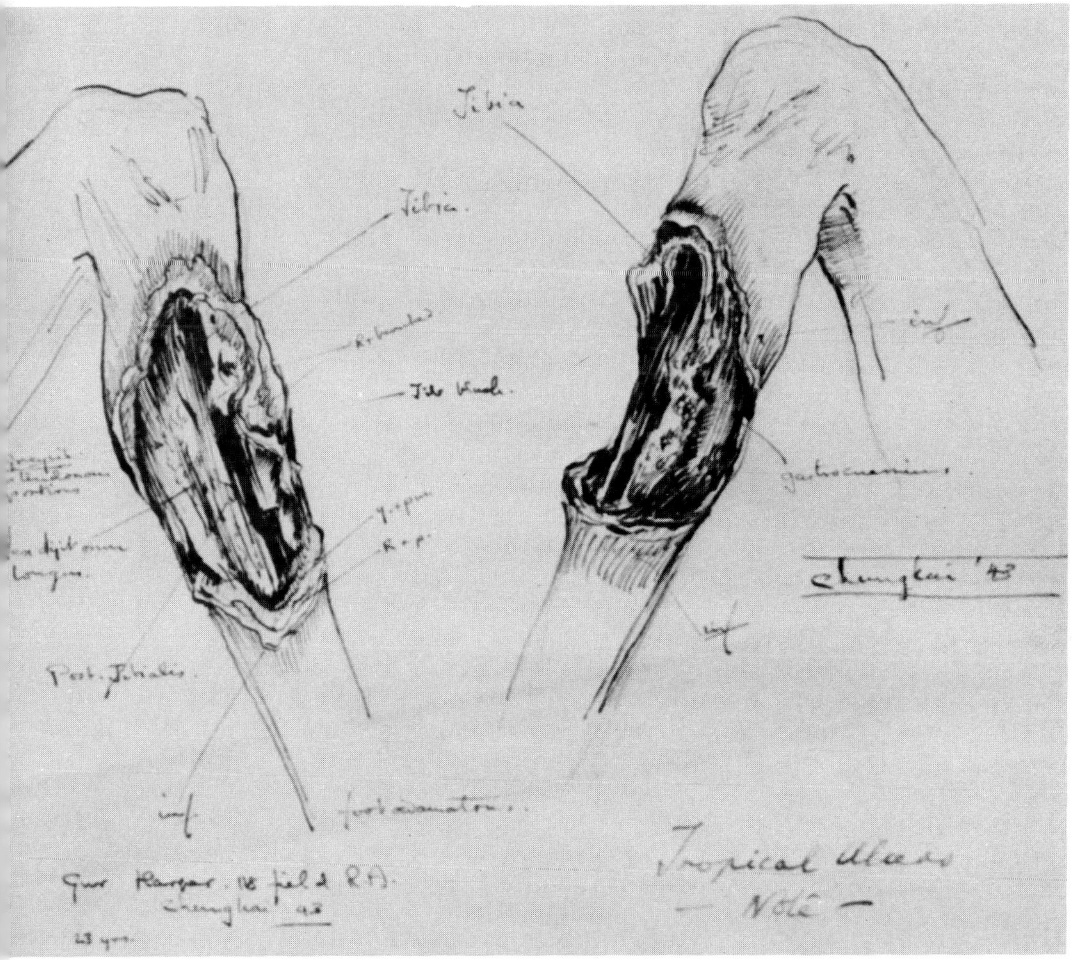

k Chalker's working drawings of a POW's tropical ulcer

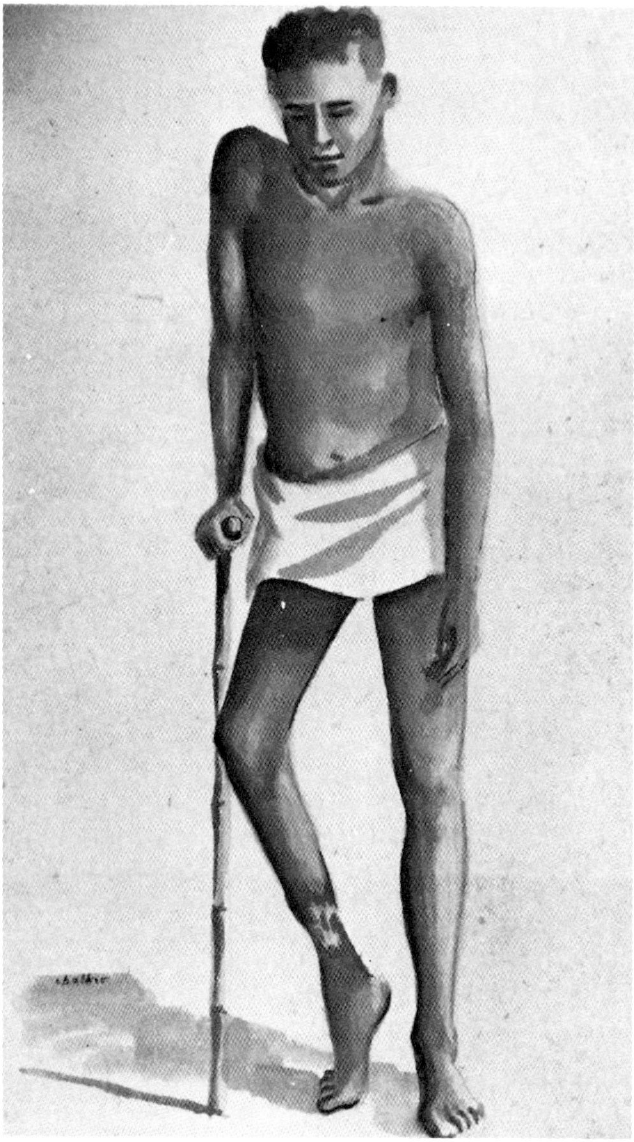

107 Hips, knee and ankle contractions following ulcer (*Jack Chalker*)

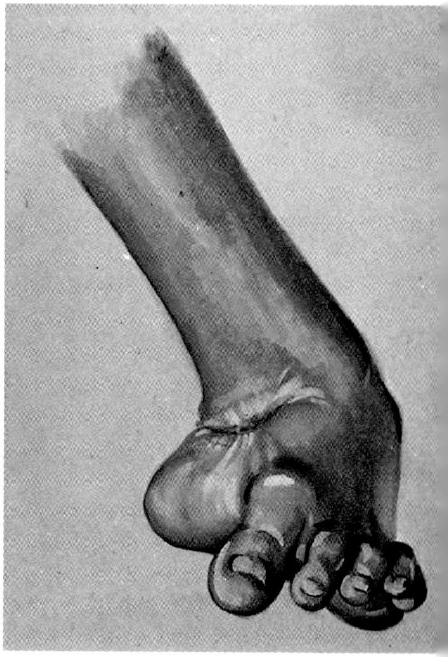

108 Foot deformity following tropical ulcer (*Jack Chalker*)

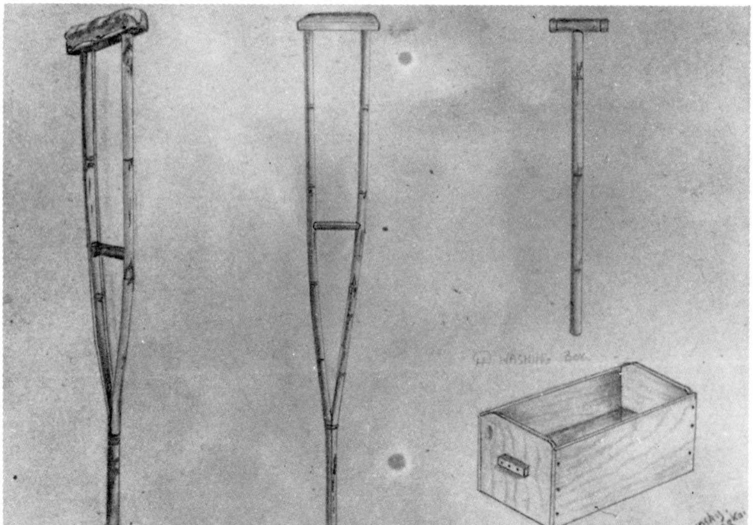

109 Crutch and walking stick mad split and round bamboo; wash (*P. Meninsky*)

10 February 1944

The skin clinic, in conjunction with the scabies clinic, is most unsatisfactory. Twenty-two men are employed in the scabies clinic and laundry, yet they deal at present with only 100 (at present 80) scabies men a day. They appear to work only in the morning and complain that shortage of wood prevents them working in the afternoon. The whole problem is confused with lack of energy and a tissue of nonsense.

The water supply of the hospital similarly is a maze of inefficiency: five people are dealing with it at the moment with no integration and a great misuse of containers and carriers.

A bombshell meeting of the Finance sub-Committee occurred today; a financial crisis is at hand owing to 'pennies from heaven' having dried up!*

Two interesting stories today: A goodly proportion of our vegetables, supplied as rations, was taken by a Nipponese soldier to feed pigs down at the garden camp! Many of the vegetables certainly are very putrid. When it was explained by the Nipponese that the vegetables looked like food for pigs, we said, 'Yes, but that is what we have to eat!' Another concerned the arrival of a party of well-dressed and healthy looking POWs, British, Australian and Dutch, who were brought from Kanchanaburi with a party plus ciné cameras, etc. These men were given specially selected roles working in the gardens, and pictures were taken under Arcadian conditions. Then squeeze boxes and band instruments were produced and further pictures taken of the men marching and singing behind the band. Finally, they sang, 'Rule Brittania' with much gusto and all went back to Kanchanaburi.

11 February 1944

I called a meeting of all MOs and laid down the stringency of the financial position. It was decided by the Finance Committee that if no more money is coming in, the officers would have to subscribe a further 2 ticals and men possibly 20 per cent of their wages. The position is to be reviewed on 10 March.

The rations in this camp seem to be better than in the other camps that I have had experience of in Thailand or indeed as a POW anywhere. The most serious defficiencies would appear to be protein, Vitamin B_2, calcium, iron and fat. The diet is not well balanced. As determined by local prices, the best buy appears to be meat. This not only is an excellent protein source but with a good B_2 value it also has good flavouring quality.

12 February 1944

Captain Simpson has analysed the expenditure by group kitchens and the various items, criticising the expenditure in some cases of flour, sugar and condiments at the expense of more valuable nutritional articles, such as meat, soya bean, towgay, coconut oil or other fat, dried fish or whitebait.

* This concerned outside negotiation.

13 February 1944

I discussed the container difficulty with Lt-Col. Riches who promised a supply from PRI of leaking tins at 30c and brought along two men who would do repair work if given some tools. I told him they could start tomorrow. Meantime, just collect all the tins outside the Q store – some of them actually given a gash in the side so that they would not be taken away!

14 February 1944

The hospital has considerably improved and haircutting and personal cleanliness is above Tarsau standards.

A financial 'flap' was on again. I am amazed at the number of long meetings we have here to discuss the financial position.

I performed several operations today, the last one late this evening on 65506, CSM. Kraanen A. NEI Army. A sequestrating right leg. His ulcer began on 4/10/43 by a blow with a chunkil and now involved tendon and bone of the tibia. Also VX 54914 Driver, Kettlewell, E.P., 105 General Transport Coy (drainage of a cervical abscess below the deep fascia of the left side of the neck) and 2876506, Pte Fraser, W., 2nd Gordon Highlanders (an acute perforated appendix).

15 February 1944

At last a disinfestor has been completed and dug in today by 2 AIF sappers over in the scabies area. If it works well, I can put in another one soon. Also most of the new fire points are now working, the container problem having been solved, partly by 'scrounging', and partly by the two workmen I acquired from Lt-Col. Riches.

16 February 1944

There was an apparently rather heavy air raid, last night, and the sound of considerable ack-ack fire. Today the Nipponese demanded more men to do work and sent a soldier down to gather up 'river men', for the most part 'bed downs' etc. who bathe and wash clothes. This soldier called for the support of 2 MPs and when dissatisfied with the fact that some men ran away and were not apprehended successfully, he beat the police up with bamboo, one being K.O'd with a blow behind the ear and the other rather badly marked. Protests were made against this step as unjust and not in the interests of camp discipline. The men were paraded and Ometzsan investigated the case. The soldier charged that when given commands requiring brisk action, the *kempis*, (camp military police) had moved with slow motion and accordingly his 'temperature rose'! Many further references were made to 'rise in temperature' and the MPs were warned that they 'must do better in the future'.

17 February 1944

I was to go to Kanchanaburi to purchase enamelware today and I received 145 ticals from Maj. Moon's Tamarkan funds. At the last minute, the Nipponese cancelled my permission and I expressed my disgust as to their lack of co-operation in medical affairs.

An operation was carried out on 2346384, Signalman Wilson F.R., Royal Corps. of Sigs. A tropical ulcer with amputation of the left leg below the knee.

18 February 1944 Friday

The morning staff conference is now a daily institution. There is still a gross shortage of tools and no materials for latrine construction. Also, Lewis has taken away five of the sanitation workers of the hospital leaving only five heavy work men.

A number of Group II personnel are to be set aside as a 'Japan party'. The present classification of men is M. & D (workers), B (light work), C (usually no work for the Nipponese but may work for the camp) and 'bed downs' (hospital). The personnel for the Japan party will all come from categories exclusive of C and 'bed down'. Lt-Col. Riches raised the point that in the case of Group II and IV, each NEI battalion shows a staggering number of C men. It is obvious that the Dutch doctors always save the men from work at the expense of the rest of the camp. Accordingly, Lt-Col. Outram and I discussed the whole problem with Overste. Metzer, the senior Dutch officer, who was sympathetic and said he would speak to the Dutch medical officers. A survey of the hospital by the Diet Committee reveals that the reduction in diets is not possible.

I attended an excellent play in the evening, *Good Morning Bill* Wodehouse. Very well cast and very funny.

19 February 1944 Saturday

I appointed Lt Bailey to the hospital staff to deal with ward equipment under Captain Hart. Bailey is a livewire and accomplished more in a single day today than has gone on for the last week. I asked him to look into the appalling delay re artifical limbs.

The Arts & Crafts Scheme has come on well. We have been able to purchase tools and the three instructors have been taken on the staff.

I have a difficult case just now – a Eurasian NEI soldier aged 21, probably dysenteric arthritis in the right hip. He is very fixed in an externally rotated position and with about 15° of flexion. He has a slight temperature daily, very little movement, bony deformity appears to be absent. There is no real shortening. I think after examining him under chloroform, I shall put him up in a double Hamilton Russell extension and a bamboo bed with 'Balkan Beams', pulleys made of tin, etc.

20 February 1944

A skin graft was carried out today on an NEI patient for a large healing ulcer of the leg.

21 February 1944

Hospital inspection on the whole was very satisfactory. Some of the beds are rough, owing to round bamboo and no matting, also some huts are in a very bad state of repair. The wards in general are clean and the patients are improving. The latrines remain disgusting. Attap palm type of urinals used here are being used to dump refuse and are obviously breeding flies.

Some rumours of a move of Group IV personnel now and particulars taken of my Christian names, etc. today.

22 February 1944

I saw the new Nippon interpreter today – an American accent and mentality and very courteous – and explained the difficulties about tools and construction. A sympathetic reception and very business-like action taken: he states that this will be HQ of No. 2 Group and it will then be easier to get things done, as at present all questions of expense have to be referred. Lt-Col. commanding No. 2 Group is having a house built in the camp.

23 February 1944

With Lt-Col. Outram, I again saw the interpreter about urgently required construction, particularly rebuilding of amoebic dysentery ward, wards 7 and 8, repairs or rebuilding of wards 20 to 9, a new operating theatre, a Q store medical inspection rooms, Groups 2 and 4, shelters over fire points and scabies centre, a shelter for the Arts & Crafts workers and latrine construction. Some amusement re the opeating theatre which term was taken as 'theatre' for a time. (Apparently, this expression was not used in America.)

I inspected the hospital kitchens today; kitchen hygiene is poor with no proper supervision of ablution, washing of, and sterilisation of food; the containers are almost non-existent; there are far too many scraps of food lying about, and flies. The food distribution is shockingly unhygienic. Of latrines, the least said the better! We will always associate these with Thailand, I fear.

I gave a 'pep' talk to the amputation cases to try and interest them in Arts & Crafts work. There is no difficulty in getting workers but I wanted them to have first choice at the scheme.

24 February 1944

There was an air raid alarm today during the afternoon, planes overhead, but no ack-ack fire. Pay arrived for the officers, $30 of which received: the rest went into the hospital (still have to pay 50c for RAMC welfare). Owing to having had two eggs daily last month, my bill for the month was 10 ticals to the mess, so it is a ticklish budget to make – no more eggs!

The skin grafts which were performed on a Dutch soldier were taken down and inspected. An area 3 in. in diameter which was covered with Reverdin grafts and then iodoform sprinkled: the take was 100 per cent. A similar area grafted with sulphanilamide sprinkled resulted in about 90 per cent. I am convinced that iodoform is the answer to skin grafting for these ulcers. Unfortunately, we now have practically none; for days I have been scratching along with the last dust in my bottle.

A very heavy wind and dust storm developed tonight at about 2230 hours and, as expected, the defective amoebic hut blew down and others were damaged. My hut nearly went also. The dust was rather choking. Fortunately, very little rain followed so that the patients did not get a ducking and were got under some sort of cover for the rest of the night.

25 February 1944

Shoals of complaints from the hospital about C diets (ration of 3.6c per day); the kitchen does not appear to be delivering the goods. The welfare officers think that the messing officer of the kitchen has lost his interest a bit. The amputees, in particular, are complaining bitterly.

A soldier who did not move to his barrack quickly enough during an air raid alarm, yesterday was beaten about the head by a soldier, Menamisan. When complaint was made to the commander, Kukabu, he promised there would be no more hitting by soldiers: the offenders are to be brought to him to decide punishment. This is a good arrangement and may allow passions to cool a bit.

26 February 1944

The plan for rebuilding the amoebic ward which has blown down was approved by Nippon HQ. We are going to try longitudinally running beds, a single row on each side with a double in the centre, also longitudinal, and a few single beds at one end for sick cases. Obviously much better for examination and nursing than this damned lateral arrangement with everyone presenting their feet to you!

The camp accomodation at present is rather congested and there have been several changes of plan re new huts going up in the eastern side of the camp. At present work has stopped. The latrines remain in a shocking state and refuse disposal is deplorable – much into open pits close to the kitchen. This also brings rats, and it is known that there are a rat plagues at Bampong, Kanchanaburi, and also, I believe, at Kinsayok, although I have not heard of soldiers affected as yet.

I have introduced a system of précis slips for patients on discharge similar to the Tarsau ones.

27 February 1944

I fortunately find plenty of work to keep me busy from dawn until dark. I seem to be thoroughly acclimatised to the tropics and never notice the heat. Today, some elimination contest in the RAMC Company in preparation for the sports. I was asked to compete in the jumps, long and high. There was a horrible drain in the run up for the long jump and I could not hit the 'board', so was close second to a man named Gill. I have never high-jumped before but won that at the 5 ft 5 in. stage, so have blistered feet now. Bare feet render athletics difficult.

It was arranged to put more barbers on the hospital to shave and cut patients' hair and that they be allocated definitely to wards rather than touring around periodically as a team. Tools are the trouble and I have had to undertake the expense of buying extra razors and clippers. Barbers are actually paid 40c. a day.

28 February 1944

Today, the camp commander, Kukabusan, when swimming in the river, saw some Chinese cabbage and other vegetables, quite suitable for consumption, floating down. Naturally, he was very angry and some of the camp commanders went into his office where he spoke of the expense and difficulty of bringing vegetables to the camp only to be wasted by the cooks. The messing officers, approximately twenty in number, were held responsible and were paraded. The commander then gave orders to his QM Sergeant as to their punishment. They were 'done over' the face and the neck with his belt, one who flinched being knocked down. Then orders were given that the whole camp was to have no meat or vegetables for three days. When Lt-Col. Outram draw attention to the 3,000 odd sick in the area, the commander kindly allowed an exception to be made in their favour; and the interpreter who sent for me very sympathetically discussed the question and made this arrangement. While no doubt a waste of vegetables under these circumstances was deplorable, there is a feeling that they may not have come from our own cookhouse. Most men in the camp are acutely food conscious. It is all very unfortunate.

29 February 1944

We picked a new site for a cookhouse urgently required for Takanoon personnel coming in on the east side of the camp. It seems that the area is to be evacuated to here and also a Japan party from there is to be quartered here temporarily. Great difficulty today as orders are out that no more refuse is to go into the river, but into pits which have to be dug. There ae not sufficient tools and these open pits are a deplorable health hazard because of flies and rats. I hope agreement will be reached to cart refuse out of the camp. Parties of men today have to dredge all bones out of the river.

There are no vegetables and no meat so the sports plan was cancelled.

Out of iodoform and rather worried about some of the ulcer cases. I cannot get fresh supplies.

1 March 1944

Two parties of 233 arrived from Takanoon; 87 were admitted to hospital. Owing to the amoebic dysentery ward having been blown down, we have had a considerable squeeze up round the hospital to find room for them. They are mostly malaria cases and tropical ulcers. These have been excised and are coming down nice and clean. They have had a little iodoform and, of course, Max Pemberton who has been in charge of the hospital, is a very sound and thorough fellow.

Capt. Calderwood has reported on shortages in the dispensary. The handling and accounting for drugs by the QMS in charge has been shockingly slack. His unsatisfactory showing in this investigation and his slovenly past conduct is such that he has been today relieved by me of his duties and returned to the lines.

2 March 1944

Maj. Graham arrived with a party of 253 of which 54 admitted to hospital. Lt Leslie's party 100 of arrived also (admitted to hospital 2).

The Arts & Crafts work on making buffalo hide into sandals is going well. They are sold to officers at 1.50 ticals and to hospital staff and ORs for 50c. Tailoring is working well. I have asked Lt-Col. Outram to request work for them in his orders. Sapper Thomas of the 'Sandal & Broom Manufacture Firm' is going to come into the hospital workshops and I wish to get them all on a salary of 20c per day.

Today I heard that a Nipponese sergeant major was going to Bangkok and asked for the purchase of certain essential drugs and dressings. A list was supplied: we would find the money somehow but I reminded them that they owed us 500 ticals out of 1,000 ticals previously given them. I was told that the new policy was that the Nippon HQ would supply all drugs, etc. and we must get special permission for any purchase. This was secured from the commander via the interpreter and I gave him 500 ticals from our funds. However, this 500 and the 500 owed to us were returned. I do not know whether the purchase will be made or not.

The dressing situation, in particular, is rather desperate. The four bolts of cotton cloth, 38 yards each, purchased for 500 ticals is now completedly used up.

3 March 1944

Accommodation of RAMC personnel is changed and there is a great deal of shifting about the camp to accommodate the newcomers. These are divided into 'red' force which consists of the Takanoon Japan party plus fit men from Takanoon and the 'blue' force which is the sick of Takanoon. The latter come on to strength today.

4 March 1944

A number of letters have come into the camp recently and many people have been cheered by these. I have not had any and I don't think any Java party men have had any luck. I arranged today for the Takanoon area to open an M.I. room of their own. The hospital is extremely full. Skin grafting today with the iodoform technique T/5186226, Pte. Lockhart, A., RASC aged 25.

5 March 1944

Deaths 1; Total in hospital 2242.
I arranged for puchase of milk from outside via Capt. Bill Adams. Adams also does meat purchase. Permission was obtained from the Nippon HQ. The probable price is 2 ticals per beer bottle of goat's milk. We are suggesting 20 bottles per day as our order.

A visit from Lt-Col. A.C. Johnson, (his soubriquet 'Ackers Crackers')* who collects butteflies and orchids assiduously. He told me that he has recently seen a good deal of Maj. Bruce Anderson, AAMC, who is in a Tamil camp and who is

* He put on a rather subtle, eccentric act.

burying about 30 Tamils a day. Now some Javanese are arriving to replace them. Tamil coolies, etc. have suffered terrible casualties on the lines.

6 March 1944

The new amoebic dysentery hut is practically complete; it will take in a few bacillary cases as well. The ward will also take in amoebic convalescents.

7 March 1944

Planes overhead and anti-aircraft fire in the early morning. Information was received re the 2/2 Pioneer Bn, Java: 160 have died as POWs to date. Some 29 were missing from action and must be presumed to be dead. This included Lt Cliff Lang, my old friend. Lt Lamb, G.H. ('Hammy') is amongst those who have died as POWs.

8 March 1944

Planes were overhead again last night. I passed an order to the Camp HQ re the prevalence of ear infections. Water is to be shaken out of the ears as much as possible after swimming.

9 March 1944

Death, 1.

10 March 1944

Captains Petrowski and Longbottom, Lewis and Brown are going off with the Japan party, 2 to each 750. Their equipment to set out: 200 tabs. quinine; 50 g iodine solution; 50 tabs. aspirin; one bandage; one packet of gauze; 2 bottles of creosote pills, anti-diarrohoea tablets, a supply to each 150 men. There were no anaesthetic materials, instruments or other stores issued so they are rather worried. It was finally arranged with Max Pemberton to do the lion's share of outfitting them, giving them some morphia, magnesium sulphate, syringes, local anaesthetic, iodoform, sulphur ointment and a few surgical instruments. They seem very cheery fellows. The clothing issued to these departing soldiers is assorted but fairly comprehensive: coats – airforce, hospital blue, or Indian pattern with a heavy shirt; trousers – trews of tartan, hospital blues, battle dress or khaki drill, anti-malarial pattern; long woollen underpants, a cotton singlet and a blue canvas rubber boots of Nipponese pattern with thin white cotton socks. Some patients with big feet, 11s and 12s, were supplied by taking footwear from the hospital patients. The officers and W/Os were given a kit of battle dress, British army pattern. The party departed today, quite a colourful turnout and in good spirits; 750 in the first party. Several soldiers told me that they were glad to have a chance to see Nippon.

11 March 1944

Concert with a good deal of classical music including Schubert and Chopin.

12 March 1944

Up betimes and on parade and ready to go to Takanoon. There is a most impressive monument to those who have lost their lives in making the Thailand/Burma Railway. A party to attend consists of 20 British, 10 Dutch, 10 Australians and we were told to send well-dressed soldiers! This we did by free borrowing. We marched across between two rivers almost two miles to the monument – a tall, substantial cenotaph of concrete with some marble slabs for inscription set in a square of approximately 20 metres with four right-angled corner bastions of stone and cement, each inscribed on the inner side with languages of the people concerned: Nipponese, Thai, Hindu, Malay, etc. The English caption read, 'May they rest in peace' which indeed they deserve. The monument was adorned with fruits and vegetables, bottles of saki, lampangs of tobacco and such good things. A table in front with a white cloth had upon it a brass urn in which three sticks smoked. Also some candles.

We were drawn up before the monument with a hollow square arrangement, a N general and higher staff officers on the left, many other N officers of high rank and many Thai officials and higher service officers on the right. In the centre were the various native groups to the right, the British, Americans, Dutch and Australians on the left.

A N priest, a 2-star private with bayonet at side, did most of the initial ceremony which was complicated and impressive.

The N general then approached and read a scroll with his message and this was interpreted in several languages. Thai officials and many Japanese officers paid their respects then any religious persons approached the monument, paying their respects and reading scrolls. Brigadier Varley also read a scroll after advancing and saluting the cenotaph. 'They shall grow not old as we that are left grow old. In the morning and at the going down of the sun, we will *remember* them.'

Many pictures were taken, including cine films. Huge numbers of colourful wreaths were grouped about the central cenotaph. It was extremely hot and this interesting ceremony took about two hours. I wish I understood more of it. Afterwards, all men were given a tin of biscuits and allowed to go to the Tamarkand camp for lunch.

On arrival 'home', I was disconcerted to find that we have two cases of clinical cholera today; one returned from work at Kanchanaburi today and was immediately taken ill, the other was from Group II – a worker feeding from No. 11 kitchen.

13 March 1944

I discussed the cholera situation with Yasanosan and we were asked to give up a drum today to go to the garden for the pigs. After explaining the needs of the hospital patients in the prevention of cholera, he kindly agreed to waive his demands. Thus, we were able to give drums out to the hospital kitchen for sterilisation of gear, particularly food containers. We asked for extra vaccine for innoculation, also for disinfectants, chloride of lime etc. This, he said, he would request from Nippon HQ by telephone. I do not think it would be wise to put the river out of bounds for swimming since skin conditions are rife. A general blitz on hygiene is recommended.*

14 March 1944

Another case of cholera today: one of my ulcer patients on 'C' diet.

15 March 1944

Cholera innoculations are going on; there are four cases in isolation. I have been feverish again with headache and malaise for two days; my blood film is positive for B.T. malaria and my spleen enlarged, so off again on a quinine course. What a country!

16 March 1944

Cholera precautions are still being stressed but camp hygiene is bad. The weather is very hot and sultry.

17 March 1944, St Patrick's Day

Conversation today with interpreter and Yasamosan re hygiene difficulties. Consent is given for a party of 10 to go out to get the jungle-wood for timber to cover latrines. This is a big forward step.

18 March 1944

A skin graft was carried out on Pte Castle, W.R. aged 35. 5th Beds. & Herts. on the back of the left leg.

* At this time our need for those large drums was desperate. I explained to Yasano that for 2,500 sick, we had only one drum to fetch water and one drum to boil it. We badly needed them to make disinfestors too. (I was aware that there was a large pile of unused drums in the Japanese area of the camp.)

When he threatened to remove one for pigs, I perhaps unwisely said that if he did, I would have him hung one day! I won minor concessions which however did not meet our grave need. I determined upon the risky project of a night raid on the Japanese lines.

With blackened face and hands, I crawled into the compound carrying one of the old, long, heavy, army torches though I did not envisage needing it. I succeeding in transporting four drums and was returning with a fifth when I was startled by a challenge from 'O'!, a N guard who was identified by me by the patchy loss of hair (syphilitic alopecia) and loose, foul rat-like teeth. Shocked, I dropped the drum and inadvertantly shone the torch which gleamed on his bayonet and revolting visage. Acting impulsively, I clobbered him over the head with the torch and ran, bobbing and weaving and expecting a bullet.

Reaching my bunk, I threw myself under a blanket with a fast beating heart and a mood of resignation and despair. I felt sure that O. would have recognised me and that even if he had not, I would have to own up to save the camp from inevitable reprisals. It was a wretched uneasy night. Incredibly, nothing happened and the next day was uneventful. O did not appear. However, on the following day, there he was conducting a parade with an obvious lump raising his cap. Puzzled, I suddenly realised the friendly intervention of 'retrograde amnesia' – the memory loss preceding concussion. He must have awakened with the conclusion that another Nipponese had attacked him as he was in his own lines and no doubt confused.

Cautiously, I introduced the drums into service separately, with splendid results. I made a mental note to avoid in future pushing my luck too far!

19 March 1944

Four cases of tropical typhus arrived in camp today from a new camp on the other side of Kanchanaburi (8 miles). These troops came recently from Kinsayok and report that there are now less than a hundred men left there. Only one medical officer. Maj. Corlette, captains Parker, Godlee, and all MOs less one, also lieutenant-colonels Lilly, McEachern, James and Hugenon and Maj. Wearne are said to be building some 200 huts in another large camp. I would very much like to see them again.

20 March 1944

The convalescent wards are very crowded at present. The hospital maintenance section is doing excellent work repairing roofs, making new beds, etc. Hospital equipment is vastly improved by the work of the workshop section. Major Graham, IMS, is doing very good work on the hygiene side.

21 March 1944

There is keen competition and interest at present in the extraordinary human race meeting to be held on 23 March. The idea is to make money for the hospital and provide amusement. The owners enter a horse at approximately one tical each to give prize money and the bookmakers pay 10 ticals for a stand on the course. Various enclosures have entry fees. A tote to pay 10 per cent. I am entered under the name of Manfred by Bill Ongley, an astute racing man. Secret trials are being held. My jockey being 'Punchy' Powell. It is believed that good time for the 100 yd will be 18 seconds. My trials up to date are about 19 seconds but I have malaria and am not trying very hard. A terrific weight of Australian bookings has promply pushed my odds down to evens, starting from 5:2 – most amusing nonsense is going on about trials and times.

Skin grafts: Pte Crooks B., 4th Suffolks, aged 23, Pte Oliphant G., 10630177 A.C.C. attached to the 1/5 Sherwood Foresters.

22 March 1944

The Nipponese have agreed to give me enough bamboo to put down deep revetted latrines for the dysentery wards.

23 March 1944

Spring meeting of the Chungkai Race Club. The first race was at 1830 the tote opening at 1800. The course was in the dry, dusty area of Group II lines, fairly flat going with a few depressions. A very large crowd consisting of most of the camp population. Various enclosures and some important looking race officials! There were six events. The Canberra Maiden Stakes, 75 yd; The Officers' Stakes, 100 yd; The Stayers' Stakes, 150 yd; The Chungkai Invitation Stakes; 100 yd; The Newcomers' Stakes, 100 yd; The Thailand Stakes, 75 yd; The affair was conducted with considerable pageantry. The 'horses' and jockeys first parading around the course, the 'horses' wearing numbers, the jockeys very diminutive and for the most part in suitable costume, peaked cap and colours, etc.! As 'Punchy' Powell had his tobacco factory on me, he withdrew as a jockey and I was presented with a new boy, a little over 7 stone. Much amusement from the crowd during the parade for The Officers' Stakes owing to our contrast in size. A number of starters in the Officers' Stakes included Bill Gayden and Captain Hetred, RAMC, with me backed down to evens with a terrific load of AIF money in particular. I got slightly left at the start but won easily in a time of 15.25 seconds. As usual, I started to shake with laughter in the middle of the race. McMullen, the camp bugler, won the Chungkai Invitation Stakes with the same jockey in the sensational time of 14.25 seconds for the 100 yd. Otherwise, my time stood. Much AIF jubilation and 'Waler' Davidson told me that he had won 100 ticals on me! I am afraid I got a little tiddly on the local brew.

24 March 1944

This hospital and the medical organisation of the camp is a fairly big show. This is illustrated by the number of other ranks (439) on the hospital pay roll.

25/26/27 March 1944

I was involved in discussion re promotions. I cannot find any real authority for promotion under POW circumstances and there is no real establishment in a huge hospital of this sort staffed by oddments from all sorts of units. I am looking into the position.

28 March 1944

The weather at present is extremely hot and for the first time I feel an extreme langour and a complete lack of energy in the afternoons. The sun strikes one like a drawn sword more fiercely than I can remember in the last two years in the tropics. The shade temperature, I believe, has reached 115° F. and some temperatures are variously stated as 145° F. (probable) to 165° F. on the authority of 'Blue' Butterworth.

29 March 1944

Deaths 1. Hot weather continues.

30 March 1944

Deaths 0.

31 March 1944

Deaths in October were 259; November 143; December 134; January 78; February 36; March 29 = 677. There were no amputations this month and the improvement in the ulcers and skin diseases is most marked. The general morale is very good and everyone seems in remarkably good spirits.

1 April 1944

I received an intriguing little parcel this morning and tried to work out what important anniversary this might be. Eventually, the date seemed significant so

I pushed it on to Max Pemberton with my best wishes. He opened it with numerous wrappings and with much mystification and in a kapok bed found a little card referring to the date. (April Fools' day!).

Operation: 5122811 Pte. Collacott, RAOC. Appendicectomy. Skin grafts: NX 38487. Sgt Holland R.S. of 2/1 Heavy Battery AIF. Tropical ulcer of the leg. 5829613, Pte Lawrence, E. A.H.G. 4th Suffolk Regt aged 26. A tropical ulcer on the back of the right foot which has been present for four months.

2 April 1944

I was disturbed to receive a notice from Maj. Richardson, the Camp QM, that there is to be a severe reduction in rations, including rice, by order of the Nipponese HQ Singapore. This information comes via Nipponese Q, NCO Takayamasan. The position looks rather serious but there may be some catch. The scale now given is sugar ⅓ ounce, salt ¼ oz., peas ¾ oz., beans ⅘ oz., flour ½ oz., oil ⅖., tea ⅛ oz. rice 17¾ ozs., vegetables not announced. One difficulty is that no definite ration scale has been given here.

3 April 1944

In view of the proposed ration scale reduction. I have stopped all rice poulticing. The commodity is needed as food.

Owing to considerable expenditure on eggs, welfare is costing more than 1c a day. It is necessary either to put more egg supply into the hospital kitchen or to increase the welfare expenditure.

4 April 1944

Hospital finance sub-committee decided to increase goat milk from 20 to 30 bottles per day. It seems to be doing good work.

Maj. A.A. Pycock of HQ 2 Group (QM) is in rage over the reduction of rations and regards this as a purely local manoeuvre for the improvement of the Nipponese NCO! After hearing a story of the past record of our little friends, I feel convinced this is so. [Subsequent events proved Pycock to be entirely right.]

5 April 1944

A party is to go to a new area consisting of 2 Group personnel, Takanoon Force. 'Red Group' 130; 2 Group Chungkai 170. We will supply the medical officer and other ranks required for the party.

Two soldiers were caught by the Nipponese bringing in Thai whisky to the camp! After rather painful interrogation and standing before the Guardroom, an ingenious punishment was devised by Kukabusan. After retreat and the evening meal, they had to march around the camp accompanied by a small organised band, squeeze box, etc. with large matting placards tied on their back and front: 'Private "X". "'Sentenced to seven days in cells for bringing Thai whisky to the camp"'. Our money has been confiscated and given to the hospital. 'The I.J.A. will not tolerate further violation of orders.'!

One I.J.A. soldier took the party round – the two delinquents and the band –

the latter playing 'Colonel Bogey', 'Roll out the Barrel' and other appropriate tunes. The profit to the hospital – $30!.

Poor Pte Collicott died today.

6 April 1944

Many of the huts leak badly and some are so decrepit they are apt to come down altogether. This has just happened to the cholera ward. Fortunately, nobody was seriously injured; the patients were returned to the ordinary wards as the danger of serious infectivity is past. It is difficult to get any construction done at present unless the huts actually fall down and even then there are many delays. There is no clear data as to the departing party. The fitter of the young captains of No 2 Group cut the cards; Captain Robson cut lowest and was then detailed.

7 April 1944

I decided to send the strongest 'horse' I have amongst the MOs, Maj. Reed, who volunteered for the job. A party of IV Group, 200 strong with five officers, departed today for Tamuang down near Kanchanaburi. W/O Draper was one of this party and through him I made an effort to get in touch with Lt-Col. McEachern and his party.

Today the hospital had a purge of a few soldiers who as patients or orderlies use the hospital as a cloak for trading and underhand 'through the fence' activities. Books could be written about the careers of some of these 'merchant princes' and the activities of some sound like the Arabian Knights entertainment, Ali Baba, etc.! Some accumulate hundreds of dollars by being an intermediary, never themselves running any risk. Most of those dealt with today were NEI soldiers.

Easter Friday today. Even a shot at hot cross buns made out of rice.

8 April 1944

An operation on Sgt Brislin, J.F., F.M.S.V.F. A rodent ulcer of the nose, this being the sixth, all the previous ones having been treated by X-ray. The Nipponese said it was not possible to get radium treatment in this country.

[Years later, he sent me a picture with presentable appearance.]

9 April 1944

Easter Sunday. I received an Easter egg from Lt-Col. Outram who is at present laid up with ulcers of one foot.

Somehow, I seem to have lost all emotional depths these days and am living in a drab way without much thought or feeling or reaction to anything. Worst of all, one's sense of beauty and appreciation of beauty seems to suffer. 'Love and the old dreams of life remind me of dry violets between the leaves of a book.' These must have existed but one can't feel very much any more. Further, I can't react very much to physical suffering or death. The tragedy of death only becomes apparent when you see the stricken face of a relative or dear one. Perhaps even they will have become so used to us being away that the suffering will not be very great when many fail to return. I think one should not be a prisoner for more than two years in fact.

10 April 1944

Deaths: 1.

An amusing story of a 'geisha' who came per barge for the pleasure of Commander Kukaboo! It seems that on the way in she was apprehended by Ometz and was enjoyed by Ometz and three British other ranks for the sum of 15 ticals.

11 April 1944

The RAMC service today with Padre Webb – this was requested as an Easter service by the company.

12 April 1944

Camp sports today, in which I competed in the high jump, the long jump and the hop step and jump. I won the latter but came third in the other two. The medical officers were busily engaged in making a provisional list of Group 2 personnel for evacuation to Nakom Patom. There is very little guide as to to policy in evacuation. Provisionally, all amoebic convalescents are being included although some are fairly well at present. Some are political parties; officers. No unanimity here.* Medical personnel I do not want included unless they are actually sick in hospital at present.

13 April 1944

One death. Two extensive skin grafting operations.

14 April 1944

Akimotosan approached me today about a rather favoured operation by the Nipponese – circumcision! I obliged with local anaesthetic.† These soldiers rather haunt us at present, the main complaint being VD which is almost universal. I am at present looking after an unfortunate who reports cryptically, 'Kanburi go. Much wine. Sleep with Thai girl. No "zig-a-zig". Not understand!!' Like most soldiers they seem very much afraid of their own medical service!

* The plan designed to keep together officers who would constitute a headquarters staff to take command when Japan collapsed. There was no clear authority and competing views. I was nominated for the medical staff.

† The affair Akimoto was not uneventful. Poor fellow, his adventures in Bangkok caused ravages to his person, leaving him with two apertures instead of one. He repeatedly begged me to tidy things up. I demurred and said, 'If I cut cut – you no guard duty go – trouble.' He struck his chest and said, 'I guard duty go.' There came an evening when he appeared bearing a bottle of credible Thai brandy which he dangled before me as 'big presento'! I weakened. Maybe I had been too severe! I consumed the brandy in the moonlight with one or two choice companions including 'Drunken Duncan' Black. Life seemed tolerable and we sang nostalgic songs. In the morning, Akimoto's operation effected, I clapped him on the back like a marshall with a favoured cadet and said, 'You brave soldier – guard duty go.'

Alas, some two hours later, the sword of Damocles fell. I was summoned and escorted to the Commandant, Kukabusan. He was seated on a bamboo stool, legs crossed, immobile, silent, his face dark with wrath like a teak god. On the table, gleaming in the sun, his moonwhite bare samurai sword which was reputed to have cut down two prisoners. My *kiotské* and *keré* were

16 April 1944

Maj. Moon and I have an interesting weekly blood match at bridge, partnered by Lt Hirsch and Taylor respectively. These two are of international standing. The stake is usually an omelette. These two excellent players have vast amusement from our performance.

I complained to the N NCO that offal was not being sent in for the sick (actually it is in part sold to the Thais). He very kindly took me out to the slaughteryard where the beasts are killed. The nearby trees were laden with vultures and a ring of Thai people made up the human equivalent. I went on to the garden site and also an enclosure full of pigs fed by our refuse. These live in a happy symbiosis with crows, who ride merrily on their backs. Picking off their ticks.

17 April 1944

Via the Thais I have managed to purchase two bolts of 38 yd of flimsy muslin for dressings at a cost of 310 ticals. The cloth is now practically unprocurable.

18 April 1944

The Camp Finance Committee Meeting.

Financial position as at 17 April 1944: credit balance of 5385.50 ticals. It is calculated that on present expenditure, there would be a balance of 7567.95 ticals at the end of May. Accordingly, the proposition is to increase the expenditure on troops messing in the lines from 2.5c to 4c per head per day.

How to divide money when parties of troops march out cause some spirited controversy.

19 April 1944

Lt-Col. Stitt of the Gordons' has compiled a book of oddments written by amusing camp personalities: it contains, amongst other things, information as to foods and wines in various parts of the world, no doubt of great interest to gourmets and epicureans. One, Jerry Perez who was castigated as a bridge partner, got him in on a dish called the 'Caucasian Stroganoff'. This includes amongst other ingredients a Caucasion bear's foot! red Caucasion wine, oysters,

faultless. Minutes ticked by as I reflected about naval court martials and the forbidding sword. Suddenly, the brooding god dropped his legs to the floor, seized the sword and pointing an accusing finger, said "Dunrop *chusa*, you despise me – I will kill you.' No doubt referring to disregard of orders. Without more ado, he swung the sword back in a wide arc and it then swished down. I remained rigid, may be petrified, but the blade stopped quivering against my neck. With a disarming gesture, he handed the sword to me and said, 'No, here is my sword, please honour me by killing yourself.' I took the sword gingerly and began talking very fast.

'Kukabusan, in my country we have many problems. All sorts of dreadful things happen. We lose our money, wives run away, homes burn down, we may know disgrace, humiliation, defeat, but all these things must be born – there is no *hara-kiri*.' My eloquent flood was stopped by the stunned incredulity in his fierce brown eyes. In contempt he spat out, 'You mean that you are such a great coward that you will not kill yourself!'

I replied, 'You are dead right about one thing. I shall not kill myself.' I was then thrown into the 'box house' with the offending Akimoto. I pointed the finger: 'You rat – no guard duty go.' He replied, 'You did not tell me "cut cut" so much pain.'

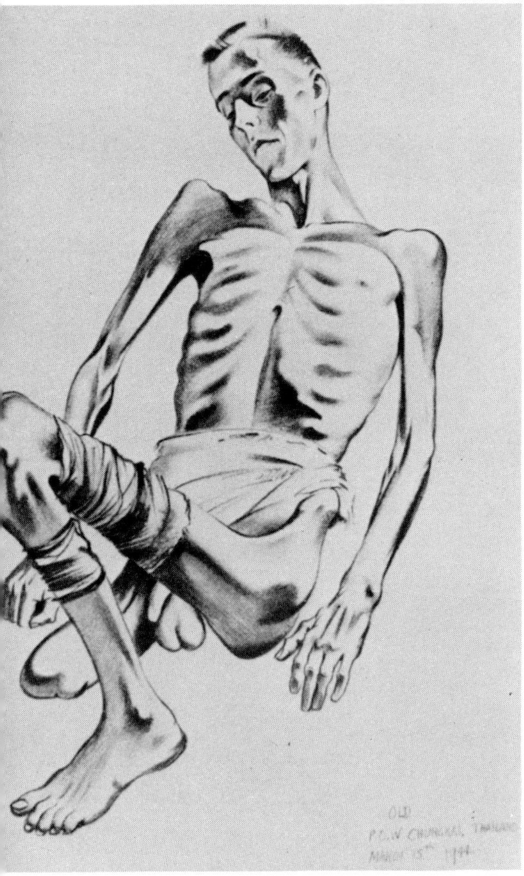

110 Extremely debilitated British soldier – amputation and multiple diseases, Chungkai. Recovered (*Old*)

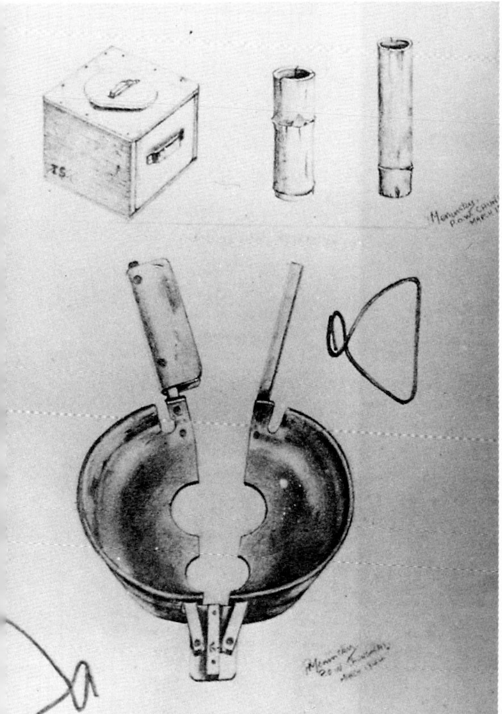

ɪnverted dish amputation shield, leg or arm; bedside box, .mboo urinal and water bottle (*P. Meninsky*)

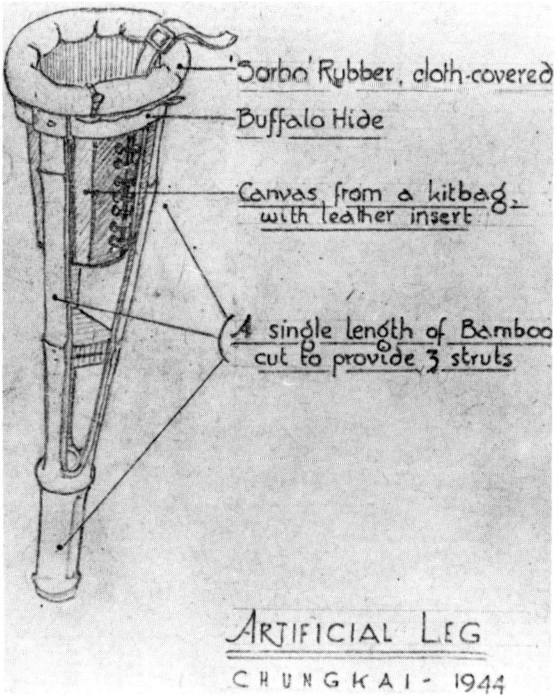

112 Bamboo and timber artificial leg for amputees improvised by Maj. Alan Woods (*S. Gimson*)

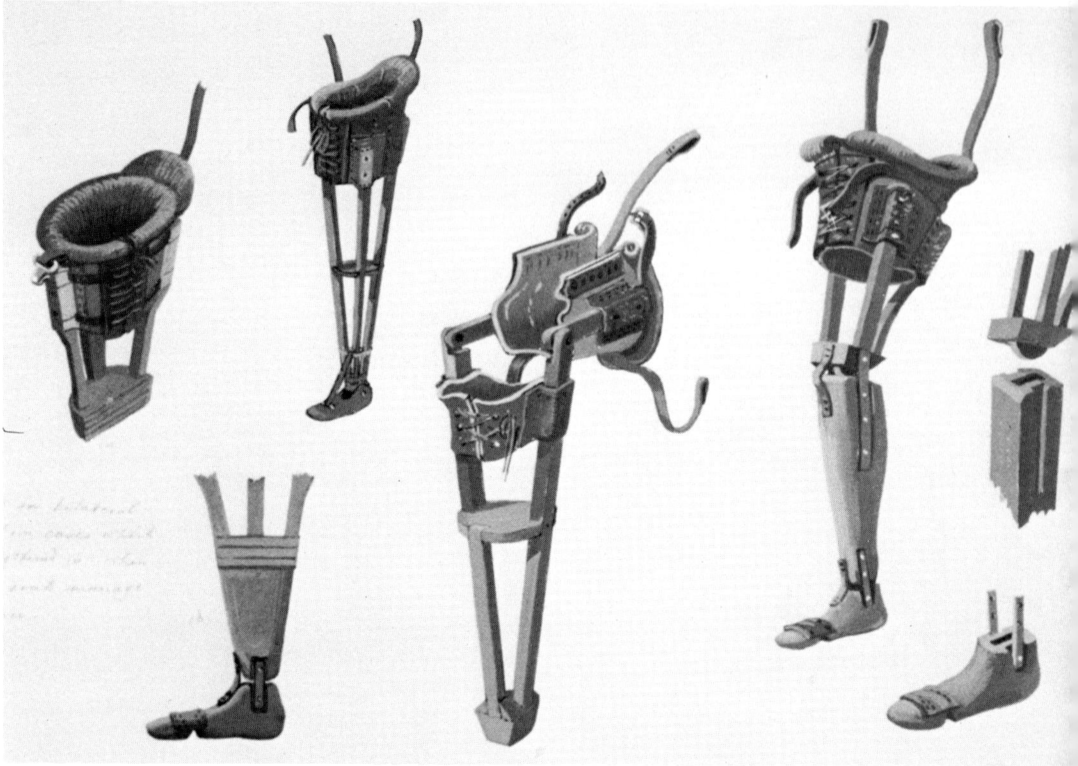

113 Artificial limbs made at Nakom Patom base hospital camp. Some with the 'solid' lower leg were hollowed out and mater
hidden within them under a wooden plate! This group includes short stumps and attachments for bilateral amputation
(*Jack Chalker*)

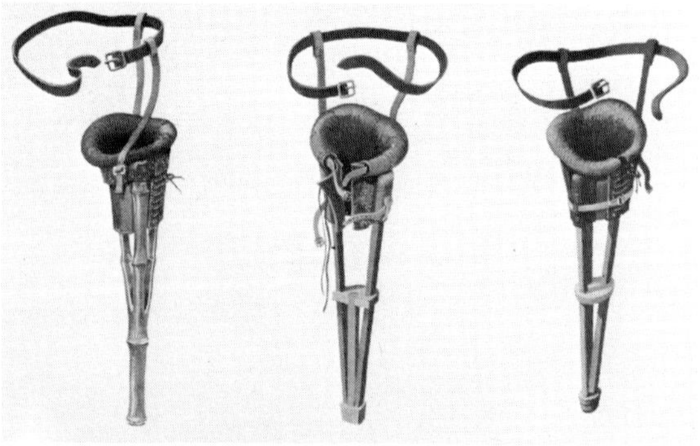

114 Artificial limbs. Progression in design from left to right, from split bamboo stump onwards. Buckets from old army webbing packs, kapok stuffing, hide from animals for lacing patches, laces etc. These were made largely by Australian legless for themselves and other amputees; the work was begun in Chungkai and continued in Nakom Patom base hospital camps 1943–5 (*Jack Chalker*)

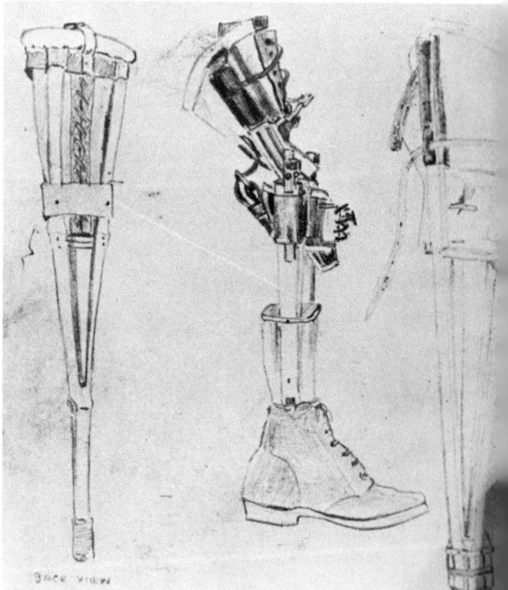

115 Pylon and prosthesis for amputees (*P. Meninsky*)

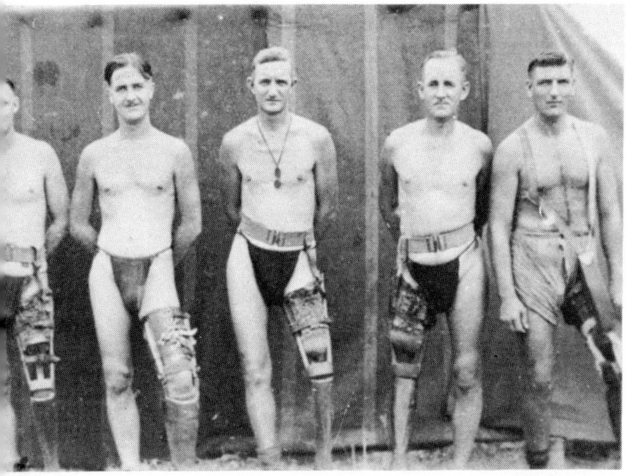

116 Amputee with prostheses. Left to right: thigh ball type, box type 4 kg; thigh stand type 3.75 kg; roller type 4.5 kg. Photograph taken at Nakom Patom after the war

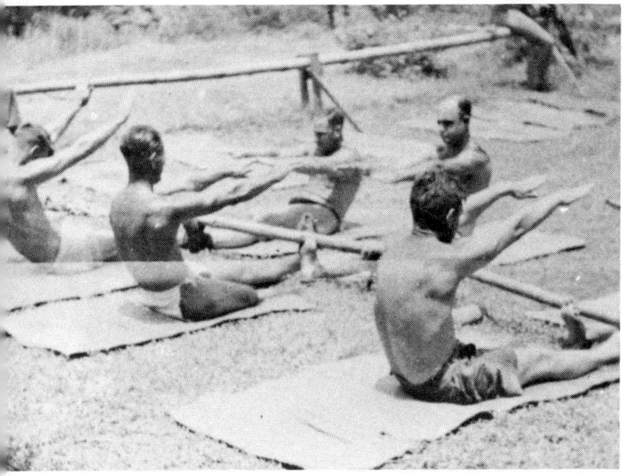

117 Low bar for amputees for toning up, breathing and stretching

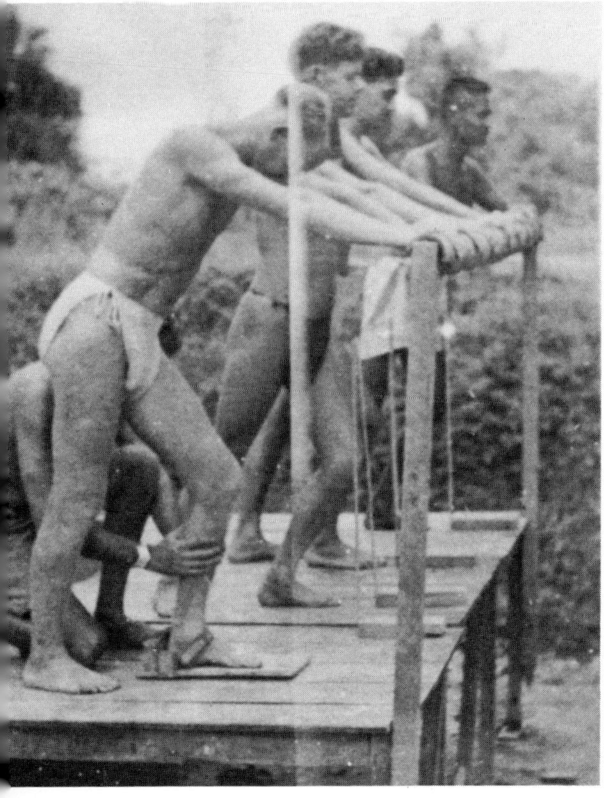

118 Rehabilitation, Nakom Patom. Ankle contraction treated by massage, heel strapped down, over-reaching exercises

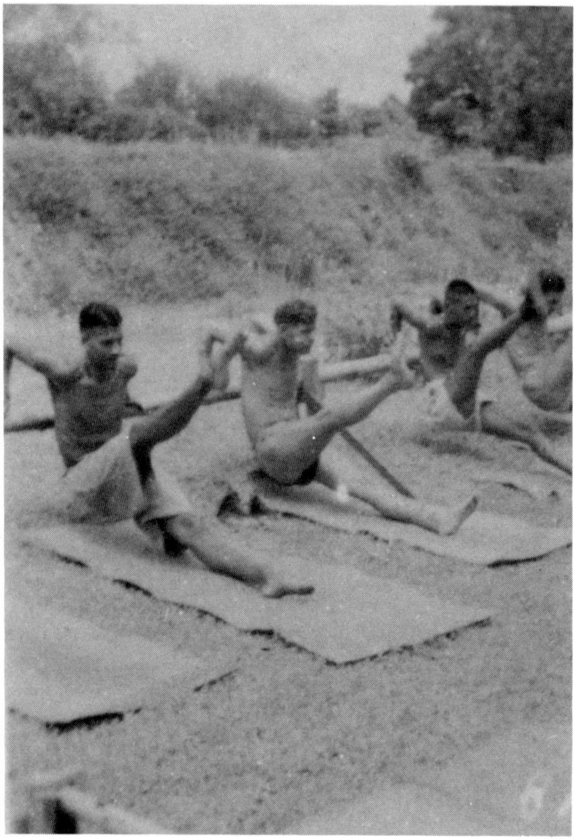

119 13-inch bar for abdominal exercises, breathing and stretching. After the war

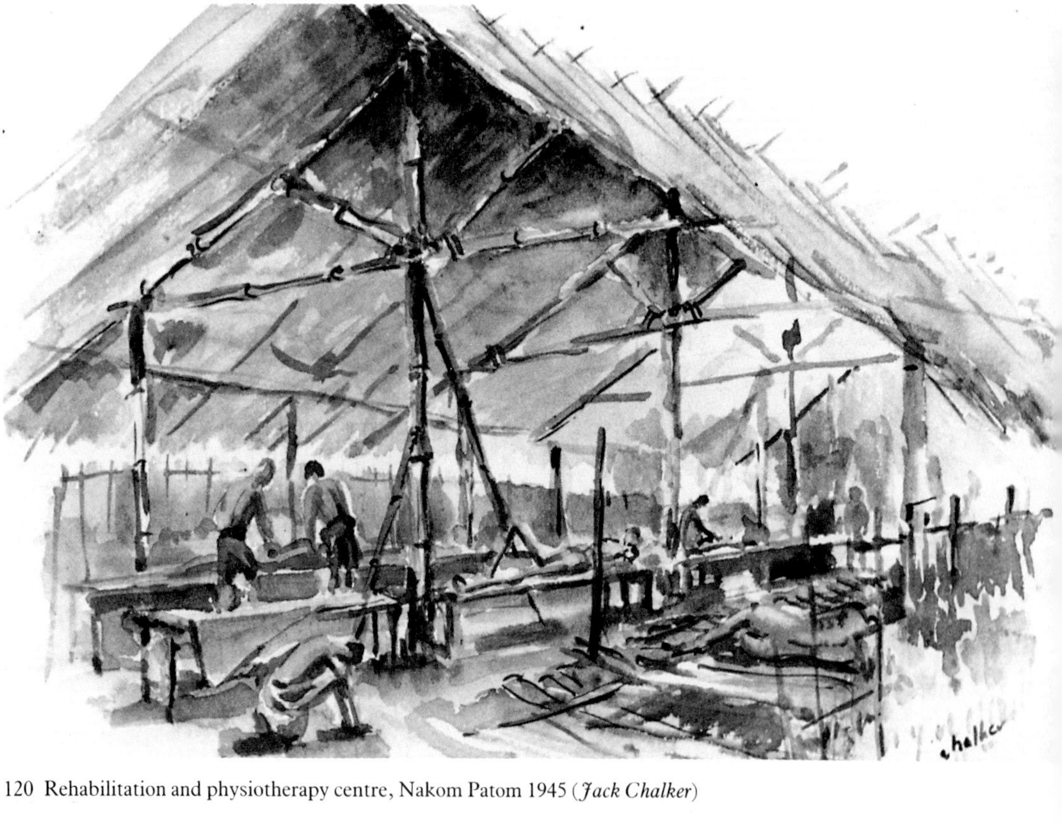

120 Rehabilitation and physiotherapy centre, Nakom Patom 1945 (*Jack Chalker*)

caviare, 20 peppercorns, whipped Caucasion cream, etc.! The directions begin: 'Take a bear's foot. Cut into 1 cm. cubes. Place in dish.' Finally one is advised that the dish is of such rarity and takes so long to prepare that in London, Paris and Shanghai where it is obtained, one must give 24 hours notice in ordering!*

20 April 1944

A further 'leg' of the Camp Finance Meeting today. A scheme of distribution of finance for outgoing parties approved: where parties were known to be going up river, an extra 50c a head will be allotted.

21 April 1944

A Hollandsche cabaret called *Circus Cavaljos*. The costumes and props were strikingly good and reflected artistic qualities and very hard work. A most appreciated item came at the last just as a heavy storm worked up: 'The Legend of the Lotus'. The holy temple of Ammon Ra in Egypt; a giant lotus from which a dream woman appears and dances before the God; a rather grotesque ugly little man gains entrance to the temple and watches. The figure and classic grace of the dancer was most convincing and you could have heard a pin drop until she at last disappears again into the flower, representing beauty, haunting and unobtainable, just beyond the grasp of the mind and heart. The little man sinks to his knees and bows his head in his arms, weeping. As we left the threatre area, the storm broke, lashing the camp in considerable fury. As luck would have it, the building which came down this time was the block with the operating theatre, blood transfusion unit, dispensary, dental centre and pathology room. It looks as if something will come down with every storm from now on.

22 April 1944

We appealed to the Nippon HQ today, Yasanosan, re the urgency of the situation. 'Could we temporarily have a portion of a hut in the Red Group area?' 'No,' and again, 'No.' Then with Lt-Col. Outram to Odachisan who eventually put our case to Yanagite *chusa*, the colonel-in-charge. He was sympathetic and gave us the temporary use of the hut in question.

200 men are requested from 4 Group. Those to go it is thought to Tamuang then possibly up river. I called on Yasanosan tonight to 'thank him for speaking to Lt-Col. Yanagite re the hut'! This was accepted smilingly. I found him vaccinating the last of about a hundred Nipponese soldiers with a watchglass containing a puddle of vaccine and blood, a glass rod and a scalpel with which he cut them and dabbed some of the puddle on the arm as they passed. I said, 'Yasanosan, you No. 1 vaccinator!' He flushed and in this sun of appreciation, said, 'You', and seizing me by my right arm he vaccinated me by cutting me in four places with the scalpal and applied the last of the blood puddle. I thanked

* This quite imaginative dish subsequently was also quoted in Countess Mountbatten's book of famous recipes!

him and slunk away hoping that an opportunity would occur later for me to have my Wasserman done!

23 April 1944

I called to see Captain Novasawa; he was very polite and asked me for particulars of all medical officers and what they were doing at present. I made a plan of the hospital and the allotment of duties. Group 2 personnel (the Takanoon party) are busy dealing with large questionaires which invite criticism,both constructive and destructive re previous treatment of POWs in Thailand. Complete frankness is required, with such questions as, 'What do you think of the Nippon engineer service?', 'What is the most detestable, deplorable, etc. incident that you have seen?' 'What is the kindest action you have seen by a Nipponese soldier?' Then opinions on all matters of camp administration were called for. As regards kindest act by Japanese soldier, one officer offered the following: an occasion when, before beating him, the soldier let him take off his spectacles and did not use a crowbar!

24 April 1944

Departure of Maj. Reed and party up river today. Part of the pathology and theatre hut blew down. Capt. McIntosh and Capt. Hardy, our pathologists, have been required to work in the N hospital. Stools, slides, etc, have to be taken a long way. N ideas of microscopy are very vague.

25 April 1944 Anzac Day

Anzac Parade assembled at 1915. There were approximately 700 AIF in the camp well over 400 were able to be present. I had to take the parade as senior AIF officer. A large crowd was watching and the lads turned out very well borrowing clothes were necessary and as a concession to the occasion, I borrowed 'Blue' Butterworth's slouch hat. We stood for one minute at attention to think of comrades who had by their sacrifice furthered the lustre of the name ANZAC, then marched to church by companies. The first AIF soldiers were leading. Padre Thompson, an Australian, took the service and rather gave us all a rocket that we only turn up to church in large numbers on this one day! This was borne out by the fact that we did not seem to remember the words of 'Rock of Ages' at all well and the only flaw was that he forgot to mention New Zealand in the sermon!

26 April 1944

I have considered the whole question of a hospital establishment under those Other Rank personnel worthy of promotion or other recognition and will shortly promulgate an order.

27 April 1944

An operation with spinal novocain on Capt. Morgan, J. FMSVF, aged 40. He has amoebic dysentery and an appendicostomy was performed accompanied by a transfusion of 450 c.c.s defibrinated blood.

28 April 1944

Hurried returns were asked for by the Nipponese today in answer to telephone calls.

29 April 1944

The Emperor's birthday and a holiday for the Nipponese, most of whom are going into Kanchanaburi where they are putting on a show in competition with other areas. All have to sing, dance or perform in some way. They have borrowed all our theatre props and have had the threatre staff working very hard to produce costumes and effects for them. Thus our show is off this week.

As martyrs to the Roman holiday, Dunlop and his MOs had to play 'Angela' Bobby Spon and her boyfriends in a soccer match of burlesque type. The actors' team appear in all sorts of weird costumes, including the Dutch clowns. One armed with a heavy wooden hammer at full back. The band played lively airs – a fairly successful do.

Sulphur emulsion has given good results in the treatment of scabies. Method: wash the patient with hot water, descab if needed, apply the sulphur emulsion with a shaving brush and rub in well. Repeat in three days.

I am dissatisfied with the detailing of parties for up river, etc. The tendency is for groups and battalions to hang on to some duty personnel and to send less fit people away. Capt. Gottla's party contain inumerable B & C category personnel and even two 'bed downs'. Yet, medical officers were not consulted. A Group 4 party which left yesterday was made up of M. & D 69, B 123, C 23: Total 195.

30 April 1944

Officers 46; surgical 86; skin 212; ulcers 416; avitaminosis 180; acute amoebic dysentery 155; malaria 71; medical 213; convalescent amoebic dysentery 600; amputations 49. Deaths 2. *Total*: 2028.

1 May 1944

Anti-malarial work is urgently required in this area since recent rains have caused some stagnant water. A meeting of work administration officials to discuss the unsatisfactory way parties are detailed for up country at present. In future, MOs in charge of MI rooms are to keep separate full rolls of categories of sick. (Extra clerks to be supplied from the officers.); The Group Medical Officers are to be notified at once and to confer with the adjutant about the selection of parties. The party, when assembled, is to be medically inspected and MOs are to attend the following N inspection, and categories M & D are to be revised each two weeks, others weekly. Only M & D categories and to be detailed for parties.

2 May 1944

The Nipponese are still stalling on the rebuilding scheme, probably because of impending movements.

3 May 1944

Norman Smith, our bulky band leader and musician, was called in to give his physical support to control an ale-stricken N soldier on the return barge journey from Kanchanaburi where the band was performing. First, the Nipponese soldier extravagantly dived into the river over one side of the barge, then, when pulled back, over the other side where there was no water at all – only mud. As he gave great difficulty to his fellow soldiers, Norman was called on to restrain him, which he did by sitting on him all the way home while he begged, 'Please, please Sir, let me go'. Some excreta was squeezed out of him. Eventually, he was carried by Norman up to his quarters and a few days later he sent a most apologetic message of thanks and 10 ticals! The soldier explained that he was still in hospital and could not come himself. He apparently considered that he had been saved from a much worse handling by his fellows.

4 May 1944

Promotions: I have done a survey of the whole hospital and have tried to bring the whole place up to a very reasonable establishment. The principle is that a Ward Master should be at least acting sergeant and Assisting Ward Master at least acting corporal. Where however a promotion has already occurred since a soldier became a POW, he is left on the same rank. These promotions were promulgated in part 2 orders by Lt-Col. E.E. Dunlop, AAMC, Officer commanding POW Camp Hospital, Chungkai, Thailand. . . . The above promotions were considered necessary for the efficient functioning of the medical personnel under difficult conditions. Chungkai POW Camp is a hospital camp of approximately 8,000 men with 2,000 to 2,200 being in hospital at any one time. Many of the others, however, require treatment in the lines. Under normal circumstances, the above promotions would be made within an establishment with pay. As the personnel concerned have shown exemplary devotion to duty and by their splendid work under appalling conditions have been the means of saving many lives, it is hoped that the War Office will subsequently grant pay from the date of promotion.

*E.E. Dunlop, Lt-Col. AAMC**

5 May 1944

Anti-aircraft fire and planes overhead in the morning.

6 May 1944

Information today is that 4 Group movement to start by barge tomorrow. Directions for movement given by Ometz to Capt. Jenkins and from his to 4 Group adjutants, etc. I tried to discuss this movement with Capt. Novasawa, asking especially that there be some liaison between ourselves and Tamuang by a party of one medical officer and one orderly accompanying the sick and that the sick men be allowed to go down on stretchers. He sent me with a 4 Group

* I subsequently did my best to make the promotions stick but the Australian Government did not accept them. The same also applied to the 11 British soldiers concerned.

soldier known to the AIF as the 'High Breasted Virgin' to see Ometz. This was a painful affair. I was dragged around and given a sound bollicking by several powerful officials. O. unfortunately had been awakened from sleep and took me to an NCO who was at bayonet practice. After much argument, O. said that I could go down myself just once and then come back. No one to come up and down with the party. This was a small concession but much appreciated. These movements can be a nightmare with nothing known as to accommodation, staff, equipment or transport at either end.*

TOTAL SICK FOR MOVEMENT

	Hospital	Lines	Total
Heavy sick	746	483	1229
Light sick	181	1463	1644
Total sick	927	1946	2873 + 400 = 3273

We are now called upon for the list of the first 1,000 heavy sick Group IV, a nominal role to be finished by the morning of the 8th.

7 May 1944

I reported to the Nippon HQ this morning re Ometz' promise to let me go down with the sick. This was not confirmed. Yasano was very angry and said, 'You are not to go because you have done bad things!' I endeavoured to put the point that it was not a personal matter but a desire that someone should go. He refused. I then wrote a letter to Lt-Col. Harvey telling him the number of various types of sickness and how they had been accommodated, the number of officers and men as set out above. The first to move to be the 1229 heavy sick. I said I would send some medical officers as soon as possible and gave him particulars of 4 Group medical personnel employed here or sick.

* The N NCO in the bayonet fighting gear, Sgt Sukarno, 'The Slug', had an evil reputation as a 'basher' who had already broken the jaws of two officers for deficiencies in saluting. Ometz said he was the Movement Control Sergeant. Periodically, he charged like an inflamed rhinoceros, roaring whilst he transfixed a straw 'body' with his bayonet.

Politely, I referred to him as 'No. 1 Movement Control Sergeant – you speak, all men do – quickly, quickly!' I then outlined my request. To this he replied, 'Sick men no work – the more sick who die the better.' After further responses along these lines, I finally lost all patience and prudence and said, 'Then you are a black-hearted villain and one day I will have you hanged!'

The insult registered slowly and then he went quite beserk, charging suddenly at me with the bayonet, seemingly to substitute me as the target. To my astonishment, the one-star private, the outwardly effeminate 'High Breasted Virgin' coolly stood in front of me facing the maddened rhino. The latter drew back a little and charged again with the same result, and yet again. Finally, sulking, he returned to his bayonet fighting course.

The 'High Breasted Virgin' had meantime pushed me back, each time interposing his body and, finally, at a safe distance he admonished me. 'We 4 Group men. 2 Group men are very bad. You are unwise to say such things to them. When you come back to 4 Group it will be better!'

8 May 1944

In all 110 cases were evacuated today after much waiting in the sun.

As it is Arthur Moon's birthday on 17 May, our bridge quartet, Dunlop, Moon, Taylor, Hirsch, held their last Chungkai session last night. There was a cake for Arthur and we gave him a marvellous card done by Old with a border of 42 little moons and a picture of 4 silently playing for the weekly omelette.

9 May 1944

No sick were evacuated today, though 200 were required to wait for hours. Talk of evacuation by trains the day after tomorrow.

A new cholera suspect cropped up today. I requested cholera vaccine and more disinfectants.

Novasawasan stipulates that on my departure, Maj. Pemberton to be No. 1 medical officer, Chungkai. I pointed out that he was not the most senior officer, but the ruling was upheld. Max is a strong-willed fellow who will make a very good CO.

10 May 1944

There was an awful flap about movement of 2 Group 1,000 lying sick and stretcher cases; 353 require stretchers. A barge party of 180 got off today, including Maj. Marsden, RAMC. There was the usual grim struggle complicated by a private feud of the soldier in charge of the barge evacuation, and the soldier in charge of repair to the steps down to the river.

11 May 1944

A search of the camp occurred.

Departure of two parties of 123 and 180. These included Maj. Moon along with cases of heavy ulcers and skin grafts, surgical cases. The orderlies also going off in small batches. It really was a terrific storm last night we were all up trying to hold the huts up. Avitaminosis Ward came down with a heavy crash. Another suspect cholera today.

12 May 1944

I have never experienced before the personal antipathy of the Nipponese that I have met with in this camp. Evacuation by barge 200, including Maj. Lendon, RAMC, Capt. Ross, RAMC.

There was a most excellent promenade concert, Eric Cliffs conducting, including Schubert's *Unfinished Symphony*', Beethoven's *Minuet in G*, Mozart, Tchaikovsky, etc. At times, looking on the stage with its white-shirted orchestra, white music stools, and Spanish Mission stage effects, together with the dark blue of the huge audience giving rapt attention, I was taken right away to things normal and almost forgotten. Just fancy the ability of these musicians to orchestrate such music, largely from memory, and to improvise the instruments! Another suspect cholera today – much the most convincing one. In view of movement, the N attitude is rather peculiar. Told as regards cholera, 'Must observe secrecy!'

13 May 1944

Movement of Group IV continues.

14 May 1944

Poor Capt. Daly, FMS VAF, Field Ambulance QM, died today – acute exacerbation of amoebic dysentery.

15 May 1944

A difficult struggle today re 'immoveables', but finally Novasawasan very kindly ruled that 5 men likely to die on the trip might be replaced by fitter men.

16 May 1944

Some Red Cross stores of food and 7 cases of Red Cross medicines were received. Operation of caecostomy for chronic amoebic dysentery was carried out: Lt Sherlaw, P.W., 2 FMS VF, aged 41. His ailment dated back to 1934. He had been treated in the famous London Hospital for Tropical Diseases under Manson-Bahr. He had deteriorated during his stay in Thailand and had a temperature swinging high and a leucosyte count of 30,000. His bowel actions were extremely frequent with much blood and mucus. We had systematically needled his large liver, but obtained no pus. He settled down extremely well. [In August, 1944, I had a letter saying he had not looked back since the operation.]

17 May 1944

All cases for departure tomorrow, numbering 478, to have rectal swabs taken today; they are to be loaded directly on to the train at this camp.

18 May 1944

Movement of sick began: 200 ORs were available for carrying sick and gear. All ranks had rations and a haversack and tea was provided before they left. Accommodation was in box trucks (25 per truck) with little enough space when two or three stretchers were put aboard.

This is the first time I have experienced any issue of Red Cross medicines. The seven cases contain some useful stuff, including clinical thermometers and syringes and badly-needed drugs.

18 May 1944

2/2 Aust. CCS Personnel Evacuated Tamuang

Heavy Sick		*To Duty*	
Pte Simpson, F.C.	9/5/44	Maj. Moon, A.A.	11/5/44
Cpl Roberts, L.P.J.	9/5/44	Sgt Haddon, R.	11/5/44
Pte Cameron, J.	10/5/44	Cpl Brown, A.A.	11/5/44
Pte Gray, T.J.E.	11/5/44	Pte Ambrose, W.	11/5/44
Pte Crowley, J.	16/5/44	Pte Murphy, J.B.	13/5/44
Pte Powell, K.A.	16/5/44	S/Sgt Harrison, W.	13/5/44
Sgt Walker, K.H.	17/5/44	Cpl Binns, K.	13/5/44

Remaining
Lt-Col. Dunlop, E.E.
S/Sgt Gibson, S.A.
Sgt Lawrence, A.G.
Pte Butterworth, M.

19 May 1944

I was up very early re the departure of 2 group second party for Nakom Patom, 522 all ranks. This party consisted mainly of amoebic dysentery and avitaminosis cases, the lying patients on stretchers (46) sitting cases (25). Everything went smoothly except for a few walking patients who went astray and had to be checked. The only catch was that at 1900 hours, the train having left at 1330 approximately, the train-load of patients was notified to us as still being at Kanchanaburi, so they may have had a rough night. Bed pans and a few essential containers were spread over all the trucks fortunately. Future moves are by train and to be complete by the twenty-third of this month. One stretcher case is ?cholera.

20 May 1944

The hospital was rearranged yesterday into five huts and the medical staff regrouped.

21 May 1944

Saying farewells; strange to see the hospital with less than 400 patients. I have handed over papers and discussed administration with Maj. Pemberton. A final game of rugger today in very wet conditions. I came to an 'ice-skating' crash with someone falling on my left leg. The result – my left knee painfully strained and worse still, left lumbar and sacroiliac region damaged with difficulty in getting up or turning over when lying.

10 Nakom Patom

May 1944

22 May 1944

Farewell to Chungkai. On parade at 0930, 500 men, parties of 100. One sick stretcher case in my party and an acute dementia, Pte Skillingslaw. Left between 1300 and 1400 in box trucks, approximately 27 per truck. The line crosses the river at Tamarkan and so to Kanchanaburi – the first sight of even semi-civilised buildings for well over a year then on again through much flatter country with some paddy fields – very hot.

Arrived at Tamuang Station in mid afternoon and lined up for a march of about 2 miles. We were speedily on a gravelled road with a good deal of motor transport traffic and passed through a fairly large village with some shops. The camp site is on undulating plains in the river valley with some areas perhaps rather low. There is a good deal of vegetation and shady trees, particularly tamarinds and mangoes, and banana groves are all about.

The hospital is much closer to the river than the general camp. This distance from the river leads to some difficulties, since to be handy to the water supply, the kitchens are down at the river end and men have about half a mile to walk to mess and bathe. In the morning, the slippery tracks have to be traversed in darkness.

The layout of the camp is otherwise good. The huts are uniform and well constructed, the usual bamboo and attap with continuous platform beds of rough round bamboo, the hardness being somewhat countered by bamboo matting. Rafters are rather low for this person and other tall people!

Hygiene is very promising: the latrines are much the same pattern as Kinsayok – deep trench pattern with bamboo and earth superstructure covered by neat huts and little cubicles made by a lattice fencework of bamboo. It has not been possible as yet to get covers for the individual rectangular apertures. For some curious reason, urinals have been forbidden, though I believe they are to be introduced soon. As the deep pits have not been revetted, (the issue of bamboo being turned down) all this extra fluid is serious and I fear that the walls of many latrines will soon collapse.

Fuel is very short and there is very little wood or bamboo to be scrounged in the area (this will be the bugaboo of these camps down on the plains). Water shortage is largely due to lack of containers and the distance to carry.

The troops were kept about two hours on the parade ground in the hot sun with much counting, *kiotské – keré* etc. Eventually, checking being complete, the Commandant, Capt. Susuki, appeared on the dais for *kashira naka* (the general salute from the troops) so that all might recognise him to avoid future mistakes! Hatori San is 2 I/C, Osukisan, adjutant (now promoted *chui*), Tanaka San deals directly with POW administration, Hirumatz San ('the Tiger') does building construction.

The Camp Administration on the POW side, by Nippon direction: Lt-Col. Knights Camp POW Commander (Lt-Col. McEachern commanded prior to his arrival). The general organisation is based on British, Australian and Dutch groups. The British OC being Lt-Col. Lillie; Australians, Lt-Col. McEachern; Maj. W.W. Wearne is 2 I/C of the Australian group and Capt. Hands, the adjutant. Lt-Col. Knights appears almost run off his legs by constant demands and I fear suffers a good deal from the jungle jealousy and parochialism of various camp and battalion groups.

I am probably to go the hospital in a day or two but meantime to live in the lines and by invitation mess at the HQ mess.

I am pleased to see that everyone here goes in for food container sterilisation. It was most pleasant to see old friends again – Billy Wearne, Jock Clarke, Alan Woods, Ewan Corlette and Hector Greiner and many others I have not seen for a long time.

22 May 1944

The daily routine is reveille at 0645 (crack of dawn); breakfast immediately after that. A.m. roll call and works' parade at 0830 with work approximately 0900 to 1230. Mid-day meal is at 1300. P.m. work 1500–1800. Evening meal 1800. Evening Roll call 2000. Lights Out 2230.

Every battalion seems to be clinging to its own finance and has its own ideas about welfare etc. I talked to some AIF battalion commanders about some attempt at pooling resources and settling a uniform basis of messing and welfare, but these ideas are not popular. There are great possibilities in this camp if everyone gets together in the utmost co-operation; there is very little sign of this as yet.

Commander Alexander with the remainder of the Chungkai Group arrived very late in the evening in darkness.

A finance meeting was held today with Col. Lilly in the chair. I was told that the camp finance officer, Lt. Barrett and Lt. Ross (dealing with hospital finance.) were excluded and Lt-Col. Harvey was ex officio. This was a pity as Barrett and Ross were the only people in possession of all the facts, including knowledge of what finance was being transferred from Group IV Chungkai. This actually amounted in all to some $8,000 with due allowance for officers' subs not yet collected at Chungkai owing to officers having left (yet it was vaguely computed as $2,500)! The chief purpose of the meeting was to decide on officers' subs for the month.Owing to rather chaotic conditions of settling in, no opportunity to check up on individual medical officers and diet orders, and lack of information as to goods available and their prices, Major Corlette has only been able to put forward maximum and minimum estimates for hosptial requirements for the month. As would perhaps be anticipated, he was allowed his minimum estimate only, $10,000. I cannot see this being enough in view of the disparity between the ration of the hospital and lines. The hospital receives about 150 grams of rice less than the camp – 550 as compared with 700; half the vegetable issue, half the meat issue. The hospital staff are allowed full rations but many patients are required to work and receive only the low hospital ration. The whole diet and financial position requires a most careful survey to get firm figures. I discussed battalion funds with Lt-Col. McEachern, Billy Wearne, Alan Woods and others and told them I thought they should at least settle on a common basis for all A.I.F. and that I hoped other groups would fall into line. All the battalion commanders I can see oppose giving up funds and individual welfare. This is the result of transition from village to city life, I suppose!

I handed over battalion funds to Maj. Wearne for O and P battalions $475 (I took $700 to Chungkai, $200 additional to AIF funds and $25 for some purchase of emetine.

Great delight today to see Red Cross stores coming into the camp – this the gift of the American Red Cross to the International Red Cross Committee.

25 May 1944

Harvey, Marsh and I went over to see the Camp HQ with a view to try to get some of the milk from Red Cross boxes set aside specially for invalids, but the parcels are to go out intact – the chief reason being that 'The men should have the pleasure of opening the packages themselves'. Also, one or two rather sinister references to the health of hospital patients and the fact that we only see the sick man's point of view! I moved into the hospital area today. Ewan Corlette and Jack Marsh (officer in charge of administration, directly responsible to Lt-Col. Harvey) are anxious that I take over some admin. work.

26 May 1944

A conference of medial officers in the afternoon and the following required of them:

1 Shortage of surgical instruments: Each MO to submit an inventory of instruments held by him. So far as possible, surgical sets will be kept intact. MO's instruments to be kept in his own ward.

2 Diets: Committed to majors Corlette, Moon, Lendon and Peddie.

3 Amoebics: arrangements made to examine the stools of convalescents, three tests each. If free from symptoms for three months and stools negative, discharge to lines. No employment in cookhouses, etc.

4 Officers & Other Patients: the policy – if not receiving any special treatment and unfit to attend parades, return to lines, e.g. people with hernia.

5 Blood Transfusion Centre to be established in the theatre block, the Chungkai officer technicians to be used. Defibrinated blood technique to be employed.

6 Massage: under general supervision of Maj. A. Moon, Capt. Parker to have direct charge. S/Sgt Harrison, NCO I/C. At present many of the masseurs are in hospital as patients and have a diet problem.

7 Dispensary: issues on a daily basis to wards. On requisition, signed by medical officer, account for receipts and issues to be made.

8 Sick in lines, MI room: The British group, Maj. Bennett, Capt. Ellis, Capt.

Lodge and Capt. Bartlett to live in the lines. Capt. Allen, Capt. Matheson, Capt. Smith and Capt. Hewatt also to see appropriate battalions in the lines.
9 Welfare Officers: Terms of reference likely to be extended to that of MO's adjutant in all non-medical matters.
10 Sick Parade Times: 1 at reveille 0730. 2 at 1415. 3 after roll call 2045 to 2100. Emergencies follow the present routine. Discharges from the hospital at 1430 and admissions 1500.

A request was made to the Nipponese for cholera vaccine 100 × 50 cc ampoules to innoculate the rest of the camp. Portable sterilisers for the theatre must be made; we need bottles for transfusion in the cholera season, etc. I asked Lt Bushell to manufacture two extra stills, giving three for the cholera season, to function near the dispensary.

27 May 1944

There was a flutter caused last night by a microscopic examination of the blood of eight men who were potential donors; the blood of six contained worms ?microfilaria. Somewhat depressed by the thought of these worms infesting most people, I examined my own blood and found this also contained worms. I spent the most miserable night contemplating the thought of most of us going home with swollen legs and carrying our scrotums on a barrow! However, fortunately, the following day I thought of having a look at the saline which I had used to dilute the blood and found that it was contaminated with strongyloid worms.*

It was a notewrothy week owing to the arrival of letters – one lovely one from Helen dated February with mention of numerous people who had written, including Walter Macallum, Ben Rank, John Colebatch and Mr. Zwar. No letters had been received from any of them. Boyd, Helen's brother was home for Christmas. Lucky dog! Two letters from Mother and Father, the latest being May, 1943.

28 May 1944

With Captain Clymer (Camp Building Officer) I went to see Hirumatzsan, 'the Tiger', and provisional approval was given for building a hospital laundry, the site to be near the dysentery wards – not, as we suggested, near the river.

29 May 1944

I inspected the hospital kitchens and sanitation with Lt-Col. Harvey. We discussed the allocation of eggs to canteens, hospital and camp. The requirement of the sick (diet kitchens) are to be met first and the rest split between the canteens on a *per capita* basis. The hospital at present consumes about 3000 daily with special diets above, and only about 4500 daily are received.

* It was many years later that I found out just how dangerous in the long term infestation with these strongyloid worms could be.

30 May 1944

Capt. Moroko inspected the hospital today, preliminary to an inspection by the Camp Commander on 1 June 1944. He notified us of the evacuation of heavy sick (1,000) to Nakom Patom to begin on 10 June 1944. There are approximately 1500 awaiting evacuation. We are to begin completing rolls as quickly as possible, submitting lists, of lying, sitting (stretcher cases) walking, amputation cases to go. To be prepared in groups of 50 with approximately equal numbers of lying and sitting cases in each group.

31 May 1944

An orderly Medical Officer is to be appointed daily, his duty to be available for emergency calls where MOs are not available, to visit the kitchen before midday and evening meals to inspect the food of patients, to investigate messing complaints along with the administration orderly officer.

1 June 1944

A big inspection of the camp by the Camp Commander and staff.

2 June 1944

Chiefly notable for the escape of Skillycorn, the acute mania, who eluded his watchers, swam the river at a rate of knots and escaped stark naked! Eventually, he was apprehended paddling a Thai canoe along the river gaily. Everyone was given a fearful rocket by Okada. It is commanded that a very strong 'box house' be made in one of the wards to contain three lunatics with six guards to be posted day and night. Jack Marsh asked why a 'box house' for three, since only two lunatics, and was told that the other place was for him (Okada)!

3 June 1944

'Japan parties' are being assembled at Tamuang – the Australians to send approximately 900. Unfortunately Ray Denny and Henry Boys of 2/2 Aust. CCS must go. Instructions: the avoidance of unboiled water and uncooked foods. Sterilisation of eating gear. Cleanliness of the hands and general measures to combat flies and filth.

Lt-Col. James' figures for the mortality in Tarsau, Kinsayok, Tonchin and Konyu-Hintok show that the worst deaths occurred in Konyu-Hintok with 20.6%. However, the great interest of all this is that it breaks down the deaths according to English, Australian, Dutch, USA and a small number of Indians, and the remarkable thing is that in the wash-up, the percentage of deaths in each national group was about the same. I think this has got to be understood in the fact that no matter how much spirit and endurance a man might show, he was simply sent back to the human grindstone until he was totally finished. These deaths, which covered all groups in Thailand, gave a total of 7,626 deaths and 43,085 alive.

Extract from Tamuang Hospital Bulletin Equipment: The provision of equipment for Tamuang Hospital has not been an easy matter. Tarsau Hospital, having despatched the best of its equipment to Nakom Patom, arrived here with 1,000 patients to increase within a fortnight to 2,500, including a large number of seriously ill patients. The amalgamation of POW hospitals, Tonchin, Tampis, Tarsau, Chungkai, Kinsayok, did not produce sufficient equipment for our needs. For example, over 480 buckets are required to run a hospital this size and out of necessity over 100 were taken from patients with appropriate varying compensation. All patients are fed in wards and 12 water points are maintained for the supply of boiling water throughout the day. Ten artificers have been constantly occupied, making buckets, bed-pans, trays, sterilisers, etc. and the provision and control of over 100 different items of hospital equipment has called for considerable ingenuity, labour and resource. Purchased tools, tins, solder, etc. have made these things possible. We have now to supply over one third of available hospital equipment for the party of 1,000 patients moving to Nakom Patom where conditions for provision or purchase are believed to be even more difficult. After this large move, Tamuang Hospital will probably contain 2,000 patients and even with less heavy sick, a large variety of equipment is necessary. The financial aid of officers together with occasional collection in lines of old tins, cloth, bottles, wire, nails etc. is 60 per cent of the battle won.

With an increasing shortage of drugs and standard equipment, improvised treatment with home made articles is more than ever necessary. The extensive diet scheme can only function fully with sufficient containers and kitchen equipment.

6 June 1944

Medical details for the Japan parties are now as follows:

The Australian party: The MOs are Hinder and Parker, party approximately 900. The NCOs Sgt MacDonald, Lt-Col. Robinson and Sgt Adams, privates Denny, Boys and Haste. Reg Newton will be in charge of the AIF party and is a stout fellow. No officers of field rank are to go; probably Capt. Hands and Capt. Gaydon (who is sick) will go. NX 44915, Padre Thorpe, H.R.B of 2/29 Bn, who is labelled a 'Pte, non-combatant chaplain' is to go. He asked me for a letter re his work in Thailand and I gave him one to testify to his splendid work and qualities.

8 June 1944

Since arriving here, I have endeavoured to get the hospital position put on some comprehensive scheme of diets and finance. Seven diets were considered adequate for our purposes, the whole hospital being surveyed and patients selected. Costing them followed simply and it seems that if the Nipponese continue to supply 1000 eggs daily for heavy sick of the hospital, the cost will be approx. 13c per head per day. The diets are well worked out and I think adequate. The diet kitchens could now be sectionalised and all food issued through the kitchens.

I have drafted a letter for Lt-Col. Knights asking the Nipponese for a more adequate hospital ration, also for extras for the very sick (invalid foods).

I put forward the full dietary scheme and its costing at a finance meeting and accordingly asked for more money for the month than the previous minimum allotted. After some discussion, this was passed. My request for extra money for the 1000 heavy sick for Nakom Patom was turned down on the grounds that Thomas had only asked for $2 a head. He must have found a gold mine at Nakom Patom!

I have done my best for N.P. by including as many officers as possible in the party. Lt-Col. James and Lt-Col. McEachern are sending down all possible money from battalion funds; the AIF have pooled money and are sending down 5 ticals a head for all AIF in this party. The defect in financial arrangements in this camp is that there is no central fund control or easy break-up of funds on movement. After some effort however on behalf of Nakom Patom, I was a little shattered when I was asked 'Who's is going to N.P. amongst the doctors?' Bill Harvey said only one was known and this was Lt-Col. Dunlop! I do not regard this as more than chatter at present and certainly it was not known to me.

12 June 1944

Depature of the first 500 for N.P. This camp is rather aflutter with departures at the moment. What with this talk of the Japan Party probably about 900 A.I.F., 200 'White Dutch', 1500 + British. All the troops seem to be quite happy about the movement, many being keen to go along with their pals. I had a rather moving farewell to O and P Battalions. I addressed them on parade briefly and retired very discomforted by three very loud and embarrassing cheers which I feared the Nipponese might regard as a demonstration.

Everyone is up in the air because the N interpreter says that the invasion of France began a few days ago; 16(?) divisions of British, and about 80 divisions of Americans are said to be ready and the bridge head already successfully made on the peninsula. No doubt as to the truth of this momentous news! Success to Montgomery and his lads!

Later: The party for N.P. now definitely laid down by the Nipponese as Lt-Col. Dunlop, Maj. Marsden RAMC, Capt. Hewatt RAMC, Maj. J.E.R. Clarke AAMC Dental, S/Sgt Gibson, Sgt Wiseman, Cpl (Local Sgt) Lawrence, Pte (Local Cpl) Brown A.A., L/Cpl Bourne J.D., Pte Butterworth, Pte Tarran and Pte Murray J.B. Patients include Pte (or local S/Sgt) Harrison, Cpl Roberts, Pte Gray T.J.E., Pte Ambrose, W., Pte Crowley, J.D. and Pte Knighton W. The actual strength laid down as at Nakom Patom: 3 medical officers and 13 ORs per 1,000 patients, ORs to be 3 NCOs and 10 privates. Five of the privates are RAMC.

* * * * *

The diaries from this date were kept spasmodically for a number of reasons, as I explain in the next section.

* * * * *

Nakom Patom Hospital

I arrived at this huge hospital camp on 14 June 1944 accompanying 500 sick of IV Group (of which approximately 1000 were being transferred). The hospital area was on flat land of the Bangkok Plains adjacent to the impressive bell-like temple.

The long hutments were built of wood instead of the ubiquitous bamboo, with reasonably well-constructed attap roofing. There was the same pattern of continuous bed platforms for the sick with a central pathway, but with a smooth wooden surface instead of slithering and rather irregular bamboo. The sick lay with their feet presenting centrally, an average of three men to a 2-metre space. The huts were even provided with window apertures, covered not by glass, but by wooden frames which could be raised.

Bedding was usually at least a personal blanket. There was practically no provision of the utensils and gear which normally are provided to care for the sick, such as bedpans, urinals, sterilisers, water containers, bucket, bowls etc., let alone more sophisticated equipment. Instruments were either possessed as treasured possessions, such as my own set, or improvised. Utensils were also improvised by POWs.

This base hospital designed to take 10,000 sick and broken survivors of the railway debacle arrived too late. The main battle for mens' lives had already been fought in the ghastly conditions of jungle hospital concentrations such as Kinsayok, Tarsau, Chungkai, Tamuang, Non Pladuc and Kanchanaburi.

There was now a great plethora of officers amongst the patients, staff, and administration. Medical Officers included Lt-Col. Coates AIF, Lt-Cols Malcolm, MacFarlane and Barrett, RAMC, and Lt-Col. Larsen (Netherlands Indian Army Medical Corps).

I found myself in an embarrassing position, since some senior British officers from the Thailand camp were dissatisfied with the combatant administration and desired to reorganise the camp with a new commander. They had evolved great confidence in me as regards hospital organisation and the involvement of all in the care of the sick. The overall administration was combatant, with the hospital administered through the Chief Medical Officer, Lt-Col. Coates.

Coates had been in Burma and was less well known to the work force in Thailand (initially 45,000 to about 15,000 in Burma). The Camp Commander, 'the Saint', was a controversial character who proved sharply disapproving of me, and critical of my schemes to tax camps to provide central funds for care of the sick. Lt-Col. Albert Coates was immensely my professional superior, a veteran of Gallipoli, who had taught me in medical school, and whilst my military rank was actually higher as Lt-Col. T/Col., there was no way that I could be induced to 'pull rank' on him. He had become legendary in Burma and Sumatra.

'Bertie', later Sir Albert, had my implicit loyalty and I was entrusted with heavy responsibilities of the Surgical Block and ultimately the rehabilitation centre. Amongst other jobs I was Medical Economics Officer (17/6/1944), with the delicate task of handling 'sources of income', these partly from outside underground threads, and by negotiating tax levels for officers and paid workmen. Keith Bostock, Australian Red Cross Commissioner, and I were also engaged in seeking help from group funds and private sources, and in attempts to get more financial help from the Japanese. This responsibility eventually involved control of camp canteen activity. The canteen balance sheet, 18 April 1946, was 35984 ticals, with a credit balance of 3000 ticals.

When the non-medical officers were removed from the camp on 23 January, 1945 I was regarded as the officer responsible for POW internal discipline – and ultimately of our own guards and picquets on release.

In my dealings with other ranks I could not have had a better and more experienced warrant officer than W/O Austin Fyfe who had served in a Highland Regiment, commencing as a boy in World War I aged 22, rising to Major DSO, MC. His patriotism was such that he re-entered the army regarded as too old to be commissioned, and was W/O in the 2/3 Machine Gun Bn 2 AIF. Eventually I was happy to have the MBE added to his major decorations. Quite a character: equally at home with British and Australian soldiers and able to handle those of any race.

There was considerable surgical talent available in Maj. Syd Krantz (Adelaide), Capt. ('Monty') J.S. McConachie (Fellows in general surgery), Maj. Alan Hazleton (eye specialist) and Capt. Jacob Markowitz, a Canadian physiologist from Toronto, who had been part-time Professor of Experimental Surgery with a background of the Mayo Clinic.

I combined much surgical and clinical work with administration, as did Bertie, the chief, whose enthusiasm for surgical work and teaching was indefatigable.

On the medical side there were valuable physicians in Maj. Edward Fisher, RAAMC, Capt. Cyril Vardy, RAMC (with much tropical experience), Lt-Col. L. MacFarlane, RAMC, and Lt-Col. (Overste.) Larsen, Netherlands Indian Army, both experienced in tropical disorders.

I acquired a gifted artist, Gunner Jack Chalker of the British Army, ostensibly to do physiotherapy work, but invaluable for record purposes. Certain members of my old 2 Aust. CCS, such as S/Sgt Alan Gibson and my batman, Pte 'Blue' Butterworth, remained closely attached and indispensible.

Markowitz I found to be a rare companion, able to compose Latin poetry in the style of Horace, and an authority on Keats and Housman. He became later a president of the Canadian Literary Society.

At first those two stalwarts of my earlier 'Force' command Maj. (Bill) W. W. Wearne OBE, and Maj. F. A. ('Boots') Woods remained my intimate helpers and counsellors. Alan Woods had a quite remarkable ability as a general handyman, born of his station, Silver Spur, in Queensland. He was cobbler in leather, tinsmith, carpenter, and jack-of-all-trades. Amongst his products were excellent pylons and artificial legs, physiotherapy and surgical equipment, and an ingenious theatre light. Two elderly privates, Bob Fox and Steve Wade, survivors of Hintok, skilled in carpentry, worked with him.

Life in Nakom Patom was more sophisticated than in the jungle, but I missed the calling birds and beasts and the grandeur of the mountain and river country. There, too, stress and tension, mounted, as the war moved to a critical climax.

Diary writing was severely curtailed in view of my *kempi* supervision, and occasional entries were for the most part buried. In the closing stages, tension bottled within was almost unbearable. So much suffering, but were we going to make it?

20 July 1944*

Deeply immersed in a tense rubber of bridge lit feebly by a coconut oil lamp, the lights out bugle was ignored by our four: Moon, and Dunlop (lightweights), Derek Hirsch and Bill Taylor. The sound was heard of my non-medical block administrative officer, Commander van Orden splashing water over his body outside the hut. Suddenly an angry accusing sentry projected a bayonet into our game. *Tenko* sentry : 'Why out of bed?' I was anxious for van Orden to regain his bed space, which he did by a crawling side entrance. I then took the blame as the senior officer of the block: 'Big mistake – did not hear the bugle: other officers were not responsible.'

'O.K. you report to guardo – half past eight o'clocko.'

I borrowed a pair of thick socks to help my shins and in due course reported well before the time with almost respectful *kiotské* and *keré*. I was ignored by the guard and remained rigidly at attention for some hours in a boiling sun. During this time there developed individual action. One by one a long sequence of orderly NCO's and guards marched up to me or rode up on bikes, and kicked or struck me, wielding rifle butts and sticks.

This became punctuated by the guard sergeant giving an ever-expanding recital of my crimes in which it seems I was out of bed hours after lights out, and had come contemptuously hours late to report to the guard. When I protested that I had come early and seemingly was not seen, the charge was added that I had been insolent to the guard.

Finally, after midday, it seemed that I had been out of bed almost all night, had come to report nearly a day late, and had been insolent to the guard beyond belief. 'Really *chusa*, if this goes on you will have to be punished'!

At this stage, ill-advisedly, I forsook my rigid position of attention and my stoicism broke. I waved my hands and yelled. 'God Almighty, do you not think it punishment standing in this sun and being kicked and beaten by a pack of bandy legged baboons!'

It took a minute before the interpreter achieved some approximate translation of this seemingly incredible insolence. *Nunda*? *Nunda*? Then all hell broke loose. With angry bellowing the guard, led by their commander, fell upon me in a fashion recalling an otter hunt or the hounds cornering a fox. They belaboured me with rifle butts, chairs, boots, etc. whilst I rolled in the dust trying to keep in a ball, my elbows protectively over my large fragile spleen, face against my chest.

Eventually I was motionless beyond resistance, lying face down in the dust, conscious of broken ribs and blood from scalp wounds. I was gathered up, dazed and rubber limbed, and trussed and roped backward kneeling with a large log between my seat and knees. As my head cleared there was the intolerable pain due to rough ground pressure on the knees and the weight and pressure of

* This account was written later than the actual date.

the log. Breathing was sharply painful with fractured ribs. Slowly the pain ceased in my legs because they had no circulation. How long to gangrene in the tropical heat? Could I last four hours? I squared my shoulders and stared in disdain at the guard.

As the sun became low there was at last a final summing up. 'Out of bed days after lights out, came days late to report to the guard, and finally guilty of appalling, heinous insolence to the guard. If we were so forgiving as to release you, would you have hard feelings against the guard?'

I considered this cautiously and replied 'Hard feelings against what guard?'

This was apparently accepted as a more reasonable attitude. My ropes were released. With a desperate heave, I disengaged from the log, but my legs were functionless. Slowly, painfully, with the return of circulation, I found I could move them and feel my feet again. At last, a little drunkenly, I was on my feet. I stood to attention, bowed and said, 'And now if you will excuse me I shall amputate the Dutchman's arm who has been waiting all day.' I was determined to show them that Australians were tough!

To prove the point I went to the operating room, watched by some of the guard. Poor Dutch patient, confronted by a surgeon covered with caked blood, sweat, and dust. I think that he would have preferred to run, but was too sick. I steadied my tremulous hands, injected the brachial plexus and removed the totally paralysed smashed up and infected limb with the patient still on his rough stretcher (Klein Nolenkamp NEIA). I patted his pale sweating head, muttered some reassuring Dutch words, and *tot van morgen* to take my leave. A bow to the Japanese and stiffly back to my bed space for the luxury of a groaning collapse.

My fellow bridge players eventually gave me an amusing card summarising the misadventure as follows:

'The Colonel takes out Hearts'

After lights out take a dekko
at the Colonel playing cards
Quite indifferent like the gecko
To Nippon laws and Nippon guards.

Suddenly bright torch appears
Holder voice most unbenigno
Calls him 'very big buggero'
'Come to guard house half past nine'

Early bird deserves the wormo
Adage old by Nips not heard
Early into late o turno
Early wormo gets the bird!

Battered by assault infernal
'No resentment,' was the cry –
'No I like it' from the Colonel
'You will suffer more than I.'

10 November 1944

The eve of a great armistice. I wonder if such an event seemed as remote to the toiling millions of the last war some twenty-six years ago, as it does to me now. Those millions who had become 'insentient engines pumping blood'.

During those appalling days of last year most of us went to some desolate bourn beyond that: to bones. A valley of dry bones. It comes back to me with the memory of Harry Thorpe's sermon 'Shall these dry bones live'. This has become a devastating experience and I speculate frequently as to whether many who have experienced it will be so resilient as to find a sweet harmony in things normal again.

There is a defensive mechanism in suffering, in that there slowly develops a palsy of the emotions, and a deadness of the imagination. In the early months of our prison life, almost all thinking men realised that there was much valuable experience to be gained from our predicament. Interest in humanity was quickened, and the intellectual processes stimulated: our intellectual 'escape' from captivity. There is a tendency for that resource to fail. One has to fight a deadly apathy of the spirit.

Here we have many blessings to count. Food is reasonably adequate though not particularly appetising, but one has learned the supreme importance of this factor. Huts are waterproof, and weather conditions so much more pleasant. We have now probably just finished the heavy rains of the monsoon season; although multitudinous restrictions necessarily control our activities, there is sufficient laxity to permit a busy working day, keen interest in professional matters, and some relaxation. Best of all one is not continually confronted with the utter misery and ill health of ones fellows, and deaths have become reasonably infrequent. Drugs, though scarce enough, permit one to relieve the more urgent problems of disease. Clothes are a minor problem when appearances don't matter at all.

'Blue' has recently solved my personal problems by having my large 'trench coat' cut up, thus providing me with two pairs of shorts and sundry garments to other people. Minor discomforts, such as the myriads of bed bugs which swarm in the area, the mosquitoes, recurring attacks of malaria, the heat at night, the ludicrous and uncomfortable beds, rice foods for ever eaten with a spoon out of a mess tin, lack of reasonable lighting, the early hour of retiring, no comforts, scant knowledge of world events, the utter lack of any personal privacy – all that does not really mean a thing compared with a mental factor. This is a compound of boredom and a sense of inadequacy and loss. Life is too sweet, too transient, not to grudge these dragging years. How full they might have been of service, of lovely things and loving, compared to this vegetable death in life. Perhaps the fault in my armour is that I have not got the old-fashioned belief in immortality to reinforce a conviction of deity, and a stubbornly retained view that there is more beauty in the world than ugliness. One needs that even to live.

But courage, *mon ami*: That is the real foundation of life. When this black page turns I shall find enchantment somewhere, somehow. 'To every action there is an equal and opposite reaction.' That is why violence is so futile. Nothing is so destructive to a cause as violence wielded on its behalf. We have learned much of the inadequacy of material things, much of tolerance, much of endurance, even if it be only to endure failure in the commerce of life hereafter. There is plenty of courage all about us even in the most maimed and damaged human beings.

But, to return to the topical events and daily scribbling which I have not been able to do since arriving in this camp. . .

The gorgeous moonlight in the earlier part of the month has been conductive to much night raiding in this part of the world, and there is also some daylight reconnaissance* Raids are usually heralded by the beating of the village 'tom tommy' drums and a thin wail of a siren. Not infrequently we hear and see low-flying planes at night, and there is sometimes a shuddering crump or two plus some ack-ack action.

Locally, stores are dispersed in special small revetted huts, and there are some IJA shelters. As far as we are concerned, there is nothing much in the way of ARP. We have some drains and a little scheme for carrying out and dispersing bed patients in the event of attack, but somehow there is not much expectation of that. No use is made of Red Cross markings or lighting. [Not permitted by IJA]

Lt-Col. Coates does the lion's share of operating these days and is much too keen to indulge in much delegation. All controversial problems drift his way. I was somewhat annoyed about a very chronic empyema case (Childs – chronic empyema, broncho-pleural fistula left base 5 months). He remains sick and debilitated, club fingers, pains in the joints and is very anaemic. He has intermittent bouts of fever, and profuse discharge, and has been several times nigh unto death. The consultant physician (T.F.) frowns upon surgery, claiming some evidence of bronchiectaris, and advances complex arguments against producing a collapse over a bronchiectatic lung. 'Pheumonectomy or nothing!'

This is, of course, appalling nonsense: the poor devil is crying out to have a septic cavity in his chest closed and will never be a candidate for major lung surgery here. In disgust I handed him over to the 'old man' who did a phrenil avulsion today as a first step. He needs a Roberts' type of operation.

Today I did an epididymectomy upon a patient, Tunnecliffe, almost certainly TB epididymitis, but curiously the sinus was on the front of the scrotum.

In Thailand there is much non-specific infection of the genital organs†

12 November 1944

There is much flutter at present over constant 'fence breaking' of the camp by invalid merchant princes who have Arabian nights adventures in the local town apparently. This practice has become more and more prevalent. Several have been caught and treated rather leniently with just a week or two in the local cells. Recently there was a theft of N QM. clothing which was promptly

* Described by one of my guards, 'The come quickly, look see, go back, speak Churchill plane'.

† I recall the dictum of Osakisan: 'In Thailand much prostitution. Not good after marriage!' Alas, POW genital disorders have little to do with sex.

'flogged'. An ultimatum was issued that either the delinquents own up or the whole camp, including medical staff and those patients able to do so, must stand outside on parade all night.

This was eventually rescinded by Lt Wakimatsu after two hours. But ultimatum: 'Either find tunics or the culprits, else all night stand.' Now one of these delinquents has been caught returning over the fence, and if others do not come forward the same proposition is offering. Reprisals, what!'

13 November 1944

An ileostomy was carried out by Lt-Col. Coates on a sick dysentery case. He is very keen on it despite the striking results that have been obtained by the minor procedure of appendicostomy.*

Alan Woods and his workshop have just produced a most ingenious little foot suction pump at my request. He has also made a very good theatre light, so far as these things are possible, with tin and coconut oil lighting. There are four oil burners, a polished rectangular frame suspended from the roof with counter balance. This will greatly help emergency operations at night.

14 November 1944

Bombshell of the day is that the western and sections of huts 1, 2, 3 surgical are to be evacuated. These constitute the 'salient' in the fence breaking, so we are all shifting here and there down as far as hut 7 where the Dutch ORs are concentrated all in one hut. This presents staffing difficulties, with five huts to be staffed instead of four, which is bad economy. One faint blessing is that there is talk of stopping the insistence on a fixed bed space for all personnel which is terribly restrictive in dealing with really sick men and permits no segregation of the very sick from others.

15 November 1944

Still no pay this month; none since 30 September. Now completely broke. Many letters are arriving, some getting 12–20. As usual none for this fellow. There has also been a small consignment of Red Cross stores, food and a few medical supplies. The IJA are even asking what we want these days. Suggestion made that a few beds be provided for surgical patients, in lieu of the floor, which frequently causes devastating bed sores.

Yesterday I helped Lt-Col. Coates remove the left kidney of a very sick case of urogenital TB (Pte Denman). There was severe infection of the prostate, seminal vesicles and bladder, and he was urinating every few minutes. His general condition was very poor, the left kidney very large and tender, the right just palpable and a little tender. There is a right apical lung lesion.

* Subsequent surgery of sick dysentery patients largely fell to me. My 21 patients (appendicostomy 12, caecostomy 2, ileostomy 7) all made good progress, but one ileostomy patient died later from another condition.

24 November 1944

In the evening the poor illumination leads to much semi-wasted time, bridge playing, gossiping, etc. In addition to the routine of work emergency calls, operations etc. fill up the day so that there is not much time for rest, and of course there is the administration of the block.

Birds cause considerable amusement around here. Very showy in the mornings, the rather silent little drongos with slender bodies like a willy wagtail, forked tails and astonishing manoeuvrability, pouncing on flies and turning in their own length. Multitudinous cheeky little mynah birds hop about on the ground a great deal and are occasionally raided by another type of almost black mynah with a little tuft above the beak – all shrilling at each other in a hostile way. The magpie robin is still evident, also smug little doves, naturally usually in pairs, and our show-piece, the golden oriel. There are scarlet-crested woodpeckers and, ever watchful above the camp, innumerable vultures and crows. Lastly multitudinous extremely small birds, not forgetting the rather pretty egregious sparrows, which gave the entrance to our hut the name coined by Billy of 'The Gate of Happy Sparrows'.

25/26 November 1944

Settling down to the new order of things and dispersion of patients and staff.

27 November 1944

Large daylight air raid today with three flights of approximately 10–12 planes in full view, and there was a thundering vibration of many bombs over Bangkok way. No air raid warning given, many at first thinking that the planes were Nippon.

29 November 1944

Night air raid with numerous planes and the sound of bombs last night. There are no slit trenches at present and only a few cautious people including many Dutch ('Remember Rotterdam!') get out of bed.

The IJA doctor saw all the hernia patients today treating them very ruthlessly. If unwilling for an operation they must go. If they are quite unsuitable for operation, they still must go, though many are quite unwell with other conditions. Equally annoying is that those who have had operations are kicked off before three months elapse. Forcing men to have operations under these circumstances is reprehensible. Operative conditions are not all that good, suture materials are wretched, malaria is rife, and the patients have to convalesce on bare boards with one blanket. The IJA supplies no special food for any type of sick man. I believe that these things should be contested more strongly.

30 November 1944

The freshly segregated permanent disability patients were under review by the IJA doctor today. He is pathetically ignorant of internal disease, and in any case gives short shift to the external. The occasional deserving case is given a curt 'oosh', just for 'face', indicating rejection. He never examines the body other than cursory inspection, a most pleasant fellow withal!

Lt-Col. More ('Mackie' of Konyu) had his liver needled by the O.M. today at my recommendation.

It is rumoured that there were 19 killed and at least 30 injured at Tamarkan POW Camp in a recent raid.

1 December 1944

Our much esteemed 'laughing Colonel' Ishi is to depart today, being replaced by Lt-Col. Yamagita of Chungkai etc. Unlike Ishi he is a man with a humane reputation. Things 'up river', as one would expect, are not frightfully bright. One party of 250 British, 250 AIF who went to Tomajoe near Conquita have 240 in hospital and 14 deaths, what with cerebral malaria and scanty quinine. The following AIF deaths recently: Smith, T. 2/2 Pioneer Bn; Outrim 2/4 M.G. Bn; Mooney 2/19 Bn; Willy 2/3 M.G. Bn. and poor 'Mick' Hornibrook RAAF.

So the sad wasting process goes on.

2 December 1944

Amongst the minor annoyances of life at the moment, the IJA doctor has stopped *post mortems*. He points in a line from the neck to pubis: 'Cut, No Good!' Barbarous people we are, I suppose desecrating the dead and offending the fine sensitivities of our hosts! Always there have been pin pricks about lectures, even those given in the medical centre, IJA compound. Now they have been stopped except for the clinical meeting. This includes Captain Markowitz's interesting physiology series, and lectures to nursing orderlies and volunteers.

Diet provision this month: 7637 ticals for special diets. General messing present provision is 5c per head per day. In assessing my own block diets for this month it is pleasing to note that with the improved ration 'minor' avitaminosis of the month, scrotum etc. has almost cleared up, so that the small E diet (5c peas and one salt fish) is now required only in a few cases. The tendency is to give ample food to a few bad cases, and to discontinue the small diets. It has been my practice to place post-operative cases of any severity on milk and ovaltine twice daily and B diet for at least a week (2 eggs and 60g of peas daily).

Today performed an ileostomy on F.M.S.V.F. soldier, Charles Hilterman. He is desperately ill.* I had planned an appendicostomy but the appendix had sloughed away and the caecum was pathological. I performed an ileostomy with some trepidation since the other three done in the camp have died. (They were not my patients.)

Lt-Col. McKellar arrived at N.P. from Tamuang with probable carcinoma of

* Charles made a good recovery as did a number of subsequent patients upon whom I operated. Subsequently, he became Managing-Director of Rothmans in Australia. We were good friends until his death.

the stomach, escorted by Lt Moroko. He brought with him a bombshell as regards IV group personnel. The medical party who came with me are still IV group and not N.P. personnel, and apparently Lt Moroko wants us back soon. There is some opposition to the departure of Jock Clarke (dentist), Maj. Marsden (pathology) and me, but the O.M. has warned me that I am likely to go. Perhaps to some new civilisation in the jungle again – what!

Meeting today. Lt-Col. Coates reported on the submission to the IJA. They have promised to equip two wards at least on a more suitable scale for sick men. The ban on meetings and post mortems was referred to and we are now only to have one clinical meeting a fortnight.

3 December 1944

Lt-Col. Coates did a laparotomy on Lt-Col. McKellar with L.A. Hard mass on lesser curve of stomach high up, regarded as cancer of stomach; a gastrostomy performed, since inoperable, and he unable to eat. A special high calorie diet has been arranged. Gastrostomy feeding – 8 eggs, 2 pints double strength milk, cod liver oil, orange judice, liver purée, vegetable soup and multiple vitamin tablets.

Many planes over this evening. Three waves of giant four-engined bombers flew almost over the camp in the direction of Non Pladuk. 12, 10, 9. Ack-ack fire, bomb impact and fires clearly seen. It is rumoured that Non Pladuk has had the 'big stick': reported POW casualties 9 killed, 3 injured only, due to slit trenches.

Night checks by the IJA have been introduced. Because one man (Price) was out of surgical, all patients and staff were turned out in the cold to be checked ('bed patients' to remain in bed). Considerable loss of sleep an annoyance to everyone.*

In accordance with the controversy over my party and group IV claims, all medically 'fit' men were paraded and inspected by the IJA doctor today (we must be popular).

Special diets for December: The IJA have made exhaustive enquiries into our finances and are apparently discontented with the fact that these are for the most part provided out of salaries of officers and Red Cross personnel. Their suggestion is that we give the meat and certain more suitable foods to the very sick, and other men eat rice! They have placed our money under lock and key and we have to obtain permission to spend it. The canteen is being closely scrutinised too.†

5 December 1944

T.A.B. vaccine available for vaccinations of staff, 1cc for all those requiring re-innoculation. I am having it myself purely to encourage *les autres* as I have lost count of the number I have had since becoming a POW. Those who have not had any T.A.B. since becoming a POW are to have 1cc.

* Price was caught 'fence jumping'.

† They are probably aware that some money is 'underground'. Camp command is naturally very disturbed.

The system of night checking in operation is a bloody bore at present, resulting in disturbance three or four times a night, even if only to be awakened by pidgin English interrogation as to numbers, or having your toe tugged through the net to make sure that you are there! This is bad for patients but I suppose that the excessive zeal will cease soon.

7 December 1944

Discussed remedial and massage centre with Maj. Clive Wallis and Capt. Gatford. Without medical supervision this show is rather at sixes and sevens and much energy is being misapplied. In addition there is a good deal of personality conflict. Jack Chalker is to be made clerk and check the records of work and attendance and on the remedial side, Sgt de Goey is to replace another Dutch soldier, van de Roer. Organisation is to be more tightly arranged and cases are to be distributed over masseurs and experts according to medical classification which will now be given by me: for example, ulcer contracture, fractures, joint diseases, fibrositis, flat feet, nerve lesions etc. If cases are sorted out into groups, treatment can be standardised and carried out by the most suitable person.

We will watch carefully the present curious predominence of NEI soldiers receiving treatment over all others, despite their minority in the camp. In contrast to the Railway, where going sick offered little refuge, loss of pay and loss of food under Nakom Patom conditions, being sick meant protection against return to working parties and remote camps.

There was an outbreak of a curious disease in NEIA termed *Muis Patti*, in which the legs seemed paralysed. I encouraged attempts at leg exercises and subtle competition seated with medicine ball teams. One day in the middle of an intense game there was an air raid. A remarkable restoration of power took them hurriedly all to cover. Alas, every man has a breaking point I suppose.

8 December 1944

We are now going in for slit trenches all around the buildings, and have a system of bugle alarms and all clears not very intelligible to any one. The IJA say that this place has been notified to the allies as a Red Cross Institution and that an attack is not considered likely. It is reassuring of course that someone might regard this place as a *Red Cross* Institution.

9 December 1944

Today and yesterday the IJA doctor is carrying out an inspection of alll sick in this block, both as regards the 'bed down' permanent disability costs for NP Block and of men fit to move out of camp.

I have a heavy cold and malaria yet again. I began to rigor yesterday during the IJA inspection. It is cold now and one does not feel very warm at night naked on canvas with one blanket and a coat. Mosquito nets are very short and I don't know how people sleep without them as when I lend mine to patients I have a lousy night. One good thing about the cold – the mosquitoes are rapidly fading out.

10 December 1944

The men marked to leave the camp soon include 89 from this block.

11 December 1944

A strange story of a POW who had a 'bird' as a pet and taught it tricks. The O.M. and 'The Chief Scout' ordered it to be killed and buried since unhealthy, and those concerned to leave camp.*

12 December 1944

A disinfecting and laundry scheme has been introduced in the camp at last, using large mudded boxes over *cwalis* as disinfectors. This will enable large numbers of men to have their gear put through daily and disinfection on a hut basis.

Enterprise is often blunted by meddlesome guards. Our kitchen and several others recently introduced ingeniously devised mud ovens. The guard commander of the day had them destroyed.

13 December 1944

(Note 11 December, 1944.)

News at the moment is largely of local origin and nobody knows the progress of the war.

14 December 1944

Today the heaviest 'Bomb Bomb' ever known around here. Large numbers of planes came over repeatedly in the latter part of the morning and about midday with thunderous and repeated showers of heavy bombs. These unloadings were very prolonged with an uncountable number of thuds, but the actual planes were almost out of view most of the time. This bombing would be heavy by any standards that I have experienced.

The acute quinine crisis of October is back again. Unless the patient is suffering from a most serious concomitant illness or is a known malignant tertian, he is simply given such palliatives as there are available (Dovers Tabs. etc.), charted, and spleen and general condition watched. Some settle for the time being after a few rigors, but I find that most go on with soaring rigors, becoming progressively exhausted. If they have five rigors unchecked usually quinine can be cajoled from the medical 'quinine barons' (Fisher and Larsen).

Things are made more difficult by great shortage of stains, so that malarial staining is used only for the most difficult cases – and now my thermometer (the last one in the block) is broken, and we can't record temperatures.

For those who detest the bitter taste of quinine it is established: better the painful bitterness of quinine than the bitter pains of malaria without quinine! Blood transfusion is used to sustain some of those grossly anaemic men, with no dearth of gallant donors of precious blood. We have evolved the technique of

* This was a wireless set carrying of course risks of death to those concerned and camp reprisals, especially against the commander.

whipping the blood with a whisk, like whipping eggs, to remove fibrin since there is no citrate! It is then strained through sterile cloth.

Tim Woodley – man of many troubles – secondary epithelioma (cancer) glands in the neck, amoebic abscess liver and lung, is today very sick. Old Tim shows amazing spirit in adversity.

15 December 1944

I am rather amazed that Jack Chalker, one of our young artists with a head resembling Rupert Brooke, has asked to do a sculpture of my head. I did not have the necessary assurance to refuse. So he comes along and works at this model. I am being continually non-plussed by this three dimensional art and being asked to turn this way and that. He is a very nice fellow, Chalker – one of the massage team.

18 December 1944

Lt-Col. Bill Harvey arrived today with a small party of sick from Tamuang. Lt-Col. McEachern informs me of two further deaths of AIF men at Tamarkan: Pte Bandinette, K.N., 2/40 Bn and Pte Hart, A.G., 2/20 Bn (both cerebral malaria).

Ewan (Corlette) has had ear and other troubles, but reports himself fairly well, also that 'my colleague Moon still endeavours to postpone the ravages of time by diligent application of various herbal ingredients to his scalp'!

Disturbing rumours that the party with Jack Marsh and Bill Mitchell was bombed on the rail journey up to Tamarkan – ? 18 killed.

19 December 1944

Conference with O.M. re a special diet kitchen for the whole camp. This is already ordered by the IJA in consequence of their recent keen interest in food matters.

20 December 1944

The IJA with their usual brisk celerity and enthusiasm for an idea have ordered that the two new wards for 'very sick' are to become a *fait accompli*: 'Shift today – speedo speedo!' The rationale of these wards is to provide special facilities and special equipment to treat the very sick such as beds, bedding etc. However, no fresh equipment is available and the wards are like all others in the hospital except that they are in the worst possible site as regards distance from the special centres of the hospital, and their whole location is immersed in mud and water in the wet season.

The new commander is showing great enthusiasm for P.T. and has ordered as many POWs as possible to do P.T. on the main central road after *tenko* in the mornings. We are asked to get 2000 out.

21 December 1944

Beds for the special new sick block are to be obtained by confiscating all the crude bamboo and timber scrap bunks scrounged or improvised here and there.

(Officers' camp beds held before capitulation are kindly exempted.) These wretched structures when deprived of the odd bits of canvas, rice sacks, etc. possessed by individuals will not much help the very sick.

There is to be another race meeting on Christmas Day (a poor choice of day) and I am expected to perform as usual as a horse. I have had two or three mild canters with my jockey who is under 7 stone. The usual strict secrecy prevails as to form and bookmakers and punters are active. My equestrian capacity has become a sort of ridiculous legend so that the 'books' either won't give quotations for me in the first race or else 10, even 15 to 1 on. It will be for me a sort of blood match with Maj. Clive Wallis, an International Rugby player, who has captained the army at times. He is nearly my size and seems very fit. I ran one trial today, not at all flat out. 100 yards in 16 seconds (my record time at Chungkai was 14 2/5 secs). I think it will be a good race. I will be Col. Coates nominee for the steeple chase. Pheidipedes by Marathon out of Greece!

23 December 1944

The IJA yesterday showed some interest in case histories and asked to see specimens, then said 'continue as before' – but again, they had no paper to supply. They particularly approved of the principle of using our envelopes of correspondence from home, and if we could not get enough of them they volunteered to confiscate them before the letters were delivered (or, I suppose, sorted)!

24 December 1944

Christmas Eve. A quiet day; all theatre work ceased except emergencies. *Tenko*, 1900; church services, 2000–2100; carol singing parties, 2100–2230; travelling entertainment, 2030–2230, parties visiting sick in huts 9, 10, 19, 20, 22, 27, 31, 50.

After roll call there was a training gallop for Christmas Day race meeting on the main road to show horses and jockeys to the prospective punters. Lights out, 2300 (half an hour extra).

25 December 1944

Christmas Day. Everyone surprisingly cheerful. Food does make a difference. IJA donated 1 tical a man for Christmas feeding.

Menu:

Breakfast	Sweet ground rice porridge
	Fried egg on rice biscuit
	Scrambled egg in cup with fish and prawn
	Sweet Marmalade square
	Sweet coffee
Lunch	Roast meat and mashed potatoes
	green peas
	Meat, onion and beef tea gravy

	Pork Pie Tamarind jam cup Cake Tea
4 p.m.	Sweet tea and Christmas cake
Dinner	Fried steak in egg batter Boiled beans and chips Cabbage Meat, onion, beef tea gravy Ginger jelly and peanut square with milk and egg sauce Tea
10 p.m.	Shortbread and tea.

Christmas Day Programme
Church

C. of E.	Roman Catholic	Free Church
0810 Holy Communion	0810 High Mass	1100 Service
1015 Church Service	0930 Massa Cantata	1200 Holy Communion
1215 Holy Communion	1100 Adoration Benediction	

Father Christmas toured the sick wards with a retinue from 1120 onwards. There was morning entertainment for sick wards.

Race Meeting & Open-air Concert (Band)	1500–1730 hours
Open Air Pantomime *Alfs' Ring*	2100 hours
Lights Out	2400 hours

The morning was spent making calls here and there; most people seemed to dig up a little crude alcohol for various 'cups'. The huge lunch did not do much to improve racing form. The race meeting had all the merry incongruity of a Thailand POW race meeting. My odds in the first race, 'the Colonel's Sprint' were just fantastic and, as I feared, I flopped. I drew the outside running which was rough and stony. I jumped away to lead and at about half-way hit a rock hard with a bare foot stripping most of the flesh from under a big toe. I rocked in my stride and got my jockey unbalanced just as Good Old Clive Wallis cracked on a tremendous sprint and passed me. I failed to recover the lead and he won by 1–2 feet with the Flying Dutchman, a fine physical specimen third. (My first and only horse racing defeat.) Clive is a magnificent looking fellow aged 31 with a big stubborn jaw, trains like hell, never smokes and is always fit. He is International at rugger, and a fine boxer.

A lad from the *Perth*, James, won two excellent races, winning easily in good time. I was determined to win the final race of the day, 'The Grand National', a steeplechase event arousing much interest. The first obstacle was a water jump over a large 10-feet drain with a high take-off alighting to a sharply sloping bank. This was followed by a bamboo fence, an attap palm hurdle and a double fence of bamboo. The water jump was approached by a side lane and the course then turned upward towards the crest of a metalled road.

Geoff Weismann strapped my toe up so well that I was almost without a limp but my odds were now down considerably to 6–4, even that, I think, mostly due to the blind faith of the AIF.

I drew the position outside Clive and was faced with losing time on the outside turn into the road, but as it turned out I cleared the water jump with a foot to spare and just ran away from the field, since no one else got clearly over. The Flying Dutchman should have been an easy second but fell at the last fence and Clive came in second after twice losing his jockey. My greatly pleased owner, Lt-Col. Coates, took me along for two impressive restorative 'snorts'.

In the evening we rose to the dignity of a dinner table plus a little more 'cup' derived from rice distillate and various sources. Billy Wearne and Allan Wood were both present and there were one or two visitors!

26 December 1944

Tired and frightfully footsore.

27 December 1944

I did a further appendicostomy today for chronic dysentery and a Thorek descent of an undescended testis, together with a hernial repair (Pte Hocking). This went well.

29 December 1944

Weather now lovely with the moon becoming full. It becomes intensely cold at night as the moon wanes.

30 December 1944

The atmosphere of the camp bow greatly improved since a 'falling out' in high places. 'Flinch' has been sacked as Camp Adjutant in favour of Capt. Headley who is a very nice fellow. The O.M. announced today that the IJA have now decided to take over the feeding of hospital patients entirely, including 'special diets'. Naturally we are all agog to find out what comes of this.

Incongruously, I was asked to captain Australia in a 'Test' match (cricket) Australia *v.* England.* It was played with a tennis ball and odd local rules. Single wicket, 18 yard pitch, no running, no stumping, 8 per side. All scoring by strokes to particular objects, over the hut 'six and out' etc. We got the father of a hiding, licked by 4 wickets, an innings and about 60 runs. The English team included 'Fizzer' Pearson and Norman Smith (Yorkshire 2nd Eleven and Colts). Fizzer Pearson, the star turn, absolutely annihilated us with his fast bowling. There was an awed silence as I went to the wicket and some talk of 'an international' (Rugby!). I ingloriously just broke my duck both innings and almost entirely shed the remaining skin on my blistered feet from the horse race. Now I can hardly walk.

* This test match was actually recorded in Wisden by E.W. Swanton subsequently.

The pantomime in the evening with Norman Smith's band and Fizzer Pearson's cast was a striking success. Fizzer and Eric Griffiths-Jones are awfully good comedians. Just how they go on improvising costumes now we have almost nothing left, I don't know. Most of the feminine costumes were made out of green mosquito netting and silver paper.

Letters arrived – all very old but how welcome. They included three adorable ones from Helen (1942–3) and poor George Bennett (5.3.42) POW Germany in Poland suffering from intense cold 33° below. (George – my batman in Greece – I had thought evacuated with a broken arm.)

31 December 1944

New Year's Eve and a special social gathering of the Nakom Patom Clinical Society organised by Syd Krantz. A very happy affair with many amusing speeches and anecdotes. I suffered a curious after reaction of profound depression. Somehow the nostalgic songs of the evening, the pathetic little drinks, the gathering darkness lit by flickering oil lamps left me with a profound melancholy: 'We are bats in an endless cage!'

I ran into that hearty Korean 'AIF, Joe' who gave me a 'Happy Christmas!' which I returned without enthusiasm. He looked in my face, sobered and said, 'Ah, it is not very happy for you.' I said, 'No Joe, how about you get me something to drink.' He shook his head and said 'Not possible'. I thanked him and sought out my 'strapper', Geoff Weisman, the hospital dispenser. I said 'Geoff, you must have something here we could drink?' He said 'No.' I interjected, 'What about that acriflavine and spirit?' We made a cocktail which seemed tolerable.

Later, after retiring, I had cause to rise to ease my bladder and looked up at the brilliant sky. There, written clearly on a saffron coloured heaven was an immortal ode, stanza by stanza. I thought, 'not even Homer, not Shakespeare can equal this, I too am immortal.' Back to my wretched bed bemused and in the morning could not recall a word of it.*

1 January 1945

Billy announces that all field officers, though probably not medical officers, will leave the camp soon. Those who are in offical positions in the camp are to make arrangements for handing over. This will be a big blow to me as far as Billy and Allan are concerned. We have long been together and are very close.

2 January 1945

Order today that *all* staff and patients are to go on parade at 0730 hours, no one exempted except acute wards 9 and 10. This was impossible and in the Surgical Block alone 44 had to remain 'bed down'. Notified today that watches and valuables are to be registered and handed in to the IJA. Certain registered watches may be allowed to be retained by medical personnel and block officials.

* It has been my one experience of the dipsomaniac urge leaving me with some enduring comprehension of the miseries of the spirit and the brief exultation of the alcoholic.

Cigarette cases, rings, plus possible weapons all to be handed in. The IJA doctor is doing a further inspection of N.P. Group today (permanent disabilities and chronic sick). Several waves of large bombers swept over today in daylight.

3 January 1945

Helped O.M. do a gastro-enterostomy today on a Dutch patient with a large duodenal ulcer penetrating the pancreas. He has been vomiting and in great pain. His acidity is high.

6 July 1945

Before turning in I did a round of patients and with a sense of horror the last thing I saw was the grim spectacle of two patients suffering from paraplegia (spinal paralysis from the waist down) following operations with spinal anaesthesia a few days before. One had undergone a toilet (scraping out) of a tropical leg ulcer by Capt. Markowitz, and the other a hernia operation (Lt-Col. Coates). Both had developed bladder paralysis. Looking at their shrunken pallid faces and desparing eyes, my words of comfort had a hollow ring.

After reaching my bed space a full realisation of disaster slowly dawned. The spinal anaesthetics of the hospital had changed from my old individually made novocaine preparation for each case to Percaine (Nupercaine). As the latter was mostly used in very low concentration, 1/1500, it had for economys sake become expedient to make it up in bulk 60-dose bottles with a rubber cap so that 1cc could be drawn off with a needle each time.

There were no scales in the camp sensitive enough to make individual preparations. Problems had been encountered with moulds growing in bulk solution and this led to introduction of small amounts of phenol, and later tripaflavine, under the careful supervision of Capt. Markowitz, who claimed no problem with 1000 personal cases in Chungkai.

In alarm I began going over in my mind all the patients I had operated on with bulk spinal, I felt hardly able to wait for the morning to check their condition, but night examination was hardly practical, and after my previous log torture episode for being out of bed after lights out, scarcely prudent. I fell into a restless sleep and a hideous nightmare in which I saw all my patients beckoning me in piteous misery.

Getting up in half light of dawn in a numb, sweating mixture of nightmare and apprehension, I began feverishly examining patients. The first, Gnr Jones, upon whom I had operated four days before for chronic osteomyelitis of the leg following tropical ulcer: He presented a distended bladder with partial retention, a 'saddle anaesthesia of buttocks and thighs', and some muscular weakness of the legs. Horror! I proceeded to examine some 28 patients and about one-third had signs and symptoms suggestive of meningeal irritation and minor disturbances of sensation, or bladder function. It seemed likely that there was a time lag in the development of a catastrophe.

With no conceivable appetite for breakfast, I sought out Lt-Col. Coates and shook his shoulder. I poured out my tale of horror, referring to his own disastrous case and that of Markowitz. The Colonel stirred painfully, sat up, dropped his legs over the platform of his bedding and slowly charged and lit a very foul pipe.

'Weary,' he said reflectively, 'do you remember the Budaberg tragedy?' 'Yes,' I said, 'just a bit. Case of a lot of children vaccinated with staphylococcal infected vaccine. Fatal results.' 'And Weary, do you remember the affair in Berlin in which sulphuric acid was dropped in 80 babies eyes?' 'Yes, dreadful affair.' There followed reference to a third notable world medical tragedy which happily was before my time, but did little to comfort me. 'Well,' said 'the Boss', 'that's what we are up against; what are we going to do?'

I said 'We are, alas, going to have to have a Court of Inquiry* and they are never very pleasant.'

12 July 1945

My thirty-eighth birthday marked by extraordinary gestures of affection on all sides and some interesting greeting cards.

The great wat of Nakom Patom still has clinging to its tower above the bell-like body some remnants of the camouflage, which has slowly been swept away by wind and rain. Some have prophesied that the war will not end until the last bit is gone. I discern a mounting tension in the situation, with highly sinister overtones. The Japanese display little change in their behaviour other than a rather trigger happy alertness and a lower 'boiling point'. The Koreans seem moody and disturbed, some more ingratiating, some like 'AIF Joe' inexplicably less pleasant. One important source remains.†

I was surprised when Z, one of the Korean guards who seemed bright and intelligent, began to make furtive contacts with me and to give me sensitive information about the war which I checked with other sources as likely to be correct. Naturally, I was worried that he was an agent of the *kempi*'s who continued to 'monitor' me from time to time. I encouraged his confidences, but gave little or nothing in return. He was pessimistic as to any hope of our being recovered alive. Invasion he felt would be met by massacre and death marches. The wall and *bund* of our camp, with the built-in machine guns facing *inwards*, lent ready credibility.

The attitudes of most of the senior officers of Nakom Patom trouble my mind. In general there is a feeling that the IJA have swung towards some acceptance of the Geneva Convention with better food and some Red Cross supplies, and that we who for years have sought underground contacts and help are now endangering this fragile trend. I am cautioned against seeking even monetary help which can be difficult to inject into camp schemes unnoticed by our captors.

* This Court of Inquiry, completed on 17 July 1945, was not very conclusive. There was a strong suspicion that the disaster was due to chemical irritation produced by the additives and not fungal contamination. Their use was discontinued. I personally felt that under the grave difficulties attending the production, some error in concentration may have occurred. Full recovery of all patients, except the initial two, resulted.

† My contraband now became an embarrassment to me not only as regarded the IJA, but from our own side by those who didn't want trouble or incidents. My wireless was passed to Clive Wallis after *Kempi* episode.

Further my record and previous arrest by the *kempis* causes unease. I fear that I am regarded as dangerous.

21 July 1945

An interesting side-light with humerous overtones. 'Ernie' of 2/2 Pioneers, a singular, muttering, wild figure with a black Rasputin beard and a 'Jap Happy' for clothing, is deputed by the Japanese to go out of the camp to a slaughteryard to collect offal to bait our nauseating fly traps, and he carries on his arm a pass for the purpose.

When, however, he approached the sentry gate and saluted he found that his pass was missing. By pantomime he depicted his role with mimicry of sharpening knives and throat cutting, by drawing an imaginary knife across his throat. The Japanese, interpreting this as a noble gesture of *hara kiri*, at once cried out in dissuasion, 'No no – not *hara kiri* – tomorrow, tomorrow, all men shake hands!'

This idyllic end is certainly not in keeping with Z's grim information as to our impending fate.

25 July 1945

Alas I have little doubt that the crisis deepens. The pattern seems to be a death march of 'fit' men ahead of any invasion with initial concentration at Nakom Nyak. The rest to be bumped off.*

The talk of Red Cross amelioration gaining more acceptance takes little account of the deadly earnestness of the Japanese, and the Götterdämmerung darkness as the Gods desert them. I am now even scared to be seen by some of my brother officers using my blade razor to shave, lest it be said that I was provoking reaction by the IJA to a forbidden article.

I have compromised by selecting 10 NCOs of high courage and discretion, each to select 10 men not otherwise chosen.† Each man to devise a weapon such as a stone. In any crisis, leaders are to alert their men and report to me. Secrecy is essential, and to be absolute. My own armoury, carefully hidden, consists of two 'Molotov Cocktails' devised from saki bottles and petrol stolen from trucks. I have plotted our desperate breakout as frontally towards a machine gun post in the wall which can be approached with visual cover to either side from enfilading fire, by parallel hutments up to the last 50 metres.

It would no doubt be easy to pre-empt an IJA massacre by a sortie; but this would be morally unacceptable as it could be the excuse for a general massacre.

How I miss the professional guidance of the good soldier Bill Wearne, but Austin is a tower of quiet strength and authority. The object can only be to get some men out to tell the story if they survive, but I am not going over the wall myself. My proper fate must be here with my patients and 'Bertie'.

* This pattern clearly emerged in Borneo with the Sandakan March.

† These men become the basis of my guards and piquets when suddenly we were required to control the camp at the end of the war.

31 July 1945

Three hundred men were ordered out of the Camp today.

1 August 1945

Caun, the Dutch interpreter, who seems to have friendly relationships with the Koreans, has had his movements in the IJA area restricted. Very likely the IJA suspect their loyalty at this stage. The feeling of tension persists.

10 August 1945

Eight truckloads of Red Cross stores arrived and were put in the IJA store.

11 August 1945

Six truckloads of these stores left the camp.

13 August 1945

An actual issue of Red Cross stores: 30 kilos of soya beans, 4 boxes of milk, 1 box malted milk, 200 boxes of soap. This in itself was reassuring, but still more so the furtive communication of Z re reports that the Russians to have entered the war, and it would seem that an Allied Conference in Berlin has given an ultimatum to the Japanese Government. Pte Caun NIEA brings similar information from Korean sources.

I can imagine the critical and tense discussions going on in Japan with the fanatical warmongers urging fight to the death. It must be a tight-run thing with our future depending on Japanese capitulation at home.

14 August 1945

All senior officers now except Lt-Col. Larsen feel we should take steps to protect the troops in the camp. Late tonight it was decided that I be appointed to ensure this with the title APM, which normally implies control of military police by a senior combatant officer. Capt. Meldrum RAMC, a pleasant capable Scot, my assistant. At once I contacted my god-given 100 emergency men.

In a conference, Capt. Vardy, Capt. Meldrum and I worked out details for disposal of guards, picquets, patrols and the posting of senior NCOs guarding stores. We are working on the basis of doing our best to enforce discipline upon the camp at a time when exuberance, or failure to maintain coordination and order, could be fatal. This we term a 'camp security scheme'. Hope is rising in my head, but who knows to the last minute what will be decided in Japan?

15 August 1945

We are ready for 'action stations'. At noon to clamp on 'camp security', but we await the critical moment. There are now mild and persistent rumours that the war is over.

16 August 1945

Oh incredible day!

There seemed no doubt that the Koreans believed the war to be over. Some

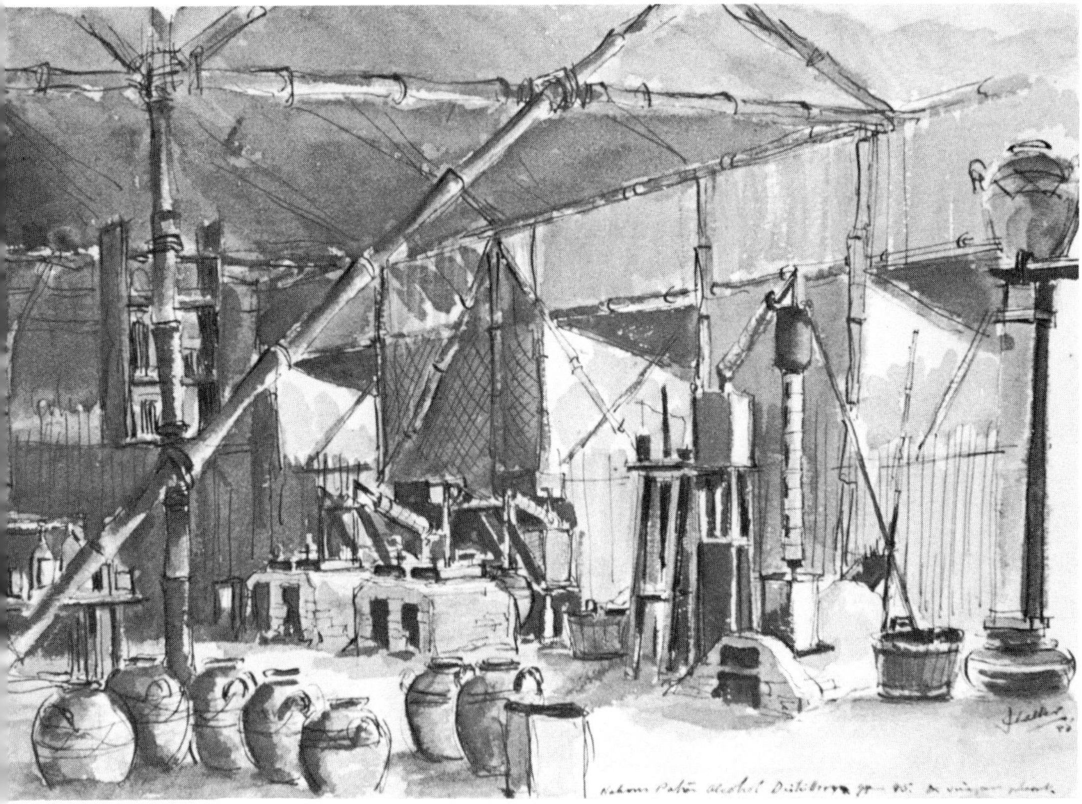

rude alcohol distillery and vinegar plant (*Jack Chalker*)

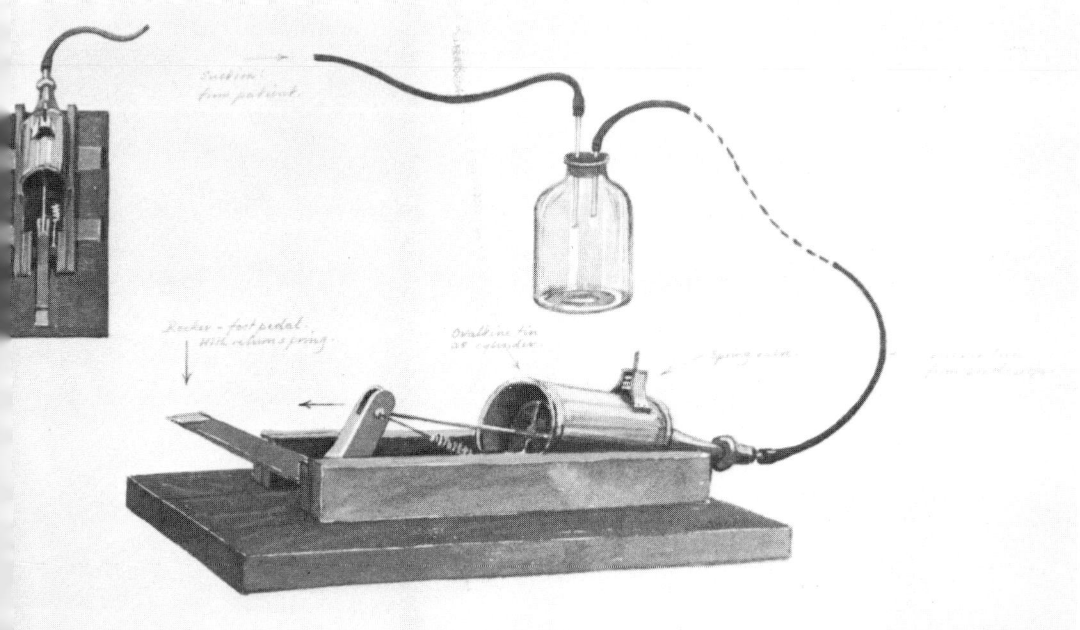

uction apparatus for use in operating theatre made from wood, odd scraps of metal and hide (for plunger backing) – and an valtine tin. Nakom Patom (*Jack Chalker*)

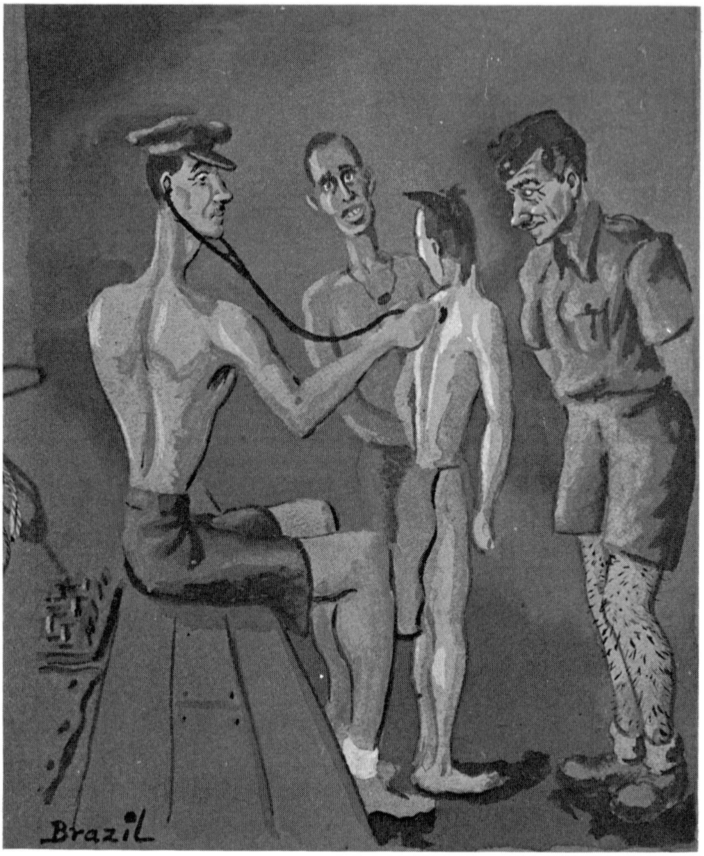

123 Birthday card, Nakom Patom, 12 Jul
1944. Col. Dunlop examining a patie
who is between S/Sgt Gibson and Lt.
Taylor (*Brazil*)

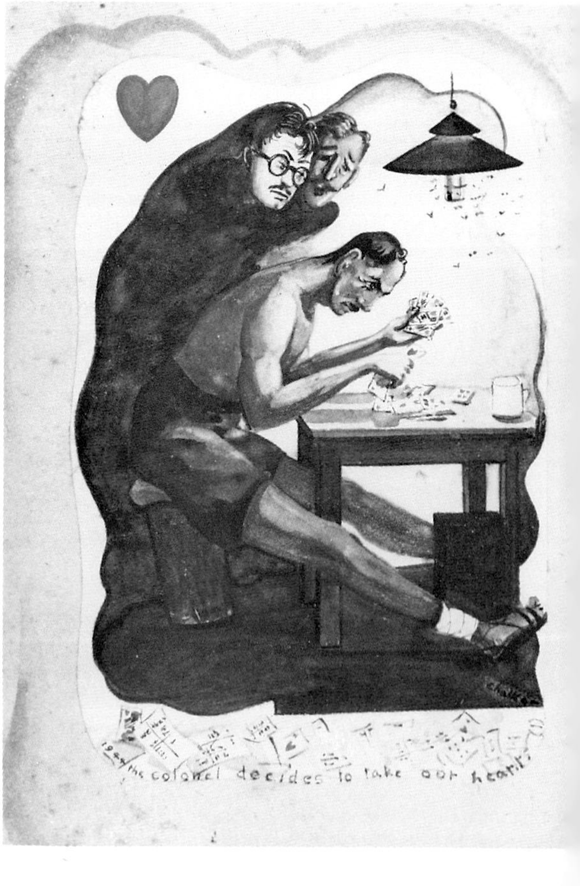

124 'The Colonel takes out Hearts' watched by D. Hirst and 'Fizzer' Pearson. Birthday card, 12 July 1944

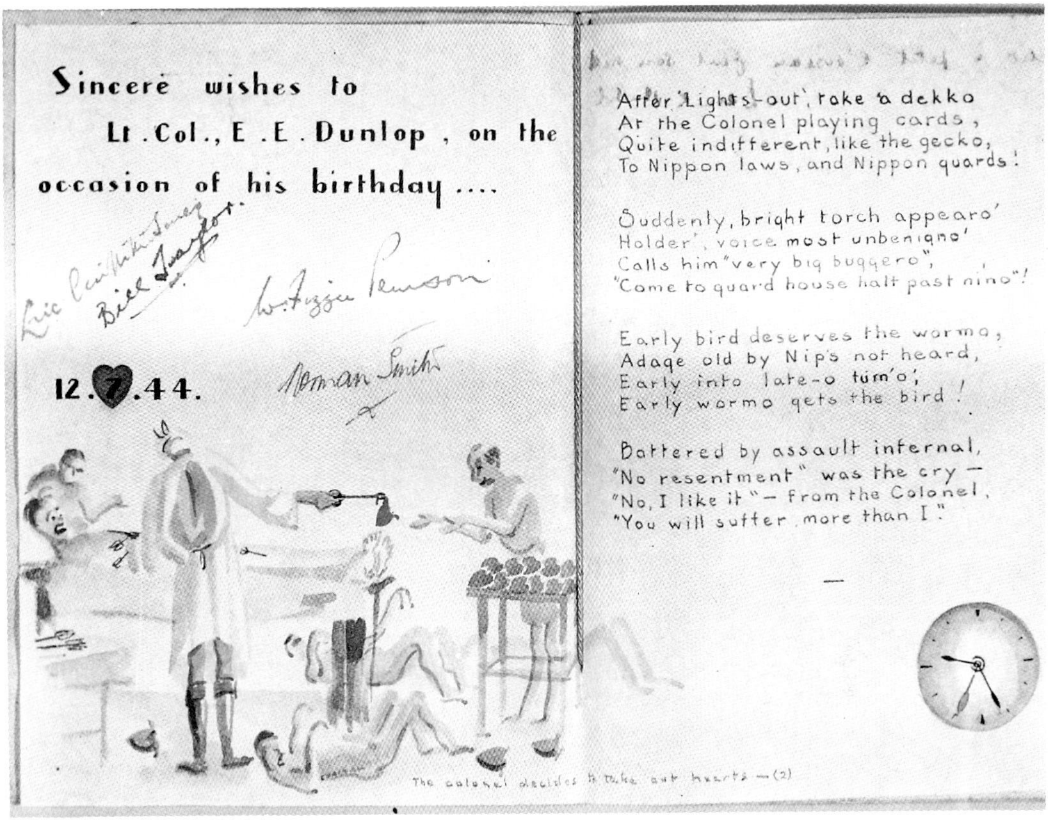

125 Interior of the card

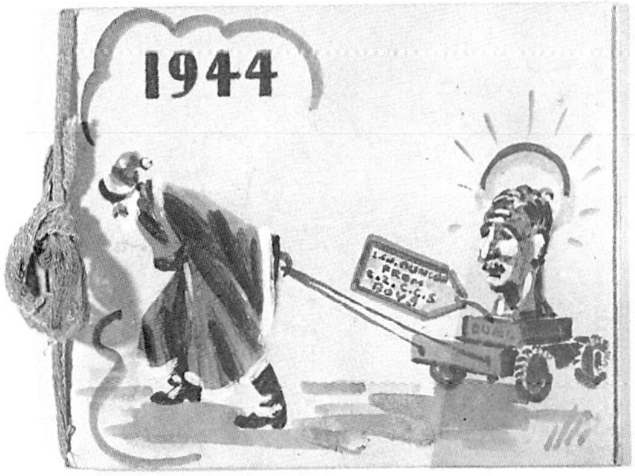

126 Christmas 1944. Front of card shows Chalker's clay head of E.E. Dunlop and inside, horse racing

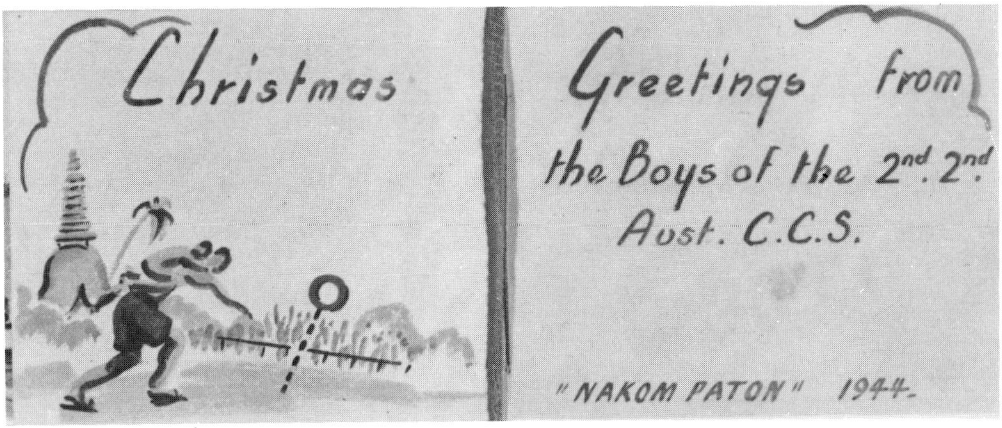

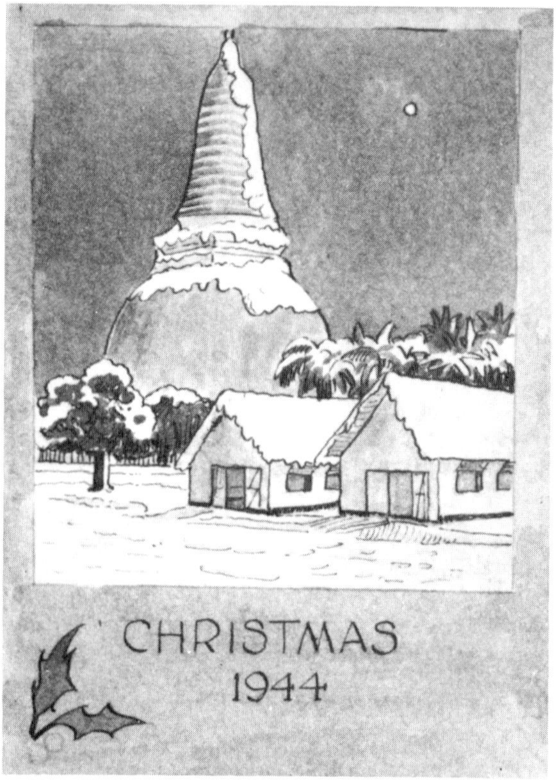

127 Card from Pte L. Lever RAOC: 'The Great Wat, Nakom Patom, shedding camouflage'

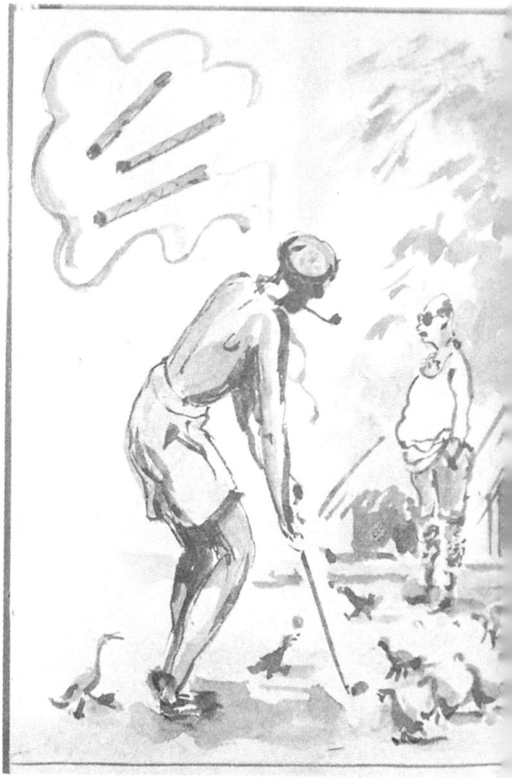

128 Birthday card, Nakom Patom, 1945. Putting competit cheroots *vs* Capt. Hamilton-Gibbs RAMC

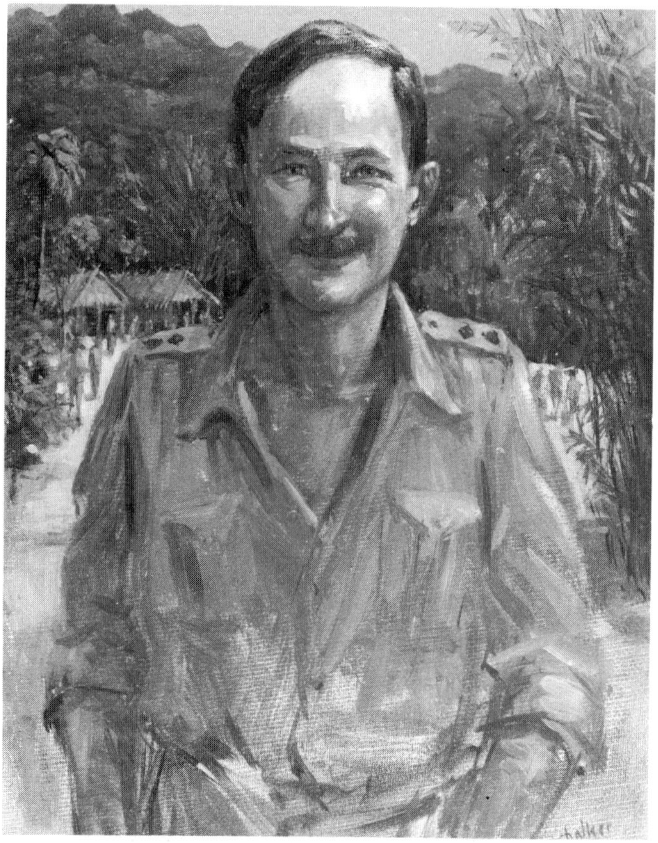

129 Portrait by Jack Chalker of Lt-Col. E.E. D as he was up country in Thailand as a POW Burma-Thailand Railway project

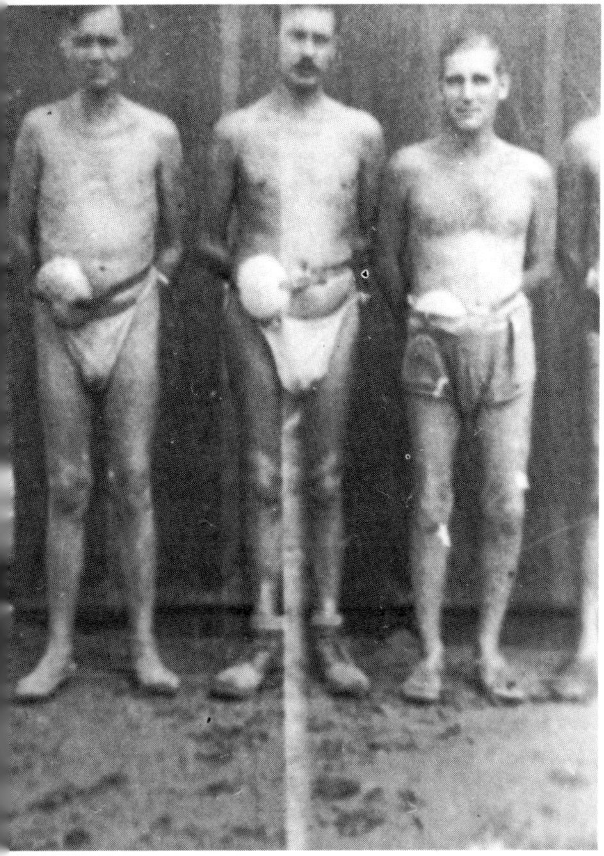

130 Dysentery. Iliostomy patients wearing adapted Dutch watch bottles as drawn in plate 92.

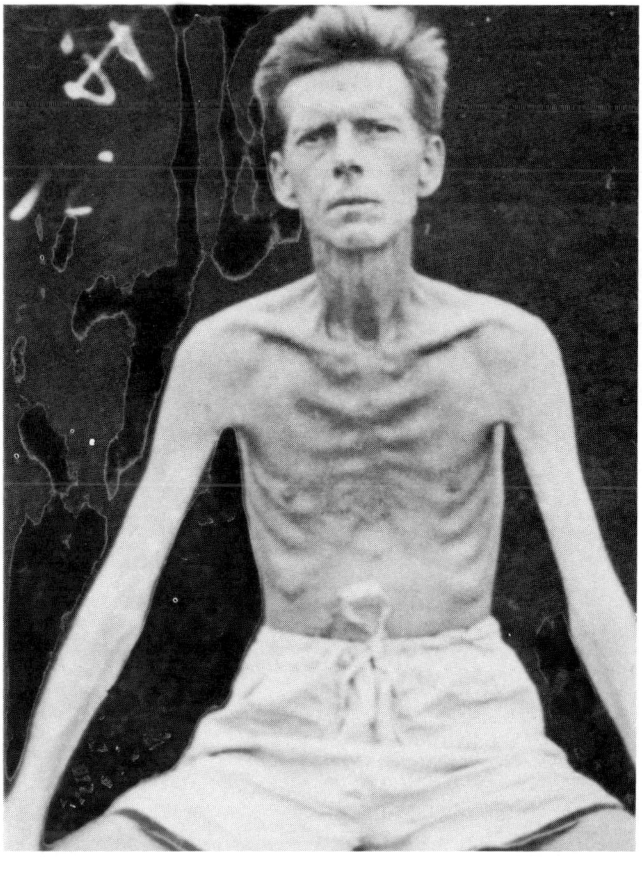

131 Typical emaciated man repeatedly sent to work. Dysentery and malnutrition

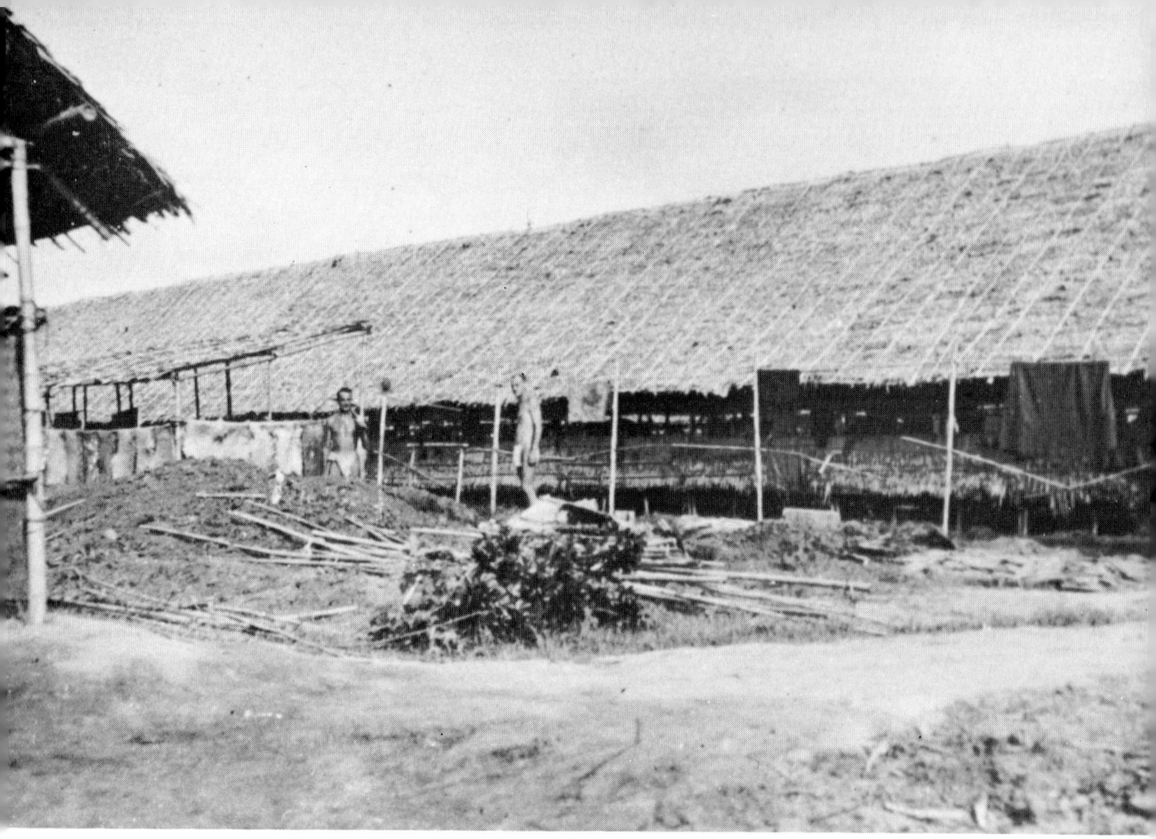

132 Kanchanaburi dysentery ward with latrine 15 in. from ward

133 Transfusion clinic, Nakom Patom. Donor and patient in preparation for transfusion

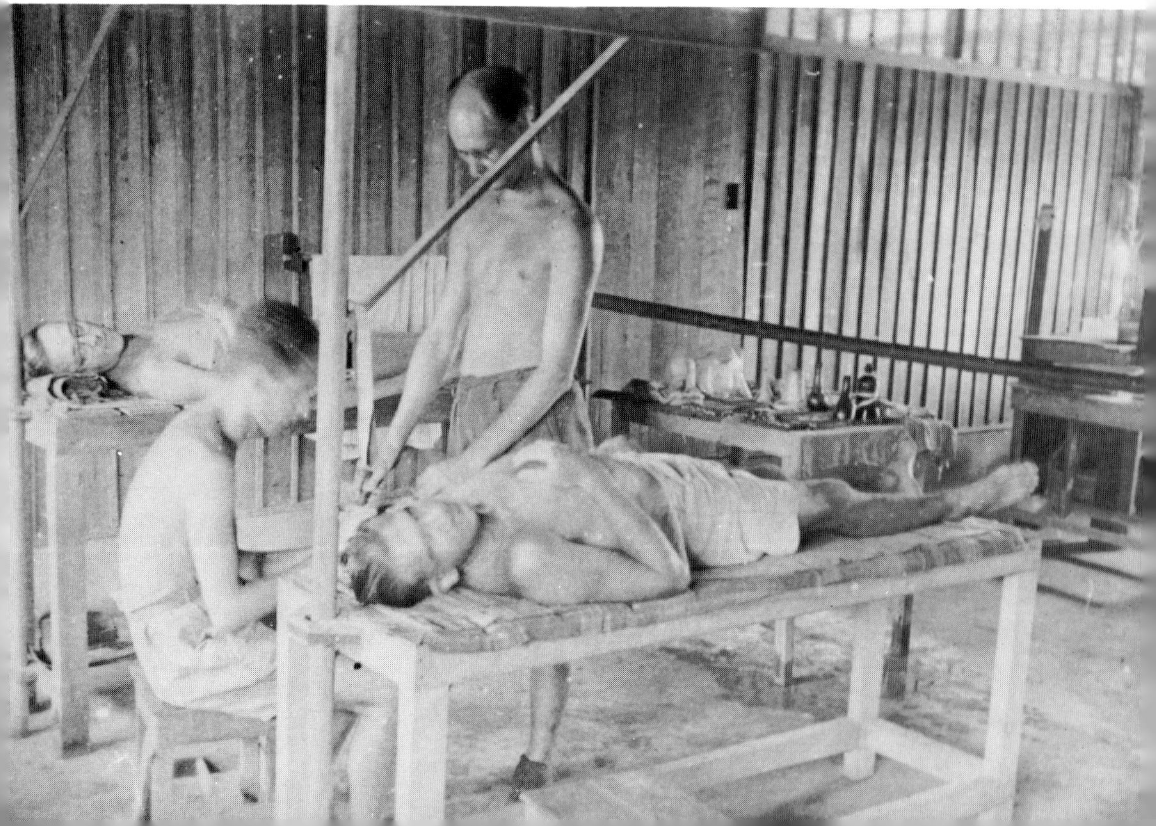

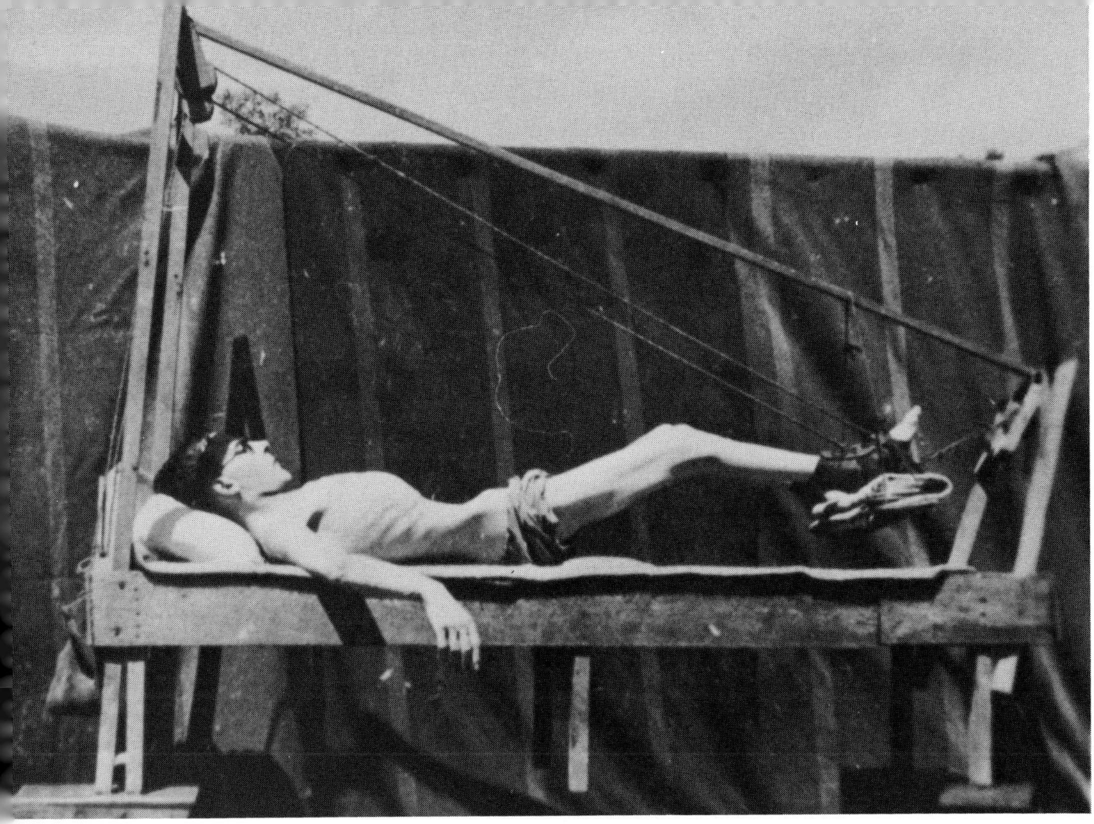

Traction bed. Contracted joints – hips, knees, ankles – post beriberi

Ward, Nakom Patom hospital 1945

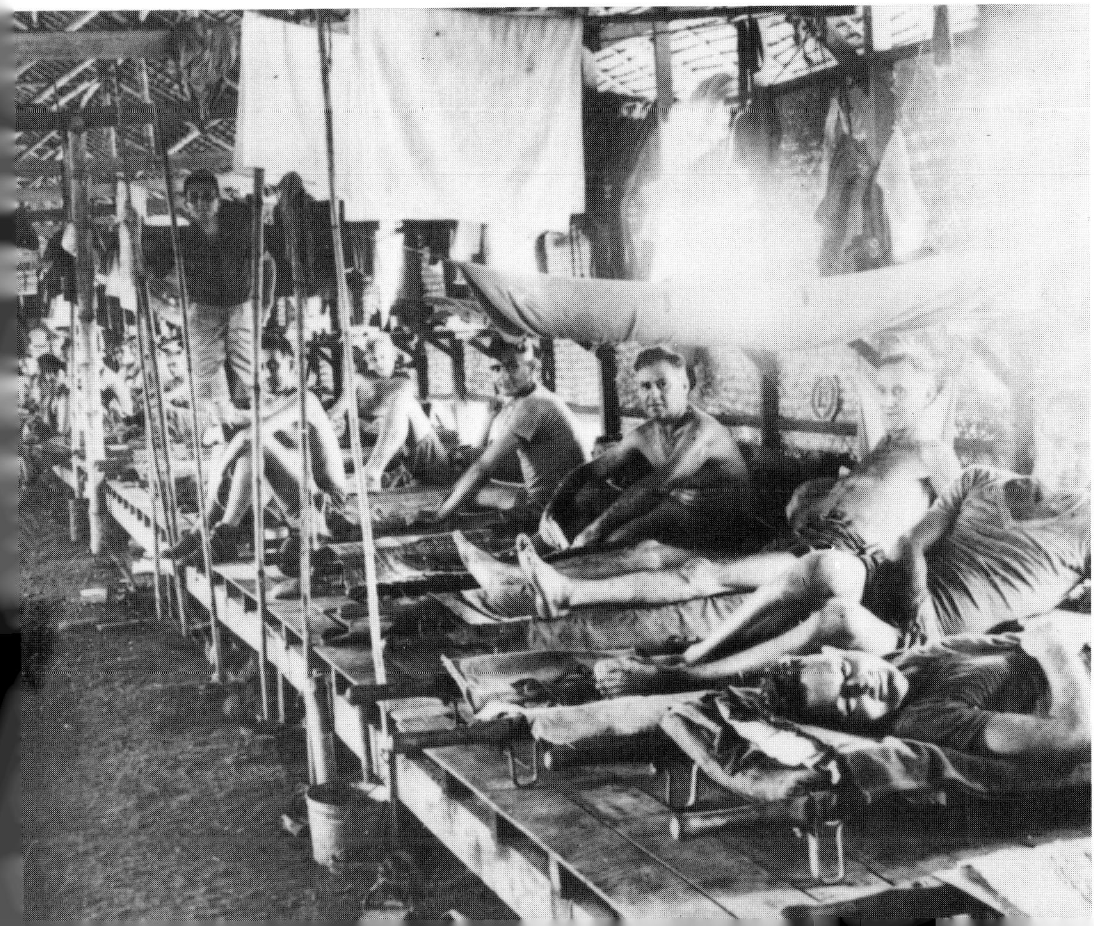

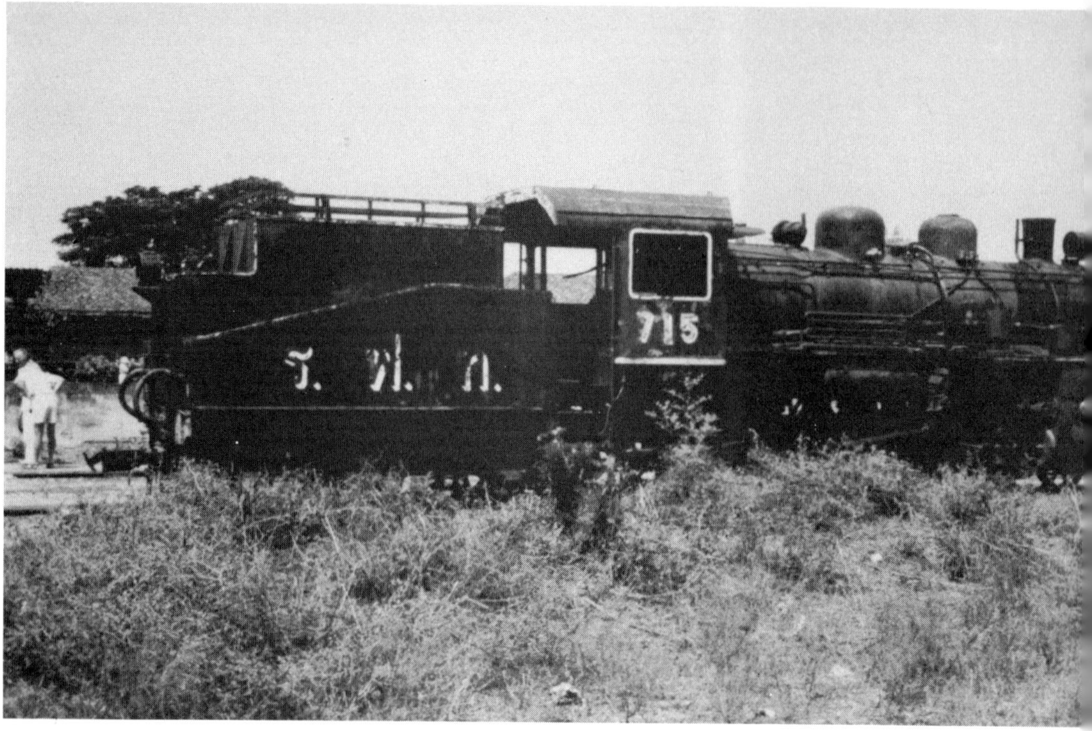

136 Engine used on railway during the war

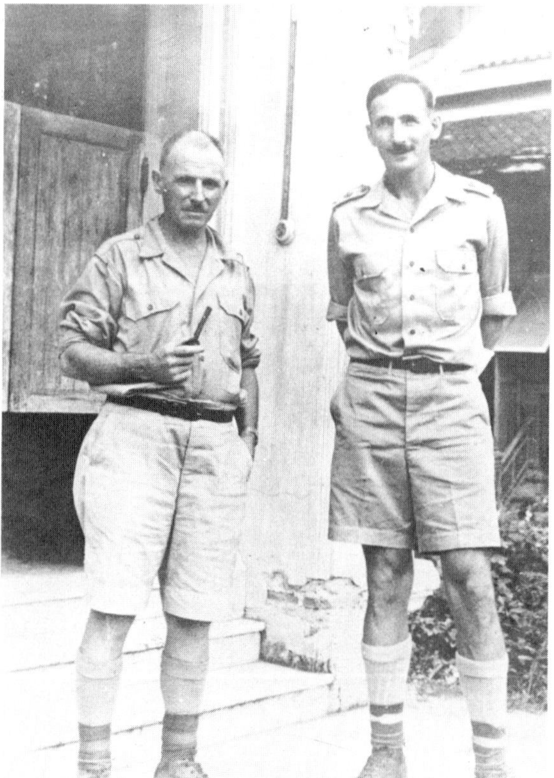

137 Lt-Col. Albert Coates and the author, British HQ, Bangkok, September 1945

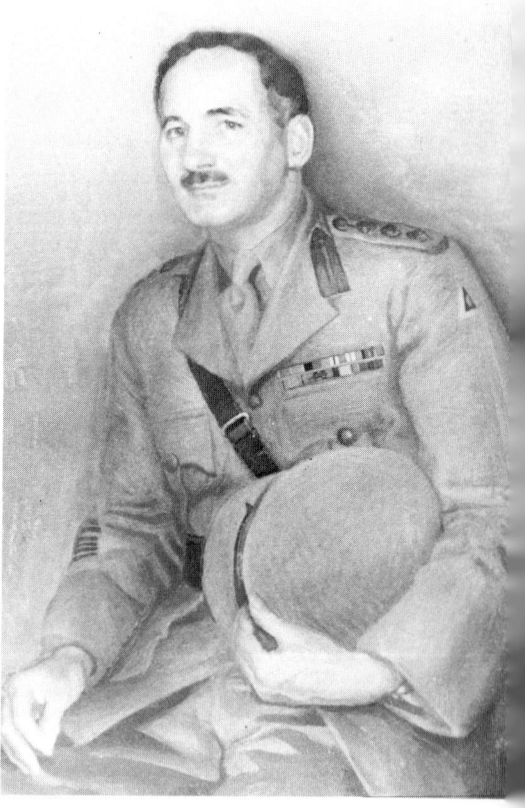

138 Portrait of the author by Murray Griffen in the Austra War Memorial

were tearful and scared. The IJA were surly and elusive. In the afternoon an IJA major arrived by car and there was a conference of their officers.

Just after 1800 hours we senior officers were surrounded by Korean Clerk Kanakowa and taken to the IJA compound. We were met at the gate by Lt Wakimatsu, who looked most unhappy. Almost immediately afterwards Lt-Col. Yamagita arrived, accompanied by Mr Monaka, the interpreter. Lt-Col. Yamagita spoke in Japanese, his momentous statements translated sentence by sentence.

'An armistice is now being held between all nations. All fronts are at peace and we have received instructions that we are to cease to regard you as POWs. Therefore we cease to guard you. The maintenance of discipline is your own responsibility. Your repatriation will be soon. I advise you to keep your health, and to cultivate the papaya trees!'

In further discussion it was arranged that we ex-POWs would guard and administer all the area inside the bund; but that the IJA would guard the operating theatre, the clinics, and our drugs which were within their compound, these to be handed over to us tomorrow.

Returning to our lines, I at once arranged with Capt. Meldrum and W/O Fyfe that the guards and piquets take over to guard the area. I stressed the delicate and 'jumpy' state of affairs, and that for the present, no one was to be allowed out of camp without special authority. Precious lives could be lost all too tragically at this stage.

There followed a general assembly of all ranks, British, Australian, Dutch and American. Lt-Col. Coates in English, and later Lt-Col. Larsen in Dutch, announced the historic, almost unbelievable, events of the day. Immediately, long-hidden and cherished flags – the Union Jack, Australian, and Dutch – were hoisted to the accompaniment of cheering, shouting, and in many cases, unashamed tears. Those flags seemed to fly proudly in a cleaner, fresher air, charged with deep, overwhelming emotion, a boundless joy still trailing robes of sadness.

So many had suffered and died; some even now would never see home; but the momentous day had come.

Looking at the gaunt, rapt, and mostly tear-stained faces about me, I recalled my light hearted entry into the war from St Mary's, London, and the happier days of the Middle east War. Wellington's apt comment crossed my mind that there was only one worse thing than winning a battle (or I suppose a war), and that was to lose it.

This has been a war against monstrous things, but one for which we all share responsibility because of the selfish pre-occupations which allowed matters to reach such hideous proportions.

There will be an enduring bonus for us all in the deep affection and comradeship which has evolved, not only between we Australians, but with men of several nations who have shared this long dark night of capitivity.

There will be strenuous and exciting days working to get the last of these maimed and damaged men on their way home.

I have resolved to make their care and welfare a life-long mission.

Postscript

I remained in Thailand for some time after the end of the war, playing a major role in the organisation and setting up of the evacuation programme for the former prisoners-of-war. There was still a great deal of work to do before men could be sent home.

I arrived back in Australia in early October 1945.

The diaries themselves were written on whatever I could find: there are a number of small black notebooks and a pile of Japanese exercise books. The originals are in far greater detail than has been published here. There is a lot of repetition, because the same symptoms, diseases, problems and emergencies kept recurring; each time, of course, the circumstances were slightly different. I have chosen not to include the many long and clinical descriptions of the numerous operations performed, the mass of statistics relating to men, rations, finances and the sick. I kept a careful record of all this, and of the deaths, including place of burial and grave number. In my diary were copies of numerous letters and reports written for our captors.

One aspect of our imprisonment only touched on in the diaries (and that only in relation to our time in Java) is the number of artists for whom we managed to procure paper, ink and watercolour paints. Their paintings and drawings add an extra dimension to the story of our prison life and form an invaluable record of the years between 1942 and 1945, when we were far from home and cut off from the world outside. The one camera that came into the camps with us had to be destroyed together with the film – the artists' work is the only visual record of these times in my camps.

I decided not to re-write the diaries, although it was a great temptation to improve the writing. The diaries were written up whenever I could snatch the time and the somewhat staccato style, with many abbreviations, was forced on me by the conditions in which I lived. A more elegant style could have been imposed on this raw material, but in the end I decided that the diaries have an immediacy which would be lost in extensive editing. These are the diaries of a working doctor, written up each day as a record which, as a Commanding Officer, I was bound to keep.

Appendix I

New Diet Scheme
Chungkai 31 January 1944

Diet A = Light Diet No. 1: Acute diarrhoea, post-operation cases, and acute fever cases.

Breakfast	0830	Soft rice porridge with sugar Sweet tea
	1100	Egg & milk custard
Lunch	1300	Soup, steamed fish Sweet tea
	1500	Soya bean milk
	1800	Soup, rice pudding with egg & sugar Sweet tea
	2000	Sweet tea

Diet B = Light Diet No. 2: Recovery diarrhoea cases, Recovery Surgical, Medical cases

Breakfast	0830	Soft rice porridge & sugar Sweet tea
	1100	Egg & mik custard
Lunch	1300	Fish & potato pie or potato or pumpkin soup or diced tongue & mashed veg. or poached egg, soft rice. Sweet tea
	1500	Soya bean milk
Supper	1800	Soup, slices of tongue or minced tender meat, mashed vegetables Sweet tea
	2000	Sweet tea

Not allowed:
Fries, green vegetables, soya bean or dhal, tough meat, peanuts, rice polishings, highly seasoned dishes or dry rice.
Allowed:
Soft rice or porridge, steamed or baked fish, vegetables or soya bean water, peeled potatoes or pumpkins, tender meat, soya bean milk, egg dishes, jam (if not too acid), very mild seasoning only.

Diet C – Ordinary Diet

Breakfast	0830	Porridge with sugar or rice and baked fish or rice and beef tea.

Lunch	1300	Vegetable stew with 2 oz meat or nasi goreng or fish mash, rice, tea.
Supper	1800	Meat and veg. stew with 4/5 oz meat or Meat and vegetable mash, Sweet. Savoury. Rice. Tea.

(This diet is based on an expenditure of 3.6c per day, 1.6c being spent on meat.)

Diet D – Amoebic Diet, Convalescent and Dysentery Cases
This is similar to Diet 'C' except the following are not allowed: Soya beans, dhall, peas, peanuts, green vegetables.

Diet E – Nutritional Diet (Medical, surgical, dysentery, avitaminosis, cases requiring optimum nutritional diet.)

Breakfast	0830	Porridge witth sugar Liver stew 4 oz liver/offal Boiled, poached, scrambled egg Roll or biscuit with dripping Rice. Tea..
Lunch	1300	As for ordinary diets with addition of meat rissole. Sweet
Supper	1800	As for ordinary diet with addition of blood pudding or liver savoury. Fruit, if available, provided by welfare officers.

Diet F – Nutritional oedema cases

Breakfast	0830	Creamed potato or pumpkin 2 poached or fried eggs, or omelette Liver stew Fish & potato rissole Sweet tea
Lunch	1300	Soup. Fish & potato pie or Scotch egg or shepherds pie or or meat and vegetable stew or steak and chips. Sweet. Sweet tea.
	1500	Soya bean milk
Supper	1800	As lunch with addition of blood pudding or liver savoury. Fruit, if available, via welfare officers.

The Approximate Cost

DIET A
1½ eggs – 12c; 1 pint soya bean milk – 2c; 8 spoonfuls of sugar 8c; 4 oz fish 4c; TOTAL = 26 cents

DIET B
2½ eggs 20c; 1 pint soya bean milk 2c; 8 spoonfuls of sugar 8c; TOTAL = 30 cents

DIET C
3.6 cents.

DIET D – as for ordinary diets 3.6c plus added vegetables 0.4c.

DIET E – Extra over rations and ordinary diet:
1½ eggs 12c; 2 oz cooking fat 8c; 3 oz meat 2c; 3 spoons of sugar 3c; TOTAL = 25 cents
Allow ordinary diet 3.6c – TOTAL OF 28.6 cents

DIET F – Extra over rations and ordinary diet.
6½ eggs 52c; 2 pints soya bean milk 4c; 6 oz fish 6c; 2 spoons sugar 2c; 1 oz cooking fat 4c; TOTAL 68 cents
Plus the ordinary diet allowance of 3.6c gives 71.6 cents.

ESTIMATES (for 2,000 men requiring these diets – daily expenditure of 199.52c, say 10c per person per day.)
Actually when cases were selected by MOs, the cost worked out at approximately 11c per man per day and this figure was accepted. 1c per man per day for welfare.

Appendix II

DISEASE RETURN FOR IJA 24 JANUARY 1944: 'HEAVY SICK' CHUNGKAI

	Hosp.	*Lines*	*Total*
Amoebic dysentery	714	–	714
Bacillary dysentery	2	–	2
Chronic diarrhoea	30	74	104
Ulcers	330	129	459
Skin diseases	115	139	254
Avitaminosis	197	141	338
Chronic Malaria	18	145	163
Limbless	55	–	55
Post Op. & Injuries	3	19	22
General Debility	34	299	333
Respiratory diseases	7	10	17
Fractures	4	–	4
Cardiac	–	29	29
(Some smaller disease groups omitted)	1,535	1,081	2,616

Appendix III

The table on the following page is reprinted from 'Medical Experiences in Japanese Captivity' by E.E. Dunlop, published in *British Medical* Journal, 5 October 1946, Vol. ii, p. 481.

Australian Patients Admitted to Author's Working-camp Hospitals June 1942 to October 1943

Camp	*Malaria*	*Dysentery*	*Enteritis*	*Cholera*	*Diphtheria*	*Pneumonia*	*Bronchitis*	*Avitaminosis and Malnutrition*	*Injuries*	*Tropical Ulcers*	*Other Skin Diseases*	*Other Diseases*	*Totals*	*Deaths*
Bandoeng, Java (June 14–Nov. 7, 1942)	37	129	7	–	–	2	2	17	8	3	25	58	288	1
Makosura, Java (Nov. 7, 1942–Jan. 4, 1943)	14	28	1	–	–	–	2	18	1	2	20	27	113	–
Changi, Singapore, south area (Jan. 7–June 20, 1943)	7	29	–	–	–	–	–	38	6	1	12	16	109	–
Konyu (Jan. 25–Mar. 12, 1943)	166	153	21	–	–	–	3	5	5	7	12	18	392	–
Hintok, Mountain Camp (Mar. 13–Aug. 23, 1943)	916	558	340	93	11	18	38	194	113	209	221	171	2,882	57
Hintok, River Camp (July 20–Sept. 18, 1943)	590	98	56	57	–	1	4	78	38	104	213	95	1,334	25
Kinsayok (Sept. 10–Oct. 23, 1943)	288	17	22	–	–	1	–	2	26	49	31	10	446	–
Totals	2,018	1,014	447	150	11	22	49	352	197	375	534	395	5,664	83
Deaths	–	10	–	63	–	1	–	3	1	–	–	5	83	–

Notes.–1. Most cases of enteritis were of pellagrous origin. 2. The figures bear little relationship to total disease, since almost all troops worked through illness, and malaria and pellagra were almost universal. 3. Where several disease were coexistent only the principal one was recorded. 4. Avitaminosis and malnutrition column: 50% were serious pellagra cases, the remainder cases of protein oedema and beriberi. 5. The low death rate at this time was quite exceptional, and is in large measure due to the fact that most of these troops were seasoned Middle East veterans of very fine physique. Large numbers, however, died at a later date in base hospitals.

Appendix IV

EXTRACT FROM CHUNGKAI HOSPITAL BULLETIN JAN, FEB, MARCH 1944. FACTS AND FIGURES ABOUT YOUR HOSPITAL

In order that personnel of Chungkai POW Camp may be fully informed as to the affairs of this large Base Hospital, it is proposed to publish a bulletin of current facts and figures from time to time.

Considerable progress is being made, and there has been a steady improvement in the health of the hospital patients, but it must be remembered that this was initially one of the most ill-equipped hospitals in the world, that drugs and dressings are very inadequate, and that the damage done to the health of many patients has been prolonged and most severe.

Accordingly, it is very necessary that you continue to give the same enthusiastic interest and support which has made this progress possible. . . .

HOSPITAL WELFARE ACTIVITIES

The hospital patients and medical staff owe a debt of gratitude for the excellent and comprehensive work carried out by the welfare staff.

This has included the supply and distribution of foodstuffs, soap and other articles, the arrangement of lectures, concerts, entertainments, readings, and an educational programme; as well as the arduous miscellaneous activities of general welfare.

In March 1944 welfare officers were officially appointed to the hospital staff as adjutants to the ward medical officers, with particular responsibility for such non-medical duties as supervision of patients' messing, discipline of patients and staff, cleanliness of wards, and ward equipment. This arrangement has worked smoothly.

Life in hospital is necessarily rather dull and restricted and a lively interest in patients by camp members is much appreciated by all. Particular thanks are due to the Band and Concert parties for their entertainment of sick, both at concerts and around the wards. . . .

HOSPITAL LAUNDRY AND SCABIES CENTRE

A steam disinfesting plant was introduced early in February, and as a result, the efficiency of this centre was greatly increased. Approximately 3000 patients have received treatment for scabies in February and March. The laundry service has been a great boon to the hospital.

Skin diseases have been greatly diminished, but the co-operation of the camp is still specially requested in matters of regular bathing, routine cleansing and sunning of bedding and bedslats, and washing and disinfestation of clothing.

Scabies infection results largely from uncleanliness of clothes and person and overcrowding.

BLOOD TRANSFUSION CENTRES

The work of this centre has been extremely valuable, and is worthy of the highest praise. As well as the impressive number of transfusions carried out, great strides have been made in routine blood grouping of camp members. (Jan. Feb. Mar. 1942 – no. grouped 2998; total to 15 April, 3168.)

Particular thanks must be expressed to all ranks who have given their blood so freely, and without thought of their own health. This sacrifice on their part has saved many lives.

The production of distilled water and saline manufacture has been increased to meet increased demands, and the possibility of further cholera epidemics.

HOSPITAL WORKSHOPS: ARTS AND CRAFTS CENTRES

The need for hospital equipment is second only to food and drugs. Despite the extreme shortage of materials, most ward and other hospital equipment is being made in the hospital.

Articles made in quantity include urinals, bedpans, commodes, surgical beds and pulleys, feeding cups, washbasins, irrigators, sterilisers and small stoves, disinfestors, stretchers and stretcher beds, back rests, legrests, oil lamps, brooms and brushes, trays, tables, orthopaedic appliances, surgical instruments, artificial limbs and eyes.

Skilled labour is available, and a high degree of improvisation is possible, but materials are extremely difficult to obtain. For example, five artificial limbs have been made and this work can be rapidly expanded, but there is a desperate shortage of such essentials as screws, wire, Sorbo rubber, elastic or rubber bands, old braces, soft leather or webbing. Artificial eyes can be made from white mahjong pieces. More of these are required.

As part of a rehabilitation scheme for limbless men and long-term invalids, a self-supporting arts and crafts industry was established, the main activities being woodwork and carpentry, tailoring, cobbling and tinsmithing.

You can help this industry by purchasing the following articles or services which are available at low price: wooden clogs, sandals, brushes, brooms, woodwork and woodwork repairs, tailoring.

The following articles are urgently needed: tins and containers of all sorts, solder, flux, nails, wire, screws, sorbo rubber, scraps of clothing, hose tops and old socks, string, webbing, scraps of leather, rubber tubing (for transfusion purposes), glass bottles of all sorts, glass tubing, canvas, elastic or rubber strips, wax, Mahjong pieces, tools of all sorts.

Nothing is too old, nothing is too small!

Glossary

Japanese Commands

Bango	Number
Hadaré make hadaré	Left turn
Hadaré narai	Left dress
Kashira hadaré	Eyes left
Kashira migi	Eyes right
Kashira naka	Eyes front
Keré	Salute
Kiotské	Attention
Mae e susumé	Quick march
Mawarré e susumé	About turn on the march
Mawarré migi	About turn
Mawarré migi mae	About turn
Migi make migi	Right turn
Migi narai	Right dress
Naoré	From salute to attention (as you were)
Wakaré	Dismiss
Yasumé	Stand at ease

Other Japanese Terms

Arigato	thanks
Benjo	latrine
Buntai	brigade
Chusa	lieutenant-colonel
Chutai	company
Chui	lieutenant
Ichi ni san	one, two, three
Katakana	Japanese alphabet – phonetic expression
Keicho	lance corporal
Kebetai	command post, guard house
Kempi	military police
Kura	rude demand with outstretched right hand, i.e. 'Come here you so and so!'
Makan	food
Mushi mushi	quickly
Roku ju ni	sixty men

sama sama	the same
Shoko	officer
Socho	
Tenko	parade
Tomadachi	friend

ABBREVIATIONS

AAMC	Australian Army Medical Corps
AAOC	Australian Army Ordnance Corps
AASC	Australian Army Service Corps
ADMS	Assistant Director Medical Services
AIC	Australian Instructional Corps
AIF	Australian Infantry Forces
APM	Assistant Provost Marshall
ATS	Australian Transport Service
Bn	battalion
CCS	Casualty Clearing Station
CO	Commanding Officer
CQMS	Company Quarter Master Sergeant
D	Dutch
DADMS	Deputy Assistant-Director Medical Services
DCM	District Court Martial
DGMS	Director General Medical Services
DMS	Director Medical Services
GCM	General Court Martial
GOC	General Officer Commanding
IJA	Imperial Japanese Army
LD	Light duties
LO	Liaison Officer
MI Room	Medical Inspection Room
MP	Military Police
N	Nippon, Nipponese
NCO	Non-commissioned Officer
NEI	Netherlands East Indies
ORs	Other ranks
QM	Quarter Master
RAMC	Royal Army Medical Corps
RAOD	Royal Army Ordnance Depot
RAP	Regimental Aid Post
RMO	Regimental Medical Officer
RO	Routine Orders
RQMS	Regimental Quarter Master Sergeant
RSM	Regimental Sergeant Major
SMO	Senior Medical Officer
3 M.T.	Third Motor Transport
VAD	Voluntary Aid Detachment

Index